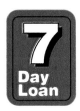
HOBBS'
Food Poisoning and
Food Hygiene

HOBBS'
Food Poisoning and Food Hygiene

7th edition

Edited by

Jim McLauchlin
Christine Little
Health Protection Agency Centre for Infections, London, UK

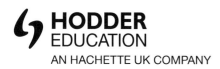

HODDER
EDUCATION
AN HACHETTE UK COMPANY

First published in Great Britain in 1953 by Arnold
Sixth edition 1993
This seventh edition published in 2007 by
Hodder Arnold, an imprint of Hodder Education, an Hachette UK Company
338 Euston Road, London NW1 3BH

http://www.hoddereducation.com

© 2007 Edward Arnold (Publishers) Ltd (Chapters 1–10 and 12–32)
© 2007 Alec Kyriakides (Chapter 11)

Hachette UK's policy is to use papers that are natural, renewable and recyclable products and made from wood grown in sustainable forests. The logging and manufacturing processes are expected to conform to the environmental regulations of the country of origin.

Whilst the advice and information in this book are believed to be true and accurate at the date of going to press, neither the author[s] nor the publisher can accept any legal responsibility or liability for any errors or omissions that may be made. In particular (but without limiting the generality of the preceding disclaimer) every effort has been made to check drug dosages; however it is still possible that errors have been missed. Furthermore, dosage schedules are constantly being revised and new side-effects recognized. For these reasons the reader is strongly urged to consult the drug companies' printed instructions before administering any of the drugs recommended in this book.

British Library Cataloguing in Publication Data
A catalogue record for this book is available from the British Library

Library of Congress Cataloging-in-Publication Data
A catalog record for this book is available from the Library of Congress

ISBN   978 0 340 90530 2

3 4 5 6 7 8 9 10

Commissioning Editor:	Georgina Bentliff/Naomi Wilkinson
Project Editor:	Clare Patterson
Production Controller:	Lindsay Smith
Cover Designer:	Laura DeGrasse
Indexer:	Liz Granger

Typeset in 9.5 on 12 pt Berling Roman by Phoenix Photosetting, Chatham, Kent
Printed and bound in India.

Photo credits: Part 2 opener (pages 166–167), © Guy Cali/Corbis; Part 3 opener (pages 348–349), © Sam Diephuis/Zefa/Corbis.

Figures 2.1, 2.2, 2.5, 2.6 drawn by Debbie Maizels, Zoo Botanica.

What do you think about this book? Or any other Hodder Arnold title?
Please visit our website: www.hoddereducation.com

Contents

Dr Betty Hobbs, an appreciation   *xi*
Contributors   *xiii*
Preface   *xv*
Acknowledgements   *xvii*
Abbreviations used in this book   *xviii*

PART 1: The role of microbiology in food poisoning and foodborne infections

1. **Introduction**   **5**
   History of microbiology and food hygiene   5
   The science of microbiology   8
   Foodborne diseases   8
   Microbiological examination of foods and in-process control   13
   Importance of foodborne disease and arrangement of subsequent chapters   14
   Summary   15
   Further reading   16

2. **Introduction to microbiology**   **17**
   Microbes and microbiology   17
   Bacteria   21
   Parasites, algae and fungi   26
   Detection and identification of microbes   29
   Summary   38
   Sources of information and further reading   40

3. **Life and death of micro-organisms in food, spoilage and preservation**   **41**
   Growth, survival and death of micro-organisms in food   41
   Spoilage   42
   Using heat to kill and injure micro-organisms in food   43
   Control of microbial growth   45
   Factors used to control microbial growth   46
   Preservation strategies   57
   Summary   58
   Sources of information and further reading   58

4. **Microbial agents of food poisoning and foodborne infection**   **59**
   Foodborne pathogens and toxins   59
   Infections   61
   Intoxications   81
   Prion disease   90
   Summary   91
   Sources of information and further reading   92

5. **Food types, reservoirs, vehicles of infection and ways of spread**   **94**
   Introduction   94
   Animals and humans   95
   Food types   100

Summary	112
Sources of information and further reading	112

6.   Epidemiology — 114

Surveillance and epidemiology	114
Surveillance systems	115
Field investigations and descriptive studies	124
Analytical studies	125
Attribution	129
Evaluation	131
Policy development	131
Burden of illness	132
Factors contributing to outbreaks of food poisoning	133
Examples of outbreaks and incidents	133
Summary	143
Sources of information and further reading	143

7.   Water supply, waterborne infection and sewage/sludge disposal — 146

Water as the most important food resource	146
Worldwide burden of disease related to water for drinking and agricultural use	148
Disease emergence related to water, food and food animals	149
Infections transmitted through water	149
Contamination of foods by water	153
Standards and legislation	155
Sewage, animal waste and risk	160
Problems with *Cryptosporidium*	162
Water use in food production, retail and households	164
Summary	165
Sources of information and further reading	165

PART 2: Food hygiene in the prevention of food poisoning

8.   Personal hygiene of the food handler — 169

Food handlers as a source of contamination	169
Hands	169
Nose and throat	170
Gastrointestinal tract	170
Prevention of food contamination by food handlers	171
Personal cleanliness and protective clothing	173
Food handlers' fitness to work	175
Training	178
Summary	179
Sources of information and further reading	179

9.   Food preparation, cooking, cooling and storage — 180

Introduction	180
Preparation	180
Cooking	181
Cooling	194
Storage	196
Summary	199
Sources of information and further reading	200

10. Food hygiene in modern food manufacturing   201
     Introduction   201
     Risk analysis, risk management and HACCP   201
     Prerequisite programmes   202
     HACCP   205
     Summary   207
     Sources of information and further reading   208

11. Food hygiene in the retail trade   209
     Introduction   209
     General principles   210
     Transport and distribution   210
     Produce   214
     Meat   217
     Fish   220
     Delicatessen counters   222
     Bakery   225
     Take-away food and in-store restaurants   228
     Home delivery   229
     Summary   231
     Sources of information and further reading   231

12. Disinfection and cleaning   233
     Purpose of disinfection and cleaning   233
     Disinfection   233
     Sterilization   236
     Cleaning   236
     The practice of cleaning   239
     Stages in cleaning   241
     Summary   243
     Sources of information and further reading   244

13. Food premises and equipment   245
     General principles   245
     Catering   246
     Food storage   259
     Cleaning equipment   260
     Staff room   261
     First aid   261
     Licensed trade   262
     Food law code of practice/practice guidance   262
     Summary   262
     Sources of information and further reading   262

14. Control of infestation   264
     Legal provision   264
     Pests of premises   264
     Pests in food   273
     Summary   274
     Sources of information and further reading   274

15.   Legislation   275
Food safety legislation   276
Food hygiene legislation   282
Official controls   293
Communicable disease legislation   297
Summary   299
Sources of information and further reading   300

16.   Microbiological criteria   301
Introduction   301
Development of criteria   301
Application of microbiological criteria   304
Responsibility of food businesses   304
Role of competent authorities   305
Sampling plans, limits and analytical methods   306
Appropriate level of protection and food safety   309
Summary   311
Sources of information and further reading   311

17.   Education   313
Introduction   313
Education   314
Getting the message across   321
Keeping up to date   322
Summary   324
Sources of information and further reading   324

18.   Food hygiene in developing countries   326
Introduction   326
Climatic factors   326
Socio-economic factors   327
Significance of foodborne illnesses in developing countries   327
Childhood diarrhoea and traditional technologies   328
Street-vended foods   329
Mycotoxins   330
Parasites   331
Bushmeat   333
Summary   333
Sources of information and further reading   333

19.   Food hygiene in the wilderness   336
Introduction   336
Diarrhoeal illness associated with wilderness travel   336
Water   337
Food   343
Safe disposal of faeces   344
Summary   345
Sources of information and further reading   345

PART 3: Contribution to food poisoning and food hygiene in specific settings and by specific professional groups

20. Food service sector including healthcare and educational institutions, small retailers and domestic caterers   **351**
   The food service sector   351
   Hospitals, schools and residential care homes   351
   Small retail and catering businesses   352
   Domestic catering   353
   Sources of information and further reading   354

21. Food safety on ships and aircraft   **355**
   Introduction   355
   Home authority principle   355
   Background and relationship to inspections   355
   Ships   356
   Aircraft   357
   UK military ships and aircraft   359
   Sources of information and further reading   359

22. Food trade associations   **361**
   Introduction   361
   Role of food trade associations   361
   Membership criteria   361
   Operating standards and guidelines   361
   Horizontal and vertical organizations   362
   Umbrella organizations   362
   Who does what   362
   Incident management   362
   Information flows   362
   Conclusion   363

23. The environmental health practitioner   **364**
   History   364
   Environmental health and food safety in the twenty-first century   365
   Inspection   365
   Sampling   365
   Training and advice   366
   Response   366
   Sources of information and further reading   366

24. Seaport and airport health   **367**
   Introduction   367
   Port health authorities   368
   Airports and non-port health authority local authorities   368
   Infectious disease control   368
   Imported food safety control   369
   Other functions of port health authorities   370

25. The medical practitioner   **371**
   Introduction   371
   General practitioners   371

Clinicians in hospitals   372
Consultant medical microbiologists   372
Consultants in communicable disease control   373
Conclusions   373
Sources of information and further reading   373

26.   **The veterinarian's contribution to food safety**   **374**
The veterinary approach to food safety throughout the food chain   374
Longitudinal integrated safety assurance schemes   375
The veterinary contribution to the formulation of food law   375
Reducing the extent of exposure of consumers to foodborne hazards   376
Conclusion   376
Sources of information and further reading   376

27.   **Commercial laboratories**   **377**
Introduction   377
Functions of commercial laboratories   377
Sources of information and further reading   379

28.   **Public sector laboratories**   **380**
Introduction   380
Functions of public sector laboratories   380
Sources of information and further reading   382

29.   **Reference laboratories**   **383**
Specialist reference microbiology services   383
Surveillance, microbial epidemiology and investigation of outbreaks   384
Advice, training, research and responding to health alerts   385

30.   **Surveillance of food and communicable disease**   **386**
Communicable disease surveillance   386
Microbiological food surveillance   388
Communication   389

31.   **The Food Standards Agency**   **390**
Regulation and advice   390
Food emergencies   391
Sources of information and further reading   392

32.   **Investigation, control and management of foodborne outbreaks**   **393**
Recognition and preliminary steps   393
Investigation   395
Control and management   396
Conclusion of outbreaks   397
References and further reading   397

Index   *399*

Dr Betty Constance Hobbs, an appreciation

Dr B C Hobbs, or Betty as she was more affectionately known to those who worked with her, died on 26 September 2002. Throughout her life she was not only a dedicated scientist and a tireless advocate of food hygiene, but also gave her time to others not involved in her specific area of work. It is with deep appreciation that this book is dedicated to her memory in the hope that future generations will benefit from its original objectives and sentiments.

Dr Hobbs completed her PhD ('An examination of various factors affecting the reduction of methylene blue in milk, and the influence of cultural conditions on the yield of metabolites produced by certain species of fungi') under Sir Graham Wilson (who later became Director of the Public Health Laboratory Service) at the London School of Hygiene and Tropical Medicine in 1937. She then joined the emergency Public Health Laboratory Service (PHLS) at their Cardiff laboratory during the early years of the Second World War and remained in the PHLS for the rest of her career, retiring in 1975. She was Director of the Food Hygiene Laboratory from its inception in 1947 until retirement.

During her career, Dr Hobbs was involved with many outbreaks and practical issues concerned with the delivery of safe food. At the request of the local medical officers, she took part in the primary investigation of the 1964 typhoid outbreak in Aberdeen, and later provided information on the presence, survival and growth of *Salmonella* in corned beef. She wrote prolifically throughout her career on many aspects of food microbiology, food poisoning and food hygiene, publishing over 140 papers and articles. She is probably best recognized for her pioneering work

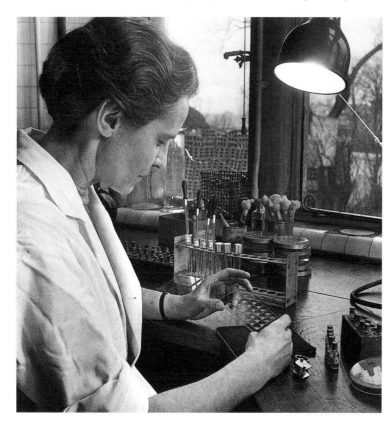

Figure 1 *Dr Betty Hobbs in 1949 (working in the laboratory)*

on establishing *Clostridium perfringens* as a cause of food poisoning.

C. perfringens was first recognized as a cause of food poisoning in the USA in 1945, where nausea and diarrhoea was reported in three outbreaks after consumption of chicken that had been cooked the day before (McClung 1945). The foods were heavily contaminated with *C. perfringens* and it was suggested that a toxin had been produced in the foods. However, in 1953 a groundbreaking paper was published by Dr Hobbs and colleagues, which established *C. perfringens* food poisoning on a much firmer basis by providing information on the epidemiology, disease presentation, diagnosis, pathogenesis and control (Hobbs *et al.*1953). This work characterized a large number of outbreaks and showed that a high proportion of food poisoning of unknown origin was due to *C. perfringens* (then called *C. welchii*). Dr Hobbs and colleagues presented vast amounts of data showing that almost all outbreaks were caused by meat which had been cooked and allowed to cool slowly: the cooking process being unlikely to kill the organism because of its ability to produce endospores with consequent heat resistance. Following consumption of the food, colic and diarrhoea but rarely vomiting occurred after 8–20 hours, which resolved after about a day. There were large numbers of *C. perfringens* in the food and the faeces of affected patients, and because this bacterium was commonly found in the faeces of animals, it represented the likely source of contamination. Human volunteer experiments were performed involving the eating of cooked meat broths. The requirement for consumption of live organism to cause disease (and not toxin) was demonstrated by the development of diarrhoea only following consumption of live culture in cooked meat broths. The disease was not produced after consumption of uninoculated broths or the filtrate from inoculated broths. It was subsequently shown that infection resulted from the production of enterotoxin in the intestinal tract during sporulation of this bacterium. *C. perfringens* food poisoning continues to be a significant problem today in both the UK and the USA, and advice on the control of this disease remains as it was given by Dr Betty Hobbs and colleagues in 1953 in their outstanding paper, now 50 years old:

> Outbreaks of this kind should be prevented by cooking meat immediately before consumption, or if this is impossible, by cooling the meat rapidly and keeping it refrigerated until it is required for use.

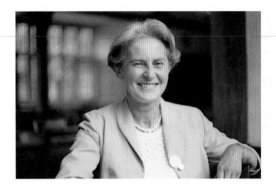

Figure 2   *Dr Betty Hobbs in 1961*

Betty's dedication to others is evidenced by her involvement with the St John Ambulance Association. She was a Sister of Order of St John. She was a committed Christian and worked for the Ludhiana Fellowship. In the early 1970s when the Christian Medical College and Hospital in the Punjab (India) was short of pathology laboratory staff she responded and gave up her holidays each year to spend time working in the laboratory. After her retirement in 1975, she spent 3–6 months each year working in Ludhiana, unpaid, at the laboratory bench.

Dr Hobbs was highly active in many other areas of food hygiene. She was a founder member of the International Commission on Microbiological Specifications for Foods, a group of expert international food microbiologists who first met in 1962 and whose primary goal was to foster the movement of microbiologically safe foods in international commerce. She was also a tireless educator and lecturer, and gave talks to a wide range of audiences, such as the Women's Institute and Townswomen's Guilds, food law enforcers, academia, and the scientific world at large, both in the UK and worldwide. One part of her educational activities was the book *Food Poisoning and Food Hygiene*, which was first published in 1953.

REFERENCES

Hobbs BC, Smith ME, Oakley CL, et al. *Clostridium welchii* food poisoning. *J Hyg* 1953; **51**: 75–101.

McClung LS. Human food poisoning due to growth of *Clostridium perfringens* (*C. welchii*) in freshly cooked chicken: preliminary note. *J Bacteriol* 1945; **50**: 229–31.

Contributors

Martin Adams
Professor of Food Microbiology
School of Biomedical and Molecular Sciences
University of Surrey
Guildford
UK

John Daniel Collins
Veterinary Sciences Centre
UCD Agriculture, Food Science and Veterinary
Medicine
University College Dublin
Belfield Campus
Dublin
Ireland

Christine Dodd
Division of Food Sciences
School of Biosciences
University of Nottingham
Sutton Bonington Campus
Loughborough
UK

Richard Elson
Centre for Infections
Health Protection Agency
London
UK

Paul A Gibbs
Food Safety and Preservation
Leatherhead Food International
Leatherhead
UK

Iain Gillespie
Environmental and Enteric Diseases Department
Health Protection Agency
London
UK

Kaarin Goodburn
Secretary General
Chilled Food Association
Kettering
UK

Melody Greenwood
Wessex Environmental Biology Services
Southampton General Hospital
Health Protection Agency
Southampton

Rob Griffin
Enforcement Division
Food Standards Agency
London
UK

Judith Hilton
Food Standards Agency
Microbiology Division
London
UK

Peter Hoffman
Laboratory of Health Care Associated Infection
Health Protection Agency
London
UK

Paul R Hunter
Professor of Health Protection
The School of Health Policy and Practice
University of East Anglia
Norwich
UK

Alec Kyriakides
Sainsbury's Supermarket Ltd
London
UK

Christine Little
Environmental and Enteric Diseases Department
Health Protection Agency
London
UK

Jim McLauchlin
Environmental and Enteric Diseases Department
Health Protection Agency
London
UK

Robert Mitchell
Environmental and Enteric Diseases Department
Health Protection Agency
London
UK

Gordon Nichols
Environmental and Enteric Diseases Department
Health Protection Agency
London
UK

Diane Roberts
Formerly PHLS Food Safety Microbiology
Laboratory
London
UK

David Tompkins
Regional Microbiologist
Health Protection Agency Yorkshire and the
Humber
Leeds
UK

Sandra Westacott
Port Health Services
Southampton City Council
Southampton
UK

Preface

This book, the seventh edition of *Food Poisoning and Food Hygiene*, retains its original tile as conceived by Dr Betty C Hobbs for the first edition in 1953. Dr Hobbs was joined by Dr Richard Gilbert (her successor as Director of the Public Health Laboratory Service Food Hygiene Laboratory) as a co-author for the fourth edition in 1978. For the fifth and sixth editions, published in 1987 and 1993, Dr Diane Roberts (Deputy Director of the Food Hygiene Laboratory) replaced Dr Gilbert as co-author.

The original aims of *Food Poisoning and Food Hygiene*, as outlined in the first edition, were to:

> bring essential facts about food poisoning and prevention to all those at work in the kitchen of every type of establishment that this work is undertaken. The facts are derived from practical experience and

knowledge gained by many workers in the field of public health during the past century. The method of preservation has been influenced by more recent experience gained in efforts to interest the food-handling public in a technical subject which should be so much their concern. It was hoped that the knowledge given in this way would lead to a better understanding of the necessity for cleanliness in the preparation and service of food, so that the incidence of food poisoning might be much reduced.

On re-reading the first edition, it is apparent that much has changed since the rather austere post-war 1953 Britain, not the least of which are the methods for delivery of messages as shown in the figure. In addition, the list of hazardous toxins, viruses, bacteria and parasites associated with foodborne (and waterborne) disease, is ever increasing as a

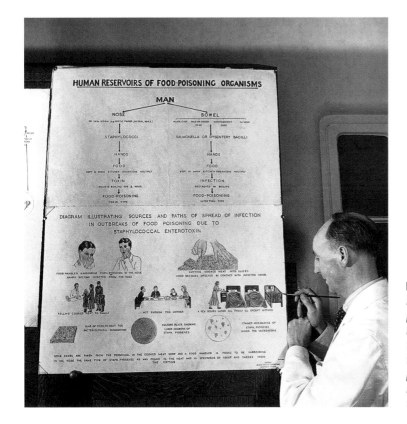

Figure 3   *The 1949 Central Public Health Laboratory chartist producing poster material used by Dr Betty Hobbs (and colleagues) for the teaching of food poisoning and food hygiene. Some of these hand-painted posters were directly reproduced in earlier editions of this book.*

result of improved scientific understanding as well as changes in food ingredients and eating habits, sourcing, manufacturing, and retailing practices. Much has also changed with respect to the professional groups involved with food poisoning and food hygiene as has legislation. It is the intention of the current editors to reflect these changes, although the principles and practices remain central and unchanged as they were in 1953. This book is dedicated to the memory of Betty Hobbs and the provision of safe food.

Jim McLauchlin and Christine Little

Acknowledgements

The Editors would like to thank all those who have contributed to the completion of this book, particularly to colleagues who provided illustrations including: Professor HV Smith (Scottish Parasite Diagnostic Laboratory, Glasgow), V Wingfield (now retired from Tesco Stores Ltd) and Dr H Appleton, Dr H Chart, MD Hampton, J Gibson, Dr NL Lang, C Maguire, C Paddon, and K Pathak in the HPA. We would also like to thank staff at Hodder Arnold for patience, support and forbearance especially to Clare Patterson the Project Editor and the Commissioning Editors Georgina Bentliff and Naomi Wilkinson. Finally we would like to thank all of the contributors for providing assistance with chapters written by other authors, particularly to Dr Diane Roberts and to colleagues within the Health Protection Agency in London. We hope that this book will provide a source of information and assistance to those with an interest in food poisoning and food hygiene, however if nothing else has been achieved, the editors have received an education through the wealth of experience and expertise from all the co-authors.

Jim McLauchlin
Christine Little

Abbreviations used in this book

Please note that throughout the text **red bold** has been used to indicate key terms.

ACoP	Approved Code of Practice		ECR	Emergency Control Regulation
AIDS	acquired immune efficiency syndrome		EEA	European Economic Area
ALOP	appropriate level of protection		EFSA	European Food Safety Authority
APHA	Association of Port Health Authorities		EFTA	European Free Trade Association
AR	attack rate		Eh	redox potential
ASP	amnesic shellfish poisoning		EHEC	enterohaemorrhagic *E.coli*
ATP	adenosine triphosphate		EHP	environmental health practitioner
a_w	water activity		EHSRs	essential health and safety
BIP	border inspection post			requirements
BOD	biological oxygen demand		EIEC	enteroinvasive *E.coli*
BSE	bovine spongiform encephalopathy		ELISA	enzyme-linked immunosorbent assay
CA	competent authority		EPEC	enteropathogenic *E.coli*
CCDC	Consultant in Communicable Disease Control		ETEC	enterotoxigenic *E.coli*
			EU	European Union
CCDR	*Canada Communicable Diseases Report*		EWRS	Early Warning and Response System
			FAFA	Food Alert for Action
CCFRA	Camden and Chorleywood Food Research Association		FAFI	Food Alert for Information
			FAO	Food and Agriculture Organization
CCPs	critical control points		FBO	food business operator
CEFAS	Centre for Environment, Fisheries and Aquaculture Science		FDF	Food and Drink Federation
			FNAO	food not of animal origin
CFU	colony forming unit		FSA	Food Standards Agency
CI	confidence interval		FSB	Federation of Small Businesses
CIAA	Confederation of Food and Drink Industries in the EU		FSO	food safety objective
			FTA	food trade association
CIBSE	Charted Institute of Building Service Engineers		GAC	granular activated charcoal
			GHP	good hygiene practice
CIEH	Chartered Institute of Environmental Health		GMP	good manufacturing practice
			GP	general practitioner
CMM	consultant medical microbiologist		HA	Home Authority
CPD	continuous professional development		HACCP	hazard analysis critical control points
DALYs	disability-adjusted life years		HAV	hepatitis A virus
Defra	Department for Environment, Food and Rural Affairs		HIV	human immunodeficiency virus
			HMRC	Her Majesty's Revenue and Customs
DH	Department of Health		HND	Higher National Diploma
DNA	deoxyribose nucleic acid		HPA	Health Protection Agency
DSP	diarrhoetic shellfish poisoning		HPA CfI	Health Protection Agency Centre for Infections
EA	Environment Agency			
EAggEC	enteroaggregative *E.coli*		HPR	*Health Protection Report*
EC	European Commission		HPU	health protection unit
ECDC	European Centre for Disease Prevention and Control		HSE	Heath and Safety Executive
			HTST	high temperature short time (pasteurization)
ECHO	enteric cytopathogenic human orphan (virus)			
			HUS	haemolytic uraemic syndrome

ICMSF	International Commission on Microbiological Specifications for Foods		PrP	prion protein
			PSP	paralytic shellfish poisoning
IFST	Institute for Food Science and Technology		PT	phage type
			QA	quality assurance
IHR	International Health Regulations		QAC	quaternary-ammonium compounds
IID	infectious intestinal disease		QMRA	quantitative microbiological risk assessment
ILSI	International Life Sciences Institute		RASFF	Rapid Alert System for Food and Feed
ISO	International Standards Organization		REHIS	Royal Environmental Health Institute for Scotland
JP	Justice of the Peace			
LA	Local Authority		RIPH	Royal Institute of Public Health
LACORS	Local Authorities Co-ordinators of Regulatory Services		RNA	ribose nucleic acid
			RODAC	replica organism direct agar contact
LISA	longitudinal integrated safety assurance schemes		RR	relative risk
			RSPH	Royal Society for the Promotion of Health
LTH	low temperature holding			
MCA	Maritime and Coastguard Agency		SARS	severe adult respiratory syndrome
MHI	meat hygiene inspector		SCID	severe combined immunodeficiency
MMWR	*Mortality and Morbidity Weekly Report*		ser.	serotype
			SfAM	Society for Applied Microbiology
MoU	Memorandum of Understanding		SFBB	Safer Food, Safer Business
MPN	most probable number		SGM	Society for General Microbiology
MRA	microbiological risk assessment		SIV	simian immunodeficiency virus
MTC	Meat Training Council		SMEs	small- and medium-sized businesses
NHS	National Health Service		SOFHT	Society of Food Hygiene Technology
NLV	Norwalk-like viruses		SOPs	standard operating procedures
NS	not (statistically) significant		sp.	species (spp. is plural)
nvCJD	new-variant Creutzfeldt–Jacob disease		SRM	specified risk material
NVQ	National Vocational Qualification		SRSV	small round structured viruses
OCT	outbreak control team		subs.	subspecies
ONS	Office for National Statistics		SVQ	Scottish Vocational Qualification
OR	odds ratio		TSE	transmissible spongiform encephalopathy
OV	official veterinarian			
p	probability value		TVC	total viable count
PA	port authority		UCAS	University and College Admissions Service
PC	performance criterion			
PCBs	polychlorinated biphenols		UHT	ultra heat treated
PCR	polymerase chain reaction		UKAS	United Kingdom Accreditation Service
PFGE	pulsed-field gel electrophoresis		UV	ultraviolet
PHA	Port Health Authorities		vCJD	variant Creutzfeldt-Jakob disease
PHLS	Public Health Laboratory Service		VLA	Veterinary Laboratories Agency
PMI	poultry meat inspector		VRQ	Vocational Related Qualification
PO	performance objective		VT	verocytotoxin
PoAO	products of animal origin		VTEC	vero cytotoxin producing *E. coli*
ppb	parts per billion		WHO	World Health Organization
ppm avCl	parts per million available chlorine		WSP	Water Safety Plan
ppm	parts per million		WTO	World Trade Organization

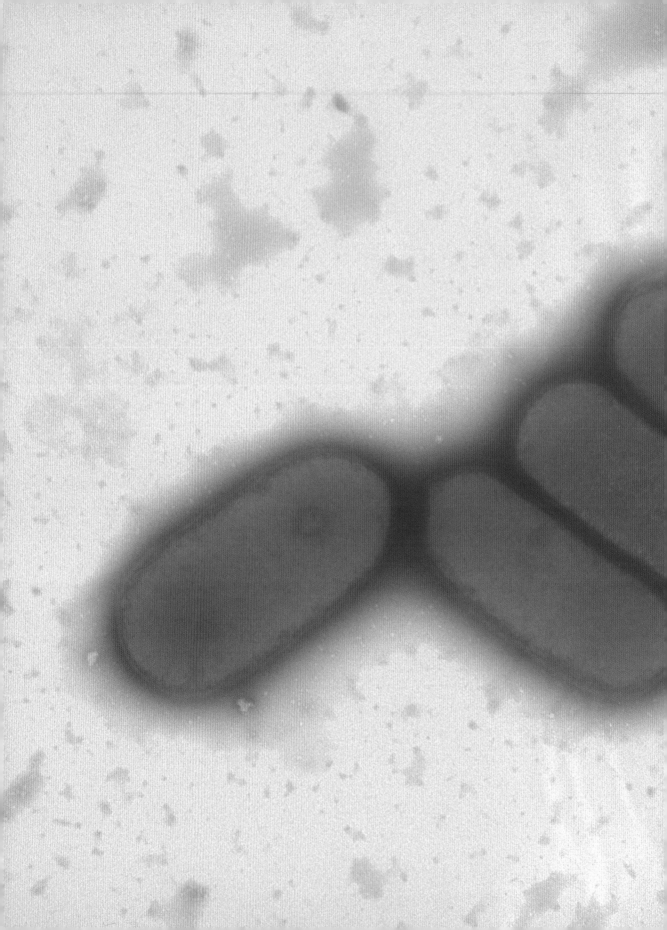

THE ROLE OF MICROBIOLOGY IN FOOD POISONING AND FOODBORNE INFECTIONS

The chapters in Part 1 provide an introduction to microbiology with descriptions of the general characteristics of micro-organisms, the agents concerned in food poisoning and other foodborne disease, the common food vehicles in which the organisms are consumed, the behaviour and ecology of the organisms in food and the environment together with their epidemiology and examples of outbreaks. A chapter on the control of microbes' survival and growth (including how spoilage occurs) together with how food is preserved is also included. This part concludes with a desciption of the importance of water in food poisoning and food hygiene.

1

Introduction

Diane Roberts

History of microbiology and food hygiene	5	Importance of foodborne disease and arrangement of	
The science of microbiology	8	subsequent chapters	14
Foodborne diseases	8	Summary	15
Microbiological examination of foods and		Further reading	16
in-process control	13		

Food should be nourishing and attractive, and free from noxious substances such as poisonous chemicals, toxins or pathogenic micro-organisms.

Food hygiene The study of methods of production, preparation and presentation of food that is safe and of good keeping quality. Thus, food hygiene is a subject with a wide scope covering not only the proper handling of food and drink, but also the correct care of premises, utensils and apparatus used in food preparation, service, storage and consumption.

Food poisoning Any disease of an infectious or toxic nature caused by, or thought to be caused by, the consumption of food or water.

Noxious substances in food give rise to **food poisoning** that usually presents as gastro-enteritis (vomiting, diarrhoea and/or various other abdominal disturbances), although other forms of illness can occur. To reduce the occurrence of food poisoning, food should be processed in such a manner that any adverse risks that may compromise safety are eliminated or reduced to acceptable limits. The most important principles behind the production of safe food are:

- the initial food quality, including the microbiological quality of raw products and additional components of composite foods
- the hygiene and care employed by all those involved in the handling of food prior to its consumption with particular reference to the prevention of cross-contamination between raw and cooked foods
- the provision of adequate conditions of storage at all stages during food preparation and service, including time, temperature and hygiene, that together with other preservation strategies, prevent the growth of micro-organisms in food
- the general design, cleanliness and maintenance of food preparation and storage areas together with associated utensils and equipment.

HISTORY OF MICROBIOLOGY AND FOOD HYGIENE

Historical beginnings

Food poisoning and food hygiene are not new. The production of safe food and drink by alcoholic or acid fermentation, and preservation by drying and the addition of salt, have been well known throughout human history. Foodborne diseases have also been recognized throughout the ages. The historical laws of the Israelites contain detailed information on foods to be eaten and those to be abhorred, as well as on methods of preparation and cleanliness of hands. The book of Leviticus records that Moses made laws to protect his people against what are now recognized as infectious diseases. Hands were to be washed after killing sacrificial animals and before eating. Laws were given about edible animals of all kinds and prohibited the eating of swine (now know to harbour pathogens such as the bacterium *Salmonella*, and being a reservoir for the parasitic 'worms' *Taenia*, the tapeworm, and *Trichinella*) and small creatures such as mice, rats, lizards, snails and snakes (also all known to harbour salmonellae). Of the inhabitants of water, only those with fins and scales could be eaten, which eliminated sea mammals, shellfish and crustaceans that live and breed in polluted coastal and estuarine waters. Among the birds there was a long list of prohibited species known to be scavengers, including vultures, eagles, seagulls and herons. Quails were edible, but when the Israelites disobeyed instructions not to store or gather more than a day's supply, and dried them all about the camp, they were struck with a 'deadly plague'. Even the dead bodies of the prohibited creatures were said to defile those who touched them.

Food poisoning was recognized by civil law in the tenth century. Emperor Leo VI of Byzantium forbad the eating of blood sausages prepared by stuffing the stomach of a pig and preserving it by smoking. The cause of the problem is not recorded but may have been botulism, which has been historically associated with this type of product. Poisoning by spoiled grain was recognized by the early Greeks and Romans, and ergot poisoning caused by toxin produced by the growth of the fungus *Claviceps purpurea* in grain was recognized in the sixteenth century. Epidemics of ergot poisoning occurred during the Middle Ages in Europe, Russia and elsewhere. However, despite the use of good traditional practices for the preparation of safe food, and the recognition that food can, on occasion, cause people to become ill, there was little understanding of the science of food hygiene, infectious disease or microbiology.

Birth of microbiology

Micro-organisms were first seen and described in 1675 by Antonie van Leeuwenhoek, a linen draper in Delft, Holland. He made lenses and magnifying apparatus and mounted these together to form a primitive microscope that revealed the presence of tiny 'animalcules' as he called them in samples from various sources including pond water and scrapings from his teeth. He also examined his own faeces during an episode of diarrhoea and described objects likely to have been *Giardia* (a disease-causing protozoan genus) and was therefore likely to have been the first person to have seen a pathogenic micro-organism.

The importance of van Leeuwenhoek's observations was not appreciated for nearly 200 years until the nineteenth century when Louis Pasteur, the great French chemist and bacteriologist, demonstrated the role of bacteria in fermentation processes in 1859. He developed the methods of growing bacteria, necessary for detailed investigations. Pasteur studied the silkworm plague that threatened to ruin the silk trade in France. He showed that the disease was caused by a bacterial infection of the silkworm, and suggested measures for its control. Pasteur investigated diseases of man and animals, including rabies and anthrax, and he is also famous for providing sufficient understanding to control these diseases by vaccination. Another aspect of his work was the study of food hygiene. He showed that the theory of spontaneous generation, that is, life arising from the inanimate, was false. Thus, if food was sterilized by heat, bacteria would not reappear unless introduced from a contaminated material.

At about the same time Robert Koch, working in Germany, proved that anthrax, tuberculosis and cholera were caused by bacteria, and he also devised methods of growing these bacteria. In Europe, America, Japan and other parts of the world microbiologists established the causative microbes of gonorrhoea, diphtheria, typhoid, dysentery, plague, gangrene, boils, tetanus, scarlet fever and many other diseases. Thus, after hundreds of years the cause of infection was revealed and studies on the relationship between microbes and diseases in man and animals were initiated. These studies demonstrated the way in which microbes spread and invade the human and animal body, and established the principles behind methods of prevention and cure. Joseph Lister applied the theory and practice of Pasteur to surgery and found that wounds became septic by the action of bacteria. He introduced the use of antiseptics and disinfectants that kill bacteria and reduced surgical wound infections.

Before 1840, when the 'Great Sanitary Awakening' began, sanitary conditions in Britain were poor.

In 1842, Edwin Chadwick's report on the sanitary conditions of the labouring population of Great Britain was published. Chadwick was a lawyer who belonged to a family with a strong belief in personal cleanliness. His report included an analysis of the most important causes of death ('consumption', typhus and scarlet fever) and their distribution, with emphasis on the squalor, inadequate sewage disposal and contaminated sources of water. This report brought about a greater awareness that the environment influences the physical and the mental well-being of the individual. The connection between dirty conditions and disease was gradually understood and measures were taken to control the disposal of sewage and the purity of water supplies.

The ptomaines are basic chemical substances (alkaloids) formed by the breakdown or digestion of putrefying tissues and were previously thought to be poisons formed in tainted foods. Hence food poisoning was assumed to be associated with taint. However, it is now recognized that even food that is heavily contaminated with food poisoning micro-organisms may still be normal in appearance, odour and flavour. Investigation into food decay led to much interest in the use of thermal processing as a means of food preservation, albeit in the absence of a basic understanding.

In 1805, Nicholas Appert, a Paris confectioner, developed a method of preservation that involved filling wide-mouthed glass bottles with food, and corking and heating the bottles in boiling water. In the same year, Peter Durand, in England, patented the use of tin cans for thermally processed foods. The process was further improved by raising the temperature and pressure for the heat process. However, it was not until the development of microbiology as a science that these processes were fully understood.

Public health microbiology and the prevention of disease

London in the nineteenth century was very overcrowded, and from 1831 onwards there was a series of severe outbreaks of cholera. At this time it was generally believed that cholera (together with other infections) was spread by 'miasma' in the atmosphere. In 1854, a London physician, John Snow, became interested in the idea that cholera 'commences with disturbances of the functions of

the alimentary canal . . . spread by a poison passed from victim to victim through sewage-tainted water.' He identified and closed a water pump that was delivering sewage-contaminated drinking water to Londoners and thus showed that a direct intervention could be used to control an infectious disease. Shortly afterwards in 1856, William Budd, also in England, concluded that typhoid fever was spread by milk or water polluted by the excreta of infected people. Snow and Budd were among the earliest epidemiologists to search for the sources and chains of infection, even before the discovery of the causative organisms. In 1874, an outbreak of typhoid fever in the Swiss town of Lauren was traced to polluted water with the result that water supplies and sewage systems were redesigned. The chlorination of drinking water in Britain was initiated by Alexander Houston in 1905 following a typhoid epidemic in Lincoln, and this development helped to drastically reduce waterborne diseases in the UK and other countries.

Milk was first incriminated as a vehicle of disease transmission after an outbreak of typhoid fever in Penrith in 1857. By the end of the nineteenth century the danger of infection from milk was well recognized, and in cities such as London heat treatment of milk by pasteurization began. This process kills most bacteria in milk, including those that are harmful. Milk was further recognized as one of the vehicles for the transmission of poliomyelitis virus in England in 1915, and later for the transmission of hepatitis A virus. Almost all foods and food types present a potential food poisoning hazard and have, at some time, been incriminated as a vehicle for transmission of food-borne diseases. The role of different food types in disease transmission is discussed in later chapters.

The growth of the science of microbiology in the nineteenth century allowed identification of the agents of some of the major foodborne diseases. The German poet Justin Kerner in 1820 first described sausage poisoning, almost certainly botulism, named after *botulus* (Latin for sausage), and the causative organism, now known as *Clostridium botulinum*, was first cultured by van Ermengen in 1896 in Belgium. However in 1888, Gaertner in Germany was first to isolate a foodborne bacterial pathogen from a case of gastro-enteritis, and this pathogen is now named *Salmonella* after the American microbiologist, Dr E Salmon. In 1885 in the USA, Denys isolated the bacterium *Staphylo-coccus aureus*, associated with an outbreak of food poisoning, and this was rediscovered by Dennison (again in the USA), who identified the same organism as the cause of a food poisoning outbreak associated with cream puffs. These early beginnings were followed by the recognition of further foodborne bacterial pathogens including *Shigella* in 1898 and *Bacillus cereus* in 1906. Many more pathogens are now known to cause foodborne diseases, including *Clostridium perfringens*, the organism whose investigation Dr Betty Hobbs was closely associated with in the 1950s.

The isolation and identification of agents of food poisoning are extremely important because a specific diagnosis can thus be made in affected patients. Identification of a specific food poisoning agent allows investigators to draw on considerable knowledge to predict the likely behaviour, proper-ties and distribution of the pathogen together with the most appropriate method to control or prevent further infection.

THE SCIENCE OF MICROBIOLOGY

Microbiology is the science that deals with the study of micro-organisms, including bacteria, fungi (moulds and yeasts), algae, viruses and parasites. **Bacteriology** is derived from the Greek '*bactron*' meaning rod, because some of the first bacteria seen through a microscope were tiny straight rods. **Virology** is the study of viruses, the smallest known micro-organisms. **Mycology** is the study of fungi, **phycology** the study of algae, and **parasitology** covers organisms of different orders which parasitize man and animals. These are considered in further detail in Chapter 2. The wider field of microbiology embraces **genetics**, the study of genes and heredity and their effect on the structure and functioning of living organisms. **Immunology** is also part of the science of microbiology and includes the study of factors involved in the response of a host to a specific challenge with a foreign agent. Finally, there is **epidemiology**, the study of the spread, frequency and distribution of disease. Epidemiology is essential to food hygiene as it provides an understanding of the reservoirs of food poisoning agents and food vehicles as well as the manner of spread.

All of these microbiological disciplines provide the knowledge based on which we can predict the behaviour of noxious substances in food and which is important in the understanding of the funda-mentals of foodborne diseases. These will be discussed in greater detail in later chapters.

FOODBORNE DISEASES

Table 1.1 lists some food poisoning agents. At this stage, the reader needs to be aware that these different microbiological agents include viruses, bacteria, fungi, algae and parasites, all of which have markedly different properties. A more detailed description of the nature of these agents will be given in the following chapter. However, the next section briefly describes the two basic mechanisms by which noxious substances cause food poisoning, namely **intoxications** and **infections**, together with brief descriptions of how these diseases manifest themselves and how they are controlled.

Intoxications

Intoxications are diseases caused by the consumption of pre-formed toxic chemicals. The toxic chemicals (**intoxicants**) can be micro-biological or non-microbiological in origin. Non-microbiological toxins include substances that are naturally present in food, those that are inadver-tently present, or are present at too high a concentration and thus cause illness. Microbial toxins either accumulate in raw products from the action of micro-organisms in the environment or are produced as a result of microbial growth in food during storage. Control of toxic substances in food components is achieved by the use of good-quality raw materials or by their inactivation during the further manufacture of food. Control of toxins generated as a result of microbial multiplication is also achieved by the use of good-quality starting materials and also by the prevention or suppression of microbial growth during storage, or, more rarely, by inactivation and further processing of food.

Non-microbiological intoxicants
Naturally occurring plant material can cause illness, for example, inadvertent consumption of toxic plants such as toadstools, hemlock and deadly nightshade. However, other 'normal' food com-ponents, if consumed in excess, can be toxic and these include alcohol, monosodium glutamate and

Table 1.1 *Noxious substances that may be present in food*

Toxin	Found in foods or food components
Intoxications	
Non-microbiological	
Inherently poisonous, unintentionally consumed foods	Toadstools, hemlock, deadly nightshade
Inherently poisonous food contaminants – accumulation during storage	Insecticides, herbicides, fungicides, lead, copper, cadmium, mercury
Natural food components, which are toxic in large quantities	Alcohol, monosodium glutamate, sorbitol
Microbiological toxins	
Toxins present in raw food components	'Red tide'-associated algal toxins accumulated by filter-feeding shellfish (paralytic shellfish poisoning and diarrhoetic shellfish poisoning toxins)
	Algal toxin accumulated in large reef fish (ciguatera toxin)
	Fungal toxins (ergot)
Toxins produced by bacteria during food manufacture	Neurotoxins of *Clostridium botulinum* (botulism)
	Enterotoxins of *Staphylococcus aureus*
	Emetic toxin of *Bacillus cereus*
	Histamine (scombrotoxin) by spoilage of fish
Toxins produced by fungi during food manufacture	Aflatoxin produced by *Aspergillus flavus* and *Aspergillus parasiticus*
	Patulin produced by species of *Penicillium*, *Aspergillus* and *Byssochlamys*
	Ochratoxin produced by *Aspergillus ochraceus* and *Penicillium verrucosum*
Infections	
Viral, gastrointestinal	Norovirus, rotavirus
Viral, extra-gastrointestinal	Poliomyelitis, hepatitis A
Bacterial, gastrointestinal	*Salmonella, Campylobacter, Clostridium perfringens, Bacillus cereus, Shigella, Escherichia coli, Yersinia, Vibrio cholerae, Vibrio parahaemolyticus*
Bacterial, extra-gastrointestinal	*Listeria monocytogenes, Brucella, Salmonella* (enteric fever), *Mycobacterium*
Parasitic, gastrointestinal	*Cryptosporidium, Giardia, Cyclospora, Diphyllobothrium, Taenia* (tapeworm), *Anisakis, Ascaris, Fasciola*
Parasitic, extra-gastrointestinal	*Toxoplasma, Entamoeba, Trichinella*
Kuru, Variant Creutzfeldt–Jacob disease	Prions (proteins)

sorbitol. Red kidney beans (*Phaseolus vulgaris*) have caused food poisoning outbreaks when consumed raw or in an incompletely cooked state: symptoms include nausea and vomiting followed by diarrhoea and sometimes abdominal pain, after an incubation period of 1–7 hours. The toxic factor in the beans is a naturally occurring protein known as a lectin or haemagglutinin. Apricot and almond kernels together with yams, bamboo shoots and cassava contain cyanide compounds, which when eaten are converted to poisonous thiocyanate that can interfere with iodine metabolism and give rise to goitre and cretinism. Both the bean-haemagglutin and the cyanides are destroyed by normal cooking such as boiling for 10 minutes. The skin and shoots of green potatoes contain an unusually high concentration of the alkaloids solanine and chaconine, these have occasionally been reported as a cause of food poisoning. Other undesirable food contaminants include heavy metals and insecticide residues, both of which should be prevented from entering the food chain.

Microbiological intoxicants

As mentioned above, microbial toxins can be either present in raw products or produced in food as a result of microbial growth during storage. Toxins present in raw products are exemplified by the algal toxins associated with red tides (e.g. paralytic shellfish poisoning and diarrhoetic shellfish poisoning toxins) and ciguatera toxin.

Paralytic shellfish poisoning (PSP) and diarrhoetic

shellfish poisoning (DSP) are associated with the proliferation of marine red algal blooms, although not all toxic blooms are red and not all red algal blooms are toxic. The toxic algae are accumulated by filter-feeding molluscan shellfish and, to a lesser extent, crustaceans. The symptoms of PSP include dizziness, tingling, drowsiness, headache, muscular paralysis and even death, whereas DSP presents with diarrhoea, nausea, vomiting and abdominal pain. Both DSP and PSP develop within a few hours after consumption of toxic food, and both are associated with eating marine products worldwide. Neither of the toxins responsible for DSP or PSP are destroyed by normal cooking, therefore control of these diseases can only be achieved by monitoring of suspect shellfish beds and rapid closure of harvest of those demonstrated as toxic, together with export control of products from affected areas.

Fish, mostly from warm coral seas, can cause ciguatera poisoning, and this is well recognized in tropical and subtropical regions such as the Caribbean and equatorial Pacific. Fish, in particular the larger and older specimens, accumulate ciguatera toxin as a result of eating small herbivorous fish that feed on a species of alga (*Gambierdiscus toxicus*) that produce the ciguatera toxin while growing on coral at the bottom of the sea. Symptoms of ciguatera intoxication include nausea, vomiting and diarrhoea, and may be severe. The symptoms begin immediately, or within a few hours, after eating contaminated fish. There are also neuro-sensory symptoms, in particular paraesthesia (numbness and tingling) and dysaesthesia (sensation of burning on contact with cold). In severe cases, shock, convulsions, paralysis and even death occurs. The illness is rare in countries with temperate climates, but cases have occurred after eating imported fish. Ciguatera toxin is not inactivated by cooking, so

control of the disease includes not consuming the most toxic parts of reef-fish (liver, viscera, roe, organs), avoiding larger reef fish, and export/import control of such foods. There are no specific treatments for cases of ciguatera, DSP or PSP.

Four of the major foodborne diseases are caused by the presence of pre-formed bacterial toxins in foods. These are: scombrotoxin poisoning, botulism, *S. aureus* and *B. cereus* food poisoning.

The flesh of scombroid fish (bonito, tuna, marlin, mackerel and herring) contains high levels of histidine as a normal constituent. When fish spoilage occurs, as the result of the growth of certain bacteria that produce an enzyme (histidine decarboxylase) histidine is converted to toxic histamine (Figure 1.1). Scombrotoxin poisoning presents within 10 minutes to 2 hours after consumption of contaminated food with a rash on the face, neck and upper chest, flushing, headache, sweating, nausea, vomiting, abdominal pain, dizziness, palpitations, swelling of the mouth, metallic taste, and diarrhoea, lasting from 4 hours to 24 hours. Treatment can be achieved by giving antihistamines but in most cases medical intervention is not needed. Spoilage can occur anywhere in the food chain – from catching of the fish to food service. Histamine is stable, and is not inactivated by cooking or the heat treatment used during the canning process. Control of this disease relies on the prevention of bacterial growth after catching and processing of raw fish, during storage, the canning procedure and post process. Control is achieved by refrigeration or by freezing of raw fish as well as by further processing such as canning, smoking, drying or salting.

Botulism is a severe paralytic intoxication caused by the ingestion of toxin produced by the growth of the bacterium *C. botulinum* in food. The onset of intoxication is usually within 12–36 hours of eating

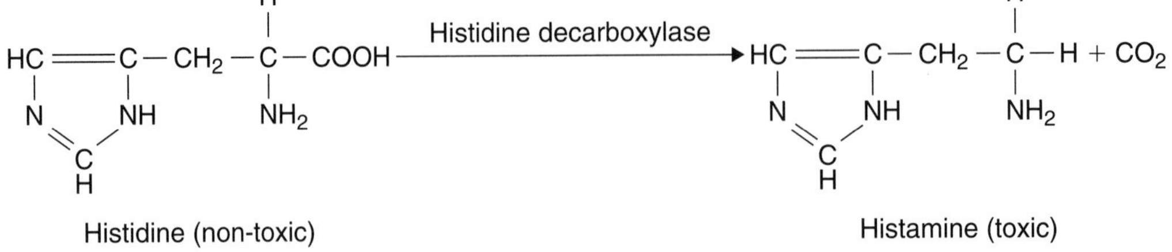

Figure 1.1   *Enzymatic conversion of histidine to toxic histamine (scombrotoxin)*

the food, and over 40 per cent of patients can die without treatment with antitoxin (antibodies). Recovery is usually within 2–8 weeks, and because paralysis of the respiratory tract is a major symptom, patients may require ventilatory support for many months. The botulinum toxins are not as stable as some of the other microbial toxins and are inactivated by normal cooking such as boiling. However, cooking is not a reliable method of control because in some procedures the temperatures achieved are insufficient to guarantee the inactivation of the toxin. Control is achieved by preventing the growth of the organism and thus elaboration of toxin by either high temperature heating such as pressure cooking or canning (this bacterium produces heat-resistant spores) or by the addition of preservatives.

Both *B. cereus* and *S. aureus* food poisoning result in symptoms of nausea, vomiting, malaise and, in some cases, diarrhoea, within a few hours of consuming foods containing the bacterial toxins. The toxins produced by these two bacterial species are quite different, but there are similarities in that both are produced as a result of excessive growth of the respective pathogens in foods, and are heat stable, i.e. are not inactivated by cooking processes. *B. cereus* is commonly found in the environment and many raw foods (e.g. soil, water, cereals, vegetables, milk, dried foods, spices and meat products). Hence food components are frequently contaminated by this bacterium, albeit in low numbers. *B. cereus* food poisoning is typically associated with cooking rice in large quantities by boiling (this allows survival of the heat-resistant spores). When such rice is dried off for several hours in a warm kitchen, bacterial growth and toxin production occurs. The toxin survives regeneration (often quick frying) and causes illness. *B. cereus* food poisoning is controlled by prevention of the growth of the bacterium in food by rapid cooling and cold storage after cooking, or by hot holding the food at more than 63 °C. *S. aureus* is present on the mucous membranes and skin of warm-blooded animals including 50 per cent of humans. Staphylococcal food poisoning is most frequently associated with contamination of food by food handlers with subsequent growth of this bacterium in processed foods during manufacture and kitchen preparation. The growth of *S. aureus* occurs only between 7 °C and 45 °C; control is achieved by storage of food outside this temperature range, by maintaining cleanliness of food handlers, and by reducing both the physical handling and the contact time between initial preparation to service and eating.

Mycotoxins are toxins produced by fungi that occur on the raw food components, or by fungal growth in food during storage. These toxins are very diverse chemically and produce a variety of toxic effects (vomiting, diarrhoea, fever, abdominal pain, hepatic and renal failure, hallucinations and cancer). Grain, peanuts and other nuts that have been inappropriately stored (usually with too much water and under warm conditions) can contain mycotoxins. Ergot poisoning from cereals in which *C. purpurea* has grown has already been briefly considered earlier in this chapter.

Infections

The second major form of foodborne microbiological disease is **infection** where invasion and multiplication by micro-organisms causes disease within the body of a host. To initiate a foodborne infection, sufficient viable micro-organisms (viruses, bacteria or parasites) (Table 1.1) must be ingested in food. There are several universal requirements for infectious micro-organisms to be classed as a **pathogen**, i.e. capable of causing disease.

- The micro-organism must be able to survive, usually in the highly acidic conditions of the stomach, before reaching the site of infection (usually the intestinal wall) where attachment and growth occurs.
- Pathogens must then be able to defend themselves and avoid being killed by the host's immune system, and compete with the large and heterogeneous gut micro-flora, most of which are harmless.
- The pathogen should be able to produce **disease** (a deviation from a normal structure or function of any part, organ or system of the body) at the site of infection, usually by elaborating a toxin (the action of which can manifest in a different part of the host's body) or invading the host's cells (including those outside the intestinal tract), or a combination of these two processes.

The properties that allow pathogens to fulfil the above criteria are known as **virulence factors**.

As previously outlined, foodborne infections that are confined to the gastrointestinal tract mostly present as a diarrhoeal disease together with vomiting, abdominal pain and discomfort. Viral gastro-enteritis (e.g. due to norovirus or rotavirus) generally have a short incubation period of 12–48 hours, followed by a symptomatic period of 1–2 days. Diarrhoea caused by bacterial pathogens (e.g. *Campylobacter* or *Salmonella*) typically show longer incubation periods (1–5 days) followed by a longer duration of illness of days to weeks. The exception to the pattern for bacterial diseases is that caused by *C. perfringens*, which produces an illness of duration similar to the viral diseases. Finally, the parasites that produce gastro-enteritis, *Cryptosporidium* and *Giardia*, usually have longer incubation periods (1–2 weeks) followed by diarrhoea of longer duration than that caused by bacteria or viruses, typically for between 4 and 6 weeks.

Foodborne pathogens can also produce diseases outside the gastrointestinal tract. Among the viruses, polio virus (or more correctly poliomyelitis virus) spreads from the gut to the blood and other parts of the body causing paralysis that usually affects the lower legs and the muscles used for breathing and swallowing; in a small proportion of patients this paralysis is irreversible. A second food-borne virus that affects sites outside the intestinal tract is the hepatitis virus; this virus targets the liver and sometimes causes jaundice. Both these viral diseases can be prevented by vaccination.

Among bacteria, several species are able to spread from the intestines into the blood and other organs; these include some *Salmonella* spp. (e.g. those causing enteric fever or typhoid), *Brucella* spp. and *Listeria monocytogenes*. *L. monocytogenes* is also able to invade the unborn baby or the brain (usually in immunocompromised adults). Infections caused by these three groups of bacteria can be life-threatening and must be treated with antibiotics. Tuberculosis is also a bacterial disease (caused by *Mycobacterium*) and spreads not only by contaminated aerosols (e.g. by coughing) but also by consumption of untreated contaminated milk. Cattle can become infected by this bacterium, which is then excreted into milk. This route of transmission is now rare in the UK, largely due to tuberculin testing and an eradication scheme for cattle, and the widespread consumption of pasteurized milk. Tuberculosis is an example of a disease transmitted from animals to humans; these are called **zoonoses**.

Infections also include extra-intestinal foodborne diseases caused by parasites. *Toxoplasma* causes toxoplasmosis which generally manifests as a mild to symptomless infection, but there can be severe brain infection especially in immunocompromised patients and unborn babies. Infection of the unborn baby (i.e. congenital infection) caused by *Toxoplasma* is very serious and can lead to long-term health problems including deafness, sight defects and mental retardation. *Entamoeba* belongs to a similar class of parasites, and not only causes a severe diarrhoeal disease (amoebic dysentery) but is also capable of travelling to the liver where it causes an abscess: this disease is largely confined to tropical regions and in the UK it occurs almost exclusively in travellers returning from abroad. *Trichinella* is a parasite found in pork or horse meat that initially causes a gastrointestinal disease but which develops into fever with swelling as the parasite migrates into muscle tissue in various parts of the body including around the eyes, hands, temples and nose, as well as the lungs. Fortunately, anti-parasitic agents are available for treatment of all three extra-intestinal parasitic infections.

Infectious agents can be present in the environment, such as *L. monocytogenes*, or reside within food components, such as the parasites *Toxoplasma* and *Trichinella* that occur deep within muscle tissue (meat). However, most of the remaining pathogens occur in the gut of either animals in the food chain or humans. There are several ways in which food becomes contaminated by the pathogens found in faeces. Infectious agents can contaminate the surface of meat directly from the animal gut contents during slaughter and further processing (e.g. the bacteria *Campylobacter*, *Salmonella* and *C. perfringens*) or via the faeces of rodents and other pests that come into contact with food. Food can also accumulate pathogens from the environment, such as when shellfish harvesting beds become contaminated by norovirus from human sewage and effluents pumped into rivers and the sea. Alternatively, indirect faecal contamination of food can result from poor hygiene via physical contact by food-handlers, utensils, other food, food contact surfaces, dirty water, flies and other pests: one or more of these factors are often associated with outbreaks of *Salmonella* infection. Food poisoning is more likely to occur if the contaminating micro-organisms are able to increase in numbers.

Examples of pathogens that grow on foods are the bacteria *Salmonella* and *C. perfringens*. The need for multiplication, however, is not universal, indeed some bacteria and all viruses and parasites are unable to grow directly in food. Hence, methods of control of infectious agents transmitted through food involve:

- processes involving heat (cooking), or more rarely, freezing that result in the death of pathogens
- prevention of cross-contamination, such as between raw and cooked foods or food handlers and food contact surfaces
- prevention of the growth of pathogens by temperature and time control together with other preservation strategies such as the amount of acid, the gaseous atmosphere and the amount of available water.

Finally, there is a group of untreatable degenerative brain disorders called 'slow viral' diseases or transmissible spongiform encephalopathies (TSEs), characterized by changes in the grey matter of the brain, which develops the appearance of a sponge. There are well-characterized TSEs in animals, such as scrapie in sheep and bovine spongiform encephalopathy (BSE) or mad cow disease in cattle. TSEs can also affect humans. The first human TSE to be identified was Kuru in 1957, which is associated with cannibalistic practices in Papua New Guinea. The rise in BSE in the UK was probably associated with changes in the rendering process in the production of animal feed, and it was also linked to the appearance of the human disease variant Creutzfeldt–Jacob (vCJD) disease. The 'infectious' agent associated with these diseases is a protein named the prion protein. Prions are probably transmitted through food and, because of their remarkable resilience, are likely to survive almost all cooking and food processing procedures. BSE has been controlled by: modification of animal feed manufacturing practices; culling of animals up to the age when they were likely to have been exposed to contaminated feed; and the exclusion from the food chain of specified offal that is likely to contain the highest levels of the prion. At the time of writing (2005), the incidence of BSE in the UK has reduced markedly and the numbers of cases of vCJD remains low with new cases being less often reported. However, because of the long incubation period before development of symptoms, the success of these control strategies or how large a public health problem this will be in the future is not yet clear.

A more detailed description of foodborne pathogens, their properties and distribution is given in the following chapters.

MICROBIOLOGICAL EXAMINATION OF FOODS AND IN-PROCESS CONTROL

Microbiological examination of food is done for many reasons. These include an estimation of their quality with respect to:

- safety
- adherence to good manufacturing practice
- keeping quality (shelf life)
- utility (suitability) for a particular purpose.

Microbiological examination can include a numerical estimation for specific organisms or groups of organisms. The approximate numbers of organisms in food are significant not only in relation to spoilage, but also to food poisoning and are used to set 'standards' for specific food groups. When microbiological criteria for food ('standards') were first formulated, it was realized that tests could not be conducted for every target organism (including all pathogens) present. Instead, those surrogate or indicator organisms were selected that were likely to reflect the quality of the sample with respect to a specific criterion. For example, the faecal bacterium *Escherichia coli* was initially suggested as a quantitative indicator of faecal contamination. This was later superseded by a much broader group (faecal coliforms) that includes this bacterium and other related organisms.

Microbiological specifications, guidelines, criteria and standards have done much to improve food hygiene and these will be fully discussed in Chapter 16. However, microbiological testing, particularly testing of the final product (end product testing) cannot assure food safety. The reasons for this are twofold:

- Tests for indicator organisms can be time-consuming to perform, and will not necessarily identify hazards at concentrations likely to cause disease.

- Microbiological examination can only be applied to a sub-sample of food. Even if perfect microbiological tests were available, in order to achieve absolute safety, the entire food product would need to be tested, thus none would remain for consumption.

To address these problems, and to provide completely safe foods for the USA space programme, the Hazard Analysis and Critical Control Points (HACCP) approach was developed in 1959; it was based on an engineering system known as the Failure Modes Analysis Scheme. HACCP is designed to ask the question 'What can go wrong?'. Central to HACCP is the identification of steps (critical control points, CCPs) in the food manufacturing process at which control is necessary for safety. To control these points, monitoring procedures are introduced to confirm and record that control has been maintained. To maintain control, monitoring should, if at all possible, be continuous, or if this is not possible, at a frequency sufficient to guarantee safety. For example, if the hazard is survival of pathogens through a cooking process for a ready-to-eat product, then the length of time of cooking, and the temperatures prior to and during cooking can be measured. Limits for these in-process controls that assure safety can then be established. During production, these critical control points are physically monitored for each batch of product.

Microbiological examination may still be performed, sometimes to verify that the HACCP process is functioning correctly. HACCP has had widespread application to almost all areas of food hygiene including the design of food premises and all functions related to food production. HACCP will be discussed in Chapter 10.

IMPORTANCE OF FOODBORNE DISEASE AND ARRANGEMENT OF SUBSEQUENT CHAPTERS

Food hygiene is of great importance to society in both the developed and the developing world. All those involved with the food chain expend considerable effort to ensure that food is safe and wholesome, but when illness does occur, this incurs considerable expense not only to the affected individuals and the health sector, but also to the food industry. A recent study in England estimated that 9.4 million people (i.e. 1 in 5 of the population) are affected each year by infectious intestinal disease at an annual cost of £0.75 billion (Anon 2000). Efforts have been made to further estimate the disease burden, and examples of this in terms of total numbers of cases as well as hospital admissions and deaths for the USA and England and Wales are given in Table 1.2. This highlights the importance of good food hygiene.

Table 1.2 *Estimated annual numbers of cases of illness and death from the five most common food-borne pathogens in the USA, and England and Wales*

	Annual numbers of cases of foodborne illness		
	Total	Hospitalizations	Deaths
USA (data adapted from Mead *et al.*, 1999)			
All cases	76 000 000	323 000	5200
Salmonella	1 341 873	15 608	553
Listeria	2493	2298	499
Toxoplasma	112 500	2500	375
Norovirus	9 200 000	20 000	124
Campylobacter	1 963 141	10 539	99
England and Wales* (adapted from Adak *et al.*, 2002)			
All cases	1 338 772	20 759	480
Salmonella	41 616	1516	119
Clostridium perfringens	84 081	354	89
Campylobacter	358 466	16 946	86
Listeria	194	194	68
Escherichia coli O157	995	377	22

*Excluding cases due to travel from other countries.

Changes made to traditional foods, such as reducing fat, sugar, salt and preservative content, may fail to take account of microbiological hazards. It is dangerous to abandon traditional and/or verified methods of preparing, processing and preserving food in favour of new untested and/or unverified methods. For example, a change in product formulation in vacuum-packed foods may affect one or more of the specific controlling factors that may well have had adverse microbiological consequences. Most outbreaks of food poisoning are local and affect relatively small numbers of patients. However, with changes in the food industry, not least being the growth of industrial-scale mass production of foods, there is an increased possibility of very large outbreaks of food poisoning. Table 1.3 shows examples of large outbreaks that have occurred over the past 15 years. In these outbreaks, large numbers of patients were affected, resulting in considerable pressure on medical facilities, which even in the developed world, can become inundated.

This book has been written for students and health professionals with an interest in food safety, and for those engaged in food handling and processing. The overall purpose of the book is to provide sufficient knowledge for an understanding of the importance, principles and nature of food hygiene. In addition, the book examines the various dangers that can occur, how they arise, and how they can be prevented. Part 1 covers general characteristics of micro-organisms; the agents concerned in food poisoning and other foodborne diseases; the common food vehicles through which the organisms are consumed; and the behaviour and ecology of the organisms in food and the environment together with their epidemiology and examples of outbreaks. A chapter on spoilage and preservation is also included. Part 2 includes details of effective preventive measures. Consideration is given to care of the hands and other points of personal hygiene, to storage preparation and cooking methods, retail sale and factory practices. In food premises the topics covered include cleaning methods, design of premises and equipment, sterilization and disinfection. Microbiological specifications, legislation and education are necessary corollaries to control the incidence of disease from food. This section also has a chapter on food hygiene outside the developed world and in the wilderness. Part 3 outlines the contributions of different settings and professional groups to food poisoning and food hygiene together with a description of how outbreaks of food poisoning are detected, investigated, controlled and managed.

Table 1.3 *Examples of very large food-poisoning outbreaks*

Year, country	Number of cases	Vehicle	Agent
1991, Egypt	91	Salted fish	*Clostridium botulinum*
1993, USA	403 000	Drinking water	*Cryptosporidium*
1994, USA	224 000	Ice cream	*Salmonella* Enteritidis
1996, Japan	7000	Bean sprouts	*Escherichia coli* O157
2000, Japan	13 420	Milk powder	*Staphylococcus aureus*
2000, Canada	2300	Drinking water	*Escherichia coli* O157 and *Campylobacter*
2005, Spain	2138	Pre-cooked vacuum-packed chicken	*Salmonella* Hador

Summary

- Foodborne diseases have been recognized throughout the ages.
- Almost all foods and food types present a potential food poisoning hazard and have, at some time, been incriminated as a vehicle for transmission of foodborne diseases.
- The two basic mechanisms by which noxious substances cause food poisoning are intoxications and infections.
- Important principles need to be followed to ensure food is produced safely: quality of the raw ingredients, hygiene and care employed by the those handling the food, adequate storage conditions (particularly temperature and time) and general design, cleanliness and maintenance of the food preparation and storage areas together with associated utensils and equipment.

2

Introduction to microbiology

Diane Roberts and Jim McLauchlin

Microbes and microbiology	17	Detection and identification of microbes	29
Viruses	20	Summary	38
Bacteria	21	Sources of information and further reading	40
Parasites, algae and fungi	26		

To understand how foodborne pathogens survive and grow in food and in food manufacturing environments, a working knowledge of microbiology is essential. In particular, it is important to understand how micro-organisms, which are extremely diverse in both morphology and physiology, are identified and detected and to know their lifecycles, distribution and habits. This information can be used to predict the properties of pathogens, and develop and implement the most effective methods for the control and prevention of foodborne disease, as well as preparation of food of acceptable microbiological quality.

Microbiology The study of microscopic life (**micro-organisms**), including viruses, bacteria, fungi, protozoa, parasites and algae.

Taxonomy The science of arrangement of organisms into groups.

Microbial morphology The shape or form of micro-organisms.

Microbial physiology The chemical processes of microbial life.

Pathogen Any disease-causing micro-organism.

MICROBES AND MICROBIOLOGY

Microbes are widespread in their distribution and their influence extends to the entire world in which we live. This influence includes a major contribution to the maintenance of the environment, allowing the production of food. However, micro-organisms, albeit rarely, cause disease in humans and in other animals, in plants, and even other microbes.

The basic building blocks of micro-organisms (and also ourselves and the food we eat) are **organic** molecules (i.e. those containing carbon atoms). These include **nucleic acids, proteins, carbohydrates, lipids,** as well as a variety of other compounds. With the exception of the viruses, all living organisms (including ourselves) are composed of **cells** (membrane-bound compartments) that reproduce. The process of reproduction involves growth and division of cells and the passing on of **genetic material** to descendents. This genetic material is encoded within a group of organic compounds called nucleic acids. Nucleic acids are composed of chains of **nucleotides** or **bases** that occur in different chemical forms, and their order in the nucleotide chain confers genetic information. This information occurs in discrete units or **genes**, that, except for viruses, ultimately resides in a double-stranded helical molecule named **DNA** (deoxyribose nucleic acid). DNA is translated to a second 'informational' molecule also composed of nucleotides, **RNA** (ribose nucleic acid). RNA is used to convert the sequences of nucleotide bases in a gene into a chain of **amino acids** (a **polypeptide chain**) of specific sequence, which provides the building blocks of proteins, including **enzymes**. Enzymes **catalyse** (increase the speed of) chemical reactions that are used by organisms to produce their chemical constituents (carbohydrates, lipids, etc.) and ultimately to reproduce themselves.

Enzymes are often named according to the substrate(s) on which they act followed by the suffix 'ase': for example lecithinases and proteases act on lecithin and proteins, respectively.

All living cells require energy, most of which is obtained by organisms through the metabolism of organic compounds. This energy is converted into a chemical carrier named adenosine triphosphate (ATP). The amount of ATP per microbial cell is relatively constant and this is degraded within a couple of hours of death of the micro-organism. ATP is relatively easy and rapid to measure, using the action of the luciferin-luciferase biochemicals responsible for the generation of light in the firefly: the amount of light produced is directly proportional to the amount of ATP present. Determination of the quantity of ATP present can be used as an 'on-the-spot' rapid method to monitor microbial contamination (and consequently measure the level of hygiene), for example, on surfaces in food manufacturing environments.

Viruses are somewhat different organisms because they do not have an independent existence, and their genetic material can be composed of DNA or RNA.

Microbes are extremely diverse in their form and function, and, although these characteristics are 'simpler' than those of plants and animals, they should never be considered as primitive. Indeed, as micro-organisms have coexisted with all other forms of life for the entire history of this planet, they are just as evolved as we are! The diversity of microbes is reflected in different disciplines within microbiology (Box 2.1).

Box 2.1 The various divisions of microbiology
- Virology – the study of viruses
- Bacteriology – the study of bacteria
- Mycology – the study of fungi (moulds and yeasts)
- Phycology – the study of algae
- Parasitology – the study of more complex unicellular (composed of a single cell, e.g. protozoa) or multicellular (composed of multiple cells, e.g. helminths, nematodes) organisms also known collectively as parasites

---

There is a another group of 'infectious' agents important in food microbiology that differ from all of the above. These are known as prions. Prions are probably composed purely of a single abnormal form of a protein that occurs naturally in mammalian neurological tissue. Prions cause a number of distinct diseases of which bovine spongiform encephalopathy (BSE) in cattle and its human equivalent (variant Creutzfeldt–Jacob disease) gained much notoriety in the UK during the 1980s. These agents are briefly discussed in Chapter 4, p. 90.

The naming of micro-organisms

Taxonomy (Box 2.2) is a branch of biology concerned with the arrangement of organisms into groups or **taxa**.

Box 2.2 The three components of taxonomy
- **Classification** – the arrangement of organisms into groups, usually reflecting the way in which organisms have evolved (**phylogenetic classification**)
- **Nomenclature** – the assignment of names to groups of organisms so that they are recognized in the same way by independent workers
- **Identification** – the recognition of new microbial isolates that determine their assignment to a pre-existing group of organisms already established by the process of classification and named in the process of assigning a nomenclature.

The system of naming living organisms is based on that devised by the Swedish biologist Linnaeus (Carl von Linneé, 1707–1778). This is a binomial system in which each distinct type of organism is recognized as a species that belongs to a wider group known as a genus. The genus name is given first (starting with a capital letter) followed by the species name: the whole name is printed in italics, for example, humans are named *Homo sapiens* and are the single surviving species '*sapiens*' within the genus '*Homo*'. The binomial names often have Latin or Greek roots that describe the organism, its habitat, or its discoverer: for example, the bacterium *Bacillus* (stick) *cereus* (wax coloured), and *Escherichia* (discovered by Professor Escherich) *coli* (associated with the large intestine).

After its first citation in a document, the genus name is abbreviated to a single letter (or more than one if there is likely to be confusion with other organisms), e.g. *B. cereus* and *E. coli*. Where there is reference to several species within a genus, or if an organism cannot be assigned to an individual species, the word species is abbreviated to sp. or spp. depending on whether reference is being made to one or more than one species. For example, *Salmonella* spp., species within the genus *Salmonella*. Names are internationally recognized and the naming of newly discovered species is governed by rules that include valid descriptions and usually the availability of an exemplar (a **type species**) that can be accessed by other microbiologists for further study including comparisons with other organisms.

Taxonomy is not a static science and names, for good reason, will on occasion change. However, changes are kept to the minimum because there is inevitably some confusion when names change. For example, in the 1980s it was realized that the bacterial species *Listeria monocytogenes* (named after Lord Lister, the pioneer of antisepsis and the cause of an increase in a type of white blood cell, the monocyte, in infected rabbits and guinea pigs) would be better classified to contain five different species that were re-named as *L. monocytogenes*, *L. innocua*, *L. seeligeri*, *L. ivanovii*, and *L. welshimeri*; however, only *L. monocytogenes* is a major foodborne **pathogen**.

Re-naming micro-organisms can also result in the bringing together of species that were previously classified into different species. For example, in the late 1980s, after consideration of the close similarity between the more than 2000 'species' of *Salmonella*, these were combined into only two species, *Salmonella enterica* and *S. bongori* (the genus is named after the American microbiologist Salmon). *S. enterica* (named because it occurs in the enteric tract) is further divided into six subspecies (subsp. *enterica*, *salamae*, *arizonae*, *diarizonae*, *houtenae*, and *indica*). The majority of human infections are due to *S. enterica* subsp. *enterica*, and because the previously named species are distinguished using **serological methods** (those based on reactions with antibodies, see later in this chapter, p. 37), these are named **serotypes**. The **serotype name** is capitalized but not italicized and is abbreviated to ser.: for example *S. enterica* subsp. *enterica* ser. Typhi, *S. enterica* subsp. *enterica* ser. Enteritidis and *S. enterica* subsp. *enterica* ser. Typhimurium. Since this is rather a cumbersome

nomenclature, these are more usually written as *S.* Typhi, *S.* Enteritidis and *S.* Typhimurium.

Viruses are classified differently. They are not usually given a binomial name, although there are some exceptions, for example the virus that causes smallpox, which is called *Variola major*. In addition, viruses are structurally quite different from other micro-organisms. The foodborne viruses will be described later in this chapter (p. 20).

Major groupings of micro-organisms

Organisms can be further classified into larger groupings (kingdoms, phyla, classes, orders and families). This classification reflects a wider and more fundamental split between organisms that have compartments or **organelles** within their cells (the animals, plants, fungi, protozoa) and are known as the eukaryotes, and those that do not and are known as the **prokaryotes** (i.e. the bacteria). An idealized representation of a prokaryotic and eukaryotic cell is shown in Figure 2.1. The organelles located within eukaryotic cells (especially **mitochondria**, which are the energy-producing organs, and **chloroplasts**, which are involved with photosynthesis in plants and algae) show many similarities to prokaryotic cells. Mitochondria and chloroplasts probably evolved from bacterial 'companions' which lived within cells (intracellularly) in the very distant past and eventually became an integral part of eukaryotic cells. Thus we probably owe our very existence and that of our natural environment to the evolution of distant bacterial ancestors.

Bacteria are almost always unicellular, i.e. they are organized as individual or single cells. However, bacteria can live in colonies on solid surfaces bound together (sometimes with fungi, protozoa or algae) by an extracellular matrix. Such collections are called **biofilms**. Biofilms are important in cleaning and disinfection because they are more resistant to cleaning agents than individual cells. In addition, cells of some bacterial species have the property of undergoing differentiation into hardy structures called **spores** that, because of their increased resistance to physical agents such as heat, are of importance in food processing (p. 25). Eukaryotic micro-organisms also form resistant spores and many have complex lifecycles involving multiple hosts. These will be briefly considered later in this chapter (p. 26).

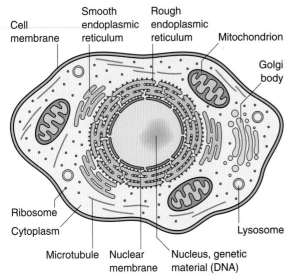

Eukaryotic cell

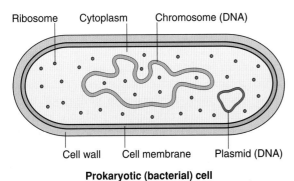

Prokaryotic (bacterial) cell

Figure 2.1   *Organization of prokaryotic (bacterial) and eukaryotic (protozoan) cells*

Size of micro-organisms

The unaided human eye can resolve at best objects of 0.5 mm in the size, and this is about the size of the largest of the protozoa. The vast majority of micro-organisms, by definition, are very much smaller than this and can only be visualized using a microscope. The use of size is rather an imprecise method of classification especially since some 'microbes' are much larger than this, for example an adult tapeworm and some seaweeds are over a metre in length. However, both of these organisms produce microscopic eggs that behave similarly to other microbes, or are closely related to much smaller forms, and are thus dealt with by microbiologists.

Size within the range of micro-organisms (bacteria, fungi and parasites) is measured in micrometres (1/1 000 000 or one millionth of a metre, or one thousandth of a millimetre), and is written as μm. Since viruses are an order of magnitude smaller, these are measured in nanometres (1/1 000 000 000 or one-thousand millionth of a metre) and written as nm.

The comparative sizes of foodborne pathogens are illustrated in Figure 2.2: from the tapeworm (1–2 m in length), protozoan cysts and parasite eggs (4–150 μm in diameter), bacteria (1–10 μm long) to a hepatitis A virus (30 nm in diameter).

VIRUSES

Viruses differ from other types of micro-organism in that they are incapable of growth outside a host. Viruses require a living cell in which to replicate and all groups of organisms are parasitized by viruses, including bacteria. Bacterial viruses are known as **bacteriophages** or phages. These have proved to be extremely useful in epidemiological fingerprinting (i.e. **bacteriophage typing**) where patterns of reactions are used to identify types (see later discussion this chapter). Viruses do not have a prokaryotic or eukaryotic cellular structure but instead have a general structure of nucleic acid (either DNA or RNA) surrounded by a protein coat or **capsid**. Viruses associated with foodborne diseases are discussed in Chapter 4, some of these viruses are listed in Table 2.1 and shown in Figure 2.3.

Table 2.1   *Foodborne viruses*

	Rotavirus	Norovirus	Hepatitis A	Poliomyelitis
Virus family	*Reoviridae*	*Caliciviridae*	*Picornaviridae*	*Picornaviridae*
Features	Triple shelled capsid, outer shell appears like spokes of a wheel	Round with cup-shaped depressions	Icosahedral without features	Icosahedral without features
Size (diameter)	70–80 nm	34 nm	28 nm	28 nm
Nucleic acid	Double-stranded segmented RNA	Single-stranded RNA	Single-stranded RNA	Single-stranded RNA

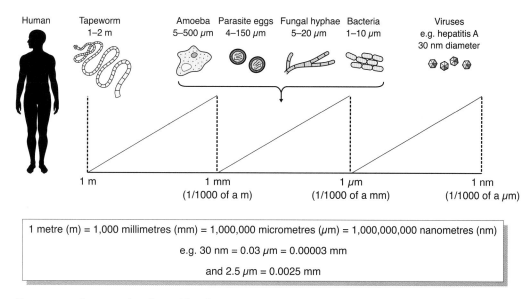

Human

Tapeworm
1–2 m

Amoeba
5–500 μm

Parasite eggs
4–150 μm

Fungal hyphae
5–20 μm

Bacteria
1–10 μm

Viruses
e.g. hepatitis A
30 nm diameter

1 m

1 mm
(1/1000 of a m)

1 μm
(1/1000 of a mm)

1 nm
(1/1000 of a μm)

1 metre (m) = 1,000 millimetres (mm) = 1,000,000 micrometres (μm) = 1,000,000,000 nanometres (nm)

e.g. 30 nm = 0.03 μm = 0.00003 mm

and 2.5 μm = 0.0025 mm

Figure 2.2 *Comparative sizes of foodborne pathogens in comparison to a human being*

Since viruses do not have an independent existence, they are incapable of growth in food or in the environment. They are transmitted through faecal/oral contact either via person to person (especially among young children and particularly noroviruses among hospitalized patients) or via direct contamination of food (especially seafood).

BACTERIA

Bacteria are a heterogeneous group of unicellular organisms that possess a rigid cell that determines their shape as **coccoid** (spherical), **bacillary** (rod shaped), **helical** or **comma-shaped** (Figure 2.4). Bacteria are divided into two fundamental groups that can be distinguished by a specific staining procedure known as **Gram staining**. Gram-stain positive (or more usually referred to as **Gram-positive**) bacteria have a fundamentally different cell wall structure and tend to be much more environmentally robust than **Gram-negative** organisms. Figure 2.5 is a schematic representation of the cell wall of Gram-positive and Gram-negative bacteria. Examples of Gram-positive and Gram-negative bacteria of different shapes are summarized in Table 2.2. Since cell walls of this type occur only in bacteria, these provide a unique target for antimicrobial agents such as the penicillins that inhibit the production of intact cell walls and prevent the production of healthy cells.

Table 2.2 *Shapes of Gram-negative and Gram-positive bacteria important in food microbiology*

	Gram-negative	Gram-positive
Coccoid (spherical)		*Staphylococcus aureus*
Bacillary (rod-shaped)	*Brucella* spp.	*Listeria monocytogenes*
	Escherichia coli	*Mycobacterium* spp.
	Salmonella spp.	
	Shigella spp.	
	Yersinia enterocolitica	
Helical	*Campylobacter* spp.	
Comma-shaped	*Vibrio cholerae*	
	Vibrio parahaemolyticus	
Rod-shaped forming endospores		*Bacillus cereus*
		Clostridium botulinum
		Clostridium perfringens

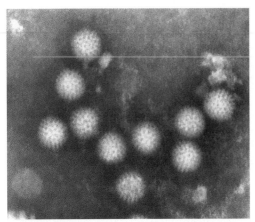

(a) Rotavirus: triple-layered icosahedral that appear like the spokes of a wheel, 70 nm in diameter

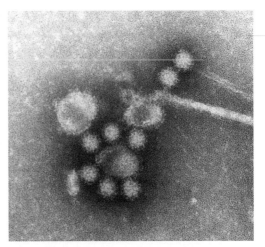

(c) Norovirus, icosahedral with cup shaped depression, 34 nm in diameter

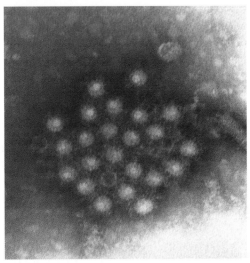

(b) Hepatitis A virus, featureless icosahedral, 28 nm in diameter

Figure 2.3   *Electron micrographs of foodborne viruses (courtesy of Dr H Appleton, Health Protection Agency)*

Surface of bacterial cells

The surface of bacteria contains structures that interface between the bacterium and its environment, and are important for influencing behaviour, the ability to cause disease, resistance to physical agents and survival. Protruding from the cell surface are long whip-like structures named **flagella** (see Figures 2.4 and 2.5) that rotate and allow the bacterium to move. Motility is important since it allows movement between environments where nutrition or protection is better (**chemotaxis**). In addition to flagella, bacterial surfaces (especially those of Gram-negatives) contain other structures including shorter and thinner **pili** (hair-like) or **fimbriae** (fringe-like) objects (see Figure 2.5) that are involved with adhesion to surfaces. These have an important role in the causation of disease as they allow the bacteria to attach to cells in the host's gut. Pili are also involved in **conjugation** (bacterial mating), when genetic material is transferred between cells. Bacteria also possess outer 'gel-like' coats known as **capsules** that are important in disease as they allow the bacteria to evade a host's immune system during infection as well as provide protection against chemical disinfection.

Flagella can be detected by their reactions with antibodies and produce 'fluffy' complexes (**agglutination** reactions): these are known as **H antigens** (from the German *hauch*). The cell wall or somatic antigens are known as the **O antigens** (from the German *ohne*), and the capsular antigens as K (German, *kapsel*). The antigenic structure of bacteria is often given after their species name, for example, to identify a particular relationship with other isolates or an outbreak of foodborne illness. For example the vero cytotoxin producing *E. coli* (VTEC) most often associated with human disease has an O antigen 157 and H antigen 7 and is written VTEC O157:H7.

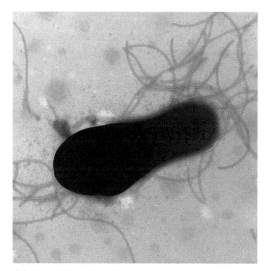

(a) Clostridium botulinum, *rod-shaped, multiple flagella and swelling of vegetative cell by spore (3 µm in length)*

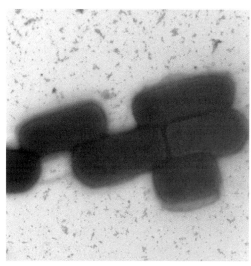

(b) Clostridium perfringens, *rod-shaped (1.8 µm in length)*

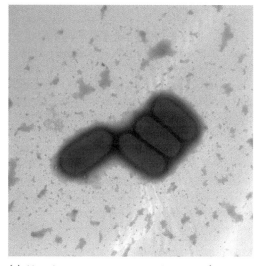

(c) Listeria monocytogenes, *rod-shaped (0.9 µm in length)*

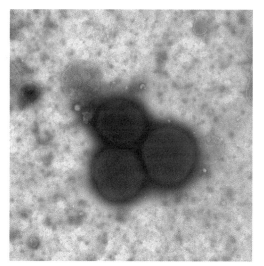

(d) Staphylococcus aureus, *coccus-shaped (0.6 µm in diameter)*

Figure 2.4 *Electron micrographs of foodborne bacteria (courtesy of Dr H Chart, Health Protection Agency)*

Contents of the bacterial cell

The internal contents of the bacterial cell are collectively known as the **cytoplasm**, and surrounding this, but inside the cell wall, is the **cytoplasmic membrane**. Gram-negative bacteria have a further membrane (the **outer membrane**) surrounding the cell wall. These membranes are **semi-permeable** and selectively allow transport of nutrients into the cell as well as secretion of enzymes and toxins out of the cell. The DNA of bacteria occurs in a single circular chromosome but some species also possess additional smaller circular genetic elements (**plasmids**), some of which can transfer genes between organisms including those for antimicrobial resistance. Also present within the cytoplasm are **ribosomes**, that are the site of protein synthesis and, in some organisms, energy storage inclusions.

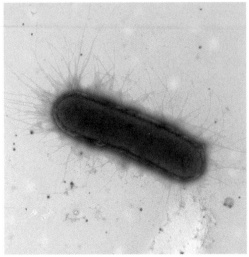

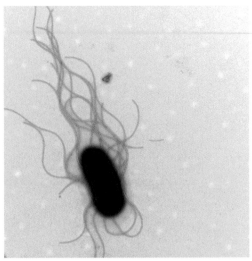

(e) Escherichia coli, *rod-shaped, with fimbriae (3 μm in length)*

(f) Salmonella enterica, *rod-shaped, multiple flagella (2.5 μm in length)*

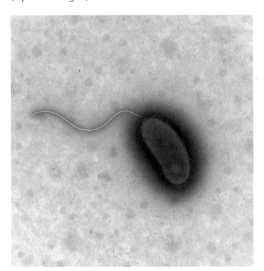

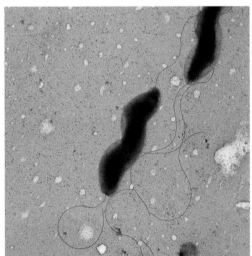

(g) Vibrio cholerae, *comma-shaped, single flagellum from the pole of the cell (2 μm in length)*

(h) Campylobacter jejuni, *spiral-shaped, single flagellum from either pole of the cell (2.5 μm in length)*

Figure 2.4 *Electron micrographs of foodborne bacteria, continued (courtesy of Dr H Chart, Health Protection Agency)*

Bacterial growth

Bacterial cells that are growing are known as **vegetative cells** and multiplication occurs by division of the cell into two. When a bacterium achieves the maximum cell size, a constriction appears at both sides of the centre axis (Figure 2.6), the membrane or envelope of the cell grows inwards and forms a septum which results in the formation of two new twin daughter cells. In some species multiplication is extremely rapid, and the time to complete a round of cell multiplication (the **doubling time**) can be less than 10 minutes under suitable conditions. Rates of growth and the effects of the external environment are considered in Chapter 3. However, it is important to further mention here that the growth of a population of bacterial cells has several different phases (Figure 2.7). First, there is a **lag**

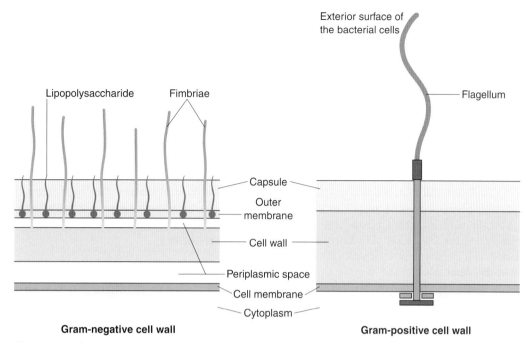

Figure 2.5   *Schematic structure of bacterial cell walls*

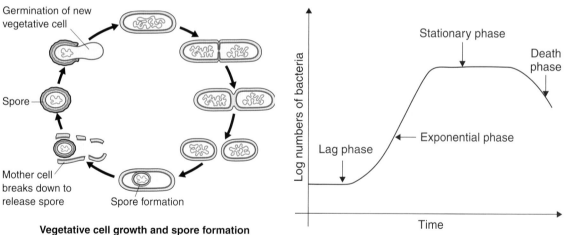

Figure 2.7   *Phases of growth of a bacterial population*

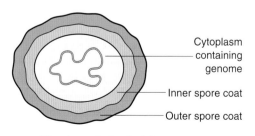

Figure 2.6   *Schematic representation of a bacterial spore and the lifecycle of a spore-forming bacterium*

phase when growth does not occur at all or occurs very slowly while the micro-organisms are adapting to new conditions. The length of the lag phase will vary depending on the environment in which the microbes have most recently been growing, the need for repair of damaged cells, the number of cells present, the medium, available nutrients (including water) as well as the external conditions including the gaseous atmosphere and temperature. Provided conditions are permissive, following the lag phase the populations of cells will double for every unit of time and this is known as the **log** or **exponential phase**. During the log phase, one cell can become over 2 million in 7 hours, and 7000 million after 12 hours continuous growth. However, this rapid increase does not continue indefinitely, and following exhaustion of available nutrients or accumulation of waste products of bacterial growth (acids, carbon dioxide, alcohols etc.) cells will stop growing, and this period is known as the **stationary phase**. The cells are still metabolically active during the stationary phase and toxins may be produced in this phase, as well as spores by species such as *Clostridium* and *Bacillus* (see p. 25). Eventually the population will decline and cells will die – this is known as the **death phase**.

To grow in food (and indeed in artificial media in the laboratory), some species of bacteria can synthesize all that they require from the simplest of components, but others will require many complicated organic compounds. However, all bacteria will require a source of carbon together with a source of water, and a permissive temperature for growth. Most food poisoning bacteria grow under normal atmospheric conditions, and in the presence of oxygen: these organisms are known as having an **aerobic metabolism**, or more simply are known as **aerobes** (e.g. *Salmonella* spp., *L. monocytogenes*, *Staphylococcus aureus*). However, some bacteria only multiply in the absence of oxygen and have an **anaerobic metabolism**, i.e. they are **anaerobes** (e.g. *C. perfringens* and *C. botulinum*). Furthermore, some organisms grow in the presence of oxygen, but only if it is at a concentration lower than that of the normal atmosphere, and thus have a **microaerophilic** metabolism, or are known as **microaerophiles** (e.g. *Campylobacter* spp.).

An understanding the physiology and distribution of bacteria is important to be able to prevent the growth of micro-organisms that lead to food spoilage or foodborne disease, as well as being able to create conditions in the laboratory to grow and detect bacteria. For example, the anaerobic spore-forming bacterium *C. perfringens* occurs widely in the environment and hence is likely to occur in food and food components found in warm kitchens. This bacterium grows extremely quickly under the anaerobic conditions found in the centre of rolled joints of meat, in poultry carcasses and in boiled masses of beef, cut up or minced, and in stews. This is because the oxygen is driven off by cooking and constituents of the meat itself will bind oxygen and create the anaerobic conditions required for the growth of this bacterium. Care must therefore be taken with adequate cooling, storage and reheating conditions to prevent regrowth of *C. perfringens* and the resulting food poisoning risk. To detect and grow this bacterium in the laboratory, an anaerobic environment must be produced, and some microbiological media (e.g. 'cooked meat broth') have similar constituents to foods most often associated with *C. perfringens* food poisoning.

Bacterial spores

In addition to production of vegetative cells, two genera of Gram-positive bacteria, *Bacillus* and *Clostridium*, produce internal spores (also known as **endospores**) within vegetative cells. Endospores are extremely robust and can survive extremes of physical conditions such as chemical disinfection and heat treatment, although there is some variation in resistance between bacterial species. Endospores can survive in dormant conditions for very long periods under adverse conditions, however when these conditions become more favourable, the spores germinate to produce vegetative cells (see Figure 2.6). Although the sensitivity of endospores to physical factors varies, some spores can withstand high temperatures for long periods. The processes for the sterilization of canned foods are based on the time and temperature that is required to destroy the most heat-resistant spores. Bacterial spores, when allowed to multiply in foodstuffs, may be responsible for spoilage (including the production of gas) as well as production of toxins that cause disease. Further information on conditions necessary to kill micro-organisms can be found in Chapter 3.

PARASITES, ALGAE AND FUNGI

An understanding of eukaryotic organisms is important in food poisoning and food hygiene since raw foods can harbour viable helminths, nematodes and protozoa that cause infections. In addition food acts as a vehicle for toxins from algae and fungi, and fungi are also of importance as a cause of food spoilage.

Helminths and nematodes (the flatworms and roundworms respectively) are a group of eukaryotic animal parasites that are also infectious to humans. The most important flatworms are the liver fluke (*Fasciola hepatica*) and the tapeworms of the genus *Taenia*. Both flatworms and tapeworms are multi-cellular organisms that have complex lifecycles involving more than one host. As these infections are more common in developing countries, these are further discussed in Chapter 18.

Liver flukes develop as 'leaf-like' animals in the bile ducts of humans, sheep and cattle (the **definitive host**) and are about 2.5 cm long by 1 cm wide. Having matured, they produce large numbers of eggs ($150 \times 90\,\mu m$) that are secreted via the bile duct into the faeces. In the environment, the eggs hatch and are not infectious to the definitive host, but they are able to infect a **secondary host**, the water snail. Here the parasite multiplies and develops, and is then released back into the environment where it is infectious to the definitive host. Liver flukes are the cause of considerable economic loss in livestock, particularly in the developing world. Infected humans develop the disease (fascioliasis) with symptoms of fever, loss of appetite with pain and discomfort in the abdomen, and abnormal liver function (occasionally with jaundice). In the UK, as a result of the distribution of the secondary host (the water snail), infection in humans used to be particularly associated with watercress consumption, although this is now, fortunately, rare.

Among the tapeworms, *Taenia solium* is associated with pork and *T. saginata* with beef. These long, ribbon-like organisms live in the intestines of humans as the definitive host, and pigs or cows as secondary hosts. The larval stages develop in tissue in the secondary host, including muscle, and produce a spotted or 'measly' appearance, hence infection to humans follows the eating of undercooked beef or pork. The adult tapeworm can live for 25 years in the definitive host (humans) and causes general irritation to the gut including nausea, abdominal pain, and weight loss: copious $32\,\mu m$ diameter eggs are released into the faeces during infection. *T. saginata* can be a more serious since the larval stages may invade other tissue in humans, and if infection of the central nervous system occurs, it is often fatal.

Among the **nematodes** or **roundworms,** *Trichinella spiralis* is probably the most important as a foodborne pathogen. Nematodes are multicellular organisms and there are many species widespread in the environment as free-living organisms but some are pathogenic to animals or plants. *T. spiralis* has no free living stage but is transmitted to humans (the secondary host) usually via consumption of poorly cooked pork (pigs are the primary host) where cysts can reside in muscle tissue. Once eaten by humans, the larvae are released from the cyst and grow in the intestines to 3–4 mm in length and cause abdominal pain, nausea and diarrhoea. A second phase follows that includes muscle pain, fever and even death as the larvae invade muscle tissue. Cysts form within muscle tissue and appear as small white specks. This infection is controlled by meat inspection (infected animals should be removed from the food chain), as well as by adequate cooking (or freezing) of pork. Infection is a greater problem in countries where wild pork is commonly eaten.

Foodborne protozoa are single-celled eukaryotic organisms that cause a variety of infections including diarrhoea (species of *Cryptosporidium*, *Giardia* and *Cyclospora*) as well as more serious systemic infections (e.g. *Toxoplasma gondii*). These diseases and their control are discussed in further detail in Chapter 4. However, it is important to note here that these organisms have complex lifecycles containing both motile and sessile 'feeding' forms (or **trophozoites**). Resistant cysts (or oocysts in the cases of *Cryptosporidium*, *Cyclospora* and *Toxoplasma* as they are produced following a sexual reproductive process) also occur. The cysts or oocysts from the protozoa are between about $4\,\mu m$ and $12\,\mu m$ in diameter, and their appearance on microscopy in stained preparations from the faeces from affected patients are the principal means of diagnosis. Cysts of other enteric parasites such as *Fasciola* and *Taenia* are also identified on microscopy of samples of faeces. Examples of cyst forms detected by light microscopy are shown in Figure 2.8.

Algal toxins and **mycotoxins** are causes of food poisoning and are discussed in Chapter 4, pp. 81 and 89. Fungi have a further important role in food spoilage. Both algae and fungi are eukaryotic organisms, the former having intracellular organelles (chloroplasts) that synthesize organic compounds by the action of light, i.e. by **photosynthesis**. Algae are familiar as seaweed that can grow to many metres in length and are well known to microbiologists as the source of agar (see p. 29). Algae are also safely

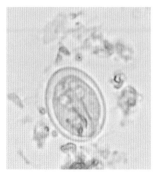

(a) Giardia duodenalis *cysts,
stained with iodine
(6–12 μm)*

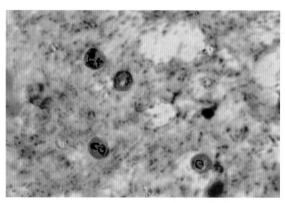

(b) Cryptosporidium parvum *oocysts stained red using
Modified Ziehl–Nielsen technique (4–6 μm)*

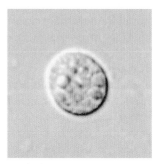

(c) Cyclospora cayetanensis
unstained oocysts (8–10 μm)

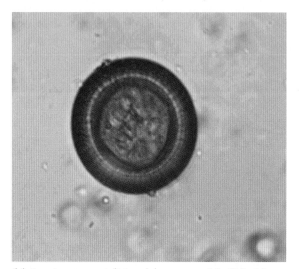

(d) Taenia *spp. cyst (35 μm) (courtesy of Dr H Smith,
Scottish Parasitology Reference Laboratory, Glasgow)*

Figure 2.8   *Spores from eukaryotic foodborne parasites*

eaten in many parts of the world. In addition to the macroscopic algae, microscopic unicellular algae exist as plankton and occur in enormous numbers, particularly in the sea: the total weight of microscopic algae and their capacity for photosynthesis in the sea far exceeds that of all terrestrial forests. One group of these planktonic algae are the dinoflagellates, so named because their motile forms have two unequal flagella, together with a complex armour-like cell wall composed of cellulose. Dinoflagellates can become so numerous that they produce 'red tides' that can be highly toxic to both fish as well as to humans when the toxins (diarrhoetic shellfish poisoning and paralytic

shellfish poisoning toxins) are consumed through accumulations in edible filter-feeding shellfish. These toxins are usually referred to as DSP and PSP respectively (see Chapter 4, p. 81). Toxins from dinoflagellates are particularly important in tropical seas where ciguatera toxin accumulates in the flesh of predatory reef fish (see p. 84).

Fungi are similarly ubiquitous and typically exhibit two phases of growth:

- The 'fruiting' body or sexually reproducing phase in which spores are produced that allow these organisms to survive periods of dormancy

● The vegetative or growth phase in which tubular filaments or hyphae of 10–50 μm in diameter are produced.

Hyphae grow from the tips and nutrients are transferred from here to the remainder of the colony. An entire mass of growth of hyphae is known as a mycelium and is familiar as the very visible woolly or hairy-looking result of mouldy spoilage of food. Not all fungi produce hyphae, and yeasts produce single spherical or ovoidal cells by their characteristic method of reproduction, called budding. Yeasts make an enormous contribution to food microbiology both as an essential component of bread, beer and wine, as well as the cause of spoilage by the production of off-flavours and taints. Yeasts also produce spores like the filamentous fungi.

Fungi are routinely cultured in food microbiology laboratories (see next section) particularly for the assessment of spoilage.

DETECTION AND IDENTIFICATION OF MICROBES

Growth of micro-organisms in the laboratory

Bacteria and fungi are routinely grown in laboratories for the assessment of food hygiene and food quality, and to investigate incidents of food poisoning. It is not possible to culture viruses, protozoa and multicellular parasites under laboratory conditions or it is so technically difficult and slow that this is unlikely to generate useful data except in research settings. However, the development of conditions required for growth in artificial media for the culturing of bacteria, and to a lesser extent fungi, by the isolation of pure cultures (the isolation and growth of a single representative strain of an individual species in artificial media in the absence of other micro-organisms) has made a considerable contribution to the understanding of foodborne disease, including the factors that lead both to its occurrence and to its control.

Chapter 3 describes the conditions for microbial growth in foods. However, growth of organisms (particularly bacteria) in the laboratory requires exactly the same considerations and these will be briefly discussed here. Culture media are nutritional environments designed for the growth of micro-organisms in the laboratory. As already mentioned earlier in this chapter, micro-organisms are very diverse in their nutrient requirements and no single medium is suitable for all uses. Media are made to suit the growth requirements of different organisms and these can have meat (peptone of beef base), yeast extract, blood, serum, milk or other proteinaceous material added to enhance growth or to allow the recognition of special attributes of specific bacteria. Culture media are dispensed in either liquid or in solid forms. Gelatine was initially used as a solidifying agent but a firm gel is now almost exclusively achieved by the use of agar, an inert carbohydrate extracted from seaweed. Agar has properties superior to that of gelatine because it melts at higher temperatures and sets at temperatures below those required for the survival of many bacteria. For the isolation of bacteria solid media are often dispensed in flat 10 cm diameter dishes known as petri dishes (Figure 2.9).

Many years of research have led to the development of culture media known as selective media that enhance the growth of certain types of bacteria while depressing the growth of others. Enrichment media are broths that contain selective ingredients that are designed to shift the growth of a mixed population of micro-organisms towards a specific species or group of organisms. Selection is achieved by, for example, the addition of salt, antimicrobial agents, detergents, and/or metals as well as by selecting specific conditions of pH, water activity, temperature and gaseous environment.

When bacteria are spread on the surface of a solid medium in a petri dish and incubated for a sufficient time and temperature (often overnight at 37 °C) cells multiply to many millions and form a visible heap or colony. On solid media, different species of bacteria produce varied and often typical colonial forms. The size, shape, colour and consistency of these colonies on particular culture media and their reactions with special media ingredients (e.g. the haemolysis of blood, fermentation of a specific sugar or precipitation of a protein), are further steps in the identification process and these are known as differential media. Chromogenic and fluorogenic media are microbiological growth media that contain enzyme substrates linked to a chromogen (colour reaction), fluorogen (fluorescent reaction) or a combination of both. The target population are

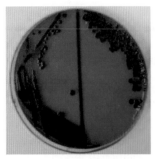

(a) Salmonella *enterica colonies on XLD agar.*
Salmonella *colonies are black and shiny (courtesy of*
Dr NL Lang, Health Protection Agency)

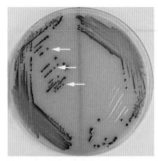

(b) Salmonella enterica *and* Escherichia coli *on*
Salmonella Chromogenic Agar. Salmonella *colonies are*
magenta (arrow), E. coli *are blue; there are no*
Salmonella *colonies present on the right-hand side of*
the plate (courtesy of Dr NL Lang, Health Protection
Agency)

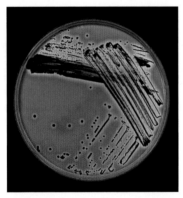

(c) Staphylococcus aureus *colonies on Baird Parker*
Agar

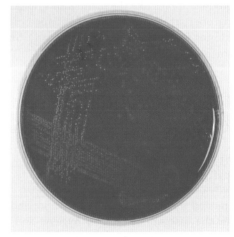

(d) Listeria monocytogenes *colonies on blood agar*

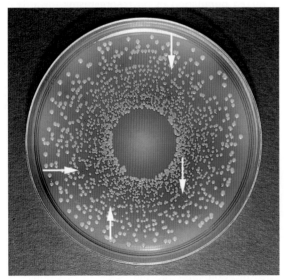

(e) L. monocytogenes *colonies (arrow) enumerated in*
the presence of other bacteria using an Oxford agar
spiral plate dilution

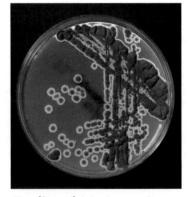

(f) Aspergillus *(fungal) colonies growing on*
Oxytetracycline Glucose Yeast Extract Agar (OGYE)
agar

Figure 2.9   *Bacterial and fungal colonies growing on solid agar media in petri dishes*

detected by enzyme systems that metabolize the substrate to release products (chromogens or fluorogens) that are easily recognized by a colour change in the medium and/or fluorescence under long-wave ultraviolet light. Chromogenic and fluorogenic media provide for more specific identification of the target organism. This in turn can reduce or eliminate the need for subculture and confirmatory tests for some organisms. Examples of commonly used differential, enrichment and selective media are given in Table 2.3.

Following the discovery of methods for the growth of bacteria in the laboratory, it soon became clear that considerable added value was obtained for the examination of food (and water) by quantifying (enumerating) both the total numbers of bacteria present, as well as numbers of potential pathogens. These are known as **enumeration methods** (Box 2.3). Enumeration methods are used extensively in food, water and environmental laboratories, although for technical reasons, no method permits the determination of the exact numbers of all organisms present. Enumerations are often given as the total number colonies that, after incubation on a suitable medium, have grown from a given volume of sample and can be written as **colony forming units per mL** or **CFU/mL**.

After the isolation in pure culture of a bacterium, in addition to the recognition of typical colonies on selective or non-selective agars, it is usually necessary to identify this culture. Identification is increasingly being achieved by **genotypic methods** (characters based on the genetic composition of an organism, see later discussion), however the majority of identifications still rely on the recognition of **phenotypic characteristics**. The **phenotype** of an organism is a reflection of the external characteristics of an organism at the time of examination and are as a result of expression of its genotype as well as its environment. Phenotypic characters include:

- The size, shape, consistency or smell of colonies growing on agar plates.
- The behaviour when growing on artificial media such as the ability to be motile or produce endospores.
- The size, shape and appearance in stained preparations examined by microscopy.

Box 2.3 Different enumeration methods

- **Pour plates** – a known volume of sample (usually 1 mL) is mixed with molten agar and allowed to set in a petri dish. Following suitable incubation, the numbers of colonies within the agar are counted
- **Spread plates** – a known volume of sample (usually less than 0.1 mL) is dispensed or spread over the surface of an agar plate. Following incubation the numbers of colonies on the surface of the agar are counted. Where drops of known volume are directly added to the agar surface, this is commonly known as a modification surface drop technique. Alternatively, a **spiral plater** may be used where a liquid inoculum is distributed over the surface of the agar in such a manner that a concentration range of 1:10 000 is achieved from the outside of the spiral to the centre (see Figure 2.9e)
- **RODAC plates** (replicate organism direct agar contact) – are used to enumerate organisms on surfaces. These are special petri dishes with a raised agar surface that are used to make direct contact, for example with a food contact surface. Following incubation, a colony count can be obtained
- **Membrane** – this is a further modification of the spread plate. Here a sample (sometimes in large volumes of many hundreds of millilitres) is passed through a membrane of a pore size (usually 0.45 µm) that allows retention of bacteria but not of the majority of the liquid being sampled. After filtration of known volume the membrane is placed on the surface of an agar plate and incubated to allow visible colonies to grow and be counted.
- **Most probable number (MPN)** – involves the inoculation of replicate tubes of an appropriate medium with different sample sizes (or dilutions). The medium is designed to indicate if the growth of a specific organism or group of organisms has occurred. By referring to tables, or now more likely a computer program, an enumeration based on a statistical probability (within defined confidence limits) of the target organism can be achieved.

- Biochemical activity such as the ability to ferment (metabolize) a specific sugar or other organic or inorganic chemical. Sugar fermentations are usually detected by the production of acid or gas. The acidity is detected by the inclusion of an indicator that

Table 2.3 Examples of commonly used differential and selective media for the isolation of bacteria and fungi

Target organisms	Name	Selective agents and indicators	Incubation conditions	Colonial appearance
Selective broths				
Campylobacter spp.	Bolton broth	Vancomycin – inhibitory to Gram-positive bacteria Cefoperazone – inhibitory to Gram-negative bacteria Trimethoprim – inhibitory to other species of bacteria Cycloheximide – inhibitory to yeasts Sodium metabisulphite and sodium pyruvate are included to inactivate growth inhibitors and to increase aero-tolerance	Aerobic at 37 °C for 4 hours then 42 °C for 44 hours Incubation at this temperature suppresses competing flora	Not applicable
Escherichia coli O157	Modified Tryptone Soya Broth (MTSB)	Vancomycin, cefixime, and cefsulodin inhibitory to other organisms Novobiocin and bile salts especially selective for *E. coli* O157	Aerobic at 42 °C for 24 hours	Not applicable
Listeria spp.	Listeria Enrichment Broth (half-Fraser, Fraser, and UVM broths)	Nalidixic acid, cycloheximide, acriflavine and cefsulodin inhibitory to other organisms Lithium chloride inhibitory to enterococci	Aerobic at 30 °C for 24–48 hours	Not applicable
Salmonella spp.	Muller–Kauffmann Tetrathionate-Novobiocin Broth	Brilliant green novobiocin and ox bile increase selectivity *Salmonella* spp. metabolize tetrathionate which allows them to proliferate	Aerobic at 43 °C for 24–48 hours	Not applicable
	Rappaport Vassiliadis broth	Malachite green and magnesium chlorite allow *Salmonella* to multiply and inhibit other organisms High salt concentration, and pH 5.2	Aerobic at 42 °C for 24 hours	Not applicable
	Selenite broth	Sodium biselenite together with cystine and phosphate enhances recovery of *Salmonellae* spp.	Aerobic at 37 °C for 24–48 hours	Not applicable
Selective agars				
Bacillus cereus	Polymyxin pyruvate Egg yolk Mannitol Bromthymol blue Agar (PEMBA)	Formulation enhances egg yolk precipitation and sporulation of *B. cereus* Polymyxin B – inhibits Gram-negative bacteria Bromthymol blue is a pH indicator to detect alkaline mannitol non-fermenting *B. cereus* colonies	Aerobic at 30 °C for 24–48 hours	3–4 m in diameter, crenated, turquoise to peacock blue, and surrounded by a zone of opacity due to lecithinase activity
	Mannitol Egg Yolk Polymyxin agar (MYP)	Polymyxin B – inhibits Gram-negative bacteria	Aerobic at 30 °C for 18–24 hours	3–7 mm, rough, dry colonies, violet pink background, egg yolk precipitation

Table 2.3 *Examples of commonly used differential and selective media for the isolation of bacteria and fungi continued*

Target organisms	Name	Selective agents and indicators	Incubation conditions	Colonial appearance
Campylobacter jejuni and *C. coli*	Cefeoperazone Charcoal Deoxycholate Agar (CCDA)	Cefoperazone – inhibitory to other bacteria, Amphotericin B – inhibitory to yeast and fungal contaminants that only grow at 37 °C	Microaerobic (5–10% oxygen) at 42 °C for 48–68 hours	3–4 mm C. jejuni – flat glossy, grey colonies with a tendency to spread C. coli – creamy grey, moist discrete raised colonies
Clostridium perfringens	Tryptose Sulphite Cycloserine Agar (TSC)	D-cycloserine Sodium metabisulphite and ferric ammonium citrate are indicators of sulphite reduction by C. perfringens Reduction of sulphite produces black colonies and if egg yolk is included detects lecithinase activity	Anaerobic at 37 °C for 24 hours in over-layered agar	2–4 mm black colonies surrounded by a black precipitate. The over-layering of the plate allows C. perfringens to grow better in an anaerobic environment
E. coli O157	Cefixime Tellurite Sorbitol MacConkey Agar (CT-SMAC)	Sorbitol is not fermented by most E. coli O157 Potassium tellurite and cefixime – inhibitory to other organisms	Aerobic at 37 °C for 18–24 hours	2.5–4 mm straw coloured colonies Other E. coli ferment sorbitol and produce pink colonies
Listeria spp.	Polymyxin Acriflavine Lithium chloride Ceftazidime, Aesculin Mannitol Agar (PALCAM)	Lithium chloride, ceftazidime, polymyxin B and acriflavine hydrochloride selective for Listeria spp. Mannitol – fermentation changes medium from red to yellow in the pH indicator phenol red The black colour is due to the hydrolysis of esculin	Aerobic at 30 °C for 24–48 hour	2–3 mm, grey green colonies; 2 mm, black sunken centres with a black halo. Colonies of all Listeria spp. have a similar morphology
Listeria monocytogenes	Agar Listeria according to Ottaviani and Agosti (ALOA)	X-glucoside chromogen cleaved by β-glucosidase Lithium chloride, nalidixic acid, polymyxin B and ceftazidime, suppress the growth of other bacteria Lecithin added to detect lecithinase activity	Aerobic at 37 °C for 24–48 hours	2–3 mm, only Listeria monocytogenes are green-blue surrounded by an opaque halo
Salmonella spp.	Brilliant Green Agar (BGA)	Brilliant green increases selectivity for Salmonella, but if present in small numbers may be missed Xylose, lysine and desoxycholate	Aerobic at 37 °C for 18–24 hours	2 mm, red-pink-white opaque coloured colonies surrounded by brilliant red zones in the agar
	Xylose Lysine Desoxycholate agar (XLD)	Salmonella spp. ferments xylose and decarboxylate the lysine, the pH becomes alkaline Sodium desoxycholate – inhibits other coliforms At near neutral pH Salmonella can produce hydrogen sulphide from the reduction of thiosulphate and produce black-centred colonies	Aerobic at 37 °C for 18–24 hours	2–4 mm red colonies with black centres (see Fig. 2.9a). Some Salmonella spp. do not produce black centres (e.g. S. Paratyphi A) and appear similar to Shigella spp. that also grows on this medium and produce red colonies

Table 2.3 *Examples of commonly used differential and selective media for the isolation of bacteria and fungi continued*

Target organisms	Name	Selective agents and indicators	Incubation conditions	Colonial appearance
Staphylococcus aureus	Baird–Parker Medium (BPM)	Highly selective due to tellurite and lithium chloride Tellurite suppresses coliforms and is also reduced by *S. aureus* to telluride giving typical black colonies Glycine and sodium pyruvate are used by staphylococci as growth factors	Aerobic at 37 °C for 48 hours	2–3 mm grey-black shiny surrounded by a zone of clearing (2–5 mm) (see Fig. 2.9c)
	Rabbit Plasma Fibrinogen Agar medium (RPFA)	Rabbit plasma – to detect coagulase activity Fibrinogen – enhances the coagulase reaction Trypsin inhibitor – prevents fibrinolysis	Aerobic at 37 °C for 48 hours	1–3 mm white or grey-black colonies, surrounded by opaque zone of fibrin precipitation, i.e. the coagulase reaction
Vibrio spp.	Thiosulphate Citrate Bile-salt Sucrose agar (TCBS)	Inhibits most enterobacteriaceae Yellow colonies due to acid production from the fermentation of sucrose and pH indicators	Aerobic at 37 °C for 20–24 hours	2–3 mm yellow (*V. cholerae*) – may revert to green at room temperature 2–5 mm, blue-green (*V. parahaemolyticus, V. vulnificus, V. mimicus*) 3–4 mm, yellow (*V. metschnikovii*)
Yersinia spp.	Cefsulodin Irgasan Novobiocin agar (CIN)	Cefsulodin, irgasan and novobiocin selective for *Yersinia* spp Mannitol fermentation produces acid in the centre of the colony resulting in a red 'bull's eye' appearance	Aerobic at 30 °C for 24 hours	1–2.5 mm although size varies between *Yersinia* spp. *Y. enterocolitica*, dark red 'bulls eye' surrounded by a transparent border
Yeasts and moulds	Dichoran Rose Bengal Chloramphenicol Agar (DRBC)	Chloramphenicol inhibits bacteria Rose Bengal dye colours the colony and inhibits spreading	Aerobic at 25 °C for 5–14 days	Yeasts – 1–2 mm creamy white Moulds – 8–14 mm, colour varies depending on species, appear 'fluffy' although strains such as *Aspergillus* will appear flat
	Oxytetracycline Glucose Yeast Extract Agar (OGYE)	Oxytetracycline – inhibits bacteria Medium has a neutral pH to increase counts of yeasts and moulds from a range of food	Aerobic at 25 °C for 5 days	Yeasts – 3–8 mm creamy white, although this may vary depending on the strain e.g. *Rhodotorula rubra* is pinkish Moulds – 1–5 mm, colour varies depending on species e.g. *Penicillium* are blue/green and *Aspergillus niger* is yellow with black centre (see Fig. 2.9f)

changes colour as the pH falls. Gas production can be detected by the inclusion of a collection vessel (a small inverted test tube) within a broth in which bubbles will be trapped and readily recognized.

- The susceptibility to chemicals such as antibiotics.
- The presence of specific enzymes, for example the action of catalase can be detected by adding bacterial growth to hydrogen peroxide and observing the generation of bubbles as oxygen is liberated.
- The production of a specific bacterial toxin such as a **haemolysin** that is able to lyse (break open) red blood cells.
- The reaction with antibodies (serotyping), for example those reacting with O, H and K antigens.

Non-cultural methods for detection of micro-organisms

In addition to methods that rely on the growth and recognition of microbial colonies on artificial media, methods are also available that are independent of this process and these are often referred to as **rapid methods**. These can involve direct visualization of the micro-organisms using a light or electron microscope (see p. 36), or the detection of substances that are specific for their presence. These substances can indicate simply the presence of micro-organisms, such as the detection of ATP (see p. 18). Alternatively, detection can be based on organic molecules, especially proteins or nucleic acids, that specifically indicate the presence of an individual species or even strain of micro-organism.

Specific proteins can be detected either by their biological activity such as enzymic or toxic activities, or by their antigenicity (see next paragraph). Toxic activity will be considered in the following section, but the presence of specific enzymic activity can be useful for the detection of some microbes. For example, most enzymes (including those from plants and animals) are inactivated by boiling. However *Staphylococcus aureus* produces a **nuclease** (an enzyme that degrades nucleic acid) that is heat stable. Hence the detection of nuclease activity in foods that have

been boiled (which can be easily performed in the laboratory) indicates that this bacterium was present at high levels in the food at some time during its life and hence is likely to have been poorly stored with respect to temperature and time, and is a potential risk for causing staphylococcal food poisoning. This heat stable nuclease (also known as a **thermonuclease**) can be demonstrated in a food in the absence of viable *S. aureus* cells because the enzyme is less susceptible than the bacterium to physical conditions and the bacterial cells may have died during the life of the food, for example, as a result of the effects of heating or acidification.

Proteins that are produced by, for example, viruses or bacterial can also be detected with antibodies using various techniques collectively known as **immunoassays**. **Antibodies** are proteins which are produced by mammals that have the property of specifically recognizing other proteins by virtue of their shape. The moieties recognized by antibodies are called **antigens** and these have proved extremely useful in the recognition of different types of bacteria (for example different serotypes of *Salmonella*) as well as for the inactivation of toxins for the treatment of disease such as botulism (see Chapter 4, p. 85). Antibodies can also be 'labelled' with enzymes and bound to solid surfaces such that when they react with an antigen their presence can be detected using a substrate of the conjugated enzymes: an example of such an immunoassay is an enzyme-linked immunosorbent assay (**ELISA**).

Microbes can also be detected by the presence of specific DNA sequences. The most common way of achieving this is by the use of the **polymerase chain reaction (PCR)**. DNA is made up of four chemically different nucleotide bases that occur in specific order or sequence. The two strands of DNA are bound together by the nucleotides in a specific way, and this is known as **complementary hybridization**. PCR relies on short sequences of DNA that are synthesized in the laboratory and known as **primers**. These are designed in pairs to span DNA sequences of choice, for example that which encodes a bacterial toxin or a sequence that is common to all members of a given bacterial or viral species. Primers bind by complementary hybridization to each end of the desired DNA sequence at **primer binding sites** and hybridization, or annealing, takes place at between

40 °C and 60 °C. When the temperature is then raised to 72 °C, this initiates synthesis of the entire primer-encompassed complementary DNA strand by the presence of a DNA polymerase enzyme named the *Taq* polymerase: the name is derived from the bacterium *Thermophilus aquaticus* from which this enzyme was originally isolated. *Taq* has the remarkable property of being stable at the temperature at which complementary hybridization is reversed, usually at about 95 °C. If a sample is cycled, usually up to 40 times, between these three temperatures (machines to do this are known as **thermocyclers**), then enormous amplification of the original DNA sequence can be achieved. PCR products are identical copies of the original target DNA sequence that can be detected by a variety of methods including gel electrophoresis (see following section) or by using further pieces of complementary DNA (known as **reporter probes**) within the amplified product. These probes are chemically labelled to fluoresce (emit light when excited by UV light) when binding occurs. Because these labels allow the detection of PCR products during the reaction, these methods are known as **real-time PCR**.

ELISA and PCR tests can be used for the detection of individual pathogens in enrichment broths, especially by commercial food testing laboratories that analyse multiple samples of similar food types for a narrow range of pathogens (see Chapter 27).

Detection of microbial toxins

Detection of microbial toxins has most often been done in specialist testing laboratories. Since toxins, by definition, have a biological activity that has a toxic effect, these were often originally detected by the use of experimental animals. However for both ethical and technical reasons, animals are now, fortunately, rarely used, although they still have a role in some toxin investigations, for example in the detection of *C. botulinum* toxins. Alternatives to animal assays include the detection of toxic effects by the observation of mammalian cells growing in tissue culture, for example vero cells were originally used to detect the verocytotoxic effects from *E. coli* O157 (see Chapter 4, p. 67).

Protein toxins are now most often detected by immunoassays and the presence of toxin genes by PCR. However, both immunoassays and PCR have the disadvantage that neither detects the presence of biologically active toxin. Immunoassays may detect inactive toxin and PCR can detect toxin genes that are either not expressed or are not expressed as active toxin. Microbial toxins, particularly those that are non-protein in nature (e.g. histamine and mycotoxins, see Chapter 4, pp. 88 and 89), can be detected by chemical means.

Microscopy

The limit of resolution of the light microscope is about 0.2 μm, and is clearly insufficient to resolve viruses. However, in unstained or, more usually, stained preparations, bacteria, fungi, protozoa, and other parasites can readily be visualized. Viruses can be observed using an electron microscope which is able to resolve to about 1 nm. However. biological material cannot be directly visualized by electron microscopy and must be dried and stained using electron scattering atoms such as tungsten or uranium. Examples of food poisoning organisms visualized by light or electron microscopy have already been shown earlier in Figures 2.3 and 2.4, pp. 24–4. As previously mentioned light and, to a lesser extent, electron microscopy has an important role in determining the phenotypic morphology of micro-organisms. Microscopy, particularly when combined with staining procedures (such as the Gram stain) often provide primary diagnostic criteria for their identification.

Characterization methods

Since the nineteenth century when techniques first became available for the culture of micro-organisms, microbiologists have been faced with a 'simple' question when more than one isolate is obtained: 'Are these isolates from the same or different origins?'. The need to answer this question led, in part, to methods for identification of species and genera of foodborne pathogens (see previous discussion). The detection of the same species of pathogen in food and from specimens from affected patients is sometimes sufficient to establish a causal link between them. However, because foodborne pathogens can be widespread in their distribution within the food chain (see Chapter 5) further subdivisions within species of '**types**' or '**strains**' are necessary. Methods to further subdivide species and characterize diversity within populations of micro-organisms are known as **typing** or **fingerprinting** techniques. These techniques can generate a high degree of complexity since micro-organisms (as well as almost all biological systems) are constantly changing, and some of the categories generated will be somewhat artificial. All typing systems rely on recognition of diversity within a species and the success of these systems are influenced by:

- **Typability** – the proportion of isolates that can be tested to give an unambiguous positive result; isolates that do not produce a positive result are designated as **non-typable**.
- **Reproducibility** – the ability of a typing system to quantitatively or qualitatively repeat the same result in independent assays.
- **Discrimination** – the amount of variation the typing system recognizes within a population under study, i.e. the number of types recognized.
- **Ease of performance** – the ability to test sufficient numbers of cultures to obtain results in a sufficient timely manner.

Typing is usually done in national or international reference laboratories; these are further discussed in Chapter 28. Typing has been invaluable in:

- elucidating routes of infection between different isolates collected within food-poisoning outbreaks
- tracking routes of contamination and hygiene problems within food manufacturing environments and the entire food chain
- identifying or confirming reservoirs of infection
- distinguishing between pathogenic and non-pathogenic variants of the same species
- providing evidence for the success of intervention strategies to prevent infection
- indicating causal links between long-term trends and changes
- identifying emerging pathogens.

Characterization based on phenotypic methods has already been briefly mentioned and includes:

- **Biotyping** – differentiation based on metabolic characters such as fermentation of sugars, resistance to heavy metals or antibiotics. Patterns of susceptibility to antibiotics are known as **antibiogrammes**.
- **Serotyping** – differentiation based on the reaction of antibodies with O, H or K antigens. The antigenic structure is known as the **serotype**.
- **Bacteriophage** (or **phage**) **typing** – susceptibility to panels of bacterial viruses or bacteriophages. The patterns of susceptibility to phages are known as the **phage type**, and are particularly used for *S. enterica* serovars including *S.* Typhi, *S.* Typhimurium and *S.* Enteritidis.

With advances in molecular biology and the widespread ability to manipulate DNA, genotypic methods are used increasingly for fingerprinting. These can be based on:

- detection of plasmid DNA
- amplification of specific toxin genes by PCR
- characterization of DNA fragments
- establishing DNA sequences of both small or entire genomes.

The size of DNA fragments can be determined by separating them within an electric current in an **agarose** (a type of highly purified agar) gel, a process known as **electrophoresis**: larger DNA fragments travel more slowly within the field than smaller fragments. An entire bacterial chromosome can be cut up or digested into specific DNA fragments using a **DNA-restriction enzyme**. These fragments can give a characteristic banding pattern when separated by electrophoresis. One particular type of electrophoresis, known as **pulsed-field gel electrophoresis** (PFGE; Figure 2.10), has, together with other techniques including serotyping and phage typing, been highly successful in providing discriminatory typing of bacteria in national centres allowing exchange of data between networks of laboratories around the world (e.g. PulseNet network in North America and Enternet in Europe). Such networks have allowed the recognition of international outbreaks of food poisoning where the same contaminated food was sold in different countries.

Experience of the discrimination and reproducibility of different methods can be of great advantage in reducing the total amount of work by application of different typing methods. These methods are often applied in a **hierarchical fashion**, such that technically more straightforward methods

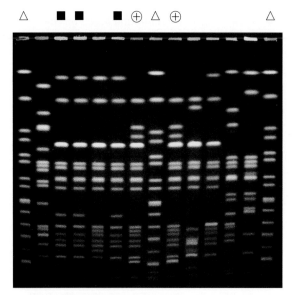

Figure 2.10 *Pulsed-field gel electrophoresis gel for fingerprinting bacterial pathogens (courtesy of C Maguire and M Hampton Health Protection Agency). Profiles from 14 Salmonella enterica cultures are shown: the profile in each vertical single line is derived from DNA culture. Those cultures with indistinguishable patterns are indicated by △ (pattern 1), ■ (pattern 2), and ⊕ (pattern 3)*

are applied to a greater proportion of isolates. The results of these initial tests allows more discriminatory, and often more time-consuming, methods to confirm, or refute, the identity of a smaller number of representatives from specific groups. Unfortunately, nomenclature for the interpretation of typing is often different for each group of organisms, but assistance should be available to do this from national or international reference centres. Multiple isolates identified as a single type or indeed strain are usually described as 'indistinguishable', emphasizing that the analysis depends on the system used and that alternative systems may reflect a different interpretation.

Summary

Microbes are diverse, and a variety of techniques are used in microbiological laboratories for the examination of food (a typical scheme for examination of food samples from a food poisoning outbreak is shown in Figure 2.11). Microbiology and microbiological techniques are vital to allow an understanding of:

- how micro-organisms are detected and identified
- how micro-organisms survive and grow in food, water and in food manufacturing environments
- the properties of both spoilage organisms and pathogens
- the most effective methods for the control and prevention of foodborne disease
- the preparation of food of acceptable microbiological quality.

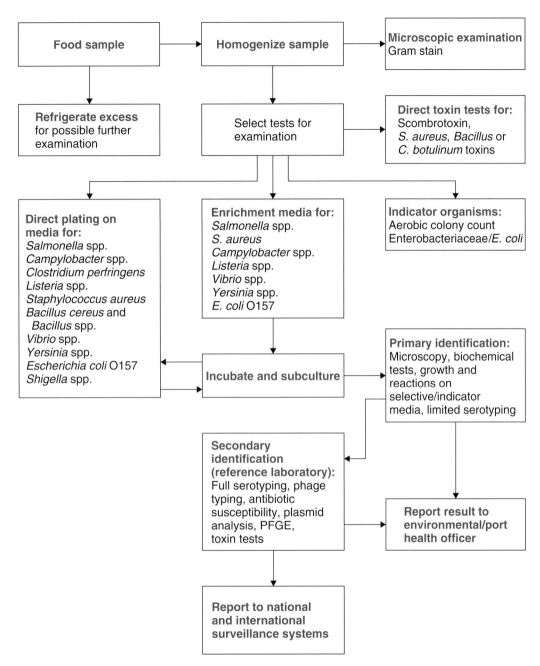

Figure 2.11   *Outline of available procedures for the examination of food samples from a food poisoning outbreak*
PFGE, pulsed-field gel electrophoresis

All websites cited below were accessed in December 2006.

SOURCES OF INFORMATION AND FURTHER READING

Adams MR, Moss MO (2000) *Food Microbiology*, 2nd edn. Cambridge: Royal Society of Chemistry.

Anon (2001) US Food and Drug Administration. *Bacteriological Analytical Manual* (available at www.cfsan.fda.gov/~ebam/bam-toc.html).

Doyle MP, Beuchat LR, Montville TJ (eds) (1997) *Food Microbiology: Fundamentals and Frontiers*. Washington: American Society for Microbiology Press.

Fisher IS, Threlfall EJ, *et al.* (2005) The Enter-net and Salm-gene databases of foodborne bacterial pathogens that cause human infections in Europe and beyond: an international collaboration in surveillance and the development of intervention strategies. *Epidemiol Infect* **133**: 1–7.

Garbutt J (1997) *Essentials of Food Microbiology*. London: Arnold.

Jay JM (2003) *Modern Food Microbiology*, 6th edn. New York: Kluwer, Plenum Publishers.

Manafi M (2000) New developments in chromogenic and fluorogenic culture media. *Int J Food Microbiol* **60**: 205–18.

Roberts D, Greenwood M (2003). *Practical Microbiology*, 3rd edn. Oxford: Blackwell.

Swaminathan B, Gerner-Smidt P, Ng LK (2006) Building PulseNet International: an interconnected system of laboratory networks to facilitate timely public health recognition and response to foodborne disease outbreaks and emerging foodborne diseases. *Foodborne Pathog Dis* **3**: 36–50.

3

Life and death of micro-organisms in food, spoilage and preservation

Jim McLauchlin

Growth, survival and death of micro-organisms in food	41	Control of microbial growth	45
		Factors used to control microbial growth	46
Spoilage	42	Preservation strategies	57
Using heat to kill and injure micro-organisms in food	43	Summary	58
		Sources of information and further reading	58

Pathogenic viruses, protozoa, parasites and some bacteria are incapable of independent growth in food, but provided they (or their toxic products) survive the food manufacturing process, they can cause food poisoning. Many food poisoning bacteria cause disease only when eaten in the large numbers that result from multiplication in food but which does not usually alter the appearance, taste or smell of the food. Spoilage of foods is the beginning of the complex natural process of decay; it is subjective and often associated with individual taste. The growth of bacteria and fungi is a major component of spoilage. Food preservation encompasses a series of strategies to prevent spoilage and the growth of pathogens. The control of microbiological survival and growth is often identical regardless of whether considering spoilage organisms or potential pathogens. The most common processing factor used to control micro-organisms in foods is temperature.

Spoilage A process whereby changes occur in food, which are unacceptable to consumers for reasons of smell, taste, appearance or texture.

Contamination The presence of unwanted and undesirable substances, including pathogens, toxins and foreign bodies, in food.

Decay A natural biological process that involves the recycling of the elements in animal or plant tissues back into the environment.

Organoleptic Changes that alter the texture, flavour, colour, etc. of food.

Preservation An active process whereby decay (spoilage) and the growth of pathogens are inhibited by modification of the physico-chemical nature of a food or the environment in which it is stored.

GROWTH, SURVIVAL AND DEATH OF MICRO-ORGANISMS IN FOOD

Food poisoning is caused by pathogenic micro-organisms or toxins present in food. Since these agents do not usually alter the appearance, taste or smell of the food, it is generally impossible to determine by visual inspection whether or not a food is contaminated with food poisoning organisms. Viruses, parasites and some bacteria are incapable of independent growth in food, but provided they (or their toxic products) survive the food manufacturing process are capable of causing food poisoning. However, many of the food poisoning bacteria cause disease only when eaten in large numbers which result from multiplication in food. The types of bacteria that breakdown food, particularly protein, so that spoilage or putrefaction is detectable by smell do not usually cause food poisoning. The early onset of obvious spoilage can be a safeguard against the consumption of food heavily contaminated with pathogens. However, control of both microbiological survival and growth is identical regardless of whether spoilage or microbiological pathogens are being considered.

Control of the growth, survival and death of microbes in foods and beverages is essential for production of a safe and wholesome product. Apart from the barriers that separate food from microorganisms in the environment (such as cans and other hermetically sealed packages), most microbiological control is achieved by physical factors, i.e. the application of specific treatments together with modification of food and food components. The most common physical factors are:

- temperature (both heat and cold treatments)
- amount of available water
- acidity
- gaseous environment
- available nutrients.

Methods of food preservation utilizing these factors are summarized in Table 3.1. These methods are applicable for controlling both food poisoning and food spoilage organisms.

Foods are heterogeneous ecosystems in which complex interactions between their chemical, physical and structural characteristics markedly influence microbial growth and survival. Bacteria and fungi will live and multiply in many foodstuffs; indeed some types of food, and the atmospheric temperature and humidity of the kitchen, provide conditions similar to those used for their cultivation in the laboratory.

As outlined in Chapter 2, (Fig. 2.7, p. 25) microbial growth can be considered in terms of lag, exponential, stationary and decline phases. These phases are identical for microbial growth in foods and in the artificial media used in the laboratory. The nutritional requirements of microbes have been briefly considered in Chapter 2. Bacteria will multiply in certain food products when they are stored in the shop or kitchen without refrigeration; in the same way, they multiply in specially prepared media inoculated in the laboratory and incubated at warm temperatures. Thus food poisoning occurs more frequently in summer than in winter.

SPOILAGE

A spoiled food is that which is unacceptable to a consumer for reasons of smell, taste, appearance, or texture. The concept of spoilage, however, is subjective and associated with individual taste,

Table 3.1 *Food preservation procedures*

Procedure	Factors influencing growth and survival
Pasteurization at 60–80 °C	Heat inactivation of vegetative spoilage and pathogenic organisms
Heating at <100 °C (baking, boiling, frying, grilling, blanching)	Heat inactivation of vegetative spoilage and pathogenic organisms (may also improve digestibility of food, reduce spoilage by inactivation of enzymes and expulsion of oxygen)
Drying/concentration at <100 °C	Reduction of water activity to delay or prevent growth
Appertization at >100 °C	Elimination of micro-organisms to achieve commercial sterility
Cooling at 0–10 °C	Reduction of temperature to prevent or retard growth
Freezing at <0 °C	Reduction of temperature and water activity to prevent growth
Drying, curing, conserving	Reduction of water activity to delay or prevent growth
Vacuum and modified atmosphere packaging	Reduction of oxygen tension to inhibit aerobes and delay growth of facultative anaerobes. Inhibition of growth by carbon dioxide
Addition of acids including lactic fermentation	Reduction of pH to retard or prevent growth
Emulsification	Compartmentalization and nutrient limitation to reduce or prevent growth
Addition of other preservatives	Retardation or prevention of growth
Irradiation	Delivery of ionizing radiation to inactivate organisms
Hydrostatic pressure	Pressure inactivation of organisms

Adapted from Adams and Moss (2000). With permission of the Royal Society of Chemistry.

cultural values, personal preferences, ethnic origin and family background. For example, the chemical and bacteriological changes associated with hanging game make the food unacceptable to some but a delicacy for others. Bananas that have become brown and sugary are considered over-ripe and therefore spoiled by many but are perfectly acceptable to others.

The major reason for spoilage is the changes brought about by the growth of micro-organisms. However, chemical changes also cause spoilage. These include: oxidation of fats, producing rancidity; browning of fruits and vegetables in contact with air; freezer burns; 'staling' of biscuits due to changes in water content; over-ripening of fruit or vegetables; and taints due to contamination by sanitizers.

Bacterial spoilage of bread, which is due to the growth of the bacterium *Serratia marcescens*, has led to 'miraculous' claims. This spoilage results in the production of a bright red pigment known as 'bleeding bread' and has led to the erroneous claim that the bread is reflecting the blood of Christ.

Spoilage caused by micro-organisms

Growth of micro-organisms in foods causes spoilage and is the start of the natural process of decay. Foods spoiled by micro-organisms can be safe to eat, indeed some spoilage is identical to fermentation and ripening processes used to produce certain foods. However, spoiled foods in which organoleptic changes have occurred can be hazardous.

The distinction between 'spoilage' and 'pathogenic' bacteria is not always clear, and some organisms can be included into both groups. In general, contamination by food poisoning organisms gives no indication of their presence in food by the common signs of spoilage such as off-odours and tastes, or changes in appearance, for example, colour, consistency or gas production.

The pathogen *Clostridium perfringens* can grow to concentrations sufficient to cause illness without generating organoleptic changes including the generation of gas. *Bacillus cereus* is common in the environment and in uncooked cereals such as rice and flour. Levels of *B. cereus* in cooked rice and other foods which have caused food poisoning without producing organoleptic changes are usually greater than 10^6/g, often 10^8–10^9/g. However, *B.*

cereus and *C. perfringens* can cause spoilage in cream and milk with 'off' flavours and the appearance of 'bitty' particles. The levels at this stage may be too low to cause food poisoning, but the toxin produced by *B. cereus* is unlikely to be consumed because of the appearance of the milk. Spores of the bacteria *Bacillus subtilis* and *Bacillus licheniformis* can survive the baking process of bread. They can germinate and spoil, producing a stringy brown mass, particularly in the middle of the loaf, called 'ropy bread'. Consumption of ropy bread causes diarrhoeal illness.

USING HEAT TO KILL AND INJURE MICRO-ORGANISMS IN FOOD

The processing factor most commonly applied to foods and beverages to kill and injure micro-organisms is heat. Other food processing factors also lead to microbial death, and these are considered later in this chapter. As outlined in Table 3.1, heating of foods is variously described as baking, boiling, frying, grilling, blanching, pasteurizing and appertizing. Appertized foods are those in which only non-pathogenic organisms survive the process and are incapable of developing within the product during its shelf-life under normal storage. These products are termed 'commercially sterile', and have a long shelf-life and are stored in ambient temperatures. Other terms associated with heat treatments are:

- **Sterilization** is a treatment designed to destroy vegetative cells and spores, for example, canning and bottling procedures of non-acidic foods. As outlined on p. 44, this is not an absolute state.
- **Pasteurization** is a heat process of shorter duration at lower temperatures than those used for sterilization. It will destroy most vegetative cells but not spores. Spoilage is delayed, but cold storage is necessary to delay growth even if preservatives such as salt are used, as in the production of pâté. Pasteurization of milk, originally designed to destroy tubercle bacilli, also eliminates the vegetative cells of other pathogenic organisms.
- **Blanching** is a quick heat treatment applied to foods for reasons other than for destruction of

organisms, such as for blanching of vegetables before freezing to slow oxidative changes. This process is also used to loosen the shells of crustaceans and shellfish.

Higher temperatures and longer heat treatments result in the elimination of the most heat-resistant organisms. Heat resistance varies enormously between organisms (Box 3.1).

Box 3.1 Heat resistance of micro-organisms

- Psychrotrophs are less heat resistant than mesophiles which are less resistant than thermophiles
- Gram-positive bacteria are more heat resistant than Gram-negative bacteria
- Vegetative bacterial cells are more heat sensitive than endospores
- Viruses, parasites, yeasts and moulds are often of similar sensitivity to vegetative bacterial cells
- Spores and cysts of yeasts, moulds and parasites are only slightly more heat resistant than their vegetative cells

---

Bacterial endospore inactivation is the principal concern in producing appertized or canned foods, so much higher temperatures are used in this process. The heat resistance of organisms is often measured in terms of **D values**. The D value is the time taken at a given temperature for the surviving population of a given organism to be reduced by 90% (i.e. 1 $\log_{10}$). D values for a range of organisms are shown in Table 3.2.

It is not possible to predict how many decimal reductions a heat process must achieve to produce a product with no viable organisms (i.e. sterile) because of the relation between heat and the death of an organism. This relation means that as the time of a specific heat treatment is extended, the number of survivors will reduce to 10^{-1}, 10^{-2}, 10^{-3} (i.e. 1/10, 1/100 and 1/100) of an organism. It may initially appear absurd to consider a fraction of an organism, however this means that with the 10^{-1}, 10^{-2}, 10^{-3} survivors, there will be a probability of one survivor occurring in 1 in 10, 1 in 100, and 1 in 1000 occasions.

The D value for a specific organism varies, especially between growth phases and under different growth conditions for vegetative cells. For example, stationary phase bacterial cells are generally more heat resistant than exponentially growing cells,

Table 3.2 *Microbial heat resistance*

	D value* (minutes)
Vegetative cells at 65 °C	
Salmonella Seftenberg	D_{65} 0.8–1.0
Staphylococcus aureus	D_{65} 0.2–2.0
Escherichia coli	D_{65} 0.1
Listeria monocytogenes	D_{65} 5.0–8.3
Yeasts and moulds	D_{65} 0.5–3.0
Bacterial endospores at 121 °C	
Bacillus stearothermophilus	D_{121} 4–5
Bacillus coagulans	D_{121} 0.1
Clostridium botulinum	D_{121} 0.1–0.2
Clostridium sporogenes	D_{121} 0.1–1.5

*The D value is the time taken at a given temperature (denoted in the subscript) for the surviving population of a given organism to be reduced by 90% (i.e. 1 $\log_{10}$).
Adapted from Adams and Moss (2000). With permission of the Royal Society of Chemistry.

and cells generally show greater heat sensitivity when growing above pH 8 and below pH 6. However, the D value concept has proved extremely useful, especially in the canning industry where the 12-D concept has long been used. This is the time taken to achieve a 12-log reduction in the numbers of the most resistant *Clostridium botulinum* (the causative organism of botulism) spores (i.e. the time taken to reduce the probability of one spore surviving from an original population of 10^{12} cells), and provides a generally acceptable margin of safety for the production of these types of food. D values can also be used for other processes which kill micro-organisms, such as ionizing and ultraviolet radiation.

Microbes are able to undergo repair following cell injury. The process of repair is, however, complex and highly dependent on the environment in which the cells occur. There is a second state which differs from injury and repair whereby microbial cells are alive but unable to grow in artificial media: this state is known as **viable but non-culturable**. These two states are important because pathogens may be present in a food but are not detected by conventional cultural methods which rely on demonstration of microbial growth.

To understand the process of food poisoning it is also important to consider the heat resistance of toxins produced as a result of microbiological growth. For example, the neurotoxins produced by *C. botulinum* are readily inactivated by heat. However staphylococcal enterotoxins together with diarrhoetic shellfish poisoning (DSP) toxin and paralytic shellfish poisoning (PSP) toxin will survive boiling whereas *B. cereus* emetic toxin and scombrotoxin (histamine) can withstand 121 °C for 90 minutes, as used in the canning industry. The heat resistance of toxins and how these cause disease will be further considered in Chapter 4.

Examples of temperature and time combinations for the treatment of milk are shown in Table 3.3.

CONTROL OF MICROBIAL GROWTH

Living plants and animals, when freshly harvested, are usually sterile inside but have a mixed microflora on the outside. Spoilage, and sometimes the growth of food poisoning organisms, occurs during storage when bacteria and/or fungi grow to unacceptable levels. The numbers and types of organism depend on the nature of the food, how this has been processed (including any contacts with the environment), storage time and temperature.

The levels of spoilage organisms which are associated with organoleptic changes will depend on the kind of food and the predominant organism. However, not all organisms present in a food are associated with the spoilage process. Spoilage flora is almost always dominated by just a few and sometimes only one species of organism. Components of the microflora compete with one another for the

Table 3.3 *Temperature and time combinations for the treatment of milk*

Treatment	Temperature	Time
Pasteurization*		
Low temperature for a long time	63 °C	At least 30 minutes
High temperature for a short time	72 °C	At least 15 seconds
Ultra high treatment (UHT)*	+135 °C	In combination with a suitable holding time[†]
Sterilization	100 °C	20–40 minutes

* Commission Regulation (EC) No 2074/2005 of 5 December laying down implementing measures for certain products under Regulation (EC) No 853/2004 of the European Parliament and of the Council and for the organization of official controls under Regulation (EC) No 854/2004 of the European Parliament and of the Council and Regulation (EC) No 882/2004 of the European Parliament and of the Council, derogating from Regulation (EC) No 852/2004 of the European Parliament and of the Council and amending Regulations (EC) No 853/2004 and (EC) No 854/2004.
[†] But not less than 1 second.

available nutrients and the organism(s) that grows the fastest under a particular set of conditions will be dominant and give rise to the spoilage (Box 3.2). The growth of a dominant species in a food is not a static situation. As the dominant species grows it can cause changes in food or food environments that makes the food a more suitable environment for the growth of another contaminating species. This process is called **succession**.

> **Box 3.2 Factors determining dominance**
>
> Which component of the microflora becomes dominant is determined by a complex interaction between:
>
> - components of the contaminating microflora (**implicit factors**)
> - storage environment (**extrinsic factors**)
> - physico-chemical properties of the food (**intrinsic factors**)
> - physical and chemical methods for food manufacture (**processing factors**)

Implicit parameters (interactions within the microflora) are the least well understood of the factors that influence the growth of microorganisms in foods. Extrinsic factors include:

- temperature at which the food is stored
- gaseous atmosphere surrounding the food
- relative humidity of the atmosphere surrounding the food
- time.

Examples of intrinsic factors are:

- nutrient content of the food
- any natural antimicrobial substances present
- pH of the food and its ability to resist pH change
- oxidation reduction potential (Eh) of the food and its ability to resist redox change
- water activity of the food
- salt concentration
- mechanical barriers to microbial invasion.

As mentioned above, the most common processing factor applied to foods and beverages is heat. Higher temperatures and longer heat treatments result in the elimination of the most heat-sensitive organisms. However, high heat treatments will also result in environments with very few microflora. These are more easily subsequently colonized by organisms such as staphylococci, which compete poorly with food flora. Other processing factors include cooling, freezing, drying, irradiation, high pressure and addition of preservatives. Understanding and controlling these factors is essential for food preservation.

Foods are regarded as **perishable** when their constituents and moisture content allow the growth of micro-organisms. **Non-perishable** foods are those unable to support the growth of micro-organisms, often because of the storage temperature, the acidity, or the amount of available water. Non-perishable foods which can be stored at room temperature are described as **shelf-stable**. **Semi-perishable** foods are those that are slow to exhibit microbiological changes, for example, those protected by curing salts. These, however, are not absolute terms and will vary between food types and different storage conditions. In addition, chemical changes can also be important in how perishable a particular food is.

It is also important to recognize that food can be highly heterogeneous and contain several distinct micro-environments. For example, C. botulinum is an obligate anaerobe and will only grow in the absence of oxygen (air). However, this bacterium can grow and produce toxin in the centre of some foods under aerobic conditions because the oxygen levels there are low, either because of the growth of the surface microflora, or as a result of being driven out by cooking. This is an example of a **nested micro-environment**.

Food is a complex environment and multiple factors are almost always present that affect the growth of microbes and therefore the shelf-life. A single factor may be insufficient to control microbial growth, however, the combination of several factors may provide sufficient safety and stability in a food product – this is referred to as **hurdle technology**. For example, if an intrinsic factor is increased, then other parameters tend to move closer to the optimum. If the conditions move away from the optimum for a number of factors then growth may cease well before the minimum for any one factor is reached. Each suboptimal growth parameter in effect becomes a hurdle, slowing the growth rate and increasing the length of the lag phase so that a combination of hurdles will eventually prevent growth. The concept of hurdles is important in preservative systems used for foods in which the interaction of growth parameters is associated with

slowing or preventing spoilage and preventing the growth of food poisoning organisms. In preservative systems that use chemical preservatives, further interactions occur between the preservative, pH, water activity and temperature that will determine whether a particular organism will grow. The preservative in effect becomes an additional hurdle to growth of micro-organisms present in the food.

There are three methods of analysing the combined effects on microbial growth when developing new food products or investigating processes that have failed. These include:

- **expert judgement** and interpretation of published literature
- **challenge testing** which involves inoculating organisms into foods under model conditions, usually under extended storage or temperature abuse
- use of **mathematical models** that predict the growth of specific organisms under a range of conditions.

FACTORS USED TO CONTROL MICROBIAL GROWTH

Refrigeration and freezing

Overall, bacteria and fungi are capable of active growth at temperatures below 0 °C and above 100 °C. However, individual species have a far more restricted temperature range, and their growth can be considered in terms of the:

- **minimum** temperature – below which no growth occurs
- **optimum** temperature – at which the organism grows fastest
- **maximum** temperature – above which no growth occurs.

The growth range of an organism can be further used to subdivide bacteria and fungi into five groups: mesophiles, obligate psychrophiles, psychrotrophs, thermophiles, and extreme thermophiles. These are defined as follows:

- **Mesophiles** grow at moderate temperatures, and are often adapted to living on humans and other warm-blooded animals, and in the soil and water in tropical and temperate climates. An important characteristic of mesophiles is their lack of growth at chill temperatures (−1 to 5 °C). Many, but not all, have an optimum temperature for growth of 37 °C (human core body temperature). Many spoilage organisms as well as food poisoning organisms are mesophilic, hence the utility of refrigeration as a strategy for food preservation. Examples of mesophilic food poisoning organisms are *Salmonella* spp., *Campylobacter* spp., *C. perfringens* and *Staphylococcus aureus*.

- **Psychrotrophic organisms** grow at low temperatures and are found in water and soil in temperate parts of the world. Minimum temperatures recorded in this group are as low as −6.5 °C for bacteria, −10 °C for moulds and −12.5 °C for yeasts. Psychrotrophs that cause spoilage of chilled foods are represented in a wide range of bacterial, yeast and mould genera. The food poisoning organisms *Listeria monocytogenes*, *Yersinia enterocolitica* and *C. botulinum* type E, even though their optimum and maximum temperatures for growth are more characteristic of mesophiles, are considered to be psychrotrophic because their minimum growth temperatures are below 5 °C.
- **Obligate psychrophiles** only grow at refrigeration temperatures and below, and are an important group of organisms that cause spoilage of foods held at chill temperatures (−1 to 7 °C).
- **Thermophilic organisms** grow at high temperatures. Thermophiles are active in

soils heated by sunlight, compost heaps and silage, where the temperature can reach as high as 70 °C. Others (**extreme thermophiles**) are found in hot springs and ocean steam vents, where temperatures may be above 100 °C. Thermophiles are probably responsible for the spontaneous combustion of straw and hay.

The minimum, optimum and maximum growth temperatures for these five groups are shown in Table 3.4. Some examples of food poisoning organisms (from these groups) are shown in Table 3.5. These categories are artificial, with many organisms not fitting exactly into one particular group. For example some microbiologists recognize a sixth category, **facultative thermophiles**, i.e. organisms that have an optimum in the mesophilic zone but can grow well at temperatures in which thermophiles grow rapidly.

As mentioned previously with respect to hurdle technology, factors affecting growth are inter-related and the minimum and maximum temperatures for

Table 3.4 *Categorization of micro-organisms based on growth temperatures*

Group	Growth range (°C)		
	Minimum	Optimum	Maximum
Obligate psychrophile	−10	10–15	20
Psychrotroph	−10	20–30	42
Mesophile	5	28–43	52
Thermophile	30	50–65	70
Extreme thermophile	65	80–90	100

Adapted from Garbutt (1997). With permission.

Table 3.5 *Growth temperatures of some bacteria that cause food poisoning*

Species	Minimum °C	Optimum °C	Maximum °C
Bacillus cereus	10	28–35	48
Campylobacter jejuni	30	42–45	47
Clostridium botulinum A/B	12.5	37–40	50
Clostridium perfringens	20	37–45	50
C. botulinum type E	3.3	35	45
Salmonella spp.	5.3	37	45–47
Listeria monocytogenes	−0.4	30–37	45
Staphylococcus aureus	6.7	37	45
Vibrio parahaemolyticus	10	30–37	42
Yersinia enterocolitica	−1.3	28–29	44

Adapted from Garbutt (1997). With permission.

growth under optimum conditions are likely to be affected by pH, water activity, etc. For example deviations in pH and water activity away from optimal growth conditions will result in an increase in the minimum and decrease in the maximum growth range.

Temperature has an important effect on the lag phase of growth. As the temperature moves towards the minimum, not only does growth rate decrease but the length of the lag phase increases. This has significant consequences in relation to the preservation of foods at chill temperatures. The increase in storage life of foods held at chill temperature is associated not only with a decrease in the growth rate of spoilage organisms, but also in an extension of the lag phase. This increase in the length of the lag phase may be as important as a method to reduce growth for food preservation.

Chilled foods are foods that are stored at −1 to 8 °C. At these temperatures psychrotrophs are still capable of growth and will eventually spoil the food but as the lag phase increases, the storage life of the product is increased considerably beyond what would be expected if the food was stored at ambient temperature. Storage life will depend on the:

- chill temperature at which food is held. The optimum storage life is as near to freezing as possible throughout the chill chain from production to consumption. Even small increases in temperatures above the minimum can substantially increase growth rates and reduce storage life
- initial levels of contamination and the types of psychrotroph present
- composition of the food
- whether any other preservation methods are used in conjunction with chilling, e.g. vacuum packaging.

Not only does chilling increase the storage life of foods but it also inhibits the growth of mesophilic food poisoning bacteria, making the food safe as long as the correct temperatures are maintained throughout the chill chain. An increase in consumer demand for a range of chill foods in the late 1980s to early 1990s coincided with food poisoning outbreaks associated with these products and psychrotrophic food poisoning bacteria, e.g. *Listeria monocytogenes*, and emphasized the importance of temperature control in food safety. Foods that carry a particular risk from *L. monocytogenes* should be held at 5 °C or below during storage, transport and display. Although the organism will grow at 5 °C, growth is slow and this bacterium is considerably less likely to increase to levels that cause problems to the previously healthy consumer unless the shelf-life is excessively extended.

Microbial cells can be damaged when they are cooled from ambient to chill temperatures, a phenomenon known as **chilling injury**. Chilling injury occurs in mesophilic organisms, in particular Gram-negative rods, including pathogens, e.g. *Salmonella* spp. However, these injured Gram-negative mesophilic pathogens could still cause illness if allowed to recover and grow in food held at ambient temperature. These effects are unpredictable.

The temperature at which the environment of a micro-organism freezes depends on the concentration of dissolved solids present. Most foods freeze at temperatures between −0.5 °C and −3.0 °C. Freezing lowers the water activity through the removal of liquid water in the form of ice crystals. The water activity (see next section) of pure water is 1.0 at 0 °C; at −10 °C this is reduced to 0.907 and at −18 °C to 0.841. In an environment in which dissolved solids are present, removal of liquid water increases the concentration of the dissolved solids in the water phase, decreases water activity and inhibits the activity of micro-organisms.

Few bacteria can grow at temperatures below about −5 °C and growth appears to be limited by the water activity of their environment. On the basis of water activity alone, yeasts and moulds should be able to grow at −20 °C, but few can grow at −10 °C and only the yeast *Debaryomyces* is capable of growing at temperatures as low as −12.5 °C.

When micro-organisms are frozen, only a proportion of the population will survive, the rest undergoing changes that lead to cell death. The number that survive in foods when frozen can vary from 40 per cent to 90 per cent. The percentage surviving is difficult to predict but depends on the age and treatment of the cells in the population, the rate at which the food was cooled, the final storage temperature, the rate of thawing, composition of the food, and the time of storage. In addition, there is great variation between different types of organism with regard to resistance to freezing (Box 3.3).

Box 3.3 Micro-organisms and freezing

- Gram-negative bacteria are more susceptible to the effects of freezing than Gram-positive bacteria
- Bacterial spores and viruses are highly resistant and virtually unaffected by the freezing process
- Yeasts and moulds survive in the way as vegetative bacteria cells
- Parasites such as protozoa, cestodes and nematodes are more sensitive to freezing. These parasites are killed or survive the freezing process very poorly.

Water

The cells of living organisms have a very high water content, i.e. more than 75 per cent, and water in the liquid state is essential for their existence. This amount of water is required to maintain the cell in an active state, and without liquid water all living organisms, including micro-organisms, will not grow or reproduce. Dormant cells have a much lower water content (e.g. 15 per cent in bacterial spores) which is insufficient for active metabolism. Sufficient water in food, however, is no guarantee that microbial growth will occur. An environment with large amounts of water but not favourable for growth is one in which the water is: dissolved in solutes such as sugars or salts; is crystallized as ice; present as water of crystallization or hydration; bound onto surfaces of a food matrix.

The amount of water available in food for microbial growth is measured in terms of the **water activity** (a_w). Reducing the water available for microbial growth is an extremely important and ancient method of preserving foods, for example by drying, salting or preserving with sugar. Lowering the water activity of a food influences the growth of food spoilage and food poisoning organisms that may be present in the raw materials or are introduced during processing. Not only will organisms cease to grow at water activity below their minimum, but death may also occur at a rate determined by the method used to lower the water activity and how far below the minimum it is. The effect of reduced water activity on microbial cells varies between organisms. Each species has its own range of water activity in which growth occurs (Table 3.6). Most organisms have an optimum approaching 1.0 (pure water), and where there are also sufficient dissolved nutrients to support growth. Lowering the water activity of foods is an important method of controlling the growth of food poisoning organisms. With the exception of S. aureus, B. cereus and mycotoxin-producing moulds, food poisoning organisms will not grow in foods with water activity below 0.93 (48 per cent sucrose, 10 per cent sodium chloride). However, although growth will not occur in foods with water activity below their minimum, food poisoning organisms can survive for long periods. This is especially true

Table 3.6 *Minimum water activity (a_w) of and the effect of sodium chloride (salt; NaCl) concentration on growth of food poisoning organisms*

Organism	Minimum a_w for growth	Effect of salt
Bacillus cereus	0.91	Will not grow above 10%
Campylobacter jejuni	0.98	Grows best at 0.5%. Will not grow above 2%
Clostridium botulinum proteolytic A and B	0.94	10% inhibits growth and toxin production
C. botulinum non-proteolytic types B, E and F	0.97	6.5% inhibits growth and toxin production
Clostridium perfringens	0.93	Most strains are inhibited by 5.0–6.5%
Escherichia coli	0.93	Will not grow above 9%
Listeria monocytogenes	0.94	Does not grow above 10%, but can survive in 15% for up to a year
Salmonella	0.93	Will not grow above 9%
Staphylococcus aureus		Grows well between 7% and 10%; 15% is
Aerobic	0.86	normally considered the maximum but
Anaerobic	0.90	growth may occur at 20%
Vibrio parahaemolyticus	0.94	1–8% required for growth; optimum 2–4%
Yersinia enterocolitica	0.98	Will not grow above 5%
Mycotoxin-producing moulds	0.8–0.61	Toxin production is highest between 0.93% and 0.98%

Adapted from Garbutt (1997). With permission.

of dried foods. *Salmonella* spp., for example, will survive in dried milk powder for several months.

The action of preservatives is enhanced when growth is retarded by reduced water activity. What actually happens depends on the way in which the water is inaccessible. If the water is absorption onto surfaces, then growth is prevented but the organism tends to survive. An extreme example of this is freeze-dried and other dehydrated foods where the water activity is less than 0.1. Freeze drying removes water rapidly from microbial cells and their environment, and the organism can remain dormant for long periods. This technique is used for the production of starter cultures in the fermentation industry when organisms need to be stored or transported in a convenient form.

The water content of a food may bear little relation to its water activity. Fresh meat, for example, has a water content of 75 per cent but a water activity of 0.98. Muscle protein and fat are the bulk of the solids present. These are not soluble in water, have little surface effect, and therefore do not significantly contribute to the water activity. Water-soluble materials (glucose, amino acids, mineral salts and vitamins) are present in small quantities. Thus the water activity of fresh meat is very high.

Foods may have low salt content and low water activity. Salted butter, a water in oil emulsion, has a salt content of 2–3 per cent suggesting a water activity of 0.993–0.989. However, salt is polar and therefore dissolves in the water phase giving a concentration in this phase of up to 18 per cent. The actual water activity, as far as microbial growth in the water phase is concerned, is about 0.86.

On the basis of level of water activity, foods can be usefully divided into high, medium, intermediate and low moisture contents, and this is valuable in predicting which spoilage organism is likely to grow (Table 3.7). Fresh foods with high water activity are prone to rapid spoilage whereas those with water activity below 0.61 are microbiologically stable. In between these two extremes, spoilage rates are normally reduced and the type of spoilage that occurs is different from that of fresh food. Specific spoilage symptoms and the spoilage organisms in foods in which the water activity has been lowered depend on: the types of organism contaminating the raw materials (this includes contamination of any agent used to lower the water activity); the method used to lower the water activity; and the concentration of any agent used.

Dehydration, i.e. the removal of water, can be

Table 3.7 *Categorization of foods based on moisture content*

Moisture content	Water activity (a_w)	Food types	Most common causes of spoilage
High	0.99–0.95	Fresh foods or processed foods with little or no preservation, such as fresh poultry, meat, fruit, milk, eggs and vegetables; fruit juices; cheese spreads and cottage cheese; unsalted butter; lightly salted bacon	Gram-negative bacteria, fast growing moulds and non-osmophilic yeasts
Medium	0.95–0.90	Foods preserved by some drying or the addition of sugar or salt, such as bread; fermented cheeses; salted butter; fermented sausages; bacon; ham	Gram-positive bacteria, moulds and yeasts
Intermediate	0.9–0.61	Foods preserved by intense drying and/or the addition of large amounts of salt or sugar, such as matured cheeses; hard salami; fruit concentrates; ripened hams; dried fruits (prunes, dates, etc.); heavily salted fish; dried fish; jams; cakes; rice	Yeasts, moulds, xerophilic moulds[*], osmophilic yeasts[†] and halophilic bacteria[†]
Low	<0.61	Foods preserved by very intense drying, such as chocolate; dried soups; honey; flour; pasta; biscuits; dried milk; dried vegetables; cereals; crackers; sugar	Microbiologically stable and will only spoil if allowed to take up water from a moist atmosphere

[*]Xerophilic moulds are those which grow in dry conditions of a_w of between 0.61 and 0.85.
[†]Osmophilic yeasts, those that grow in high sugar concentrations, e.g. 20% (a_w 0.62).
[†]Halophilic bacteria, those that require >1% salt (sodium ions).
Adapted from Garbutt (1997). With permission.

achieved by using solar energy, or by tunnel and belt, fluid bed, pan, foam mat, drum or roller, spray, freeze drying and by concentration. Concentration is also a strategy for reduction of water activity and is used in liquid foods that do not reach a dry state, such as meat extract, tomato paste, fruit juice concentrate and condensed milk.

Acidity and alkalinity (pH)

Acidity is the primary factor preventing growth and survival of micro-organisms in fermented foods such as yoghurt, sauerkraut and pickles. In addition, this factor is used together with reduced water activity, heat or chemical preservatives as part of a combined preservation process. Acidity is measured by **pH**, which not only denotes if an environment is acidic, but also alkaline or neutral. pH is a result of the concentration of hydroxide (OH^-) and hydrogen (H^+) ions and a solution of pH 7 is neutral. pH values less than 7 are described as acidic and those above 7 as alkaline.

All micro-organisms have a pH range in which they can grow and an optimum pH at which they grow best. It is possible to generalize the influence of pH on the growth rate of micro-organisms: bacteria usually have a minimum pH for growth of around 4.0–4.5, an optimum pH between 6.8 and 7.2 and a maximum between 8.0 and 9.0. There are some exceptions, e.g. *Lactobacillus* spp., which are important in lactic acid fermentation, grow within the range 3.8–7.2 with an optimum around pH 5.0. Yeasts and moulds are generally less sensitive to pH than bacteria and are capable of growing over wide pH ranges, e.g. *Fusarium* spp. are capable of growing over the pH range 1.8–11.1. Yeasts have optima between 4.0 and 4.5 and moulds between pH 3.0 and 3.5. *Saccharomyces cerevisiae*, for example, has a pH range of 2.3–8.6 with an optimum pH of 4.5. pH ranges for growth of food poisoning organisms are shown in Table 3.8.

Not only does pH influence the growth rate of an organism within its pH range, but it also has an overall influence on the growth curve. At pH values below optimum, the growth rate decreases, the maximum number of cells produced drops, the length of the lag phase increases, the length of the stationary phase shortens, and the death rate increases. The effect of weak acids on microbial cells is temperature dependent. pH values that inhibit

Table 3.8 *pH ranges for growth of selected food poisoning organisms*

Organism	Minimum	Optimum	Maximum
Bacillus cereus	4.9	7.0	9.3
Campylobacter	4.9	7.0	9.0
Clostridium botulinum	4.2	7.0	9.0
Clostridium perfringens	5.5	7.0	8.0
Escherichia coli (VTEC O157)	4.5	7.0	9.0
Listeria monocytogenes	4.1	6.0–8.0	9.6
Salmonella spp.	4.05	7.0	9.0
Staphylococcus aureus	4.0	6.0–7.0	9.8
Vibrio parahaemolyticus	4.8	7.0	11.0
Yersinia enterocolitica	4.6	7.0–8.0	9.0

VTEC, vero cytotoxin producing *E. coli*.
Adapted from Garbutt (1997). With permission.

growth and cause cell death have less effect as the temperature is lowered since there is less dissociation of the acids, i.e. the antimicrobial activity is directly related to the concentration of undissociated acid. Undissociated weak acids can permeate through the cell membrane, acidify the cell interior and inhibit metabolism and growth.

Acidic compounds occur as **inorganic acids** (such as hydrochloric and phosphoric acids) or **organic acids** (such as propionic, acetic, lactic, benzoic, sorbic and citric acids) which are composed of short chains of carbon atoms. Organic acids commonly occur as a natural component of fruit, animal tissues, leaves and spices, and are often used as preservatives for reasons of solubility, taste and low toxicity. Organic acids are also end products of bacterial fermentation. The antimicrobial effects of acids vary – generally these increase with increase in length of the carbon chains, but acids with longer chain length are limited because of low solubility. Acids used in food processes in order of antimicrobial activity are: propionic > acetic > lactic > citric > phosphoric > hydrochloric. Hence the minimum pH for an organism depends on the type of acid present: generally, the minimum is higher if an organic rather than an inorganic acid is responsible.

The pH of foods varies markedly. Most are acidic, ranging from the very acidic to almost neutral. Foods are rarely alkaline although high pH will inhibit microbial growth similarly to low pH. Egg white is one of the rare exceptions, with a pH of about 9. Hakari (buried or rotten shark) is a delicacy in Iceland in which a very high pH (around

11) is generated from ammonia produced by the decomposition of cartilaginous fish.

Adjusting the pH of foods with organic acids is an important method of food preservation and controls the growth of both food poisoning and food spoilage bacteria. The pH of processed foods is often modified using organic acids such as lactic and citric acids. Acetic acid is usually included in mayonnaise and similar salad dressings either as pure acetic acid, spirit or wine vinegar. Similarly, mould spoilage of processed sliced bread can be controlled by the addition of small amounts of acetic acid or propionic acid. Benzoic acid is used in soft drinks, fruit juices, pulps, and flavourings. Sorbic acid is useful for inhibiting mould growth in flour, confectionery, cheese, marzipan, prunes and food colouring. Citric and lactic acids have moderate antimicrobial activity and inhibit microbial growth at low pH values. These acids naturally occur in food and as a result of fermentation processes. Strong inorganic acids are not often included in processed foods but hydrochloric and phosphoric acids are used in the manufacture of carbonated and non-carbonated drinks. Colas, for example, contain phosphoric acid.

pH changes in foods due to the activity of micro-organisms are common. Milk sours (becomes acidic) as a result of lactic acid production by streptococci and lactobacilli. Meat becomes alkaline when spoilage is caused by Gram-negative rods such as *Pseudomonas* spp., since this organism uses amino acids as a carbon source leading to the production of ammonia. Some foods have a higher buffering capacity that resists pH changes. This is usually associated with their protein content, e.g. meat has a higher buffering capacity than vegetables. Lactic acid production from sugars is the basis for many food fermentation processes.

Control of foodborne pathogens by regulation of pH is particularly important. Foods with a pH less than 4.2 are normally considered safe with regard to the growth of pathogenic bacteria, although there is some evidence of survival of food poisoning bacteria (e.g. *Escherichia coli* O157) below this pH. In properly prepared foods, this situation is unlikely to occur and the pH is normally determined by the presence of weak organic acids that are more inhibitory. Growth of pathogenic bacteria in foods with pH less than 4.2 is therefore unlikely. When organic acids are used to adjust the pH to just below

the minimum for growth of food poisoning organisms, there is a lag before death occurs. This has important implications for certain products such as mayonnaise and similar salad dressings in which egg is used as an ingredient and may therefore pose a potential *Salmonella* hazard. However, commercially made mayonnaise has pasteurized egg and also contain an acidifying agent(s).

In canned foods, pH 4.5 is used as the borderline between acid and low acid foods, i.e. those with pH greater than 4.5 requiring a minimum '12D botulinum cook' and those with pH less than 4.5 do not require such a severe heat treatment. The assumption is that *C. botulinum* is unable to grow and produce toxin in canned foods with a pH of 4.5 or less. Although *C. botulinum* can grow in the laboratory at pH 4.2, growth does not occur in food at this pH and no outbreaks of food poisoning due to *C. botulinum* have ever been recorded with foods with a pH of 4.6 or less in which the organism has grown.

Oxygen

As outlined in Chapter 2, micro-organisms vary in their requirement for oxygen and their response to oxygen in the environment. Conditions in which oxygen is present are described as **aerobic**, and where oxygen is absent as **anaerobic**. **Aerobes** are organisms that need oxygen to produce the necessary energy for growth. Most fungi and algae, and many bacteria and protozoa are aerobes. **Microaerophiles** are similar to aerobes in that they require oxygen to generate the necessary energy for growth, but they cannot grow in the oxygen concentration present in air (20 per cent). For example, oxygen concentrations above 10 per cent are toxic to *Campylobacter* spp., which will only grow between about 1 per cent and 10 per cent with an optimum at 6 per cent. **Obligate anaerobes** will only grow in an environment in which oxygen is absent; the food poisoning organisms *C. botulinum* and *C. perfringens* are both obligate anaerobes. **Facultative organisms** are those that can grow both in the absence and the presence of oxygen. **Facultative anaerobes** do not metabolize oxygen but will grow in its presence, e.g. streptococci. **Facultative aerobes** can grow in the absence of oxygen, but when oxygen is present they use this in their metabolism, e.g. *Escherichia coli*.

The amount of oxygen present as well as the ability of a food to react with oxygen is known as the reduction or **redox potential (Eh)**. Individual species of micro-organisms have a redox range in which they will grow that relates primarily to their reaction to oxygen in the environment. The growth of micro-organisms lowers the redox of an environment by using up oxygen, production of reducing substances or a combination of the two. When the microflora consists of a mixed population with different redox requirements, one species may lower the redox and change the environment in favour of another.

Living tissues that form the basic raw material for foods tend to have a negative redox because of their respiratory activity. Apart from the reducing substances produced by respiration, tissues can contain other materials that have reducing activity, e.g. ascorbic acid in vegetables and fruits, reducing sugars in fruits, and the sulphhydryl groups associated with protein in muscle tissue. The actual redox of a food depends on many factors:

- oxygen concentration (tension) in the environment of the food and its access to the food
- density of the food structure, which affects the ability of oxygen in the environment to penetrate
- types and concentration of reducing substance in the food that resist changes in redox towards the positive. Resistance to change in redox is **poising capacity**.
- the manner in which the food is processed
- the pH of the food. For every unit decrease in pH the Eh increases.

The surface of solid foods in contact with the air will have a positive redox whereas the interior may be negative. Processing can radically alter the redox of a raw material. Mixing a food with air at any stage during processing can increase the redox, e.g. milk during the milking and bottling processes. Mincing of meat increases the surface area to volume ratio, giving air access to the bulk of the food, and increases the overall redox. Heating drives off oxygen and may increase the quantity of reducing substances in a food. Canned foods, for example, have a negative redox. Packaging may exclude oxygen and maintain a low redox inherent in the food or produced by microbial growth within a closed environment. The situation inside packaging may be complicated by the accumulation of carbon dioxide resulting from microbial metabolism in vacuum packaged meat, or is sometimes added as part of the gaseous atmosphere in modified atmosphere packaging (see p. 54).

The growth of micro-organisms in foods in relation to redox is dominated by whether oxygen has access to the food. The surface of foods in contact with the atmosphere will support the growth of obligate aerobes, facultative anaerobes, or facultative aerobes. Foods from which oxygen has been excluded or removed by some mechanism, such as heating, and foods with high reducing activity will support the growth of obligate and facultative anaerobes. Partial removal of oxygen may allow the growth of true microaerophiles. The exact nature of the developing microflora will, however, depend on other factors such as the pH and water activity of the food, the composition of the contaminating microflora and the relative numbers of individual species present at the outset. Moulds will generally only grow on food surfaces in direct contact with atmospheric oxygen but there are exceptions, e.g. *Bacillus fulva* that can cause the spoilage of canned fruits. Some moulds, e.g. *Rhizopus* spp., will grow at low oxygen concentrations but will not sporulate unless there is direct contact with air.

As mentioned above, factors that influence the growth of micro-organisms, i.e. water activity, pH, temperature, redox and availability of nutrients, do not act independently but interact with each other to determine whether growth will occur in a particular environment. Minimum and maximum values for individual parameters are usually quoted under conditions in which the other factors that affect growth are optimal. For example, proteolytic strains of *C. botulinum* will grow in an environment containing up to 10 per cent sodium chloride but this applies only at an optimum pH of 7.2 and an optimum temperature of 35 °C. Reduce the pH to 5.2 and the growth of the organism is inhibited by 5 per cent sodium chloride.

Foods are rarely nutrient deficient and the environment for growth tends to be either aerobic (at least when growth starts) or anaerobic: the main interactions are between water activity, pH and temperature. However, as far as facultative anaerobes are concerned, an anaerobic environment becomes another interacting factor. For example, the minimum water activity for the growth of *S.*

aureus is 0.86 under aerobic conditions but anaerobically this is increased to 0.90.

Micro-organisms grown in the laboratory are normally grown as **pure cultures** (monocultures), i.e. only one species is present. The growth characteristics of the organism will depend on the composition of the culture medium, pH, redox, and the temperature of incubation. This situation also applies to industrial fermentation processes and sometimes the growth of micro-organisms in foods when a single species has survived a heat process, e.g. *Clostridium* spp. in a canned food, or when a previously sterile product has been contaminated after the process by a single organism, e.g. *Micrococcus* spp. during the packaging of ultra high treatment (UHT) milk. Fresh foods, however, are usually contaminated with a mixed natural microflora of the food animal or plant plus contaminants from the environment. A significant proportion of the microflora can survive processing or are reintroduced via post process recontamination or a combination of the two, e.g. in pasteurized milk. Given circumstances of pH, temperature and water activity under which more than one component of the contaminating microflora can grow, organisms will compete with one another for available nutrients. Organism(s) that grow fastest under a given set of conditions will usually become dominant. However, if the initial contamination level of an organism is particularly high it may maintain dominance even though it would normally be suppressed by other components of the microflora. This happens when meat is spoiled by the organism *Brochothrix thermosphacta*. Some food poisoning organisms have poor competitive ability and are suppressed by the normal spoilage microflora.

Other gases

Gases may be used to inhibit spoilage organisms and thus to prolong storage life. Carbon dioxide, ethylene oxide, propylene oxide, sulphur dioxide and ozone, are all used to kill or inhibit Gram-negative bacteria, moulds and yeasts. The ethylene and propylene oxides and ozone have some effect on bacterial spores. Safety precautions are necessary in factories where they are used.

Carbon dioxide (CO_2) at high concentrations and low temperatures is useful against a wide range of Gram-negative spoilage organisms. There is little effect against pathogens except perhaps staphylococci because of low temperature storage. Vacuum-packed fresh meats in gas-impermeable plastic film keep much longer at refrigeration temperatures than meat stored in air. There is a rapid increase in carbon dioxide in the gas phase of the package to 10–20 per cent in 4 hours to a maximum of 30 per cent and a reduction in oxygen content to 1–3 per cent due to enzymic activity in the meat. For atmospheric storage the best concentration is about 20 per cent; an atmosphere of 35–75 per cent carbon dioxide, 21–28 per cent oxygen and the remainder nitrogen has been used for transportation. Carbon dioxide inhibits moulds and yeasts in refrigerated fruit and vegetables, and it helps to control ripening in fruit. The concentration used varies according to the product, for example, 5–10 per cent for apples. The gas has an inhibitory effect on microbial growth, it also helps to maintain the physiological health of plant tissue.

Solid carbon dioxide is used as a refrigerant in the storage and transport of unfrozen eggs, meat and poultry, and frozen food such as ice-cream. The gas from dry ice helps to prevent the growth of psychrophilic spoilage organisms. Carbon dioxide allowed to accumulate naturally or added directly to a contained environment extends the storage life of millions of tons of respiring fresh plant and animal produce. Elevated levels of carbon dioxide can damage food and produce 'off' flavours, discoloration and tissue breakdown.

The carbonation of soda and fruit drinks and of sparkling drinking waters to levels of 3–5 atmospheres of carbon dioxide kills or inhibits the growth of spoilage and pathogenic bacteria. The higher the pressure of carbon dioxide and the lower the sugar content the faster the rate of death.

Sulphur dioxide (SO_2) is added to foods and beverages as liquefied gas or as salts – sulphite, bisulphite, metabisulphite. It is used extensively to control spoilage organisms, mostly moulds and yeasts, in soft fruits, fruit juices and pulps, syrups, desiccated coconut, jam, fruit yoghurt, wines, sausages and hamburgers, fresh shrimp, acid pickles and in the starch extraction process. In fruit juices and in wines it inhibits moulds, bacteria and undesirable yeasts, although it has no effect on wine yeasts. As sulphite or bisulphite in sausages it delays growth and it controls 'black spot' in shrimp.

Sulphur dioxide is also used in many foods as an antioxidant or reducing agent to inhibit enzymic and non-enzymic action or browning.

Ethylene oxide and **propylene oxide** has been used to reduce microbial contamination and to kill insects in dried foods, such as gums, spices, dried fruits, cereals and potato flour.

Ozone is used mainly for the treatment of water where it is particularly effective against the parasite *Cryptosporidium* which is resistant to the normal chlorine levels used in water treatment. Ozone decomposes rapidly in the water phase of foods such that antimicrobial action takes place mostly at the surface. Ozone (Box 3.4) is a powerful oxidizing agent and gives a rancid flavour to fats, lowers pH, coagulates protein and inactivates enzymes. It can be produced by ultraviolet (UV) lamps and is partly responsible for the killing effect of UV light in cold storage rooms. The threshold for killing and the rate depends on the amount of organic matter. In clean water, less than 10 parts per million (ppm) is bactericidal, and much larger concentrations – greater than 100 ppm – are required to repress spoilage organisms from food surfaces.

Box 3.4 Susceptibility to ozone
- Bacteria are more susceptible than yeasts and moulds
- Gram-positive bacteria are generally more sensitive than Gram-negative
- Bacterial spores are resistant

Ozone may be used as a maturing agent in ciders and wine, and to disinfect the interiors of soft drink and mineral water bottles before filling.

Irradiation

Ultraviolet light has limiting penetration, thus it is of value for thin layers of fluid only. It is used, for example, in the purification of water for the depuration of shellfish, and for the surfaces of food to prevent spoilage by moulds. Clean surfaces, given adequate exposure, can be disinfected. UV **light** has been used for the decontamination of air in filling and sterility testing, inoculating areas of microbiology laboratories, and in bakeries where it helps to control the occurrence of mould spores on bread.

Ultraviolet radiation is unsuitable for certain foods containing fat because it accelerates lipid oxidation and rancidity, for example, in butter. Also it produces spots of discoloration on the leaves of green vegetables.

Ionizing irradiation (gamma rays) (Box 3.5) has advantages over other methods used to destroy bacteria in food, and it can be used for the preservation of food. It has a high energy content, great penetration and lethality. Penetration is instantaneous, uniform and deep. At low levels there are no organoleptic changes in the food product, and even at high levels chemical changes are small. Foods may be processed in any state, frozen or liquid and in their packages.

Box 3.5 Resistance to ionizing radiation
Gram-positive bacteria are the most susceptible followed by Gram-negative bacteria and moulds, bacterial endospores and yeasts, and viruses, which are most resistant.

Process control is precise and more effective than for heat processing, and regulatory control is likely to be more strict. The few disadvantages include:

- the continued activity of enzymes in irradiated food during storage
- public acceptability.

Antibiotics

Antibiotics used in human and veterinary medicine have a limited role in food processing because of the danger of spoilage organisms and pathogens acquiring resistance. Three antibiotics are used in foods and these are natamycin, nisin and tylosin: none of these has therapeutic value. Natamycin is an antifungal agent; it is used in some countries to protect raw, ground peanuts, the surface of sausages and the rinds of soft and hard cheese against mould growth. Nisin is a naturally occurring antibiotic produced by strains of *Streptococcus lactis*. It affects Gram-positive bacteria only and may be used to prevent 'blowing' of cans and to preserve cheese, chocolate, milk and clotted cream. In addition, it is used in the preservation of green peas, beans, sauces and ketchup. Tylosin is sometimes used as a feedstuff additive.

Curing and smoking

Salt has traditionally been used as a preservative down the ages. Sodium chloride crystals and salt (brine) solution with sodium or potassium nitrite or nitrate are used as curing salts. The suggestion of a carcinogenic hazard from nitrite in food has resulted in reduction of concentration of nitrite added to cures. Sodium nitrite (50–200 ppm) may be used in specified types of cured meat and in a small concentration (5 ppm) in some types of cheese.

Additives known as **adjuvants** are used in many cured meat products. They include ascorbates for colour and phosphates, glucono-δ-lactone and sugar for pH, texture and flavour. All these substances alter susceptibility to bacterial growth. Sugar in high concentration withdraws water from the food (osmosis) and so has a preservative effect. Curing usually produces changes in the food to prevent spoilage or is done to change the type of spoilage.

The preservation and safety of a cured product is the result of interactions of many factors:

- curing salts
- microbial content of the raw product
- time and temperature of processing
- types and numbers of organisms that survive or gain access after processing
- conditions which determine growth, including pH, reduction potential, water activity,
- decreasing nitrite concentration
- packaging
- shelf-life
- temperature of storage.

Smoking is also an ancient process now used for a few products, mostly to give flavour and colour to meats and fish. Smoke contains a wide variety of organic compounds, tarry fractions and formaldehyde, as well as antioxidants and oxides of nitrogen. Natural smoke may be absorbed directly onto food surfaces. Hot smoking takes place at 60–80 °C and cold smoking at 25–30 °C. The preservative effect is present throughout small sausages and on the surface, but not the inside of large pieces of meat.

Compounds of smoke may be dissolved in water. Liquid smoke is used as a spray or dip; there is little or no antibacterial activity. Smoking is generally effective against Gram-negative rods, micrococci and staphylococci. Smoke and spice may increase the period at risk for spoilage by masking odours.

Packaging

Packaging is designed to preserve the quality of the food. Its various functions are:

- protection against water vapour, oxygen and other gases, light, dust and other dirt, weight loss, and mechanical damage
- prevention of entry of micro-organisms, insects and vermin.

It may affect the mode and rate of spoilage, and the survival and growth of pathogens. Care must be taken that the contents do not damage the pack. Packaging material, if not sterile, should introduce few organisms. Containers include cans, paper, cardboard, glass and plastic (rigid) and plastics and foil (flexible).

The most important factor is the permeability of the packaging material to oxygen, carbon dioxide and water vapour, particularly if preservative gases are used for the pack and for perishable products such as meat, poultry and fish. Film may be highly permeable so that conditions in the pack are similar to those in the unpacked product, permitting growth of pseudomonads which is inhibited by gas-impermeable film. Polythene may allow the passage of moisture, but not oxygen, and surface spoilage occurs. Within a pack the usual factors govern the growth and activity of micro-organisms such as the food medium, temperature, water activity, pH, gases and competitive flora. In gas-impermeable, hermetically sealed, evacuated or non-evacuated packages, oxygen is used and carbon dioxide forms, the pH drops and lactic acid organisms become active; the typical aerobic spoilage flora is retarded and altered so that shelf-life increases by 50 per cent. Enterobacteriaceae including salmonellae survive and sometimes grow on the surface of packaged fresh meats even when large numbers of lactic bacteria are present. Anaerobes rarely cause problems in packaged fresh meat even in vacuum packs. However, in cooked or lightly cured meat with few competitors C. perfringens and C. botulinum can grow even in the presence of gaseous oxygen. Carbon dioxide alone or mixed with nitrogen may be used to replace the atmosphere in hermetically sealed packages. A mixture of carbon dioxide and air may increase time to spoilage.

Aseptic filling and containers are used for sterile foods, for example UHT milk, so that shelf-life is increased. All packaging requires careful control of the process of production.

PRESERVATION STRATEGIES

Many foods and food components contain sufficient nutrients to support the growth of micro-organisms. Time is another factor which must be considered with respect to food preservation. The maximum growth rates of micro-organisms have been considered in Chapter 2, but it is worth reiterating here that under ideal conditions, the doubling times for bacteria can be less than 20 minutes. Hence all those involved with the preparing, storage and serving of foods must ensure that delays that allow unacceptable levels of microbial growth do not occur. Table 3.9 shows how the treatments (physical factors) and storage environments (extrinsic factors) of perishable foods can be modified for preservation.

Dairy products are a good example of how food preservation strategies are applied. The raw product (milk) is capable of supporting the survival and growth of a wide range of microbial pathogens and

Table 3.9 *Intrinsic and extrinsic parameters in the preservation of selected foods which support microbial growth*

Food (physical factors)	Extrinsic parameters (storage environment)	Intrinsic parameters (properties of the food)
Apple	Air- or CO_2-enhanced storage atmosphere Cooled or ambient temperature storage Variable relative humidity	a_w 0.98 pH 3.0 (organic acids present) Redox at surface positive Wax-coated epidermis
Apple juice in carton (pasteurized)	No gaseous atmosphere Ambient temperature	a_w 0.98 pH 3.2 (organic acids present) Redox + 400 mV
Modified atmosphere packaged minced beef	$CO_2/N_2/O_2$ atmosphere Chill temperature High relative humidity	Redox positive a_w 0.98 pH 5.2
Canned meat	Gaseous atmosphere: none in sealed container Ambient storage temperature	Redox negative a_w 0.98 pH 5.2
Haddock fillet on ice	0 °C (melting ice)	Redox positive at surface a_w 0.98 pH 6.8
Frozen haddock fillets	−18 °C (air freezer)	Redox positive at surface a_w 0.84 pH 6.8
Pasteurized milk (heated 63 °C for at least 30 minutes or 72 °C for at least 15 seconds)	No gaseous atmosphere: 4 °C (refrigerator)	Redox positive a_w 0.98 pH 6.6
UHT milk (heated to132 °C for not less than 1 second, aseptic packaging)	No gaseous atmosphere: ambient temperatures	Redox positive a_w 0.98 pH 6.6
'Sterilized' milk (filtration, homogenization, heating to >100 °C for 20–40 minutes, aseptic packaging)	No gaseous atmosphere: ambient temperatures	Redox positive a_w 0.98 pH 6.6

Adapted from Garbutt (1997). With permission.

it is not possible to obtain milk in a sterile form. Different heat treatments can be applied to milk, depending on the shelf-life and consumer preference. These treatments are (Table 3.3, p. 45):

- low temperature holding (LTH) pasteurization
- high temperature short time (HTST) pasteurization
- ultra high temperature treatment (UHT)
- sterilization.

Aseptic packaging is important for the preservation of UHT and sterilized milk because it provides a physical barrier that prevents contamination after the heat treatment. Refrigeration is extensively used as a method for the preservation of almost all diary products. Canning is used as a physical barrier for evaporated and condensed milk, which also has reduced water activity, and canned products are shelf-stable at room temperature. Powdered milk is also shelf-stable at room temperature because of the much reduced water activity. Butter is preserved by compartmentalization, but there is also reduction in pH and water activity by bacterial fermentation and the addition of salt, respectively. Sour cream, yoghurt and cheese can be preserved by reduction of the pH, which is a result of bacterial fermentation. Most cheeses use reduction in water activity as an additional preservation strategy by physical drying (including the removal of whey and by pressing) and by the incorporation of salt. Ice cream is principally preserved by freezing.

Summary

Many foods and food components contain sufficient nutrients to support the growth of micro-organisms. The control of microbes in foods and beverages is essential for production of safe and wholesome products. Control involves prevention or delay of spoilage as well as prevention of the growth and survival of pathogens. Apart from barriers which separate food from micro-organisms in the environment (e.g. canning), control of microbes is principally achieved by physical factors, i.e. the application of specific treatments together with modification of food and food components. The most common physical factors are temperature (both heat and cold treatments); amount of available water; pH; a gaseous environment; the available nutrients; and shelf-life.

SOURCES OF INFORMATION AND FURTHER READING

Adams MR, Moss MO (2000) *Food Microbiology*, 2nd edn. Cambridge: Royal Society of Chemistry.

Doyle MP, Beuchat LR, Montville TJ (eds) (1997) *Food Microbiology: Fundamentals and Frontiers*. Washington: American Society for Microbiology Press.

Garbutt J (1997) *Essentials of Food Microbiology*. London: Arnold.

Jay JM (2003) *Modern Food Microbiology*, 6th edn. New York: Kluwer Academic/Plenum Publishers.

4

Microbial agents of food poisoning and foodborne infection

Iain Gillespie

Foodborne pathogens and toxins	59	Prion disease	90
Infections	61	Summary	91
Intoxications	81	Sources of information and further reading	92

Food poisoning is caused by a wide range of noxious substances (poisonous chemicals or pathogenic micro-organisms, such as bacteria, protozoa, viruses, and toxins produced by bacteria, algae and fungi) that may be present in food. These agents are not only responsible for gastroenteritis, but can also cause disease outside the intestinal tract, as well as resulting in long-term disability and, rarely, death. Understanding the nature, distribution and occurrence of pathogenic microbes and toxins is essential for prevention and control of food poisoning, as well as understanding the principles behind hygienic food processes.

Disease Any change from a normal physiological state or function.

Morbidity Effect of disease.

Mortality Death as a result of disease.

Symptom Manifestation or evidence of disease.

Diagnosis The process of identification of disease based on the recognition of symptoms, signs and/or investigations.

Pathogen A micro-organism that has the capacity to cause disease, i.e. has the property of **pathogenicity**.

Virulence Relative degree of pathogenicity.

Toxin A poisonous substance with the capacity to cause disease.

Gastroenteritis Acute inflammation of the lining of the stomach and/or intestines characterized by a combination of nausea, vomiting, diarrhoea and abdominal discomfort. Gastroenteritis limited to the small intestine is referred to as **enteritis** and where both the small intestine and colon are affected it is called **enterocolitis**.

Endemic disease Disease that is present all the time and/or restricted to a particular region/area but the number of people affected remains relatively constant.

Epidemic disease Disease whose incidence suddenly increases in a given region/area.

FOODBORNE PATHOGENS AND TOXINS

All foodborne pathogens or toxins are agents which, by definition, must be ingested (in food) before they can cause disease. The time between ingestion and the onset of disease symptoms is known as the incubation period. Prodromal symptoms are those that indicate the start of the onset of disease, and the infective dose is the amount of the agent that needs to be present in food to produce symptoms of disease. The infective dose is established based on observations of the natural occurrence of the disease, experimental studies on animals or human volunteer feeding experiments, where ethically permissible. The symptomatic period is the time period for which disease manifests. It can be shortened or eliminated by **treatment** which may include the use of antibiotics. **Sequelae** are pathological conditions, sometimes long term, which occur as a result of disease. Chronic kidney disease, for example, is sometimes a sequela of a foodborne illness.

Reservoirs of infection are places where pathogens are present and which can act as their source via various routes of transmission. **Carrier states** occur where humans or animals (known as **carriers**) harbour a **pathogen** without exhibiting symptoms. Some individuals have **immunity**, resistance against infection. Immunity is either **innate** or **acquired** by previous exposure to a specific pathogen or **toxin**. The **incidence** is the number of new diagnoses in a given period, and the **seasonality** is a measure of how the incidence changes during different times of the year.

There are many foodborne pathogens and toxins, and hence great diversity of foodborne diseases and disease mechanisms as well as reservoirs and routes of transmission. In addition, because foodborne diseases occur over a range of severity and duration, and many diagnostic methods are in use, there are marked differences among the rates at which different agents are detected. Table 4.1 gives some estimates of the rates at which different pathogens are reported through national surveillance, detected by routine laboratory investigation, presenting to their general practitioner, and occurring in the community: these comparative differences are known as **reporting pyramids**. Furthermore, routine diagnostic tests do not identify the aetiological agents responsible for most cases of **gastroenteritis**. This is known as the **diagnostic gap**. Figure 4.1 shows rates

of laboratory reports from England and Wales for selected pathogens.

Routes of transmission vary, depending on the:

- reservoirs of infection
- type of food
- nature of the pathogen
- infective dose (and the ability of a specific pathogen to survive/grow in food)
- immunity of the host.

Many of the pathogens described below are transmitted via non-foodborne routes, including drinking water, recreational bathing, or by direct contact with an infected animal or human. It is often difficult to ascribe an exact route of infection in a specific patient. Moreover, the basic principles of hygiene and public health control measures often apply equally regardless of the pathogen or route of infection.

Asymptomatic carriage, as well as excretion after the symptomatic period is common to many gastrointestinal pathogens, hence the importance of hygienic practices for food handlers. Current food safety legislation states that (Regulation (EC) No. 852/2004 on the hygiene of foodstuffs; see Chapter 8):

> No person suffering from, or being a carrier of a disease likely to be transmitted through food . . . is to be permitted to handle food or enter any food handling area in any capacity if there is any likelihood of direct or indirect contamination.

The purpose of this chapter is to outline the characteristics of the major microbial food poisoning agents and principal means of control.

Table 4.1 *Reporting pyramids for enteric pathogens*

	Ratio of cases to reported national surveillance			
	Reported through national surveillance	Detected by routine laboratory investigation	Presenting to their general practitioner	Occurring in the community
All infectious intestinal disease	1	1.4	23.2	134
Salmonella	1	1.4	2.3	3.2
Campylobacter	1	1.5	3.6	7.6
Rotavirus	1	1.5	11.3	35
Norovirus	1	1.4	248	1562

Adapted from Food Standards Agency (2000). Crown copyright material is reproduced with the permission of HMSO and the Queen's Printer for Scotland.

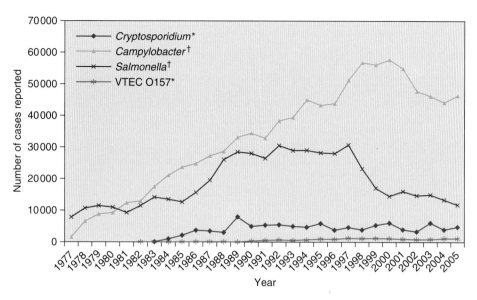

Figure 4.1   *Trends in laboratory reports of human infection from selected enteric pathogens, England and Wales, 1977–2005. *All cases; †pathogens isolated from faeces and lower gastrointestinal tract. (Health Protection Agency, unpublished data)*

INFECTIONS

As outlined in Chapter 1, foodborne microbio-logical disease requires the ingestion of viable micro-organisms followed by multiplication and invasion, leading to disease within the body of a host. Foodborne infections are caused by bacteria, viruses or protozoan parasites, which can either be confined to the gastrointestinal tract or invade sites elsewhere in the body. Each of these broad groups of agents causing microbial infections will be considered in turn. The principal features of foodborne infections are summarized in Table 4.2.

Gastrointestinal infections

Bacterial gastrointestinal infections

Salmonella (excluding enteric fever)

Salmonella is a genus of Gram-negative bacteria which was first isolated in 1888 from meat that had caused food poisoning, and named after the American pathologist D E Salmon. Salmonellas were originally grouped according to their antigenic structure and over 2000 serotypes were originally designated as different species. Most of these different 'species' were named according to the disease they caused and the predominant animal host or the place it was first isolated. However, subsequent molecular analysis classified all salmonella into two species, *Salmonella bongori* and *Salmonella enterica*, the latter being further subdivided into six subspecies. Most of *S. enterica* responsible for disease in animals and man belong to subspecies I, i.e. *S. enterica* subsp. *enterica* which can be discriminated further by serotyping, bacteriophage, and DNA-based characterization. These serotypes were referred to as *Salmonella typhimurium* and *Salmonella enteritidis*, but are now more correctly named as *S. enterica* subsp. *enterica* serovar Typhimurium and *S. enterica* subsp. *enterica* serovar Enteritidis, respectively. This is more simply named as *S. Enterititidis* and *S. Typhimurium* (see chapter 2, p. 19).

Most serotypes of *S. enterica* are widespread in nature and have the potential to act as intestinal pathogens in a variety of animals including humans. However, relatively few serotypes account for most of the human infections reported every year. Of the 84 472 laboratory-confirmed cases of salmonellosis reported in England and Wales between 2000 and 2005, 86 per cent were attributable to the 10 commonest serotypes (Table 4.3). Despite minor changes in the relative frequency of most of these serotypes, their public health importance has

Table 4.2 *Principal features of foodborne gastrointestinal infections*

Bacteria	Symptoms and possible consequences	Incubation period	Duration of illness	Likely infective dose (agent/g% food)	Microbiology and growth characteristics	Sources
Salmonella	Diarrhoea, vomiting, abdominal pain, fever; blood poisoning (septicaemia) and in severe cases death	U 12–48 hours R 5–72 hours	~10 days	U 10^5–10^6; can be as low as 10–20 cells in fatty foods (e.g. cheese or chocolate)	Non-sporing; growth occurs between 2–54 °C (optimum 37 °C); acid resistant (growth at pH 4.0–9.0); growth at a_w above 0.94; sensitive to nitrites; killed by normal cooking and pasteurization	Undercooked foods or contaminated by raw foods/faecal matter. Mainly meat (especially poultry), eggs and dairy products. Also infected food handlers and pets
Campylobacter	Diarrhoea (often bloody), abdominal pain and fever; vomiting rare; sequelae include reactive arthritis and Guillain-Barré syndrome	U 1–3 days R 1–10 days	~10 days	100 s	Non-sporing; grows at >30 °C, pH 6.5–7.5, and at reduced oxygen concentrations; does not generally grow in foods; sensitive to drying, freezing; killed by normal cooking and pasteurization	Raw or undercooked meat, especially poultry; unpasteurized milk, bird-pecked milk, untreated water and pets
Clostridium perfringens	Diarrhoea, abdominal pain	U 12–18 hours R 8–22 hours	12–48 hours	U >10^5/g	Heat-resistant spores; growth at 15–52 °C (optimum 43–45 °C), optimum pH 6–7; anaerobe	Cooked meat dishes with poor temperature and time control
Verocytotoxin-producing *E. coli*	Abdominal pain, vomiting, diarrhoea that may contain blood, kidney failure; can be fatal, young children and elderly people particularly vulnerable	U 3–4 days R 1–14 days	Two weeks in uncomplicated cases	Very low (e.g. 10 s of cells)	Non-sporing; grows at 10–45 °C; acid resistant (grows at pH 4.5); killed by normal cooking and pasteurization	Direct contact with animals and their faeces, infected people and the environment; beef and beef products; unpasteurized dairy products; unpasteurized apple juice; raw vegetables
Norovirus	Predominately vomiting and diarrhoea with occasional fever; sequelae rare	12–24 hours	1–2 days	10–100 infectious particles	Replication in the human gut but not in food or the environment; environmentally robust; inactivated by normal cooking	Infected humans; contaminated surfaces; raw or undercooked shellfish
Cryptosporidium, Giardia and *Cyclospora*	Diarrhoea, abdominal pain, bloating, nausea and vomiting; cryptosporidiosis can be chronic and life-threatening in the immunocompromised	3 days to 6 weeks	4–6 weeks	<1000 oocyst/cysts	Replication in the human gut but not in food or the environment; environmentally robust; inactivated by normal cooking and pasteurization	Other infected humans or animals; drinking or recreational water; faecally contaminated food or beverages

U, usually; R, range.

remained fairly constant, suggesting their high degree of adaptation to their predominant food animal hosts in which they proliferate but not necessarily cause illness.

Salmonella is a remarkably resilient bacterium which will adapt and grow under a wide range of environmental conditions. There is evidence of growth between 2 °C and 54 °C, although this may be strain dependent, and growth between 6 °C and 45 °C is much more typical. Growth generally occurs between pH 4 and 9 (optimum between pH 6.6 and 8.2) and at water activity above 0.94. Salmonellas are unable to tolerate high levels of nitrite or salt, and are killed by pasteurization and normal cooking processes.

The infective dose required for salmonellosis depends on the serotype, the vehicle of infection and on host susceptibility, but experimentally, large numbers (1000 to several million) of bacteria are required for infection. Illness usually occurs 12–48 hours (range 5–72 hours) after the consumption of contaminated food and is characterized by non-bloody diarrhoea, nausea, vomiting, fever and abdominal pain. Some serotypes (e.g. *S.* Dublin and *S.* Virchow) are more likely to cause invasive disease in humans and sequelae, including meningitis and septic arthritis. Salmonellosis is diagnosed by the isolation of the bacterium from samples of faeces, usually taken during the symptomatic period, and also from blood or other body fluids when systemic infection has occurred. Carriage and shedding of the organisms may occur for up to a year in children under 5 years (median 10 weeks) and for up to 12 weeks (median 4 weeks) in older patients.

Antimicrobial chemotherapy is recommended for invasive disease, but not in uncomplicated gastro-enteritis: treatment may prolong carriage of this bacterium. Some strains posses exceptional properties for acquiring resistance to antimicrobial agents used in both human and veterinary medicine as well as in animal husbandry. The increased resistance to antimicrobial agents has reduced the effective therapeutic options for treating human systemic infections (see the section on enteric fever p. 78). The mechanism of disease production by *Salmonella* is poorly understood, however, this ability involves the

Table 4.3 *Ten most common non-typhoidal* Salmonella *serotypes associated with human infection. Faeces and lower gastrointestinal tract isolates: England and Wales, 1981–2004*

Serotype (number of isolates) by year				
1981	1985	1990	1995	2000
Typhimurium (3592)	Typhimurium (5245)	Enteritidis (18 143)	Enteritidis (10 454)	Enteritidis (8267)
Enteritidis (1000)	Enteritidis (2997)	Typhimurium (5085)	Typhimurium (2349)	Typhimurium (2590)
Hadar (600)	Virchow (821)	Virchow (1133)	Virchow (516)	Hadar (328)
Virchow (597)	Stanley (255)	Newport (256)	Hadar (498)	Virchow (292)
Saint-Paul (262)	Infantis (247)	Infantis (255)	Heidelberg (209)	Infantis (161)
Montevideo (253)	Agona (190)	Hadar (237)	Newport (163)	Newport (149)
Infantis (213)	Derby (183)	Heidelberg (237)	Infantis (139)	Blockley (146)
Newport (196)	Hadar (174)	Montevideo (214)	Blockley (133)	Agona (141)
Heidelberg (150)	Montevideo (156)	Kedougou (183)	Java (128)	Montevideo (132)
Agona (137)	Indiana (145)	Agona (134)	Montevideo (120)	Java (117)
2001	2002	2003	2004	2005
Enteritidis (10 912)	Enteritidis (9968)	Enteritidis (10 128)	Enteritidis (8740)	Enteritidis (6896)
Typhimurium (2129)	Typhimurium (1949)	Typhimurium (2111)	Typhimurium (1405)	Typhimurium (1557)
Virchow (378)	Virchow (251)	Virchow (250)	Newport (655)	Virchow (362)
Hadar (250)	Hadar (209)	Bareilly (192)	Virchow (288)	Newport (188)
Newport (178)	Agona (175)	Braenderup (169)	Stanley (152)	Stanley (172)
Infantis (168)	Infantis (168)	Hadar (156)	Braenderup (117)	Hadar (164)
Braenderup (156)	Braenderup (156)	Newport (145)	Hadar (115)	Infantis (130)
Java (121)	Java (155)	Agona (139)	Infantis (103)	Goldcoast (127)
Agona (120)	Newport (124)	Stanley (121)	Agona (101)	Kentucky (102)
Stanley (93)	Stanley (100)	Infantis (120)	Java (88)	Java (85)

Health Protection Agency (unpublished data).

bacterium surviving acids in the stomach and attaching to and invading the cells lining the intestines.

The epidemiology of human salmonellosis in the UK has been dominated for the past quarter of a century by one serotype, *S*. Enteritidis (Table 4.3), and by one phage type (PT) within this serotype, PT4. The third most commonly reported serotype in England and Wales prior to 1980, *S*. Enteritidis incidence increased gradually in the early 1980s, and then rapidly in the late 1980s (from 2997 cases in 1985 to 15 153 cases in 1988). During the early 1980s, PT4 as a proportion of all *S*. Enteritidis cases increased from 37 per cent to 81 per cent (Figure 4.2). Epidemiological studies in the late 1980s confirmed an association between the consumption of eggs/egg products and this illness. *S*. Enteritidis infects the ovaries and oviducts of chickens, facilitating vertical transmission and increasing the likelihood of contamination of egg shells and, less commonly, their contents. If contaminated eggs are stored inappropriately and/or heated inadequately (or not at all, as is common in some foods) then the likelihood of illness increases.

Despite control measures introduced in the late 1980s, the disease incidence remained high, and it was not until a vaccination programme for chickens was introduced in association with reinforced bio-security measures in the 1990s that the incidence dropped dramatically from 22 254 cases in 1997 to 8267 cases in 2000. (See Box 4.1 for control measures.) No egg can be guaranteed *Salmonella*-free, and therefore for people who are particularly vulnerable to infection (young, elderly and infirm people) it should be ensured that eggs are cooked until the whites and yolks are solid. Caterers should replace raw shell eggs with pasteurized liquid egg. Where this is not possible, eggs from a reputable

---

Box 4.1 Control measures for salmonellosis

- Excluding *Salmonella* as much as possible from throughout the food chain
- Application of good standards of hygiene throughout the food chain
- Thorough cooking of meat, poultry and eggs
- Pasteurization of milk
- Reducing the risk of cross-contamination, particularly from raw eggs, meat and poultry
- Application of good temperature and time control during food preparation
- Excluding food handlers until 48 hours after being **symptom** free (first normal stool, see Chapter 8).

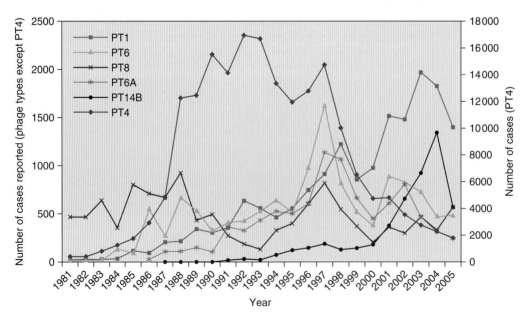

Figure 4.2 *Trends in laboratory-confirmed human infections caused by the most common phage types (PT) of* Salmonella enteritidis. *Faeces and lower gastrointestinal tract isolates, England and Wales, 1981–2005. (Health Protection Agency, unpublished data)*

source and ideally from vaccinated flocks should be used.

Although important, eggs are not the only food vehicle of transmission of infection for salmonellosis. Poultry and meat products are also associated with outbreaks as are many other products, including ready-to-eat or minimally processed foods (salad products, fruit, dried coconut, ice cream, chocolate, bean sprouts, peanuts, cheddar cheese and infant formula milk). In England and Wales, approximately 50 per cent of cases are associated with recent foreign travel. Since the potential for growth of *Salmonella* is greater during the summer (temperature control of foods is more difficult in hotter periods), and because of the contribution of foreign travel, there is a marked seasonality for salmonellosis with cases occurring more commonly in the summer (Figure 4.3).

Campylobacter

Campylobacter spp. were probably first described in 1886 by Theodore Escherich. He noted small curved bacteria in the intestines of infants who had died of 'cholera infantum'. Initially considered a cause of animal disease, *Campylobacter* spp. were first isolated from diseased sheep, cattle and pigs in 1913, 1919 and 1948, respectively. Although implicated in the United States in multiple outbreaks of gastroenteritis in prisons during 1938 and described in detail in four

symptomatic children in the 1960s, it was not until the development of reliable techniques for the growth of *Campylobacter* in the 1970s that its role in human disease was fully appreciated.

The infective dose for *Campylobacter* infection is low. Human volunteer studies have demonstrated that the ingestion of a few hundred cells is sufficient to cause illness. The incubation period is likely to be inversely proportional to the inoculum, with most illness occurring 2–5 days after exposure, although this can range from 1 to 14 days. *Campylobacter* infection usually presents as an acute enteritis, with symptoms of diarrhoea (28.5 per cent with blood in the stool), malaise, fever and abdominal pain. Abdominal pain may be so severe that *Campylobacter* enteritis can be confused with acute appendicitis. Disease is usually self-limiting with therapy limited to fluid and electrolyte replacement. Treatment with antimicrobial agents can be effective in eliminating the organism from the stool and reducing the duration of symptoms. Up to 0.2 per cent of cases develop bacteraemia (the presence of bacteria in the blood); rarely sequelae including reactive arthritis, irritable bowel syndrome and **Guillain–Barré syndrome** (a type of peripheral paralysis). Diagnosis of *Campylobacter* infection is by isolation of the bacterium from samples of faeces and from the blood of more severe cases.

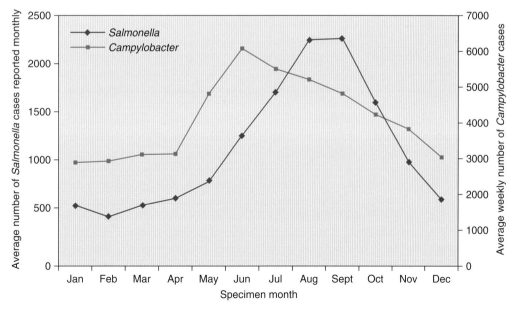

Figure 4.3 *Seasonal pattern of human* Salmonella *and* Campylobacter *infections. Faeces and lower gastrointestinal tract isolates, England and Wales, 2000–05. (Health Protection Agency, unpublished data)*

Campylobacter spp. are the most commonly reported bacterial cause of infectious gastroenteritis in most of the developed countries. Approximately 40 000 laboratory-confirmed cases are reported in England and Wales annually (Figure 4.1, p. 61), with about 90 per cent of cases due to *Campylobacter jejuni* and much of the remainder to *Campylobacter coli*: the disease produced by these two species is indistinguishable. The increase in incidence over the past 25 years (Figure 4.1, p. 61) is likely to reflect improved methods of isolation and identification of these two species, as well as increased ascertainment. Little is understood about the mechanisms by which *C. jejuni* and *C. coli* cause disease in humans. However, tissue injury can occur along the bowel from the jejunum (the small intestine from the duodenum to the ileum) to the colon (large intestine).

The epidemiology of *Campylobacter* infection remains poorly understood. Most cases are sporadic and the low infective dose, long and variable incubation period and the relatively poor routine follow-up of human cases mean that outbreaks, if they occur, are rarely recognized. Infection is highly seasonal, with a consistent annual rise in incidence in late spring to early summer (Figure 4.3). The reasons for this are unknown, although the influx of migratory birds (the avian gut is the natural reservoir for *Campylobacter*), coupled with seasonal changes in animal husbandry and human behaviour may be influential. The consumption of bird-pecked doorstep-delivered milk accounts for a small minority of cases. Foreign travel is a major risk factor for infection, accounting for approximately a fifth of cases. The highest rates of infection are observed in those returning from the Pacific islands and the Asian subcontinent, with the Iberian Peninsula the most commonly implicated European destination.

Campylobacter spp. are unable to grow outside the mammalian gut (including in food) and are sensitive to drying, freezing and disinfection. Inadequate heat treatment and cross-contamination are therefore likely to be important factors in foodborne transmission. Undercooked meats (especially poultry) have consistently been identified as major risk factors for infection, with unpasteurized milk and untreated water implicated in the few recognized outbreaks. See Box 4.2 for control measures.

> **Box 4.2 Control measures for *Campylobacter* infections**
> - Pasteurization of milk
> - Water treatment
> - Adequate cooking of meat and poultry
> - Covering doorstep-delivered milk bottles to prevent bird pecking
> - Probably most importantly, preventing cross-contamination (by hand or via food contact surfaces, particularly from raw meat, in both the domestic and commercial catering environment).

Clostridium perfringens

Clostridium perfringens was established as an important foodborne pathogen by the work of Dr Betty Hobbs in the late 1940s and early 1950s. This bacterium is a Gram-positive spore-forming obligate anaerobe and is widely distributed in the environment, in foods, as well as occurring in the gut flora in healthy humans and animals. Because of the production of robust endospores, *C. perfringens* can remain dormant for prolonged periods and survives dehydration as well as many normal cooking processes: some strains are able to survive boiling for more than 3 hours. Indeed heating actually activates the germination process, converting spores into vegetative cells. The bacterium will grow between 15 °C and 52 °C (optimum 43–45 °C) and many foods (typically cooked meats, poultry, fish, stews, pies and gravies) with high water activity and neutral pH, provide an excellent anaerobic growth medium in which rapid multiplication can occur: doubling times of 8 minutes have been described under ideal conditions.

The symptoms of *C. perfringens* gastroenteritis (abdominal pain; profuse diarrhoea; nausea, but rarely vomiting) occur 8–22 hours (usually 12–18 hours) after the consumption of heavily contaminated foods. Where large number of vegetative cells (usually $>10^5$/g) are consumed, the bacterium sporulates in the lower small intestine, produces enterotoxin, and thus causes the above mentioned symptoms. Illness usually lasts for 12–48 hours and complications are rare. *C. perfringens* is part of the faecal flora of healthy people, and not all the members of this species are able to produce enterotoxin. Hence, the isolation of this bacterium alone is insufficient to establish a diagnosis. Ideally diagnosis is achieved by the detection of enterotoxin in the faeces, usually using an immunoassay (enterotoxin is generally present only within the first 48 hours after onset), together with isolation of high (>10^5/g) numbers of *C. perfringens* spores capable of producing enterotoxin in faeces of affected patients. The same strain of *C. perfringens* should be present in the faeces of most patients affected in an outbreak, as well as occurring in high levels (>10^5/g) in foods implicated with disease.

Due to the short duration and relatively low severity of disease, most sporadic cases of *C. perfringens* gastroenteritis will not present to general practice or primary care facilities. Similarly, small family outbreaks will go unrecognized. The incidence in the community is under-ascertained by national laboratory-based surveillance by a factor of greater than 300 (Table 4.1, p. 60). An understanding of the epidemiology of *C. perfringens* gastroenteritis is therefore derived largely from general outbreaks and these tend to follow the classic pattern of infection described above. Almost all outbreaks are associated with meat and poultry produced in larger scale catering (i.e. restaurants, schools, weddings, etc.) in which temperature and time control are more difficult because of the need to cook larger quantities of foods in advance with a lack of adequate refrigeration. Furthermore, most outbreaks involve:

- inadequate cooking, cooling or reheating
- cooking too far in advance
- storage of foods at room temperature
- the use of leftovers, particularly for stocks and gravies.

C. perfringens will survive most cooking processes unless equivalent to the most stringent used for canned foods, hence control of food poisoning due to this bacterium is by adequate cool storage and reheating (Box 4.3).

Box 4.3 Control measures for *C. perfringens* food poisoning

- Cool hot food rapidly, particularly through 55–15 °C, within 90 minutes of cooking
- Thoroughly reheat pre-cooked foods to >70 °C immediately before consumption
- UK food safety legislation requires that, subject to certain exceptions, food which is likely to support the growth of pathogenic micro-organisms or the formation of toxins must be kept at or below 8 °C or at 63 °C or above (The Food Hygiene [England] Regulations 2006 SI 14, see Chapter 15).

Verocytotoxin producing *E. coli*

Escherichia coli is named after the German paediatrician Theodore Escherich who first isolated the organism from the intestines of infants in the 1880s. This bacterium forms part of the normal intestinal microflora of humans and warm-blooded animals. Most strains are harmless commensals that may have a role in vitamin synthesis. However, some *E. coli* possess specific virulence factors which allow these bacteria to cause disease in humans and animals, and foodborne transmission of these subtypes can occur.

The most important *E. coli* from a food safety perspective is **verocytotoxin producing *E. coli* (VTEC)**, which belong to the **enterohaemorrhagic group of *E. coli* (EHEC)**. This group of bacteria produces powerful toxins. These toxins are named vero cytotoxin (and Shiga-like toxins in North America because of the similarities of one of these with toxin produced by *Shigella* spp. [see following section]). VTEC was first recognized as a foodborne pathogen in the United States in 1982 following two outbreaks of a distinct bloody diarrhoeal syndrome linked to the consumption of hamburgers from a single fast-food restaurant chain. Subsequent laboratory investigations revealed sporadic infections in the United States, some with a history of undercooked beef consumption. In the UK, sporadic cases have been reported since 1982, but it was not until a large outbreak occurred in central Scotland in 1996 that this micro-organism gained public and political notoriety. For further details of this outbreak see Chapter 6, p. 135.

The consumption of as little as 10 VTEC in food is sufficient to cause infection, which occurs when the bacterial cells attach to the epithelium in the upper intestine and produce vero cytotoxins that damage the gut lining. This leads to bloody diarrhoea (**haemorrhagic colitis**) and severe abdominal pain. Serious sequelae that can occur include:

- **Haemolytic uraemic syndrome (HUS**; damage to the kidneys results in blood in the urine)
- **Haemolytic anaemia** (loss of red blood cells)
- Thrombocytopenia (loss of platelets, especially in children)
- **Thrombotic thrombocytopenic purpura** (loss of platelets and excessive clot formation, leading to damage to the kidneys and nervous system) especially in adults.

These sequelae contribute greatly to the significant morbidity and mortality associated with this pathogen. Between 2 and 8 per cent of cases develop HUS and 2 per cent of these prove to be fatal. VTEC is the biggest single cause of acute renal failure in children and those who survive are often left with permanent renal impairment and are candidates for renal transplantation. Treatment of VTEC focuses on fluid and electrolyte replacement and on monitoring patients for the development of HUS. Antibacterial chemotherapy is not recommended as studies suggest that their use increased the likelihood of HUS. Diagnosis of infection is by the isolation of the bacterium from the faeces of affected patients. However, isolation of VTEC can be difficult because of the considerable numbers of other non-pathogenic *E. coli* which occur in faeces. The detection of antibodies in serum and saliva samples has also been used to assist diagnosis.

Most infections in the UK are due to a single serotype of VTEC, i.e. O157, but other serotypes have been associated with this disease including O26, O111 and O145. This may reflect isolation and detection methods rather than true prevalence as diagnostic laboratories do not routinely screen for non-O157 VTEC or for VTEC O157 which ferment sorbitol (an important diagnostic feature of VTEC O157 is that most do not ferment this sugar). Indeed in continental Europe where immunological screening is undertaken, a broader range of VTEC serotypes are reported. VTEC O157 predominates in the United States, Japan and New Zealand, whereas in Australia VTEC O111 is reported most commonly.

Approximately 1000 laboratory-confirmed cases of VTEC O157 infection are reported annually in England and Wales and 80 per cent of cases do not form part of recognized outbreaks. The incidence in Scotland exceeds that in the rest of the UK by a factor of 3. VTEC infection is highly seasonal, with increasing incidence in spring, peak reporting in mid-summer, declining incidence through autumn and a rapid drop in incidence during the winter.

Contact with the environment, especially with animal excreta, is the important risk factor for infection. The natural reservoir for VTEC O157 is the gastrointestinal tract of animals (particularly cattle) and the organisms can be excreted in high numbers by apparently healthy animals. Since there is a low infective dose, poor hygiene following visits to farms and the countryside as well as secondary person-to-person transmission can lead to infection.

Foodborne transmission does occur – over 40 per cent of general outbreaks of VTEC O157 infection reported in England and Wales between 1992 and 2005 were of foodborne origin (in these outbreaks initial foodborne transmission is often followed by person-to-person spread). Because of the natural environment of the organism, contamination of meat during slaughter and preparation is inevitable. Cross-contaminated cooked meats are commonly implicated in outbreaks. Unpasteurized or poorly pasteurized milk is also implicated in outbreaks.

The organism exhibits remarkable survival properties. Unusually acid tolerant, VTEC O157 will survive fermentation, drying and storage for up to 2 months in a fermented sausage with a pH of 4.5, and indeed this food type has been associated with outbreaks. Other acidic foods of pH values between 3 and 4 associated with VTEC O157 outbreaks are mayonnaise and apple juice, in which the organism has been shown to survive for between 1 and 7 weeks. VTEC O157 are resistant to drying and can survive for long periods under hostile conditions. However, VTEC O157 does not have unusual heat resistance and D values at 57–64 °C are between 270 and 9.6 seconds. The organism will not survive pasteurization. See Box 4.4 for control measures.

Box 4.4 Control measures for VTEC

- Thorough cooking of meat (core cooking time/temperature combination of 70 °C for 2 minutes or equivalent)
- Pasteurization of milk
- Reducing the risk of cross-contamination by good kitchen hygiene. Because of the high rate of secondary transmission, cases of doubtful personal hygiene, nursery or pre-school children, food handlers or clinical/social care workers should be excluded until the organism has been cleared from the stool.

Other pathogenic *E. coli*

The remaining pathogenic or enterovirulent *E. coli* can be subdivided into four groups, depending on their virulence mechanisms. Confirmation of illness is through isolation of the organism from the affected person's faeces and/or other body tissues including blood. Strains are differentiated from each other and from non-pathogenic strains of *E. coli* by a combination of serotyping and testing for virulence factors known or presumed to cause diarrhoeal disease.

Recognized in the 1960s, **enterotoxigenic *E. coli*** (ETEC) cause diarrhoea in infants in less developed countries and in travellers to these regions from industrialized countries. Illness usually follows (<24 hours) the intake of 106–108 cells (less for infants) via the consumption of faecally contaminated food or water. ETEC colonizes the upper small intestine where toxin production causes excess fluid secretion. The illness is usually self-limiting (3–4 days duration) without the need for specific treatment. Antimicrobial chemotherapy can be effective if given early but antibiotic resistance is an increasing problem.

Enteroinvasive *E. coli* (EIEC) cause an invasive form of diarrhoea similar to that caused by *Shigella* spp. (see next column). The infective dose for illness is low (as little as 10 cells) and illness usually commences 12–72 hours after the consumption of food and water contaminated with faeces from other affected individuals. EIEC strains invade and destroy the epithelial cells of the lower intestine, eliciting a significant immune response and a clinical picture similar to bacillary dysentery, with bloody diarrhoea and fever. Illness is usually self-limiting but strains of EIEC occasionally cause HUS in children. Infection with EIEC is rare although under-ascertainment may occur due to confusion with shigellosis.

Enteropathogenic *E. coli* (EPEC) are pathogenic but their virulence does not relate to the excretion of typical enterotoxins. EPEC enters the body with consumption of untreated water or faecally contaminated food. Cells which survive transport through the stomach attach loosely to the gut epithelium where they cause watery or bloody diarrhoea through alteration of the microvilli brush border or acute tissue destruction (possibly toxin-mediated). EPEC is a major cause of severe infantile diarrhoea worldwide and is highly infectious to infants. The infective dose is very low, but adult disease is rare.

First described in 1987 but still relatively poorly understood, **enteroaggregative *E. coli*** (EAggEC) is increasingly recognized as a cause of diarrhoea in developing and developed countries. It has been associated with acute persistent (>14 days) diarrhoea in children and the immunocompromised. Their name is derived from the 'stacked-brick' formation produced when grown *in vitro*. *In vivo*, the bacteria adhere to cell walls and produce a heat-stable enterotoxin which causes watery diarrhoea.

Shigella

Shigella is a group of non-motile Gram-negative rods which are closely related to *E. coli* and cause **bacterial dysentery**, which is a severe diarrhoeal disease in which there is blood and mucus in the faeces. Hippocrates used the term dysentery to portray a distinct diarrhoeal disease, and the condition has been described in medical writings since the beginning of recorded history. However, it was not until the late nineteenth century that bacterial dysentery could be distinguished from that caused by amoebae. *Shigella* is named after Shiga, a Japanese microbiologist who first demonstrated that a bacterium from the faeces of patients with dysentery could be **agglutinated** (clumped) by antibodies in patients' sera. Historically, *Shigella* has played an important role in prolonged military campaigns in which unsanitary conditions led to faecal–oral transmission via contaminated water or food, and bacillary dysentery claimed more lives than the military action itself in some campaigns.

Infection with *Shigella* spp. is confirmed by isolation of the organism from faeces. *Shigella* is classified into four species, which can be identified on the basis of biochemical as well as serological reactions:

- *Shigella dysenteriae*, Group A, 12 serotypes
- *Shigella flexneri*, Group B, 6 serotypes
- *Shigella boydii*, Group C, 18 serotypes
- *Shigella sonnei*, Group D, 1 serotype.

The infective dose for shigellosis can be as low as 10 cells depending on host susceptibility and the incubation period ranges from 12–96 hours (up to 7 days for *S. dysenteriae*). The transit of viable cells to the mucosa of the large intestine leads to invasion of epithelial cells. Here cells multiply and spread to adjacent cells, causing inflammation, **desquamation** (cell shedding) and ulceration. This, plus inhibition of water absorption by the colon, leads to the clinical presentation of abdominal pain, fever and diarrhoea with blood and mucus in the faeces. Some strains within serogroup 1 of *S. dysenteriae* produce a powerful exotoxin called Shiga toxin, which causes a clinically more severe disease and can lead to HUS in children. Following infection with *S. flexneri*, some genetically susceptible individuals go on to develop **Reiter's syndrome**, an inflammatory condition that presents with arthritis, conjunctivitis and urethritis. Otherwise shigellosis is usually self-limiting with a median duration of 7 days. Antibiotics can limit excretion and shorten the duration of symptoms, but multiple antibiotic resistance has led to the advice from some that treatment should be reserved for patients with severe illness. However, as humans represent the only significant reservoir for infection and rates of person-to-person transmission are high, others advocate treatment for all laboratory-confirmed cases or cases with known bacterial dysentery.

S. sonnei is endemic in England and Wales and usually causes a mild illness of short duration. Incidence tends to be higher in infants and young children and occurs in periodic waves depending on **herd immunity** (protection from a disease conferred on a susceptible individual by virtue of a high level of immunity in a population). Over half (54 per cent) of outbreaks (65 reported between 1992 and 2005) occur in schools (40 per cent in primary and 37 per cent in nursery schools), with 14 per cent in residential institutions and 14 per cent in the community, with person-to-person transmission being responsible for 88 per cent of these outbreaks. Only five foodborne outbreaks were reported to national surveillance between 1992 and 2005. A buffet meal was implicated in one, possible links with coriander were identified in two, and green salad and iceberg lettuce in the remaining two. One hundred people were affected in the final outbreak, which was part of a Europe-wide problem in 1994. Most S. flexneri and all S. boydii and S. dysenteriae infections in England and Wales are associated with foreign travel and are more severe.

Globally shigella had a major impact, causing an estimated 164 million cases and 1 million deaths annually. Most infections (69 per cent) and deaths (61 per cent) are thought to occur in children younger than 5 years, with 99 per cent of infections occurring in developing countries, where S. flexneri predominates. Transmission may be via food contaminated by infected food handlers, or through the consumption of vegetable crops irrigated with untreated water or contaminated by infected crop workers. Flies also can have a role in transmission and infections can be acquired by drinking or swimming in contaminated water. As no vaccine for shigellosis exists, people from developed countries visiting developing countries should drink only treated or bottled water and should avoid ice unless it is known to be made from treated or chlorinated water. See Box 4.5 for control of shigellosis.

Box 4.5 Control measures for *Shigella* infections

- Sewage should be adequately disposed of and should not come into contact with vegetables and salad products
- Good personal hygiene should be exercised at all times and foods should be protected from flies
- In developing countries travellers should only eat food that is freshly cooked and piping hot. Travellers should avoid salads and eat fruit only if it can be peeled

---

Vibrio

Vibrio cholerae is a Gram-negative comma-shaped bacterium, responsible for the disease cholera. The discovery of *V. cholerae* is often credited to the German bacteriologist Robert Koch, who isolated the bacteria in pure culture while studying the disease in Egypt in 1883. However, it later emerged that the bacterium, and its hypothesized aetiological role in cholera, had been previously described by the Italian physician Filippo Pacini in 1854. Not all strains of *V. cholerae* have the ability to cause disease, as the presence of genes encoding a toxin and a colonization factor are required for pathogenesis. The term 'cholera' has ancient origins (Greek: 'a flow of bile') and is reserved for the disease caused by toxigenic *V. cholerae* strains of the O1 and O139 serogroups, although other serogroups can cause similar illness referred to collectively as the non-epidemic *V. cholerae* or non-O1, non-O139 *V. cholerae*.

Disease commences 24–72 hours after the ingestion of water or food contaminated with thousands to millions of cells. Bacteria which survive transit through the acid environment of the stomach attach to the mucosal cells in the upper intestine and produce an enterotoxin which results in the secretion of water and electrolytes into the intestinal lumen. Diarrhoea commences when the colon cannot reabsorb fluid at the rate equal to production. The disease progresses rapidly and large volumes of diarrhoeal faeces with a classic 'rice-water' consistency can be produced in a matter of hours. Additional symptoms (e.g. vomiting, cramps) accompany excess fluid loss (>5 per cent of body weight) and death can occur if fluid loss exceeds 10 per cent. Case fatality rates of 1–10 per cent have been reported and are dependent largely on access to healthcare and treatment by proper rehydration.

Treatment with antimicrobial agents (tetracyclines, ciprofloxacin, trimethoprim, erythromycin and furazolidone) is effective in severe cases of cholera in epidemics where they reduce the severity and duration of symptoms. However, rapid replacement of fluids and electrolytes forms the most essential aspect of treatment. The diagnosis is confirmed by the isolation of the bacterium from the faeces, in which it occurs in very high numbers. Because of the numbers and the distinct shape, microscopic examination of faeces provides a strong indication of the presence of *V. cholerae*.

Vibrios are aquatic organisms and survive well in riverine, brackish and estuarine water, their natural environments. Toxigenic strains of *V. cholerae* are often outnumbered by non-pathogenic forms. Pathogenic *V. cholerae* survives for prolonged periods in such environments, and this may be enhanced by associations with marine invertebrates and algae. When conditions are not conducive to growth, *V. cholerae* switches to a metabolically inactive 'viable but non-culturable' (those which are alive but in a form unable to grow on artificial culture media) form but which can cause disease in human volunteers. Although distinct reservoirs exist in the Gulf of Mexico and western Australia, cholera may have originated in the Ganges delta of the Indian subcontinent, where it probably caused sporadic infections which pre-date accounts of a similar disease in medieval India. From here it spread throughout the globe in a series of **pandemic** (widespread epidemic) waves, facilitated by increased international trade and rapid post-industrial urban development in the absence of adequate sanitation (see Chapter 7, p. 148). What is widely believed to be the eighth pandemic began in Bengal in 1992, is caused by an O139 strain of *V. cholerae*, which is, as yet, limited to the Indian subcontinent and southeast Asia.

Epidemic cholera exhibits a strong seasonal pattern, with increased incidence in hotter months, possibly linked to changes in salinity or zooplankton populations. Large meteorological phenomena, such as the El Niño effect, can also increase incidence. Humans are infected through the consumption of faecally contaminated food and water. Water is probably the major route of transmission and source of contamination for food (see Chapter 7), although the organism can multiply in food, increasing the likelihood of illness. Foodborne transmission occurs

through consumption of crops cultivated in untreated water, through washing or handling foods which receive no further processing or by the consumption of raw/undercooked seafood. Although the organism can be excreted for several weeks or months after infection, secondary transmission is rare.

Epidemics of cholera in developed countries in the nineteenth century precipitated public health and sanitary reform which eradicated indigenously acquired cholera in those countries. With occasional exceptions (see above), cholera is a disease of developing countries associated with both poor water hygiene and inadequate sewage treatment. Given the environmental reservoir for *V. cholerae*, a source of cholera is likely to exist indefinitely. See Box 4.6.

Vibrio parahaemolyticus is a facultative anaerobic, Gram-negative rod-shaped bacterium, which like *V. cholerae*, is halophilic (salt loving). The natural habitat of *V. parahaemolyticus* is coastal and estuarine waters worldwide, although the bacterium has been isolated from saline-free waters. The role of *V. parahaemolyticus* in foodborne disease was first elucidated by Fujino in Japan, who isolated the bacterium from patients and the implicated food vehicle, half-dried sardines (*hirashu* in Japanese), in an outbreak of gastroenteritis affecting 272 people (including 20 deaths) in 1950. The high disease incidence in Japan is indicative of the predilection for raw or lightly cooked seafood, and seafood is almost the sole vehicle of infection worldwide.

V. parahaemolyticus can be isolated frequently from raw fish and shellfish harvested from coastal and estuarine waters, but generally numbers are low and the majority of isolates lack the ability to cause gastroenteritis. However, the micro-organism can grow rapidly in temperature-abused seafood, and illness occurs 12–24 hours after the consumption of large numbers (10^5–10^7) of a pathogenic strain. The illness has been described as a mild form of cholera, i.e. a rapid onset of profuse diarrhoeal illness with acute abdominal pain with some vomiting and fever, lasting a few days in uncomplicated cases. Hospital admission following severe fluid loss is uncommon. The seasonal pattern of disease, increased incidence in summer and early autumn, reflects the bacterium's sensitivity to cold and its ability to grow in poorly refrigerated foods. The disease is diagnosed by the isolation of the bacterium from the faeces of affected individuals. See Box 4.6 for control measures.

Box 4.6 Control measures for *Vibrio* infections

- Establishment of minimum sanitary requirements to reduce the risk of cholera in developing countries where the disease is endemic is essential for control.
- Appropriate cold storage of raw and cooked seafood is an important factor for prevention of *V. parahaemolyticus* gastroenteritis
- Appropriate heat treatment will also readily kill *V. parahaemolyticus*

Yersinia

Yersinia enterocolitica is a facultative anaerobic Gram-negative rod to coccobacilliary shaped bacterium first described by Schleifstein and Coleman as a cause of facial lesions and enteritis in humans in the United States in 1939. The clinical spectrum of infection with *Y. enterocolitica* is variable and depends largely on the age and susceptibility of the host. Unsurprisingly, given the name of the micro-organism, self-limiting entero-colitis is the commonest manifestation, affecting over three quarters of cases, beginning usually 1–10 days after the consumption of a relatively high number of cells and persisting for 5–14 days. Abdominal pain, fever and diarrhoea predominate, whereas nausea and vomiting are reported less frequently. The terminal ileum and caecum are most commonly affected and occasionally it can be misdiagnosed as appendicitis, especially in older children. Inflammation of the lymph glands in the abdomen (**mesenteric lymphadenitis**) may also occur. Extra-intestinal infections (e.g. bacteraemia, meningitis, endocarditis) have been reported, especially in patients with predisposing conditions, and a number of sequelae, e.g. reactive arthritis, Reiter's syndrome, **erythema nodosum** (a red swelling of the skin of the arms or lower legs), can accompany the infection. Diagnosis is by the isolation of the bacterium from the faeces, and treatment with antimicrobial agents is not usually indicated unless there is bacteraemia.

The natural reservoirs of *Y. enterocolitica* include rodents, rabbits, pigs, sheep, cattle, horses and dogs and the organism has been isolated from lakes, streams, and drinking water. Pigs appear to play an important role in human transmission. The oral cavities, throats and intestinal tracts of pigs are often colonized by the serotypes most commonly causing human disease (O:3, O:9 and O:5,27 in the UK and Europe; O:8 in North America), whereas those found in other animals and the environment are often non-pathogenic and from other serogroups. It is unsurprising therefore that a history of pig meat consumption or direct contact with pigs can often be obtained from patients with yersiniosis.

The incidence of laboratory-confirmed *Y. enterocolitica* infections in the UK has declined in recent years, with only 18 cases reported in 2004. This is likely to be a surveillance artefact, as most clinical laboratories do not routinely screen for this pathogen. The Infectious Intestinal Disease Study (Food Standards Agency 2000) demonstrated that, in 1995, for each case reported to the national centre approximately 1700 cases existed in the community. However, the same study also showed that *Y. enterocolitica* could be isolated from healthy controls at a frequency equal to or greater than symptomatic cases, perhaps justifying the reduced laboratory investigation.

Y. enterocolitica grows over the temperature range –2 °C to 45 °C (optimum 22–29 °C). However the **psychrotrophic** (growing in the cold) nature of *Y. enterocolitica*, especially in foods of neutral pH, low to moderate salt and high water activity (such as meat or milk) mean that refrigeration alone is insufficient for control (see Box 4.7).

Box 4.7 Control measures for *Y. enterocolitica* infection

- Reducing contamination of raw meat (especially pork)
- Appropriate heat treatment of meat and milk (e.g. pasteurization)
- Preventing cross-contamination from raw to cooked foods.

Gastrointestinal protozoa: Cryptosporidium, Cyclospora and Giardia

Cryptosporidium, *Cyclospora* and *Giardia* are genera of protozoan parasites which infect a wide range of vertebrates. Species within these genera cause human cryptosporidiosis, cyclosporiasis and giardiasis which present as severe diarrhoea (together with abdominal cramps, bloating, nausea and vomiting) of 4–6 weeks duration. The incubation period ranges between 3 days to 6 weeks and infection is usually self-limiting. However, in the case of cryptosporidiosis, infection can be chronic and life-threatening, especially in the immunocompromised, including those with acquired immune deficiency syndrome (AIDS). These infections probably constitute the most common causes of protozoal diarrhoea worldwide and are also a significant cause of morbidity worldwide. Although particularly common in the developing world (see Chapter 18), cryptosporidiosis and giardiasis are a significant cause of diarrhoea in northern Europe and North America. There is no specific chemotherapy for cryptosporidiosis, but cyclosporiasis can be treated successfully with trimethoprim, and giardiasis with metronidazole.

None of these protozoa are able to multiply in food or the environment, hence transmission is via direct or indirect oral contact with the faeces of an infected host in which these organisms occur in extremely large numbers during infection. Infection can therefore be spread via contact with:

- other infected humans (person-to-person) or animals (zoonotic)
- faecally contaminated drinking water (or water used in food or beverage production) as well as water used for recreation
- faecally contaminated food or beverages.

All three groups of protozoa have a complex lifecycle which is completed in a single animal host. The lifecycle includes a feeding stage(s) which grow and multiply in the intestinal tract, and a resting or cyst stage which is excreted in the faeces. The **cysts** (also known as **oocysts** for *Cryptosporidium* and *Cyclospora*), or transmissive stages, are extremely robust and can survive for months, even years, in particular in cool, dark and moist environments, and ultimately infect another host. *Cryptosporidium* oocysts and *Giardia* cysts are infectious as soon as they are passed into the environment. However, the oocysts of *Cyclospora* require a maturation period (probably 5 days to 2 weeks) before they become infectious. The extreme resistance of *Cryptosporidium* oocysts to chlorine means that this chemical is ineffective at killing this organism at the concentrations used for water treatment or in food production environments. The cysts are generally sensitive to freezing, drying and mild heat, and will certainly be killed by pasteurization processes.

Cryptosporidium, *Cyclospora*, and *Giardia* are all complex genera, with multiple species, many of which are not infectious to humans. The majority of cases of cryptosporidiosis are due to *Cryptosporidium hominis* and *Cryptosporidium parvum*. All cases of cyclosporiasis and giardiasis are due to *Cyclospora cayetanensis* and *Giardia duodenalis*, respectively. *G. duodenalis* is also named *Giardia intestinalis*, and *Giardia lamblia*, all of which refer to the same group of human pathogens. *C. hominis* and *C. cayetanensis* appear specific to humans, hence all infections will involve either direct contact with another infected person, or food, water or beverages contaminated with human sewage. *C. parvum* can not only infect humans, but also livestock (especially cow and sheep) as well as other domestic, pet and wild animals. Hence cases of *C. parvum* infection can involve direct contact with another infected person or animals, as well as food, water or beverages contaminated by human or animal faeces. Less is known about the possible host reservoirs for human giardiasis. Clearly this involves other humans, but the role of *G. duodenalis* from pets or wild animals (especially rodents) remains to be established.

Contaminated drinking water has been implicated in transmission of infection in cryptosporidiosis, cyclosporiasis and giardiasis (see Chapter 7). However, as mentioned above, contamination of food and beverages is also important. Outbreaks of cryptosporidiosis have been associated with improperly pasteurized milk (see Chapter 6, p. 136), as well as freshly pressed apple juice made from fruit collected off the ground where cattle had recently been allowed to graze. In both of these outbreaks, the beverage ingredients were contaminated by animal faeces. Cryptosporidiosis and giardiasis outbreaks have occurred where food handlers were either infected, or had recently changed nappies in children. These outbreaks highlight the importance of personal cleanliness and hygiene of food handlers. Finally, in the mid-1990s, a series of outbreaks of cyclosporiasis occurred in North America associated with raspberries grown in Central America. Here the likely route of contamination was via sewage-contaminated water used for diluting the fungicide solutions sprayed on the fruit (see Chapter 6, p. 141).

Gastrointestinal viruses

Norovirus

Noroviruses are a group of small (35–40 nm diameter) single-stranded RNA viruses belonging to the family *Caliciviridae*. Their early history goes back to 1929 when Zahorsky recognized a syndrome in humans which he called 'hyperemesis hiemis' or **winter vomiting disease**, based on the main clinical presentation and seasonal pattern of disease. Numerous accounts of this syndrome were reported and ascribed different names in the subsequent four decades, but while infectivity was demonstrated, all attempts to isolate a bacterial pathogen or viral agent failed. However, in an outbreak of gastroenteritis in a school in Norwalk, Ohio, USA, a previously undescribed virus-like particle was identified as the causal agent. Subsequent outbreaks identified viruses morphologically similar to the Norwalk virus throughout the world (hence the name **Norwalk-like virus** or **NLV**). Their names were based on the geographical location of the outbreak (e.g. Snow Mountain, Hawaii, Taunton etc.). These viruses were subsequently grouped together and termed **small round structured viruses (SRSV)** in the UK based on the morphological distinctions between this group and other small round viruses found commonly in the gut, but were still known as Norwalk viruses or NLV elsewhere. Following molecular characterization, international consensus was reached and the term **norovirus** adopted.

As few as 10–100 infectious particles are required for illness, which usually commences 18–48 hours after exposure (typically 24 hours). The onset of symptoms is sudden with nausea and vomiting (which can be severe and projectile) predominating, with low-grade fever and mild diarrhoea in most cases. The disease is self-limiting and symptoms rarely last for more than 2 days, although a small number of affected individuals require hospital treatment due to dehydration. Diagnosis is by detecting the virus in faeces (less commonly vomitus) either by electron microscopy or, now more usually, by immunoassay or by polymerase chain reaction (PCR).

The host range for norovirus is limited to humans and person-to-person transmission is by far the most common and important transmission pathway for infection. This occurs usually directly via the faecal–oral route, or indirectly by the contamination of environmental surfaces and other items. Aerosolized vomitus is an additional source of transmission, especially in closed environments such as residential institutions, cruise ships and healthcare settings and in kitchens (see Chapter 6, p. 134). The low infective dose, high volumes of virus particles

shed by infected individuals and the organism's ability to persist in the environment all contribute to high transmission rates. Foodborne transmission is also important however, and occurs mostly after eating contaminated shellfish and via infected food handlers (see Chapter 6, p. 138). Waterborne transmission has been documented but occurs rarely.

Bivalve molluscs such as oysters, mussels, clams and cockles feed by filtering particles from seawater, and are often grown and harvested in estuaries. These waters can become contaminated with microbial pathogens through the discharge of untreated sewage (as well as accumulation of agricultural wastes and run-off after rain) and organic particles (including those of sewage) are concentrated by the shellfish. The processes of **depuration** and **relaying**, which involve allowing molluscs to cleanse themselves in purified water for 36–48 hours or moving them to cleaner water for 4 and 6 weeks, respectively, are used in the UK and elsewhere to remove this contamination (see Chapter 7). However, these processes are more effective at removing bacteria than viruses. Illness follows the consumption of contaminated raw or undercooked molluscan shellfish and outbreaks occur more often in winter because human viral pathogens are more abundant during this period and higher levels of the virus occurs in human sewage. Furthermore, because molluscs are cold blooded, their metabolism slows in colder water during the winter months, and depuration and relaying are therefore less effective. Finally, the romantic association between St Valentine's day in February and the consumption of oysters adds greatly to disease burden around this time. Caterers can reduce the risk of gastroenteritis linked to molluscs by insisting on fresh produce from a reputable supplier, especially if they are not going to be cooked further. Suppliers should be encouraged to grow and harvest molluscs from cleaner sea or brackish waters, i.e. class A or B beds, which are based on the presence of indicator bacteria (*E. coli*) but may not reflect the presence of the virus (Table 4.4), and discouraged from harvesting after periods of heavy rain as this has previously been linked to viral gastroenteritis in volunteers eating depurated oysters.

Norovirus is environmentally robust. It survives a pH of 2.7 for 3 hours, is not killed by heating to 60 °C for 30 minutes and can be recovered from dry surfaces for 30 days at 20 °C but less than 1 day at

Table 4.4 *Microbiological classification of shellfish harvesting waters and requirements for marketing for human consumption (Regulation [EC] No. 854/2004, Regulation [EC] No. 2073/2005)*

Class	Standard	Requirement for marketing for human consumption
A	<230 MPN *Escherichia coli*/100 g of flesh and intra-valvular flesh	May go directly for human consumption
B	<4600 MPN *E .coli*/100 g of flesh and intra-valvular flesh	Must be depurated, heat treated or relayed to meet Class A standards
C	<46 000 MPN *E .coli*/100 g of flesh and intra-valvular flesh	Must be relayed for 2 months to meet category A or B; may also be heat treated by approved method
Prohibited	>46 000 MPN *E .coli*/100 g of flesh and intra-valvular flesh	Prohibited for human consumption

MPN, most probable number.

37 °C. Norovirus can be recovered from shellfish after 1 month of storage at 4 °C and after 4 months when frozen. The virus survives well in water including sea water, but is killed by boiling. Excretion of norovirus in faeces begins a few hours before the onset of symptoms, reaches a peak 24–72 hours after exposure and can continue for 7–10 days after symptoms have resolved. Humans therefore represent the main source of further transmission and this is reflected in guidance on preventing person-to-person spread of diseases resulting from gastrointestinal infection (see Chapter 8).

Other viruses

In addition to norovirus, other enterically infecting viruses can also causing diarrhoeal illness. Although many of these are transmitted via person to person, especially during childhood, they can also be transmitted via food handlers as well as by sewage contamination of drinking water, shellfish, fruit, vegetables and salad products. These viruses include **aichivirus**, **rotavirus**, **sapovirus**, **parvovirus** and **astrovirus**. As with norovirus, there is, to varying degrees, evidence for environmental robustness which allows survival on dry surfaces, in food matrices and in water (including sea water). However, all are killed by boiling.

Extra-intestinal infections

Foodborne infection is not confined solely to the gastrointestinal tract, although invasion from this organ will inevitably be involved in the initial phase of infection. The principal features of these infections are summarized in Table 4.5.

Bacterial infections

Listeria monocytogenes

Listeria monocytogenes is a Gram-positive, non-spore producing bacterium. The disease listeriosis was first recognized by Murray and colleagues in 1924 in Cambridge (England) among breeding stock of laboratory guinea pigs and rabbits. They identified the causative organism, which they named *Bacterium monocytogenes* (now *Listeria monocytogenes*), named after Lord Lister, the pioneer of antisepsis, and because it produced a **monocytosis** (an abnormal increase in the number of phagocytic white blood cells in the blood) in the infected animals. It later became apparent that the disease also affects humans, and following a series of outbreaks in Europe and North America in the 1980s, it was established that consumption of contaminated food was the principal mode of transmission. Because of the high mortality of listeriosis, this disease is one of the major causes of death from a preventable foodborne infection.

Listeriosis most commonly affects the unborn, **neonates** (infants aged up to 28 days), the immuno-compromised and the elderly, but it can occur, albeit rarely, in otherwise healthy individuals. The disease is largely extra-intestinal, presenting primarily as abortion, septicaemia or central nervous system infections, with a high case fatality rate in all patient groups. Diagnosis is by the isolation of the organism from blood, cerebrospinal fluid (when meningitis occurs), or from samples collected from multiple sites in the newly delivered infant and its mother. Listeriosis shows a marked seasonality with the majority of cases occurring in the end of the summer and early autumn.

Table 4.5 *Foodborne extra-intestinal infections*

Agent	Symptoms and possible consequences	Incubation period	Duration of illness	Likely infective dose (agent/g of food)	Microbiology/growth characteristics	Sources
Listeria monocytogenes	Abortion, septicaemia or central nervous system infections; high case fatality rate	R 1– >90 days	NA	>10³ *	Psychrotrophic: temperature range 0–45 °C (optimum 30–35 °C); pH between 5.5 and 8 and high NaCl and nitrite; resistant to drying	Widely dispersed in nature; foods include pâtés, sliced meats, soft cheese, ice cream, cream, butter, sandwiches, vegetables and fish
Salmonella Typhi and *Salmonella* Paratyphi	Fever, malaise and headache; diarrhoea; occasional death in untreated infections	R 10–14 days	3 weeks	≥10⁴	Resistant to drying and freezing; Sensitive to 30% NaCl, 200 mg/L sodium hypochlorite and normal cooking/pasteurization	Infected humans; contaminated food (raw vegetables, shellfish, milk products) or water
Hepatitis A	Flu-like symptoms, anorexia and vomiting; darkened urine, pale faeces and jaundice; hepatic failure and death more likely in older patients	R 15–45 days	U 3 weeks Can be up to 6 months	NK	Can survive outside the body for several months depending on environmental conditions	Person-to-person transmission predominates; intravenous drug use; faecally contaminated water, shellfish, fruit and vegetables in developing countries
Hepatitis E	As for hepatitis A but often more severe; life-threatening for women in the later stages of pregnancy	U 40 days R 15–60 days	1–4 weeks	NK	NK	Faecally contaminated water in developing countries; disease in developed countries becoming increasingly recognized; risk factors unknown but potential porcine source of infection

U, usually; R, range; NA, not applicable; NK not known.

The epidemiology of listeriosis is complex, but occurs after ingestion of *L. monocytogenes* in food. The micro-organism is ubiquitous in the environment and the incubation period between consumption of contaminated food and symptoms of serious infection is long and variable (1–>90 days), making it difficult to establish links between cases and specific food exposures. Between the late 1960s and the early 1980s, the incidence was extremely low in the UK, with fewer than 100 cases reported annually in England and Wales. Between 1987 and 1989, the incidence doubled, with, on average, 250 cases reported annually. This upsurge was due largely to the consumption of Belgian pâté from a single manufacturer (see Chapter 6, p. 134). The incidence declined following dietary advice to pregnant women and the immunocompromised, in addition to withdrawal from retail sale of the implicated brand of pâté (see Chapter 17, p. 317). More recently there has been a shift in the epidemiology of listeriosis. Throughout the 1990s, the incidence was stable, with on average 110 cases reported annually. However, between 2001 and 2005, the incidence increased, to >200 cases annually: the increase is largely confined to patients ≥60 years presenting with bacteraemia (Figure 4.4). It cannot be explained by gender, regional or seasonal differences, or by the patients' underlying conditions. Clusters of cases were identified during 2001–05, associated with the consumption of sandwiches in hospitals, and butter, although these clusters did not account for the increase in incidence. The reason(s) for the rise are not known.

Worldwide, a range of food types have been associated with transmission and these include products which are based on meat (pâtés and sliced meats), dairy products (soft cheese, milk, ice cream, cream and butter), vegetable products (coleslaw, salted mushrooms, pickled olives, cut fruit) and fish (smoked fish, shellfish and roe), as well as foods with a variety of ingredients (sandwiches). Although diverse in their constituents, these foods have many common features:

- They are able to support the multiplication of *L. monocytogenes*.
- They are processed with extended (refrigerated) shelf-life.
- They are consumed without further cooking.

L. monocytogenes is able to multiply in a wide range of food types and will grow at relatively high water activity (>0.95), between −2 °C and 45 °C, between pH 5.5 and pH 8, in 10 per cent sodium chloride, and in 200 parts per million (ppm) sodium nitrite. *L. monocytogenes* also shows considerable survival properties in moist and dry environments, and has been shown to colonize specific sites in food manufacturing environments for several years.

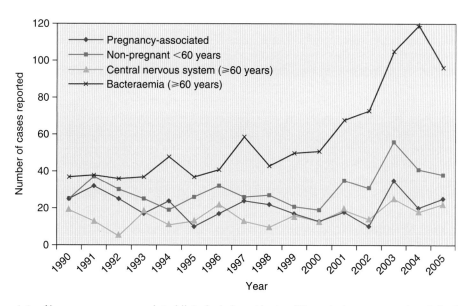

Figure 4.4 *Non-pregnancy-associated listeriosis in patients with central nervous system infections and bacteraemia alone, England and Wales, 1990–2005. (Health Protection Agency, unpublished data)*

The principal methods for the control of listeriosis are aimed at excluding *L. monocytogenes* from the food chain and prevent its multiplication (Box 4.8).

Box 4.8 Control measures for listeriosis
- Control of the quality of raw materials
- High standards of hygiene within well-designed and well-maintained manufacturing environments
- Adequate temperature and shelf-life control
- Dietary advice to 'at risk' groups, which, in the UK, involves advising pregnant women and those with impaired resistance to infection to not eat soft ripened cheese of the brie, camembert or blue-veined types and pâté, and to reheat shop-bought cooked chilled meals or ready-to-eat poultry until piping hot.

Salmonella (enteric fever)

S. enterica serovar Typhi and *S. Paratyphi* A, B and C are the causative organisms of typhoid and paratyphoid fever respectively, known collectively as enteric fever. Enteric fever occupies a special place in history, indeed reports of enteric fever pre-date Christ. Along with cholera, the disease represents the bacterial scourge following the industrial revolution in developed countries, prior to sanitary reforms from the mid to late 1800s. Prince Albert (the husband of Queen Victoria) died of enteric fever in 1861. Enteric fever remains endemic in many parts of the developing world.

Typhoid fever is often clinically more severe than paratyphoid fever but both illnesses can range from asymptomatic infection to death. Enteric fever occurs following ingestion of the bacteria via contaminated food or water, where *S.* Typhi or *S.* Paratyphi invade the lymphatic system, then the blood, followed by the reticulo-endothelial system (the macrophage system), the gall bladder and discharge back into the intestines. Classically, illness begins with fever, malaise and headache, often with respiratory tract symptoms. Typically this occurs 10–14 days after exposure but varies depending on the infective dose (on average tens of thousands of organisms) and host susceptibility. Fever increases sequentially during the first week and the patient becomes progressively toxic and apathetic. Constipation, **bradycardia** (slowness of the heart) and **hepatosplenomegaly** (enlargement of the liver and spleen) are common at this time. During the second week, patients become weaker and their mental state deteriorates while their fever may remain stable or swing. In the era before effective chemotherapy, illness progressed and by the third week the patient became uncomprehensive, muttering and disorientated 'muttering delirium' and 'coma vigil'. Gastrointestinal involvement occurred at this time (classically described as **pea-soup diarrhoea**) and death occurred from toxaemia, exhaustion or other complications.

Large numbers of the bacterium occur in the faeces during infection, which is the source of environmental contamination. In those who survive, recovery begins towards the end of the third week with a steadily falling fever, but prolonged convalescence with weakness, weight loss, and debilitation persisting for months. Relapse (often in the biliary tract) occurs in 10–20 per cent of affected individuals and a minority become carriers (exemplified by Typhoid Mary [see Chapter 8, p. 169]). Enteric fever is diagnosed by isolation of *S.* Typhi or *S.* Paratyphi from faeces, blood or urine. The detection of antibodies in serum samples may be helpful for diagnosis, but can be difficult to interpret if the patient has been vaccinated.

Chloramphenicol had been the treatment of choice for enteric fever, reducing greatly the mortality and the duration of fever but increasing the likelihood of relapse, continued or chronic carriage and bone marrow toxicity. Emergence of chloramphenicol resistance in the 1970s prompted the use of amoxicillin and trimethoprim-sulfamethoxazole as alternatives, but the efficacy of these drugs has diminished with the recent emergence of multidrug-resistance. Fluoroquinolones (ciprofloxacin in particular) have been highly effective in the treatment of enteric fevers and became the drugs of choice in the late 1980s and early 1990s. Strains exhibiting reduced susceptibility to ciprofloxacin were reported soon after its introduction, and this proportion has increased. However, ciprofloxacin is still the first-line treatment, but alternative antibiotics are available if resistance is suspected. Two effective vaccines are available, a live but attenuated oral *S.* Typhi and an injectable killed preparation.

Unlike most salmonellae which are able to the infect a broad range of animal hosts, humans represent the only hosts of *S.* Typhi and *S.* Paratyphi.

Isolation from animals is exceptional and from the environment only after human contamination. In developing countries where enteric fever is endemic, the public health infrastructure is often unable to keep pace with increases in population and urbanization and therefore the separation of humans from their sewage does not occur to the extent required to control disease (see Chapter 7). In endemic countries, risk factors for contracting enteric fever include eating or drinking contaminated food (raw vegetables, shellfish, milk products) or water, inadequate sanitation and living conditions, poor personal hygiene, and close contact with infected individuals. Incidence is higher in summer months. In developed countries modern sanitation and clean water means that the incidence of enteric fever is low and most cases are associated with travel to areas where the disease is endemic. The highest risks are for travellers to the Indian subcontinent, south-east Asia, and parts of Latin America and Africa. The seasonal pattern of infection follows trends in foreign travel to these destinations. Small indigenous outbreaks occur in the UK but are rare, and are usually linked to infected food handlers (see Box 4.9) or to contact with individuals who have travelled to developing countries.

Box 4.9 Control measures for enteric fever

- Clean water supply
- Adequate sewage disposal
  Good food processing and handling practices
- Vaccination against typhoid fever when travelling to areas where sanitation and food hygiene is likely to be poor
- As no vaccine for paratyphoid fever exists travellers should exercise good food and water hygiene.

Protozoan infections: Toxoplasma gondii

Toxoplasma gondii is a foodborne protozoan parasite which causes both mild and severe infections known as toxoplasmosis. *T. gondii* is able to complete a complex lifecycle only in members of the cat family which results in the shedding of millions of resistant oocysts in the cat's faeces. These oocysts are infectious – via oral ingestion – to any warm-blooded animals including livestock animals and humans. Once ingested, *T. gondii* is able to reproduce and invade various organs of the body (including muscle tissue) where it forms tissue cysts

also known as bradyzoites. In healthy individuals, infection is mild or asymptomatic, and when symptoms do occur, these present as an influenza-like illness with a raised temperature, swollen lymph glands, fatigue and muscle and joint pain. However, for the fetus and in immunocompromised individuals (including those with AIDS) toxoplasmosis can be life-threatening. *T. gondii* is able to cross the placenta and, if this occurs early in pregnancy, the fetus can either die, or be born with gross abnormalities including chorioretinitis (a type of inflammation of the eye), hydrocephalus (inflammation of the brain resulting in a marked enlargement of the head, 'water on the brain') and cerebral calcification. Infection later in pregnancy can be less severe, but can result in sequelae including chorioretinitis, mental retardation, ocular palsy (paralysis of the eye) and deafness. In immunocompromised patients, serious infection of the brain, heart and eyes are most common.

Toxoplasma can be transmitted to humans by:

- direct contact with the faeces from an infected feline
- consumption of food (or water) contaminated by feline faeces (although this will be domestic cats in the UK, other species of wild cats such as cougars in North America may be important)
- consumption of raw and undercooked meat which contains tissue cysts
- mother to baby transmission.

Toxoplasmosis is most commonly diagnosed by the detection of antibodies in the serum, but can also be detected by demonstration of the organism by microscopy. Since most infections are sub-clinical, treatment is usually unnecessary. However for pregnant women and the immunocompromised, a variety of effective drugs are available. See Box 4.10 for control of toxoplasmosis.

Box 4.10 Control measures for toxoplasmosis

- Meat should be thoroughly cooked, especially when consumed by pregnant women
- Good personal hygiene should be exercised at all times, especially to avoid cross-contamination between meat products
- Cat litter trays should be regularly changed and cleaned (preferably not by pregnant women, but if this is not possible, wear rubber gloves).

Viral infections

Hepatitis A

Hepatitis A virus is a spherical, symmetrical, non-enveloped RNA virus. The term hepatitis A was coined in the 1940s to distinguish this form of transmissible hepatitis acquired through the consumption of contaminated food or water (epidemic jaundice) from that associated with blood or blood products (serum jaundice caused by the Hepatitis B virus). However, descriptions of epidemic jaundice fitting the clinical picture of hepatitis A can be traced to ancient China and accounts of outbreaks were reported in Europe in the seventeenth and eighteenth century. The causative agent was identified in 1972, when the virus particle was first detected by electron microscopy.

As the name suggests, Hepatitis A causes hepatitis (inflammation of the liver), but a quarter of infections are asymptomatic and in most instances the illness is self-limiting and uncomplicated. Clinical symptoms develop typically 15–45 days after exposure and patients often experience a prodrome of flu-like symptoms, fever, chills, malaise, fatigue, anorexia and vomiting. More distinctive signs of hepatitis follow, including dark-coloured urine, pale/clay-coloured faeces and jaundice of the eyes, skin and mucous membranes. Symptoms usually begin to resolve in the third week of illness, with 85 per cent of patients recovering fully after 3 months and 99 per cent after 6 months. Disease severity is strongly correlated with increasing age. Infection in children younger than 2 years is rarely recognized clinically as hepatitis, and acute infections are more likely in older adolescents and adults. The greatest risk of fulminant hepatitis, hepatic failure and death occurs in patients older than 50 years.

Hepatitis A is distributed throughout the world and the incidence depends largely on population density, public health sanitation and sewage treatment. Three patterns of infection exist. In poorer developing countries asymptomatic infections occur early in childhood, resulting in infrequent disease in adults. In the more developed European and North American countries, childhood exposure occurs infrequently and the main burden of disease lies in older adolescents and adults. Older people are protected from infection through exposure earlier in life during more endemic times. Finally, in relatively closed communities (e.g. Greenland) previously exposed to the disease, epidemics occur in susceptible migrant adults and children born since the previous outbreak.

In developed countries transmission is usually via the person-to-person route (especially in settings where individuals are unable to maintain high standards of hygiene), in men who have sex with men, in intravenous drug users and in travellers to developing countries. Foodborne transmission is rare (see Chapter 6, p. 140). Passive or active vaccination can be used to prevent infection in the above groups or in contacts of infected individuals. However, basic hygiene (hand-washing especially) remains the cornerstone of prevention. Transmission among travellers to developing countries where disease is endemic can occur through:

- direct person-to-person contact
- drinking untreated water
- drinks containing contaminated ice
- consuming fruit, vegetables, shellfish or other uncooked foods from sewage-contaminated water or contaminated during harvesting or handling.

The risk of infection relates to length of stay and incidence of hepatitis A, and vaccination is indicated for travellers to endemic areas including the Indian subcontinent, the Far East (not Japan), north Africa, south and central America, sub-Saharan Africa and the Middle East.

Hepatitis E

Hepatitis E virus is a spherical symmetrical non-enveloped RNA virus. The existence of an enterically transmitted hepatitis virus distinct from hepatitis A was suspected following studies of waterborne hepatitis in India in the late 1970s, which found patients lacked antibody responses indicating recent hepatitis A infection. Volunteer feeding studies confirmed the theory and the disease was termed enterically transmitted non-A, non-B hepatitis. The disease was later renamed hepatitis E and the virus was identified in 1990. The clinical features of hepatitis E infection are similar to those described above for hepatitis A. However, the incubation period for infection is often longer (mean 40 days, range 15–60 days) and the disease is more severe. The case fatality rate is 0.1–1 per cent. The infection can be life-threatening in women in the later stages of pregnancy, with case fatality rates approaching 20 per cent.

The incidence of hepatitis E is highest in developing countries in tropical or subtropical areas of the world with inadequate environmental sanitation. Most disease presents as endemic or sporadic cases although major epidemics do occur affecting tens of thousands of people at a time. Serological studies in developing or endemic regions have shown a much lower seroprevalence than would be expected for an enterically transmitted virus (1–28 per cent) and an age-specific prevalence markedly different from hepatitis A, with increasing infection in older children and younger adults. Faecally contaminated water appears to be the primary source of hepatitis E infection and epidemic outbreaks are often preceded by periods of heavy rain which lead to contamination of water supplies with untreated sewage (see Chapter 7). Foodborne transmission occurs uncommonly and person-to-person transmission is rare.

Hepatitis E infection in developed countries is usually associated with travel to endemic regions. However, recent studies have identified cases with no history of recent foreign travel (termed autochthonous). In several studies of autochthonous hepatitis E infection in England and Wales, affected individuals have tended to be older (mean ~65 years), predominantly male and a putative link with either contact with pigs or the consumption of pig meat has been established. Certainly hepatitis E is endemic in British pigs and several human cases have been shown to be infected with virus strains similar to those found in pigs. These findings have been documented elsewhere. Further epidemiological and microbiological research is required to determine the true incidence of autochthonous hepatitis E infection and to better understand its potential zoonotic origins.

Polio virus

The polio virus is now, fortunately, rare, and the disease it causes has been almost eradicated as a result of the use of a highly effective vaccine. This virus is an enterovirus that initially causes a febrile illness and then crosses the blood–brain barrier to invade the central nervous system and cause paralysis, most often of the lower limbs. There are no animal hosts for the polio virus and because it is excreted in the faeces during infection, transmission is most often via faecal–oral route through water (see Chapter 7). A large-scale World Health Organization (WHO) vaccination programme is presently attempting to eradicate this disease worldwide.

INTOXICATIONS

Toxins of microbiological origin can occur in raw food materials as well as being produced during food manufacture or storage. The principal features of these toxins and their respective intoxications are summarized in Table 4.6.

Toxins present in raw food components

Toxins produced by algae in marine environments and concentrated in raw foods as a result of shellfish or fish feeding on algae present a particular problem for the food chain. These toxins, known collectively as marine algal toxins, are associated with blooms of microscopic algae which accumulate in higher animals, either shellfish or fish, or even crustaceans. The toxins are all heat stable, such that they are not inactivated by normal cooking processes. Diarrhoetic shellfish poisoning (DSP) and paralytic shellfish poisoning (PSP) may be associated with red tides where blooms contain millions of algal cells per litre of seawater, although concentrations as low as 200 cells are sufficient to produce poisonous shellfish. It should be noted, however, that non-toxic plankton species can also cause sea-water discoloration and not all toxic algae blooms are coloured. There is no specific treatment for any of these intoxications.

Shellfish poisoning

Diarrhoetic shellfish poisoning has been reported throughout the world, with most incidents recognized in Europe and Japan. The first cases in the UK were reported in 1994 when two people became ill after the consumption of imported mussels. Another outbreak occurred in 1997, in which over 50 people were affected after eating UK grown mussels served in London restaurants (see Chapter 6, p. 138). Diarrhoea, nausea, vomiting and abdominal pain occur 30 minutes to a few hours after the consumption of contaminated shellfish and last for up to 3 days. No fatalities have been recorded.

Worldwide, the most common vehicles are mussels, clams and scallops, which concentrate DSP toxins, although oysters, cockles and crab can also become contaminated. Okadaic acid (from the algae *Prorocentrum* spp.) and dinophysis toxins 1, 2

Table 4.6 *Foodborne intoxications*

Toxin	Symptoms and possible consequences	Incubation period	Duration of illness	Likely infective dose (amount of toxin/g of food)	Microbiology and growth characteristics	Sources
Diarrhoetic shellfish poisoning	Diarrhoea, nausea, vomiting and abdominal pain	30 minutes to a few hours	Up to 3 days	~40 μg of toxin	Mainly okadaic acid (from the algae *Prorocentrum* spp.) and dinophysis toxins 1, 2 and 3 (from *Dinophysis* spp.)	Most commonly mussels, clams and scallops; also oysters, cockles and crab
Paralytic shellfish poisoning	Paralysis of the mouth, throat and extremities, ataxia, dizziness and muscular and respiratory paralysis; mortality 1–12% with higher rates in children	U 3 hours R 15 minutes to 10 hours	3–4 days	150 μg of toxin	Mainly saxitoxin, neo-saxitoxin and gonyautoxins) produced by species of the *Alexandrium*, *Pyrodinium*, *Gonyaulax* and *Gymnodinium* genera of dinoflagellates	Clams, oysters, cockles, mussels, scallops and some crustacea
Amnesic shellfish poisoning	Vomiting, diarrhoea, abdominal pain, temporary or permanent short-term memory loss; paralysis and death in severe cases	<24 hours	Days to weeks	60–290 mg of toxin	Domoic acid produced by the microscopic diatom *Nitzschia pungens*	Mussels
Ciguatera	Abdominal pain, nausea, vomiting, and diarrhoea followed by neurological symptoms ranging from numbness and tingling, to respiratory paralysis; mortality of 0.1–20%	15 minutes to 24 hours	2–3 days for gastro-intestinal symptoms, neurological symptoms can recur years after exposure	>1 μg of toxin	Ciguatoxins produced by dinoflagellates belonging to the *Gambierdiscus* and *Prorocentrum* genera	Carnivorous marine fish including groupers, barracudas, snappers, and jacks
Clostridium botulinum (foodborne)	Blurred vision, aversion to light, impaired speech, difficulty swallowing Descending weakness and paralysis. Mortality up to 46% without treatment with antitoxin and 10% if antitoxin administered within 24 hours of onset	U 18–36 hours R 2 hours to 10 days	Recovery over many months	<1 ng of toxin	Strict anaerobes; growth above pH 4.5 and a_w above 0.94, temperature range 3–50 °C Some grow in 10% salt; some are extremely heat resistant	Home preserved meat, fish or vegetables
Clostridium botulinum (infants)	Constipation, feeding difficulties, decreased muscle tone (floppy baby syndrome), increased drooling, weak cry; mortality of <2%	NK	Recovery over many months	NK	Germination of spores in the immature infant gut	Honey, corn syrup, infant formula feed; dust or soil

Table 4.6 *Foodborne intoxications* (continued)

Toxin	Symptoms and possible consequences	Incubation period	Duration of illness	Likely infective dose (amount of toxin/g of food)	Microbiology and growth characteristics	Sources
Staphylococcus aureus	Vomiting; diarrhoea	R 2–6 hours	6–24 hours	10 mg of toxin	Aerobic; growth at 7–48 °C (optima 35–37 °C), pH 4–9 (optima 6–7), a_w above 0.83, 20% salt	Processed foods: cooked meats, fish and shellfish; dairy products
Bacillus cereus (emetic syndrome)	Nausea; vomiting Diarrhoea	R 1–6 hours 2–3 hours	12–24 hours	10 mg of toxin	Growth at 10–50 °C (optima 28–35 °C)	Cooked rice
Bacillus cereus (diarrhoeal syndrome)	Abdominal pain Diarrhoea	R 8–16 hours	~24 hours	10 mg of toxin	Growth at 10–50 °C (optima 28–35 °C)	Cooked meats, poultry and vegetables; soups, sauces and desserts; spicy foods
'Bacillus subtilis' group	Vomiting; diarrhoea	R 1–6 hours	12–24 hours	10 mg of toxin	Growth at 10–50 °C (optima 28–35 °C)	Various poorly stored cooked foods
Scombrotoxic fish poisoning	Rashes on the face and neck, flushing, sweating, headache; nausea, vomiting, diarrhoea; collapse in severe cases	R 10 minutes to several hours	A few hours	>200 ppm (200 µg/g of fish)	Production of histamine from histidine in fish flesh by spoilage bacteria under poor temperature control	Scombrid fish especially tuna, mackerel, bonito and sardines
Aflatoxin	Liver cancer	Long term (years)	NA	NA	Produced by *Aspergillus* spp.; require high humidity and temperature	Cereals, oilseeds, spices and tree nuts
Ochratoxin	Nephrotoxin, hepatotoxin, teratogen, immunotoxin; potential carcinogen	Long term (years)	NA	NA	Produced by *Aspergillus* spp. in the tropics and *Penicillium* spp. in temperate regions	Grain; coffee beans, beans, pulses and dried fruit, coffee, wine, beer and grape juice
Patulin	Nephrotoxin, immunotoxin; potential carcinogen (high level exposure)	Long term (years)	NA	NA	Produced by fungi belonging to the *Penicillium*, *Aspergillus* and *Byssochlamys* genera	Apples; also mouldy fruits, grains and other foods (e.g. pear juice, grape juice)

U, usually; R, range; ppm, parts per million; NK, not known; NA not applicable.

and 3 (from *Dinophysis* spp.) are the commonest of a family of DSP toxins that cause the gastro-intestinal symptoms. The less common **yessotoxin** and **pectenotoxins** cause more systemic damage.

Paralytic shellfish poisoning is an intoxication caused by the consumption of bivalve molluscs (clams, oysters, cockles, mussels, scallops and some species of crustaceans) contaminated with dino-flagellate algae. During the winter the algae occur as cysts on the seabed in waters at latitudes greater than 30° north or south, where the water temperatures are approximately 15–17 °C. Under favourable conditions they rise to the surface and proliferate, creating visible red tides. Several outbreaks have been reported in the UK, the largest being in 1968 when 78 cases were affected after consuming locally grown shellfish in the north-east of England.

Over 21 neurotoxins have been associated with PSP, but the main toxins (**saxitoxin, neo-saxitoxin and gonyautoxins**) are produced by species of the *Alexandrium, Pyrodinium, Gonyaulax* and *Gymno-dinium* genera of dinoflagellates. The onset of illness occurs 15 minutes to 10 hours (typically 3 hours) after the consumption of shellfish containing approximately 150 μg of toxin. Symptoms vary depending on the toxin involved, the amount ingested and susceptibility of the host, and include paralysis of the mouth, throat and extremities, ataxia (loss of balance), dizziness and muscular and respiratory paralysis. Estimates of case-fatality rates from outbreak investigations range from 1 per cent to 12 per cent with higher rates reported in children than adults.

Amnesic shellfish poisoning (ASP) was first described in Canada in 1987 when 107 people were ill after the consumption of blue mussels. The causative agent is a microscopic red-brown salt-water diatom (*Nitzschia pungens*) which is widely distributed in coastal waters of the Atlantic, Pacific and Indian oceans. The organism produces a powerful heat stable neurotoxin called **domoic acid**, and this toxin is concentrated in shellfish feeding on the diatoms. Symptoms of ASP intoxication occur within 24 hours of consumption and include vomiting, diarrhoea, abdominal pain, temporary or permanent short-term memory loss. In severe cases seizures, paralysis and death may occur.

Diagnosis of DSP, PSP and ASP is by detection of the respective toxin in extracts from shellfish.

All of these toxins are extremely heat stable, so monitoring of toxin levels in shellfish beds with subsequent closure when the toxin levels detected exceed statutory limits (Box 4.11) remains the principal way of protecting the consumer from illness (Regulation [EC] No. 853/2004). Import and export controls are important for products from hazardous areas and during seasonal periods where problems with this type of contamination can occur.

Box 4.11 Statutory limits for some marine biotoxins in shellfish

- PSP – 800 μg/kg
- ASP – 20 mg domoic acid per kg
- Okadaic acid, dinophysistoxins and pectenotoxins together – 160 μg of okadaic acid equivalents per kg
- Yessotoxins – 1 mg of yessotoxin per kg

Ciguatera toxin was first described in the Caribbean in 1555. The name is derived from the marine snail *Turbo pica* which was called *cigua* by Spanish migrants to the Caribbean and erroneously identified as the source. Ciguatera is commonest of the clinical syndromes associated with marine biotoxins and is a major public health problem in the Caribbean and south Pacific, particularly in areas with tropical reefs. However, increase in foreign travel and the export of tropical fish as food have made ciguatera a global concern. Ciguatoxins are powerful neurotoxins produced by marine dino-flagellates belonging to the *Gambierdiscus* and *Prorocentrum* genera. Ciguatera toxin is not easily excreted by fish and is concentrated up the marine food chain as a result of reef fish grazing on algae which are then consumed by larger subtropical and tropical carnivorous fish. Toxic levels are accumu-lated in such species as groupers, barracudas, snappers, and jacks. Other natural marine toxins transmitted by similar routes (**searitoxin, maitotoxin,** and **palytoxin**) have been associated with similar syndromes.

The incubation period and clinical manifestations vary with dose, the type of ciguatoxic fish consumed and its geographical origin. Gastrointestinal symp-toms of abdominal cramps, nausea, vomiting, and diarrhoea usually commence between 15 minutes and 24 hours after consumption and are followed by neurological symptoms such as numbness, tingling, dizziness, blurred vision, reversal of hot and cold temperature sensations, blindness and respiratory paralysis. The neurological sequelae can persist for several months and death occurs in 0.1–20 per cent of cases, with children more severely affected. Ciguatoxins are unaffected by cooking, and toxic fish appear no different from non-toxic fish. Diagnosis is by detection of the toxin in the flesh of fish, and the use of 'biological indicators' (family pets and elderly relatives) advocated by some is not recommended. Box 4.12 lists the preventive measures.

Box 4.12 Preventive measures for ciguatera intoxication

- Avoiding consumption of larger (≥2 kg) fish
- Avoiding consumption of the most toxic parts (liver, viscera, roe and other organs)
- Export control measures for produce from 'at risk' areas

Toxins produced by bacteria during food manufacture, preparation or storage

Botulinum toxins

Clostridium botulinum is a group of obligate anaerobic, Gram-positive endospore-forming rods, and their toxins cause **botulism**. Botulism has been known since ancient times, but its aetiology was only elucidated by van Ermengen in the late 1890s. On studying a large outbreak in Belgium, he demonstrated that illness was caused by the consumption of food containing a potent toxin produced by an anaerobic bacterium which he named *Bacillus botulinum* from the German *bolulismus*, meaning sausage poisoning (Latin *botulus* – sausage). *C. botulinum* is widely distributed in nature, and produces seven different neurotoxins (designated A–G) which are some of the most powerful toxins known. Types A, B, E and to a lesser extent F are associated with human botulism. These toxins stop neurotransmission by preventing release of **acetylcholine** (the chemical involved in neurotransmission) at neuromuscular junctions and thus causing paralysis. Botulism can spread by different routes, and the most common form in the UK during 2000–06 was wound botulism, which occurred exclusively among injectors of illegal drugs. Only foodborne and infant botulism will be considered here.

The symptoms of foodborne botulism occur typically 18–36 hours (range 2 hours to 10 days) after the consumption of food in which the organism has grown and produced toxin. The classic presentation is of acute bilateral cranial neuropathies with symmetrical descending muscle weakness and paralysis. Patients will often initially complain of nausea and a dry mouth followed by diarrhoea. Later the patients often become constipated. Cranial nerve dysfunction usually begins in the eyes (blurred vision, slow reacting or dilated pupils, aversion to light, drooping eyelids) and continues to the mouth and throat (impaired speech, difficulty swallowing). Muscle weakness then descends symmetrically, affecting the trunk, the upper and lower extremities. Death occurs because of paralysis of the respiratory muscles and diaphragm or obstruction of the upper airways by the weakened glottis. Symptoms may differ depending on the amount of toxin ingested. Urgent treatment can be life-saving and involves inactivation of existing toxin by administration of **antitoxin** (antibodies to inactivated toxin produced in another animal, usually in horses or sheep). Supportive treatment and assisted respiration is sometimes needs for many months. Antimicrobials should not be given because they may increase toxin release in the gut.

C. botulinum is a group of diverse bacteria with a wide range of properties for growth and survival. All members of this species are strict anaerobes, will grow in foods above pH 4.5 and water activity of 0.94, and between 3 °C and 50 °C. Some will grow in up to 10 per cent salt, and are extremely resistant to heat: 121 °C for 3 minutes is required for a 12 D kill (see Chapter 3, p. 44). These properties are among the major factors influencing the conditions for safe canning of foods. Botulinum toxins are heat-labile proteins and are inactivated by thorough cooking. Foods associated with food botulism therefore usually have been consumed with no or minimal cooking (e.g. preserved meat, fish and vegetables).

Foodborne botulism is fortunately rare in the UK, with only six incidents reported in England and Wales in the past 20 years, comprising 33 cases with 3 deaths. All but two incidents were either travel-associated or linked to the consumption of home-prepared food which had been brought into the country. Due to the seriousness of botulism, strict controls are put in place by food manufacturers worldwide for preventing growth of *C. botulinum*, especially in high-risk foods. Botulism is much more common in countries where home preservation of meat, fish or vegetables is common (e.g. southern and eastern Europe and the Inuit communities in North America) because these processes are inherently less controlled than for commercially manufactured food. In the UK, the practice of home-preserving foods is not common. Currently the worldwide incidence is highest in Georgia and the Inuit communities in North America: among the latter the practice of burying fish and the meat from marine animals in sealed containers in the ground for prolonged periods prior to consumption is a significant risk for botulism.

Infant botulism was first recognized in California in 1976 and the majority of cases reported worldwide have occurred in western USA. Due to the immature gut flora of the infant, *C. botulinum* spores are occasionally able to gain entry to the gut (possibly through the consumption of honey or corn syrup, or through contact with dust or soil), where multiplication and production of toxin occurs. Infant botulism is almost exclusive to the first year after birth (and most within the first 6 months), and the symptoms are similar to food botulism. Infants present with constipation, feeding difficulties, decreased muscle tone (hence the name floppy baby syndrome), increased drooling and a weak cry. The condition may progress to cranial neuropathies and respiratory weakness; the case-fatality rate is <2 per cent. Recovery usually starts 3–5 weeks after onset although relapses can occur. Only six cases have been documented in England and Wales since the condition was first described, with only one case reported in the past 10 years. None of these cases died. Treatment of infant botulism involves supportive care only.

The diagnosis of all forms of botulism relies on the detection of neurotoxin in serum or faeces in both foodborne and infant botulism. Isolation of *C. botulinum* from faeces is also supportive of a diagnosis, but because *C. botulinum* spores are common in the environment, these may be present in faeces in the absence of disease. In cases of foodborne botulism, toxin and the organism (at high levels) should be present in implicated foods. See Box 4.13.

> **Box 4.13 Control measures for foodborne botulism**
> - Correct processing and formulation of food to prevent the growth of *C. botulinum*. The most common cause of foodborne botulism is under-processing, especially with insufficient heating
> - For control of infant botulism, honey and corn-syrup should not be fed to very young infants. In the UK, there is a voluntary code so that a warning is given on honey jars 'Not to be fed to infants under six months of age'.

Enterotoxins

Staphylococcus aureus are aerobic, Gram-positive, coagulase-positive cocci. Their name is derived from their clustered appearance on microscopy (Greek: *staphulē;* – a bunch of grapes – and *kokkus* – berry) and the yellow pigmentation of colonies when grown on microbiological media (Latin *aurĕus* – golden). Some *S. aureus* produce enterotoxins, and 19 have been described (A–E, G–R, U, V). These toxins are heat stable, will survive some normal cooking processes, and are responsible for staphylococcal food poisoning. *S. aureus* is part of the normal human microflora, particularly of the skin, the hands and nasal passages, cause a variety of skin and wound infections (boils and furuncles) and can be transferred to foods during processing. Between 30 and 50 per cent of the population carry *S. aureus*, of which 10–25 per cent are capable of producing enterotoxin. Following consumption of food on which *S. aureus* has grown (usually to $>10^5/g$) and produced enterotoxin, there is rapid (2–6 hours) onset of symptoms which include nausea, vomiting, abdominal pain and diarrhoea. In extreme cases, dehydration and collapse can occur and intravenous therapy is indicated. Recovery usually occurs within 6–24 hours. There is no specific treatment for staphylococcal food poisoning.

S. aureus multiplies in a range of foods, generally over the range of 7–48 °C (optima 35–37 °C), between pH 4 and 9 (optima 6–7), at water activity above 0.83, and at high salt concentrations: some strains are able to grow in 20 per cent salt. This bacterium competes poorly with other microflora in food, and >90 per cent of staphylococcal food poisoning outbreaks are associated with processed foods which have a minimal microflora. The foods associated with outbreaks are:

- 53 per cent ham, meat pies, corned beef, tongue, preserved meat

- 22 per cent cooked poultry
- 8 per cent cooked fish and shellfish
- 8 per cent milk, cheese and desserts containing milk or cream.

Owing to the relatively mild and short duration of illness, outbreaks of *S. aureus* gastroenteritis are reported infrequently, with this pathogen accounting for only 2 per cent of all 1900 foodborne general outbreaks reported to national surveillance in England and Wales between 1992 and 2005. Almost two-thirds (62 per cent) of these outbreaks occurred in commercial catering premises, with restaurants and venues served by caterers commonly implicated. The disease is highly seasonal with most outbreaks occurring in the summer (especially July) since this is the time when temperature control of foods is most difficult.

Diagnosis of staphylococcal food poisoning is by detection of enterotoxin in food. In addition there should be high counts (usually $>10^6$/g) of an enterotoxin-producing *S. aureus* strain present in implicated food. However, because of the stability of staphylococcal enterotoxins, the toxins can be present in food in the absence of viable organisms since the latter may be killed during food processing by, for example, cooking or by reduction in pH as occurs during the manufacture of cheese. During an outbreak, the implicated *S. aureus* strain may be present in the faeces of affected patients, as well as of food handlers. Human carriers are the main reservoirs for *S. aureus*, therefore control of this food poisoning involves temperature and time control as well as the hygienic behaviour of food handlers (Box 4.14).

Box 4.14 Preventive measures for enterotoxin food poisoning

- Avoid direct handling of cooked foods – use suitable utensils wherever possible
- Food handlers with septic lesions should be excluded until treated successfully
- Where hand contact is unavoidable, hands should be cleaned thoroughly and disposable gloves used where practical
- Foods should be refrigerated, and displayed for time periods in line with current European food safety legislation, and disposed after such time has elapsed
- Food processes should be controlled to prevent the growth of *S. aureus* in raw materials, and in the fermentation and maturation stages of foods such as sausages and cheese

---

Bacillus toxins

Bacillus is a genus of Gram-positive, aerobically growing rods which produce robust endospores that are highly resistant to adverse environmental conditions including extremes of temperature, pH and salt. Their ubiquity in the environment means that almost all raw foods and food materials (particularly those of vegetable origin and those with soil contact) are likely to be contaminated by *Bacillus* spores. Two groups of *Bacillus* cause food poisoning:

- *Bacillus cereus*
- the '*Bacillus subtilis*' group.

The most common cause of *Bacillus* food poisoning is due to *B. cereus*. This bacterium produces two distinct types of disease, the **emetic** and the **diarrhoeal** syndromes. *B. cereus* will grow on a wide range of foods: most strains multiply between 10 °C and 50 °C, optimum 28–35 °C, with generation times of 18–60 minutes. Some strains will grow **psychrotrophically**, i.e. in the cold. The emetic syndrome is characterized by an incubation period of 1–6 hours (usually 2–3 hours), nausea, vomiting, stomach cramps followed by diarrhoea of less than 12 hours duration in about a third of cases. Epidemiological information from outbreak investigations invariably implicate the improper storage and subsequent use of cooked rice.

When rice is prepared in bulk too far in advance and then stored under the warm ambient conditions of a kitchen, *B. cereus* endospores (which can survive boiling) germinate and vegetative cells proliferate rapidly, usually to $>10^6$/g and produce a heat-stable toxin, **cereulide**. Cereulide is extremely heat stable and will survive heating to 121 °C for 90 minutes, and is the sole toxin associated with the emetic disease. Food poisoning of this type can be easily avoided by implementing suitable temperature control measures for cooked rice. However, anecdotal evidence from outbreak investigations suggests that some caterers are reluctant to do this as refrigerated cooked rice sticks together, making its subsequent use more difficult.

The diarrhoeal syndrome is characterized by an incubation period of 8–16 hours, abdominal pain, profuse watery diarrhoea and rectal **tenesmus** (straining). Symptoms usually last for longer than the emetic syndrome but generally not more than 24 hours. Disease associated with the diarrhoeal syndrome has been linked to a wide variety of foods, including cooked meats, poultry and vegetables, soups, sauces and desserts. Spices are often heavily contaminated with *B. cereus* and their use in eastern and northern European countries explains the higher disease incidence observed there. If inadequate heat treatment occurs, *B. cereus* spores germinate and grow rapidly under favourable conditions. The consumption of large numbers of cells in food $(10^5–10^9/g)$ ensures a large number of viable cells in the gut, where the production of heat-labile high-molecular-weight enterotoxin causes disease. This disease is more similar to *C. perfringens* food poisoning and not primarily due to pre-formed toxin.

Diagnosis of *B. cereus* food poisoning is by the detection of high levels of this bacterium in foods consumed by the patients. However, because cereulide is so heat stable, food vehicles may no longer contain viable organisms if growth and toxin production has occurred prior to cooking. Hence, diagnosis is confirmed by the detection of emetic toxin in food. Diarrhoeal toxin may be present in the faeces of patients with the diarrhoeal syndrome, as will be high levels of *B. cereus*. The bacterium may be present in the faeces of patients with the emetic syndrome, however for reasons outlined above, implicated foods may no longer contain viable *B. cereus*. There is no specific treatment for *B. cereus* food poisoning.

Gastroenteritis caused by the *B. subtilis* group *(B. subtilis, B. licheniformis, B. pumilis* and *B. amyloli-quefaciens)* occurs less frequently than *B. cereus* gastroenteritis. Symptoms depend on the causative organism (e.g. acute-onset vomiting often followed by diarrhoea with *B. subtilis*, diarrhoea accompanied infrequently by vomiting with *B. licheniformis*). Illness follows the consumption of a wide variety of poorly stored cooked foods containing large numbers of *Bacillus* cells $(10^4–10^9/g)$ in food. There is no specific treatment for the *B. subtilis* group food poisoning.

Due to the relatively short and mild illness, sporadic cases of *Bacillus* spp. food poisoning are likely to be grossly under ascertained. Outbreaks are also likely to be under-reported, but they do occur and are an important resource for describing the epidemiology. In England and Wales between 1992 and 2005, *Bacillus* spp. were implicated in 67 of 1898 general outbreaks reported to the Health Protection Agency. *B. cereus* was most commonly reported (67

per cent), with the *B. subtilis* group accountable for most of the rest (28 per cent). Eighty five per cent of *B. cereus* outbreaks occurred during the summer or autumn, and 67 per cent were in restaurants (40 per cent in Indian and 37 per cent in Chinese restaurants). Rice dishes were implicated in just under half of the outbreaks. Outbreaks of *B. subtilis* group gastroenteritis occurred throughout the year and were more commonly linked to restaurants (79 per cent; with 47 per cent in Indian restaurants). A wider variety of foods were implicated with cooked poultry, meat and vegetables reported either with or without rice dishes.

Bacillus food poisoning results from spore germination and excessive growth of vegetative cells. See Box 4.15 for control measures.

Box 4.15 Control of *Bacillus* food poisoning

- Foods should be eaten hot and soon after cooking
- If this is not possible, spore germination can be reduced by control of:
  - pH
  - water activity
  - or, more usually, by temperature
- Foods should be cooled rapidly and stored cold (not in bulk) or held at about 63 °C

Scombrotoxic fish poisoning

Scombrotoxic fish poisoning is an intoxication which was first described in 1830 and is recognized worldwide. The name is derived from scombroid fish from the *Scomberesocidae* and *Scombridae* families (e.g. tuna, mackerel, bonito) which are most often implicated, although other non-scombroid fish (e.g. sardines) are also involved. These dark, oily fish contain high levels of the amino acid histidine within their flesh and, as a result of bacterial spoilage (especially by *Morganella morganii* and *Klebsiella pneumoniae*), histidine is converted to **histamine** (also known as **scombrotoxin**) through the action of the enzyme **histidine decarboxylase** (see Chapter 1, p. 10). Spoilage and histamine formation by the mesophilic bacteria *Morganella* spp. and *Klebsiella spp.* occurs in non-refrigerated environments. However, histamine formation occurs, albeit much slower, at refrigeration temperatures, probably by **psychrotrophic** bacteria, especially *Photobacterium phosphoreum* which is common in marine environments. Histamine is very heat stable and survives subsequent processing (including canning), and mild to moderately severe illness follows the ingestion of fish containing >200 ppm of histamine. Diagnosis of scombrotoxic food poisoning is by detection of histamine in food and food remnants.

Illness is characterized by a rapid onset (10 minutes to several hours, probably dependent on dose) of symptoms which includes rashes on the face and neck, flushing, sweating, headache, nausea, vomiting, diarrhoea, burning of the mouth and abdominal cramps. In severe cases collapse can occur following constriction of the airways, and hospitalization rates in outbreaks have been comparable with those due to bacterial intoxications at the severe end of the gastrointestinal disease spectrum. In most instances symptoms resolve in a matter of hours without the need for medical intervention, although anti-histamines are effective at relieving symptoms if administered early in the course of the disease.

Most incidents of scombrotoxic fish poisoning occur in the United States, Japan and the UK, although this is more likely to reflect ascertainment than disease occurrence. Incidents of sporadic disease often go unrecognized due to the relatively mild symptoms of short duration. Outbreaks are likely to be under ascertained as they tend to affect fewer people than those attributed to other pathogens, possibly due to the existence of localized raised histamine levels within fish flesh (termed 'hot spots'). Between 1992 and 2005, scombrotoxic fish poisoning was identified in 61 and suspected in a further nine (70; 4 per cent) of the 1900 foodborne general outbreaks reported to the Health Protection Agency as part of national surveillance in England and Wales. These outbreaks accounted for only 0.8 per cent of all those affected but 3.7 per cent of all those admitted to hospital. Eighty per cent occurred after consumption of food prepared in commercial catering premises, most often in restaurants and hotels. Where a food vehicle was identified (68 outbreaks), tuna was implicated in 66 of these whereas one outbreak each was attributed to sardines and salmon. Outbreaks occurred in each month of the year but were most commonly in the summer, probably because temperature control is more difficult at higher ambient temperatures (Box 4.16).

> **Box 4.16 Control of scombrotoxic fish poisoning**
> - Effective temperature control to inhibit bacterial growth on fish from the moment of capture – through processing (including during canning) and food preparation
> - An awareness of this type of disease and the need for proper handling of fish by the public and caterers
> - The seasonal pattern of illness suggests control should be focused on preparation and serving.

Toxins produced by fungi during food manufacture and storage

Some fungi produce substances that are poisonous to human and animals. Not all fungi are able to produce toxins and some toxigenic fungi only produce toxins under certain conditions of temperature, humidity, etc. Toxins appear in some food due to fungal infections of foodstuffs (e.g. crops) and in others due to growth in stored products. Unlike bacterial, viral and protozoan gastroenteritis, the period from exposure to the onset of disease is invariably long (for further details, see Chapter 18, p. 326).

Aflatoxins
Aflatoxins are a group of 13 chemically similar compounds produced by certain species of the *Aspergillus* genus, most notable *Aspergillus flavus* and *Aspergillus parasiticus*. Their importance was discovered in the 1960s following a disastrous outbreak of what was termed 'turkey X disease', which resulted in the death of over 100 000 turkeys in England. The outbreak was traced to the use of imported Brazilian peanuts in feed. The peanuts were found to contain B1 aflatoxin from *A. flavus*. Subsequent animal experiments demonstrated a link between aflatoxin and the development of liver cancers. Aspergilli are ubiquitous soil organisms which primarily decompose vegetable matter. Under favourable conditions (high temperature and high relative humidity) the fungi grow on vegetation, hay and grains, and produce toxin. In developed countries aflatoxins occur in foods in low levels, so concern focuses on potential long-term carcinogenic effects. In developing countries a handful of outbreaks of severe aflatoxicosis with high mortality have been documented following

the prolonged daily consumption of high levels of aflatoxin-contaminated foods.

Ochratoxins

Ochratoxin A, B and C are mycotoxins produced by *Aspergillus* and *Penicillium* fungi. Of these, ochratoxin A, discovered in the mid-1960s, is most prevalent. It is produced by *Aspergillus* spp. (especially *A. ochraceus*) in tropical regions, and by *Penicillium* spp. (especially *P. verrucosum*) in temperate regions and is most commonly found as a natural contaminant of stored grain. It is also found in other raw and processed foods and beverages (e.g. coffee beans, beans, pulses and dried fruit, coffee, wine, beer and grape juice). Its public health significance stems from its role as a nephrotoxin, hepatotoxin, teratogen, immunotoxin and as a possible neurotoxin. It has also been implicated in the development of urinary tract tumours in humans although there is disagreement about the carcinogenic potential of ochratoxin exposure.

Patulin

Patulin is a mycotoxin produced by fungi belonging to the *Penicillium*, *Aspergillus* and *Byssochlamys* genera. Patulin can occur in mouldy fruits, grains and other foods (e.g. pear juice, grape juice), although the major concern focuses on contaminated apples and apple products. These moulds can grow naturally in and on apples and the principal risk is from use of visibly mouldy fruit flesh in the production of apple juice. Patulin has been demonstrated to cause significantly increased mortality in laboratory animals on repeated administration. There is evidence of carcinogenicity at high but not low levels, immunotoxigenicity and neurotoxigenicity but not teratogenicity or mutagenicity. Prevention is through appropriate storage of apples, the avoidance of damaged or poor-quality fruit, good manufacturing practice, and regular monitoring of levels in apple juice. A 'guideline' or a 'recommended' maximum concentration agreed with the apple processing industry is 50 µg/L.

Given the potential long-term effects of mycotoxins it is important to ensure that levels in foods are low. Control is therefore based on voluntary or statutory monitoring of mycotoxin levels in foodstuffs. Analytical methods employed for screening include thin-layer chromatography, high-performance liquid chromatography and enzyme-linked immunosorbent assays, and levels below 1 µg/kg can be detected routinely.

PRION DISEASE

Prion diseases or transmissible spongiform encephalopathies (TSEs) are a series of neurological diseases which came into prominence in the UK during the late 1980s with a large outbreak of bovine spongiform encephalopathy (BSE) together with human cases of a similar, and probably related disease termed variant Creutzfeldt–Jacob disease (later termed vCJD). The understanding of these diseases is poor, and hence the effects and effectiveness of their control is both uncertain and controversial. The TSEs are probably caused by an abnormal form of a protein called prion protein (PrP), which occurs in the neurological tissues of healthy animals. Its function is not known. Abnormal forms of PrP (designated with a suffix, e.g. PrP^{CJD} or PrP^{BSE}) can develop and are involved in some way in the transformation of normal PrP to the abnormal form. This disease is therefore believed to be due to an 'infectious' protein unlike any of the other micro-organisms or toxins discussed in this chapter. The abnormal PrPs do not contain any nucleic acids, and represent a highly unusual hazard for food processing because they can be transmitted through consumption of contaminated material, and because they are highly resistant to inactivation by physical processes such as heat.

In TSE disease, the abnormal PrP accumulates in aggregates (known as fibrils) in the central nervous system, giving a spongy appearance to the grey matter of the brain – hence the name spongiform encephalopathy. Large amounts of abnormal PrP can accumulate in animals before symptoms become evident. The agents are most easily transmissible to animals of the same or closely related species, and this restriction in infectiousness is known as the species barrier. All TSEs present with neurological disease and examples of these occur in sheep (scrapie), deer (chronic wasting disease), mink (transmissible mink encephalopathy) and cows (BSE).

In humans, vCJD initially presents as psychiatric symptoms, followed by severe neurological abnormalities including slurred speech, poor gait, tremors and involuntary movement. The degeneration is irreversible and leads to general dementia and death. The diagnosis is confirmed by clinical observations during life, and of the appearance of the neurological tissue and the presence of the abnormal PrP after death (i.e. by autopsy). The mean age at death is 29 years and at the time of writing, 194 confirmed human cases of vCJD have occurred, the majority in the UK. A similar human disease occurs in Papua New Guinea (**Kuru**) and this is also foodborne, being associated with cannibalistic rituals. The ceasing of these rituals some 40 years ago, and the emergence of recent cases illustrates the potential for very long incubation periods for TSEs.

The BSE epidemic was probably caused by the incorporation of material from bovine carcasses into animal feed, which resulted in recycling of PrP^{BSE} among cows. Until the end of 2005, over 179 000 cattle were diagnosed with BSE in the UK, and cases in other countries are probably linked to the export of either live cattle or animal feed. In 1996 it was shown that vCJD was almost certainly caused by the PrP that causes BSE in cattle and all confirmed cases of vCJD have so far occurred in people who have lived in countries where BSE has been confirmed. Following this epidemic, controls were implemented (Box 4.17).

At the time of writing, the occurrence of BSE in cattle in the UK has almost disappeared, and the annual rate of recognition of new cases of vCJD has reduced markedly. It remains to be seen how effective the measures listed in Box 4.17 are for the control of this disease.

Box 4.17 Control measures for prion diseases

- Surveillance of animals and particularly cows. All cows found to be infected with BSE are disposed off by incineration
- A ban on the use of meat and bone meal in animal feed
- A ban on the sale of meat from animals older than 30 months – as a result of the steep decline in BSE cases and the progress made in developing effective tests for the disease under the BSE testing system, from November 2005, cattle aged over 30 months that have tested negative for BSE can be sold as food
- Removal of **specified risk material** (SRM, cattle brain and spinal cord) during processing of butchering. BSE is localized to the brain and spinal cord of affected animals
- Use of such killing processes that neurological tissue should not contaminate the carcass during slaughter (e.g. through the use of captive bolts)
- Export controls from countries where BSE occurs
- In addition to these measures, controls have also involved human and animal products used therapeutically (including those used for blood transfusion), as well as decontamination and sterilization of surgical instruments

---

Summary

Foodborne infections usually occur as the result of breakdown in basic hygiene or the emergence of new pathogens. With the exception of the latter, foodborne disease is therefore largely preventable. The following are essential in reducing the risk:

- Effective separation of raw and cooked food during purchase, handling, cooking and consumption
- Ensure raw meats are cooked adequately so that they are piping hot throughout
- Being aware of the potential food safety risks associated with foreign travel and taking steps to avoid those risks.
- Handwash before and after preparing food and before consumption.

The responsibility for food safety does not, however, lie solely with the consumer. The food industry and the government must ensure as much as possible that the burden of pathogens or toxins in foods available to the consumer is minimized, especially as experience had shown that food safety advice to the public is not always heeded. This is best achieved through a hazard analysis (Hazard Analysis and Critical Control Points) approach adopted at each stage of the food production process.

All websites given below were accessed in November 2006.

SOURCES OF INFORMATION AND FURTHER READING

Carter MJ (2005) Enterically infecting viruses: pathogenicity, transmission and significance for food and waterborne infection. *J Appl Microbiol* **98**:1354–80.

Collins SJ, Lawson VA, Masters CL (2004) Transmissible spongiform encephalopathies. *Lancet* **363**: 51–61.

Crowcroft NS, Walsh B, Davison KL, *et al.*; PHLS Advisory Committee on Vaccination and Immunisation (2001) Guidelines for the control of hepatitis A virus infection. *Comm Dis Public Health* **4**: 213–27.

Dawson D (2005) Foodborne protozoan parasites. *Int J Food Microbiol* **103**: 207–27.

Doyle MP (1990) Pathogenic *Escherichia coli*, *Yersinia enterocolitica*, and *Vibrio parahaemolyticus*. *Lancet* **336**: 1111–15.

Dupont HL (2000) *Shigella* species (bacillary dysentery). In: Mandell GL, Bennett JE, Dolin R (eds) *Mandell, Douglas, and Bennett's Principles and Practice of Infectious Diseases*. Philadelphia: Churchill Livingstone, pp. 2363–9.

Feinstone SM, Gust ID (2000) Hepatitis A Virus. In: Mandell GL, Bennett JE, Dolin R (eds) *Mandell, Douglas, and Bennett's Principles and Practice of Infectious Diseases*. Philadelphia: Churchill Livingstone, pp. 1920–40.

Food Standards Agency (2000) *A Report of the Study of Infectious Intestinal Disease in England*. London: The Stationery Office.

Food Standards Agency (2005) Beef and beef new controls explained (available at: www.food.gov.uk/multimedia/pdfs/bsebooklet.pdf).

Gilbert RJ, Humphrey TJ (1998) Foodborne bacterial gastroenteritis. In: Hausler WJ, Sussman M (eds) *Topley and Wilson's Microbiology and Microbial Infections*, Vol 3 Bacterial Infections. London: Edward Arnold, pp. 539–65.

Health Protection Agency (2006) Gastrointestinal disease (available at: www.hpa.org.uk/infections/topics_az/gastro/menu.htm).

Kotloff KL, Winickoff JP, Ivanoff B, *et al.* (1999) Global burden of *Shigella* infections: implications for vaccine development and implementation of control strategies. *Bull World Health Organ* **77**: 651–66.

McLauchlin J, Grant KA, Little CL (2006) Foodborne botulism in the UK. *J Public Health* **28**: 337–42.

McLauchlin J, Little CL, Grant KA, *et al.* (2006) Scombrotoxic fish poisoning. *J Public Health* **28**: 61–2.

Miller SI, Pegues DA (2000) *Salmonella* species, including *Salmonella typhi*. In: Mandell GL, Bennett JE, Dolin R (eds) *Mandell, Douglas, and Bennett's Principles and Practice of Infectious Diseases*. Philadelphia: Churchill Livingstone, pp. 2344–63.

National Creutzfeldt–Jakob Disease Surveillance Unit website (www.cjd.ed.ac.uk).

Old DC, Threlfall EJ (1998) Salmonella. In: Hausler WJ, Sussman M (eds) *Topley and Wilson's Microbiology and Microbial Infections*, Vol 3 Bacterial Infections. London: Edward Arnold, pp. 969–97.

Purcell RH, Emerson SU (2000) Hepatitis E virus. In: Mandell GL, Bennett JE, Dolin R (eds) *Mandell, Douglas, and Bennett's Principles and Practice of Infectious Diseases*. Philadelphia: Churchill Livingstone, pp. 1958–66.

Scoging AC (1998) Marine biotoxins. *Society for Applied Microbiology Symposium Proceedings, Toxins* **84**: 41S–50S.

Skirrow MB. Infection with *Campylobacter* and *Arcobacter*. In: Hausler WJ, Sussman M (eds) *Topley and Wilson's Microbiology and Microbial Infections*, Vol 3 Bacterial Infections. London: Edward Arnold, pp. 567–80.

Wieneke AA, Roberts D, Gilbert RJ (1993) Staphylococcal food poisoning in the United Kingdom, 1969–90. *Epidemiol Infect* **110**: 519–31.

5

Food types, reservoirs, vehicles of infection and ways of spread

Jim McLauchlin

Introduction	94	Summary	112
Animals and humans	95	Sources of information and further reading	112
Food types	100		

Understanding of the distribution and ecology of foodborne pathogens and foodborne toxins, and of the ways in which they are transmitted, is vital for the preparation of food that is safe to eat. This knowledge should be used to prevent contamination of food by both pathogens and microbial toxins inhibit the growth of pathogens, and thereby prevent incidents of food poisoning.

Vehicles of infection The media by which disease-causing agents are transmitted.

Routes of infection The course or way in which disease-causing agents are transmitted.

Reservoirs of infection The usual place or host in which disease-causing agents live and multiply.

Microbial ecology The relationship between micro-organisms and their environments.

Microbial contamination The presence of unwanted micro-organisms.

Zoonoses Diseases and infections which are naturally transmitted between vertebrate animals and humans.

INTRODUCTION

Micro-organisms occur ubiquitously in the environment and the vast majority of these are harmless. However, a small proportion either produce toxic substances or are able to infect humans, animals or plants. Foodborne illness is caused by micro-organisms or toxins transmitted by one of various routes of infection (Box 5.1).

Box 5.1 Routes of infection
- Person to person
- Animal to animal
- Animal to human
- Human to animal
- Direct contact with the environment

Any of the routes listed in Box 5.1 can be responsible for transmission of infection either directly or indirectly from contaminated food, beverages or water, which act as vehicles of infection. Contamination by food poisoning agents may occur at various stages during the food chain: in raw products prior to harvesting, during slaughter or processing, in the factory, cross-contamination in the kitchen or from food handlers. To cause disease, some pathogens have to multiply during processing and storage and, in some instances, produce toxin. Others are unable to multiply in food but occur in sufficient numbers at their original point of contamination to be infectious. Toxins may be present in raw food components, and some are not inactivated during processing. The conditions for growth and survival of pathogens have already been considered in Chapter 3, and the properties of the individual pathogens and toxins in Chapter 4. The purpose of this chapter is to discuss the distribution and ecology of the agents of food poisoning, and outline how they are transmitted. The role of water, and to a lesser extent the environment, is considered in Chapter 7.

ANIMALS AND HUMANS

Bacteria were first recognized as agents of foodborne disease in the late nineteenth and early twentieth century. At first food animals were considered to be the main reservoirs for salmonellosis, and early investigators concluded that infected animals were the source of the contaminated meat eaten by those affected. Subsequently it was showed that humans and animals could harbour *Salmonella* spp. without showing signs of disease. This led to the general realization that when exposed to foodborne or waterborne disease-causing agents, both humans and other animals either become ill after a variable time (the incubation period) or resist the disease, showing no symptoms at all. The conditions provided by various organs of the human or animal body (i.e. nose, throat, bowel, etc.) allow survival of potential pathogens for considerable periods. Furthermore, pathogens can be harboured and excreted for a variable period of time by both humans and animals without symptoms of disease. The ability to harbour a pathogen without exhibiting symptoms is known as the carrier state.

Subsequent investigations in the following years showed that the initial observations were further complicated by the diversity of both foodborne diseases as well as the food poisoning agents, including toxins, which are produced following active microbial growth in food.

The human reservoir

In any outbreak of infectious disease there will be of one of five possible categories of infected individuals (Box 5.2).

Box 5.2 Categorizing infected individuals
- Those with **acute illness**
- **Ambulant cases with mild symptoms**, which may or may not be recognized or the illness is attributed to other causes
- **Convalescent carriers** who, after being in either of the above two categories, will continue to excrete the organisms after recovery from illness

---

- **Temporary carriers** or **symptomless excreters** who harbour the infecting organism, usually for a short time
- **Uninfected contacts** – individuals who are exposed to a contaminated food but have not developed infection

---

The excretion of *Salmonella* Typhi in stools may persist for many years (as exemplified by Typhoid Mary, see Chapter 8, p. 169). Other pathogens are generally excreted for a few weeks or, rarely, for months and only exceptionally for a year or more. Treatment of persistent excreters with antibiotics tends to prolong the period of excretion and encourage resistance of the organisms.

As has already been outlined in Chapter 4, there is a considerable variety of foodborne pathogens. The proportion of patients in the five categories listed above (acute illness to uninfected contacts) varies greatly depending on the pathogen, as does their ability to act as reservoirs of infection. By definition, foodborne pathogens are ingested with food, and therefore enter the gastrointestinal tract through the mouth. Because of the diversity of foodborne pathogens and the different ways in which they cause disease, infection occurs at different sites in the gastrointestinal tract, as well as in extra-intestinal sites (Table 5.1). However, it is important to note that most pathogens occur in the faeces (as well as vomitus), which can also act as a vehicles of infection by:

- direct **person-to-person** contact
- **contaminating foods** either directly or indirectly
- **contaminating sites in the environment**, which indirectly contaminates food via sewage or water.

The more fluid the stool, the greater the danger of spread. During infection, liquid stool is produced in greater volumes, is more likely to contaminate hands and the environment, and is therefore at greater risk of spreading infections than well-formed stools. Water droplets from flushing lavatories, soiled seats, door and toilet handles, as well as taps can therefore also act as a vehicle for transmitting infection from person to person, as well as contaminated hands and passing the infection to food. Most intestinal organisms are readily washed from the skin by good

Table 5.1 *Anatomical location of gastrointestinal and foodborne pathogens in humans*

Pathogen	Occurs in faeces	Infection transmitted by direct faecal contact*
Nose, throat and skin		
Staphylococcus aureus	No†	No
Stomach		
Helicobacter pylori	Yes	No
Liver and bile ducts		
Fasciola hepatica	Yes	No
Hepatitis A and E	Yes	Yes
Cryptosporidium spp. (immunocompromised only)	Yes	Yes
Salmonella Typhi	Yes	Yes
Small intestines		
Rotavirus, norovirus and Hepatitis A	Yes	Yes
Bacillus cereus, Clostridium perfringens, Listeria monocytogenes	Yes	No
Campylobacter (C. jejuni and *C. coli)*,	Yes	Yes
Escherichia coli (EPEC and ETEC)	Yes	Yes
Salmonella enterica	Yes	Yes
Shigella spp.	Yes	Yes
Vibrio (*V. cholerae* and *V. parahaemolyticus*)	Yes	Yes
Yersinia enterocolitica	Yes	Yes
Cryptosporidium (*C. parvum* and *C. hominis*), and *Giardia duodenalis*	Yes	Yes
Cyclospora cayetanensis	Yes	No‡
Toxoplasma gondii	Yes	No
Taenia solium and *T. saginata*	Yes	Yes
Trichinella spiralis	Yes	No
Large intestines		
Campylobacter (C. jejuni and *C. coli), E. coli* (EHEC and EPEC)	Yes	Yes
Salmonella Enteritidis, *Shigella* (especially *S. dysenteriae*)	Yes	Yes
Yersinia enterocolitica	Yes	Yes
Entamoeba histolytica	Yes	Yes
Skeletal muscle		
Trichinella spiralis	Yes	No
Other organs including the contents of the pregnant uterus and the central nervous system		
Listeria monocytogenes	Yes	No
Toxoplasma gondii	Yes	No

*Some bacterial pathogens transmitted by indirect contact, often following multiplication in food.
†Occurs in low numbers in healthy carriers, but can be transiently present in higher levels after staphylococcal food poisoning.
‡Requires a period of maturation and is not immediately infectious.
EHEC, enterohaemorrhagic group of *E. coli*, EPEC, enteropathogenic group of *E. coli*, ETEC, enterotoxigenic group of *E. coli*.

hand-washing with soap and water, and are therefore not harboured in the skin, except staphylococci (see p. 97). Personal and hand hygiene is dealt with in greater detail in Chapter 8, and it is sufficient to say here that patients (including food handlers) may usually return to work 48 hours after symptoms of vomiting and/or diarrhoea have ceased (see Chapter 8, p. 175). There are some notable exceptions, including those patients with verocytotoxin producing *Escherichia coli* (VTEC), S. Typhi, and S. Paratyphi. Possible routes of infection associated with human faeces are shown in Figure 5.1.

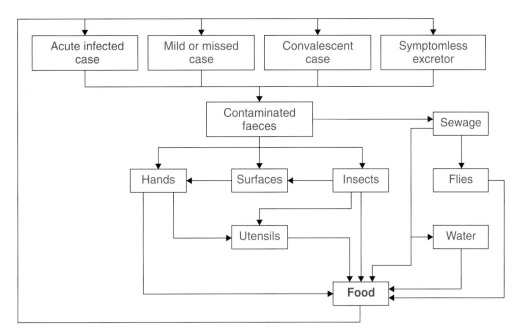

Figure 5.1   *Faecal–oral routes of infection for humans*

Human faeces (or vomitus) is not alone in acting as a vehicle for food poisoning organisms. The mucous membrane of the human nose, the hand and the skin are the primary habitat and natural home of *Staphylococcus aureus*, and 30–50 per cent of the general population carry staphylococci in the nose. In patients and staff in hospitals, nasal carriage may be higher: this bacterium has been detected on the hands of 14–44 per cent of people. As previously outlined in Chapter 4, not all *S. aureus* produce the enterotoxins responsible for food poisoning. However, in those individuals who are carriers, nasal secretions contain large numbers of bacteria, which will inevitably contaminate the hands. In addition, the pus from staphylococcal skin lesions (e.g. boils, carbuncles and whitlows), as well as septic cuts and burns, can contain high levels of this bacterium: a small speck of pus is capable of inoculating food with millions of *S. aureus*. Although staphylococcal food poisoning is now much less common then in previous decades, most outbreaks begin after contamination of foods by staphylococci from food handlers' hands. Personal hand hygiene is dealt with in greater detail in Chapter 8. As outlined later in this chapter, because foods contain potential pathogens, hands can also be a direct source of transmitting pathogens from food to food. Figure 5.2 shows the most common routes of infection for *S. aureus* food poisoning.

Inanimate objects such as towels, pencils, door handles, crockery and cutlery may serve as intermediate objects of transfer of infection, particularly when inadequately cleaned. Hot air dryers, and single-use towels and other cleaning equipment help to reduce the spread of infection. Pedal-operated water supplies both for hand-washing and for toilet flushes should be installed where practicable. The design of equipment to discourage the survival of pathogens on surfaces is further discussed in Chapters 12 and 13. However it is important to note here that home kitchens can represent a greater hazard as a reservoir of pathogenic organisms (most importantly as a result from cross-contamination from raw foods) than commercial kitchens. Mattick and colleagues (2003) noted the following in a comparison between practices of domestic and commercial kitchens.

- Domestic kitchens had poorer designs and there was greater difficulty cleaning and containing spills.
- The temperature of water used for washing-up in domestic kitchens was lower than in commercial kitchens, and dishcloths, scourers, and tea-towels were used on multiple occasions.

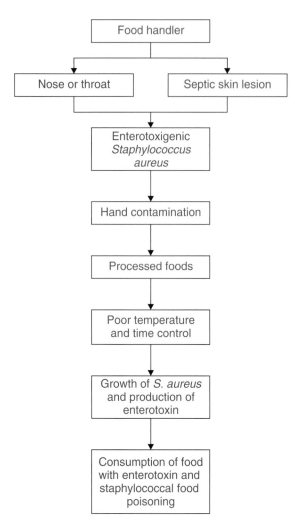

Figure 5.2 *Route of infection in staphylococcal food poisoning*

- In domestic kitchens there was greater possibility of cross-contamination with *Campylobacter* and *Salmonella* from raw chicken.
- Domestic cooks had a lower level of knowledge of food hygiene and training.

The animal reservoir

Animals (including domestic food animals, pets and wild animals) are important reservoirs for foodborne diseases. Many of these diseases are transmitted via consumption of contaminated food (or water), and are often also transmitted via direct contact with animals. As previously outlined for human gastro-intestinal diseases, foodborne infectious agents most frequently associated with animals are excreted in their faeces, and hence animal faecal wastes (e.g. livestock slurry) represents a potential source of contamination for foods such as crops, as well as being the most likely route of transmission for human gastro-intestinal diseases transmitted by direct contact with animals. In addition, the contents of the animal gastro-intestinal tract is likely to contaminate the surface of animal carcasses during slaughter, and hence meat will probably be contaminated with potential pathogens. Edible parts of food animals (e.g. raw meat and milk) may also contain potential pathogens in addition to those which are acquired during slaughter. Table 5.2 lists various food types obtained from vertebrates and the associated zoonotic disease-causing agents.

As animals are susceptible to a wide range of potential zoonotic pathogens, appropriate farming practices may prevent transmission of infections from other animals (including wild animals), and these are often referred to as **biosecurity** measures. In addition legislation and codes of practice are in place to prevent the contamination of animal feeds. Feedingstuffs contaminated with *Salmonella* may be a source of infection for animals. To reduce this risk, *Salmonella* is monitored and controlled at a number of points in the production processes. There is also statutory monitoring for the presence of *Salmonella*, *Clostridium perfringens*, and Enterobacteriaceae in processed animal protein destined for livestock feedingstuff (The Animal By-Products Regulations 2005 SI 2347 [www.opsi.gov.uk/si/si2005/20052347.htm#sch3]). In addition, a Defra code of practice provides guidelines for establishing good production practices and safeguarding the microbiological quality of finished feed for livestock (www.defra.gov.uk/animalh/diseases/zoonoses/zoonoses_reports/salmorethan10000.pdf). There are also Defra codes of practice for the control of *Salmonella* in the rendering and fishmeal industries, which recommend testing for *Salmonella* at various critical control points to facilitate risk assessment and allow corrective action to be taken. The manufacturing processes involved in the production of animal feeding-stuffs would be expected to eliminate *Salmonella* in most cases. Feed has to be tested by an approved laboratory before despatch and shown to conform to microbiological criteria for animal feeds (i.e. free from *Salmonella* and C. *perfringens*; for Enterobacteriaceae the sample fails if any arithmetic mean of duplicate plates exceeds 30).

Table 5.2 *Raw foods of vertebrate origin and selected zoonotic diseases*

Food type	Agents	Occurrence and route of contamination
Red meat	*Toxoplasma gondii*	Muscle
	Trichinella spiralis	
	Prions (bovine spongiform encephalopathy)	Neurological tissue
	Clostridium perfringens	
	Listeria monocytogenes	
	Campylobacter (C. jejuni and *C. coli)*	
	Escherichia coli (ETEC)	
	Salmonella enterica	Faeces and faecal contamination
	Yersinia enterocolitica	
	Brucella spp.	
	Cryptosporidium parvum	
	Taenia solium and *T. saginata*	
	Fasciola hepatica	
Poultry meat	*T. gondii*	Muscle
	C. perfringens	
	L. monocytogenes	
	Campylobacter (C. jejuni and *C. coli)*,	Faeces and faecal contamination
	Salmonella Enteritidis	
Eggs	*S.* Enteritidis	Internal contents via trans ovarian infection
	Campylobacter (C. jejuni and *C. coli)*	
	S. Enteritidis	Surface contamination from faeces or the
	C. perfringens	environment
	L. monocytogenes	
Milk	*Bacillus cereus*	
	Clostridium perfringens	
	Listeria monocytogenes	
	Staphylococcus aureus	
	Campylobacter (C. jejuni and *C. coli)*	Contamination from faeces or the environment,
	E. coli (ETEC)	or natural occurrence of mastitis
	S. enterica	
	Brucella spp.	
	Cryptosporidium parvum	

ETEC, enterotoxigenic group of *E. coli.*

Other animals including pets, companion animals, wild animals, and vermin

Pets, and farm and wild animals, can be carriers of gastrointestinal pathogens, and care should be taken to prevent the transmission of infections to humans. VTEC, *Campylobacter, Salmonella* and *Cryptosporidium* have been recognized as causes of outbreaks where wild or farm animals in public settings, such as in schools or open farms, were the possible sources of infection. In these settings there should be adequate hand-washing facilities available after any physical contact with animals, and these animals should be excluded from areas where eating or preparation of food takes place.

Pet animals can be of considerable benefit as companions. Pet or companion animals clearly live together with humans in households, however, no matter how clean these animals appear, they may carry possible pathogens (Table 5.3). It is recommended that:

- hands are washed after stroking animals and before preparing food
- pets are kept out of kitchens, particularly away from food contact surfaces
- pet foods are prepared separately from other foods and using different bowls and utensils
- soiled cat litter trays are cleaned every 24 hours.

Table 5.3 *Examples of gastrointestinal pathogens carried by pet and companion animals*

Animal	Pathogen
Rats, mice, guinea pigs, gerbils, ferrets	Salmonella
Birds	Salmonella, Campylobacter
Cats	Salmonella, Campylobacter, Cryptosporidium, Toxocara (round worm), Toxoplasma
Dogs	Campylobacter, Cryptosporidium, Giardia, Toxocara (round worm), Salmonella
Reptiles	Salmonella

Because of the risks of infection, special precautions should be taken by specific groups. For example, it is recommended that children under 5, individuals with weakened immune systems, pregnant women and the elderly should avoid contact with:

- reptiles, because these are frequently carriers of *Salmonella*
- baby chicks and ducklings
- puppies and kittens under 6 months old
- pets with diarrhoea.

Rats and mice can suffer from infection and become symptomless excreters of a variety of pathogens including *Salmonella* spp. These pathogens may be acquired on farms, in sewers and from garbage. Wild birds are natural carriers of *Salmonella* and *Campylobacter* spp., although the former is more common in scavengers such as seagulls and even pigeons feeding on urban waste from tips and sewage outflows.

Flies are probably important vectors in the spread of disease, particularly where animal faeces are found in close vicinity of the human population. In countries with efficient sanitation systems and where transport is mechanized, flies are probably of less concern, but there may still be direct contamination of food from animal sewage. Where sanitation is poor and intestinal disease such as dysentery and typhoid are endemic, flies in abundance are a menace. There will be ready access to infected excreta from cases and carriers and bacteria can be transferred to foodstuffs. Rivers and other waters polluted by sewage from man and animals will flood fields and vegetable crops and thus increase fly infestation.

In developed countries with good sanitation, there are still untidy dustbins with ill-fitting lids, and boxes of refuse in the back premises of private houses, blocks of flats, restaurants, hotels, canteens and other food establishments, which may be placed near the kitchen windows. Flies can feed on unwrapped food waste and regurgitate pathogens on to foods. Particles of infected material will also be carried on the feet. *C. perfringens* has been isolated from green and blue bottle flies. Other insects, such as cockroaches and ants, can carry food poisoning bacteria. In general, cockroaches are less likely to harbour infection than flies because they breed in wall cracks and paper rather than refuse and manure heaps. Similarly, wasps, bees and spiders are unlikely to harbour pathogenic bacteria because of their breeding and feeding habits. Ants in large numbers are more significant vectors. The importance of controlling vermin is further discussed in Chapter 14.

Contact with wild animals also represents a reservoir of infection similar to pets and companion animals and the actions to prevent infection should be the same as that outlined above. Risks from consumption of bushmeat are discussed in Chapter 18.

FOOD TYPES

Meat and poultry

Red meat (pork, beef, lamb, goat and other game) and poultry meat constitute a major part of the diet of the population in the UK, northern Europe and North America. As outlined in the previous section, both red meat and poultry is likely to contain potential pathogens that can contaminate their surfaces during slaughter and butchery (see Table 5.2). Most of these pathogens are of faecal origin, or come from outer surfaces of the skin, hide, hoofs or hair, etc. Cross-contamination is therefore a major hazard at the butcher's shop – between raw products, as well as the external packaging and ready-to-eat products that are also sold by these retailers. Cross-contamination can also occur in domestic kitchens (as well as during carriage from the shop to home environments) in exactly the same ways as at the butcher's. The potential for cross-contamination is illustrated by the very large outbreak of VTEC infection which occurred in central Scotland in 1996, in which cross-contamination between raw and cooked meat products was implicated and resulted in 508 confirmed cases with 19 deaths (see Chapter 6, p. 135). The surface of meat is not the only source of potentially infectious agents and the parasites: *Trichinella spiralis* and *Toxoplasma gondii* may be present in deep muscle tissue. Both will be killed by freezing and thorough cooking, but may remain viable in raw and partly cooked meat.

The spread of organisms from raw to cooked foods and the periods of storage between preparation and eating contribute considerably to contamination. If freshly cooked, roasted, boiled or fried meats were always eaten hot, the incidence of food poisoning would be considerably reduced. All raw meat may be contaminated with pathogens and the spread of infection between raw and cooked materials takes place at all stages of processing, retailing and cooking throughout the food chain. Pathogens are spread by means of hands, surfaces of equipment such as chopping blocks, cutting boards, slicing machines, various utensils and cloths, etc. Food handlers may be victims of the foods they touch and thus also become a source of infection. There are particular problems with foods prepared from minced meat. The external surface of the meat is most likely to be contaminated with pathogens during processing. When this is minced, the external surface will become part of the internal part of the minced product which is exposed to the least amount of heat during cooking. Hence the occurrence of food poisoning due to *Salmonella* spp., *Campylobacter* and VTEC with these types of product.

Cooked foods eaten cold or warmed are also vehicles of food poisoning. The spores of C. *perfringens* survive cooking, germinates and multiplies actively during long slow cooling and storage. Temperatures higher than 100 °C are required to ensure that spores are killed. Heat penetrates slowly into meat so that there is a greater hazard associated with the survival of this bacterium in large cuts, for example greater than 2.7 kg. When meat is rolled the contaminated outside will be folded inside where the temperature reached may be inadequate to destroy spores or even vegetative cells. Inside the meat rolls oxygen is driven off and the atmosphere is sufficiently anaerobic to encourage the growth of C. *perfringens*.

Meat is further processed into a wide variety of shelf-stable and perishable products which can require a further period of cooking or are ready-to-eat. Microbiological hazards include the pathogens present in the raw product that are not eradicated by cooking or processing, or those which are acquired from the processing environment. As there are many different types of processed meats and meat products, only some of these are mentioned in the following sections as examples of the range of meat products available.

Fresh processed meats (such as hamburgers and sausages)

Often these products have a short shelf-life and some (e.g. sausages) are enclosed in edible casings and blended with salt, sodium nitrite, sodium nitrate, ascorbic acid. Other flavouring and bulking materials can be included, such as bread and other grains (oats are included in haggis). Some of these products undergo a degree of cooking, drying or smoking which extends their shelf-life. Microbiological hazards are essentially similar to any raw meat, but greater care must be taken to achieve thorough cooking because the outside surface of the raw meat (which is therefore most likely to be contaminated) is in the interior of the processed product.

Salting, curing and smoking

This is particularly common for pork (ham) products and involves periodic coating of meat with salt (sometimes together with spices) and storing in cool environments where the action of the salt releases water from the meat. Cured hams or bacon are similarly processed except that sodium nitrite is also used with a lower level of sodium chloride. These processes can be combined with smoking, which not only aids in the drying, but also adds distinct flavour as well as antimicrobial phenolics to the surface of the product. These are generally a very safe product, although cross-contamination hazards may occur during storage, retailing and preparation, for example from meat slicing machines.

Perishable cooked uncured meats

Most pork and poultry products undergo thorough heat treatment to destroy all non-spore-forming bacteria. Beef products are usually processed at a lower temperature sufficient only to destroy non-spore-forming pathogens. Cooked uncured meat products are ideal substrates for microbial growth, and many are frozen prior to shipment and distribution. However, if they are held at above freezing point spoilage occurs after a few days. Microbiological hazards are associated with undercooking, and as a result of cross-contamination with raw product.

Perishable cooked cured meats

Precooked cured meats include luncheon meats, frankfurters, bologna and pâté. The heating step destroys the normal meat microflora except for spores and other heat-resistant bacteria. During chilling, holding and packaging, contamination of exposed surfaces may occur, however some processes rely on the added salt and nitrite to inhibit the growth of survivors and contaminants. On prolonged storage at refrigeration temperatures, spoilage may occur and oxygen-impermeable films are used to prolong the life of these products. As with uncured cooked meats, microbiological hazards are associated with undercooking and as a result of cross-contamination with raw product or from factory sites. The extended shelf-life is associated with hazards because of secondary growth of the surviving microflora (such as C. botulinum) or following contamination during processing and storage, for example by Listeria monocytogenes and S. aureus. A large outbreak of listeriosis occurred in the UK during the late 1980s, which was associated with consumption of Belgian pâté, which was most likely to have become contaminated from factory sites after cooking (see Chapter 6, p. 134).

Canned and pickled cured meats

Canned cured meats may be shelf-stable or perishable. Examples of shelf-stable products include canned wieners, corned beef, frankfurters, meat spreads, luncheon meat, hams, sausages covered with oil, and vinegar-pickled meats. The canned wieners and frankfurters are given a 'botulinal cook' in hermetically sealed containers. Perishable canned cured meats made from pork must be stored in the refrigerator: these contain nitrite and salt at levels used to prepare shelf-stable products but their heat treatment is inadequate to inactivate spores. Perishable canned cured meats may be shelf-stable for up to 3 years if properly processed and refrigerated. Spoilage can occur rapidly with these products

and microbiological hazards are similar to those described above due poor cooking, to cross-contamination, or growth of secondary contaminants.

Fermented and acidulated sausages

Fermented products such as chorizo, cervelat, Lebanese bologna, pepperoni, salami, summer sausage, Thuringer, depend on natural fermentation for preservation, resulting from the growth of lactic acid bacteria (with consequential lactic acid production) and low water activity. Other products do not rely on the natural lowering of the pH but are controlled by the addition of citric acid, lactic acid, or glucono-δ-lactone. Microbiological hazards include the survival of acid-tolerant organisms (particularly VTEC where poor processing may result in insufficient acid) and the growth of S. aureus.

Dried meats

Commercial dried meat products such as beef jerky includes cooking that destroys normal vegetative cells and a rapid drying step which reduces the water activity below the level at which microorganisms of concern can grow. Microbiological hazards include cross-contamination and VTEC O157 contents have been associated with jerky consumption.

Pies and pasties

These may be made with pre-cooked cured or uncured meats which include vegetables and gravies as fillings within some sort of pastry. Gelatine or aspic is also sometimes added as an additional filler or glaze. These products are baked and then eaten either hot or cold. Hazards include problems with incomplete cooking or cross-contamination as well as contamination from food handlers' hands. As S. aureus grows readily in meats with a relatively high salt content, staphylococcal food poisoning has been associated with these products.

Data complied by the Public Health Laboratory Service (which later became part of the Health Protection Agency) illustrate the range of food poisonings associated with both red meat (Smerdon et al., 2001) and poultry (Kessel et al., 2001). Between 1992 and 1999, 1426 general outbreaks (incidents affecting one or more private residences or institutions in which two or more people were thought to be exposed) were reported in England and Wales. In these outbreaks, 16 per cent of cases

Table 5.4 *General outbreaks of food poisoning associated with red meat in England and Wales 1992–99**

Agents responsible	Number of outbreaks	Number of patients		Meat type			
		Total	Hospitalized	Beef	Pork	Lamb	Other
Salmonella spp.	83	2180	128	17	35	7	24
Clostridium perfringens	99	2112	22	50	15	17	17
Staphylococcus aureus	8	73	7	2	6	0	0
VTEC	7	56	26	1	2	0	4
Campylobacter spp.	5	125	0	0	2	0	3
Bacillus cereus	2	7	0	1	1	0	0
Norovirus	3	93	0	1	1	0	1
Other and not known	21	631	2	5	11	1	4

*Data adapted from Smerdon *et al.* (2001).
VTEC, vero cytotoxin producing *Escherichia coli.*

Table 5.5 *General outbreaks of food poisoning associated with poultry in England and Wales 1992–99**

Agents responsible	Number of outbreaks	Poultry type		
		Chicken	Turkey	Other and mixed
Salmonella spp.	159	125	25	3
Clostridium perfringens	57	31	26	0
Staphylococcus aureus	10	6	4	1
VTEC	2	2	0	0
Campylobacter spp.	16	14	1	1
Bacillus cereus	2	2	0	0
Norovirus	4	2	2	0
Other and not known	16	14	2	0

*Data adapted from Kessel *et al.* (2001).
VTEC, vero cytotoxin producing *Escherichia coli.*

(n=5277) were linked to red meat and 19 per cent of cases to poultry (n=7230). Tables 5.4 and 5.5 present a summary of the agents responsible for outbreaks associated with red meat and poultry, respectively. In both studies the major factors responsible for over 70 per cent of outbreaks were inadequate heat treatment, cross-contamination and inappropriate storage.

Eggs

Eggs contain chemical and physical defences against micro-organisms. The shell, shell membranes and bacterial inhibitors in the albumen protect the white and the yolk from microbial contaminants and bacterial growth. However, when these defences are removed or breached, this protection is gone. The yolk is an excellent medium for bacterial growth and liquid whole egg or egg yolk permits rapid growth of bacteria if the temperature is appropriate.

Poultry is a major reservoir of *Salmonella* and the shells of hens' eggs may be contaminated through contact with faeces in the cloaca or in the nest, barn or cage as well as during storage, packing, processing, distribution and preparation. *Salmonella* can penetrate the shell under certain conditions of humidity and temperature. Transovarian transmission (particularly by *S.* Enteritidis phage type 4 in the UK) occurs when eggs are infected during their formation in the hen's ovaries. Eggs are therefore occasionally laid with salmonellae already present in the yolk and or the albumen. The presence of *Salmonella* in eggs is fortunately rare (Table 5.6), although a large number of recent outbreaks in the UK have been linked to eggs produced in Spain, particularly with those used in the catering industry.

Washing whole shell egg does not assure removal of all bacteria. The temperature of the wash water is insufficient to effect killing of bacteria, although its pH may affect bacterial growth. Gram-negative bacteria on the egg shell can be resistant to detergents in the wash water: even chlorine rinses of

Table. 5.6 *Prevalence of* Salmonella *spp. in eggs in the UK, 1995–2006**

Year	Eggs	Number of pooled samples of eggs‡	Salmonella detected: number of pooled samples (%)
1995/1996	UK	13 970	138 (1.0)
1996/1997	Non-UK; EC	1433	29 (2.0)
2002†	UK, France, country of origin not known (unlabelled)	726	7 (1.0)
2003	UK and other EC	5686	17 (0.3)
2003	UK	4753	9 (0.3)
2002–2004†	Germany, Spain, Portugal, UK, USA, country of origin not known (unlabelled)	2101	86 (4.1)
2005/2006	Non-UK	1744	157 (9.0)

*Data adapted from Little *et al.* (2007).
†Public health investigations.
‡ Each sample consisted of six eggs.

whole shell eggs may not prevent contamination by salmonellae.

Eggs are not only used whole, but are also processed as liquid whole egg, or as dried products. Liquid whole egg (a blend of egg albumen and yolk) is used extensively in commercial catering. Contamination of liquid egg products generally comes from the egg surface and from small particles of shell which drop into the liquid, which can be further processed by freezing or drying. One infected egg may contaminate many batches of liquid egg for freezing or drying.

In late 1963 the Liquid Egg (Pasteurization) Regulations came into force (since replaced by The Egg Products Regulations 1993 SI 1520; www.opsi.gov.uk/si/si1993/Uksi_19931520_en_1.htm#tcon). In England and Wales all liquid, frozen and dried whole egg, yolk and albumen must be pasteurized (64.4 °C for 2.5 minutes) which significantly reduces the number of spoilage bacteria and pathogens (including *Salmonella*) without affecting the functional properties of the products. Because liquid egg white may have pH between 7.6 and 9.3, its pH should be stabilized by the addition of ammonium sulphate before heating. Destruction of the enzyme α-amylase, present in the yolk of eggs, is used as a test for the effectiveness of heat treatment; a similar test is used for pasteurized milk when the enzyme phosphatase is destroyed by heat. Imported liquid whole egg must also conform to the α-amylase test. Bulked liquid egg is pasteurized in other countries, but the processing times and temperatures vary.

Pan-dried flaked albumen may be heated in the dry state at 54.4 °C for 9–10 days to kill *Salmonella*, but the treatment of spray-dried albumen by heat is unsatisfactory because of the low moisture content. As there is no α-amylase in egg white the test as used for whole egg is invalid.

Although *Salmonella* contamination of hens' eggs is uncommon, it is more common in ducks' eggs. This is not only because the oviduct of ducks, similarly to hens, may become infected, but also because ducks lay their eggs in wet and muddy places, and the egg shells are more porous and thus more susceptible to bacterial penetration than are those of hens.

Success in preserving eggs depends on preventing spoilage or pathogenic organisms from entering the egg, and maintaining egg quality by preventing loss of carbon dioxide and water. Vaccination against *Salmonella* of laying flocks has dramatically reduced contamination in chickens and an appropriate shelf-life will also maintain the quality of the eggs. Refrigeration is also effective at preserving egg quality – it slows down the loss of carbon dioxide, and slows the growth of pathogenic bacteria. Recommendations for the use of pasteurized liquid egg in uncooked and lightly cooked foods should be observed. In the UK, the 'Lion Quality' mark on both the eggs and the egg boxes (www.britegg.co.uk) is commonly used in retailing (Box 5.3).

Box 5.3 What 'Lion Quality' means

The eggs:
- have been produced to high standards of food safety, including vaccination against *S*. Enteritidis
- have been transported and stored at below 20 °C
- have 'best before' dates on them or the box of 21 days after laying.

In addition, caterers and consumers should wash their hands after handling eggs, and the eggs should be:

- kept in the refrigerator after purchase
- stored separately from other foods
- discarded if dirty or cracked
- used by the 'best before' date marked on the shell, this guarantees that they are fresher than required by law (must not exceed 28 days from the date of lay)
- eaten as soon as possible after cooking.

Cooked egg dishes should be stored in a refrigerator. The use of hens' eggs in lightly cooked or uncooked foods such as mousse and custards has given rise to cases and outbreaks of S. Enteritidis phage type 4 reported since 1987: warnings given to the public do not seem to reduce the incidence of infection until vaccination of chickens was introduced (for further details see Chapters 4 and 6).

Dairy products

Milk

Dairy products form an important part of the diet of the UK and are consumed either as drinking milk, or as processed products such as cream, butter, ice-cream, yogurt and cheese. Dairy products are mostly derived from cows, but milk and milk products from sheep, goats, buffalo and other mammals (horse and donkey) are being increasingly consumed. Historically milk was a common reservoir of infection, being linked to a range of diseases including brucellosis, typhoid and paratyphoid fever, and bovine tuberculosis: the last was responsible for 65 000 deaths between 1912 and 1937. However tuberculosis eradication programmes in cattle (including the control of this infection in wild animals, particularly badgers) with pasteurization of the majority of dairy products means that tuberculosis and now foodborne disease, in general, associated with dairy products is much rarer. However, unpasteurized drinking milk can still be legally sold in England and Wales (it was banned in Scotland in 1983), but these can only be sold from a relatively small number of registered producers that undergo annual tuberculin testing.

Milk, however, still represents a reservoir of microbiological hazards, which spread by three principal routes (Table 5.2, p. 99). First, faecal contamination of udders can occur, particularly in cows whose faeces naturally have a much more liquid consistency than that of sheep and goats, which inevitably leads to contamination of milk. The ranges of pathogens present in faeces has already been discussed earlier in this chapter and includes *Campylobacter*, pathogenic *E. coli*, *Salmonella*, *L. monocytogenes* and *Cryptosporidium parvum*. Second, animals may have **mastitis** (inflammation of the mammary gland), which can be due to a range of potential pathogens including *S. aureus*. During this infection, the bacterium is excreted in raw milk in high numbers. If the milk is not properly refrigerated, *S. aureus* can grow and produce enterotoxin. The staphylococcal enterotoxin is likely to remain biologically active even following pasteurization and subsequent processing, and a large outbreak associated with spray dried milk in Japan has been mentioned in Chapter 1. Finally, contamination can occur directly from the environment, and includes spores of *Bacillus cereus* (and other *Bacillus* spp.) as well as *C. perfringens*.

The process of pasteurization has already been described in Chapter 3 (p. 45), however, it is important to reiterate here that potential pathogens (as well as toxins) occur in unpasteurized or poorly pasteurized milk as well as in milk which may become contaminated after pasteurization. In a study of 27 outbreaks (662 affected individuals) which were reported in England and Wales between 1992 and 2000, 14 were associated with unpasteurized milk (Gillespie *et al.*, 2003). Bird-pecking of bottled drinking milk was implicated in one outbreak. The range of pathogens associated with such outbreaks is shown in Table 5.7; the majority of outbreaks were due to *Salmonella*, *Campylobacter* and VTEC, all of which could be attributed to faecal contamination. There has been a disproportionate association of infections with failure of small on-farm

Table 5.7 *Outbreaks of infectious intestinal diseases associated with milk in England and Wales, 1992–2000**

Pathogen	Number of outbreaks
VTEC O157	9
Campylobacter spp.	7
Salmonella Typhimurium	6
S. Enteritidis	2
Other *Salmonella*	2
Cryptosporidium	1

*Data adapted from Gillespie *et al.* (2003).
VTEC, vero cytotoxin producing *Escherichia coli*.

pasteurization processes in England and Wales. However, the potential for industrial dairies to cause large outbreaks is illustrated by an outbreak in Illinois (USA) in 1985 in which 16 000 S. Typhimurium infections occurred following an unrecognized pasteurization fault.

Spray dried and dehydrated milk

Milk can be subsequently treated and dehydrated by a variety of processes to produce evaporated milk and milk powder, some of which is specially prepared for babies as **infant formula** and **follow-on feed**. Dehydration of milk requires care in preparation and outbreaks associated with *S. aureus* have been mentioned above. The process of spray drying involves preliminary concentration in which water is removed by evaporation, often using pasteurization temperatures. This is followed by spraying the products through rotary atomizers into the top of a large chamber supplied with air which has been filtered and heated to 160 °C. Dry milk powder is collected at the bottom of the chamber. Problems can occur where survival (and multiplication) of bacteria occurs after the primary heating step, or where contamination occurs from factory sites. Although the hot air would be expected to kill most pathogens, rapid cooling occurs and there is good evidence for *Salmonella* to survive the spray-drying process.

As previously mentioned, spray-dried milk powder has been the vehicle in staphylococcal enterotoxin food poisoning; one large outbreak in Japan affected over 13 000 cases. *Salmonella* in dried milk has been associated with outbreaks in Europe, North America and Australasia. Most notable was an outbreak in the UK in 1985 where 76 people (48 babies, one of whom died) became infected with *Salmonella* Ealing following consumption of powdered milk from a single manufacturer. The source of contamination was probably the machinery within the spray-dryer (see Chapter 6, p. 137).

It is worth mentioning here a particular, but fortunately rare, problem recently identified and associated with the feeding of powdered infant formula milk and a Gram-negative bacterium *Enterobacter sakazakii*. This bacterium causes severe systemic infection in very young infants, particularly those who are premature and of low birth weight: in a recently reported series, more than 40 per cent of these infected babies died (Bowen and Braden 2006). The animal or environmental sources of this

bacterium are poorly understood, although it has been isolated from dry materials such as milk powder, chocolate, cereals, flour, spices, pasta and dust. Thus manufacturers should include warning labels on powdered infant formula that these products are not sterile and require proper handling, preparation and storage. In addition, infants at particular risk (i.e. those who are of low birth weight or premature) should be fed sterile alternatives.

Cream

Cream is prepared by separating a lipid-rich fraction of milk, usually by centrifugation, often also with heating to 40–50 °C. Most of the milk-contaminating bacteria are separated into cream by this process, which is performed on pasteurized milk or pasteurized after separation but before bottling. A few creameries carry out in-bottle pasteurization. Cream may be put into cartons and bottles at the creamery or may be transported in cans or churns for filling at distribution centres. Cream is usually subject to a higher pasteurization temperature (up to 80 °C) than that used for milk. The microbiological hazards of raw or post-pasteurization contaminated cream are similar to that of milk, although there are surprisingly few outbreaks associated with this product. This is possibly due to under-recognition, and because cream is rarely eaten alone, it may be more difficult to identify it as a vehicle of infection than other dairy products. However, outbreaks have been associated with S. Typhimurium, VTEC, and *S. aureus*: the latter particularly with cakes and desserts.

Butter

Butter is prepared from the lipid-rich portions of cream. There are two types of butter: **cultured butter**, which has no or limited salt and in which lactic acid reduces the pH to 4.5–5, and **sweet-cream butter** which has a higher pH (6.5–7) and a higher concentration of added salt. Butter has generally been considered a safe product because the partitioning effect between the fat and water droplets in the emulsion effectively increases the salt concentration to safe levels, which prevents the growth and survival of foodborne pathogens.

Outbreaks of listeriosis have been associated with butter consumption, probably resulting from contamination at the dairy and where temperature abuse (possibly that of heating to improve spreadability) may break down the butter emulsion. Outbreaks of food poisoning due to toxic levels of *S. aureus* enterotoxin have also been described and a single outbreak in the USA associated with *Staphylococcus intermedius* (a second staphylococcal species which also produces enterotoxin) has been reported. Under some experimental conditions, the growth of *Salmonella* and *L. monocytogenes* in butter has been detected and the general trend to salt reduction in foods may make this product more problematic not only with respect to *L. monocytogenes*, but also to VTEC and *Salmonella*, particularly because this product is often stored at room temperature.

Ice-cream

Ice-cream is prepared by freezing sugar, stabilizers and emulsifiers with either milk fat (when it is described as **dairy ice cream**) or vegetable or other animal fats (when it is just described as ice-cream). Flavourings are also added to this mix, including fruits, nuts, chocolate, etc., and some formulations also contain egg products. Prior to introduction of compulsory heat treatment for ice-cream, outbreaks due to *Salmonella* (including *S.* Typhi) and *S. aureus* were common. However, microbiological problems with ice-cream are now rare, although in other countries, *Salmonella* outbreaks are recorded more frequently.

Yoghurt

Milk is fermented to produce a variety of low pH, liquid, solid or semi-solid products that can be grouped under the general category of yoghurt. Flavourings as well as fruit, nuts and preserves can also be added. Provided the process is well-controlled, the ability to use high temperature pasteurization with a low pH (usually <4.2) makes yoghurt a very safe product. However, outbreaks of food poisoning have been known to occur, albeit rarely. Most notable was an outbreak of 27 cases of botulism (the largest in the UK) which occurred in 1989. Here hazelnut purée (in which *C. botulinum* had been allowed to grow during storage in cans) was used to flavour the yoghurt: the low acidity prevented further growth of the bacterium, but did not inactivate the toxin (see Chapter 6, p. 136).

Cheese

Cheese is a heterogeneous group of foods prepared by the acidification of raw or pasteurized milk using bacterial cultures combined with clotting, usually by the action of rennet. The curds formed in this way are further treated by heating, cutting, pressing and salting, producing products of varying water content and pH. Cheese can be classified as hard, semi-hard and soft (Box 5.4): hard cheeses having the lowest pH and water content, and soft cheeses a high water content and near neutral pH. Some fresh cheeses are eaten shortly after manufacture, but others undergo ripening, sometimes for several months or more, which can be accompanied by secondary mould or bacterial growth, imparting a characteristic flavour.

Box 5.4 Types of cheese and their examples
- **Hard:** Caerphilly, Cheddar, Cheshire, Derby, Edam, Gruyére, Gouda, Lancashire, Leicester, Parmesan
- **Semi-hard:** Gorgonzola, Mozzarella, Munster, Roquefort, Stilton
- **Soft:** Brie, Cambozola, Camembert

Microbial hazards associated with cheese can include bacterial (histamine and staphylococcal enterotoxins) and fungal (aflatoxin) toxins, both of which may be present in raw milk and survive any heat treatment, including pasteurization or are produced during production or maturation. However cheese can also serve as a vehicle of bacterial foodborne pathogens, particularly *Brucella abortus* and *B. melitensis* (now fortunately rare in the UK), VTEC, *L. monocytogenes* and *Salmonella*. VTEC is a particular problem in cheese manufacture because this group of bacteria occurs in the faeces of cows (as well as other milk-producing animals) and consequently will occur in milk. Because of the acid tolerance of these bacteria, and their low infective dose, raw milk cheeses of all types are potential vehicles of infection. Outbreaks caused by VTEC transmitted through cheese consumption have been recognized in Europe (including the UK), North America, and Australasia.

In contrast, *L. monocytogenes*, although it may be present in unpasteurized milk, is able to colonize sites within cheese and other dairy manufacturing environments. It is particularly problematic as a contaminant during the high degree of handling for production of soft cheese in which the bacterium will actively colonize and grow. The pH of hard cheese is sufficiently low to prevent the growth of this bacterium. Outbreaks of listeriosis have been associated with both pasteurized and unpasteurized soft cheeses, particularly in those with a rind generated by a mould growth. The action of the mould can also locally raise the pH in this part of the cheese and allow a more permissive environment for *L. monocytogenes* to grow. Very large outbreaks of listeriosis associated with this food type occurred in Switzerland and the USA in the 1980s, and this prompted the UK Department of Health to warn pregnant women and the immunocompromised not to consume mould-ripened soft cheese.

Salmonella will also, on occasion, be present in the faeces of cows, and consequently contaminate milk for cheese manufacture. *Salmonella* will rapidly multiple during the cheese-making process and survive in curds unless a high degree of acidity is reached. During ripening, although there will be an initial decline, small numbers of *Salmonella* will survive storage at the lower pH range of cheese, even for many months. A very large outbreak of *S.* Typhimurium occurred in Canada in 1984 in which an estimated 10 000 cases resulted from consumption of contaminated cheddar cheeses. A fault in the process was identified such that raw milk was allowed to contaminate pasteurized product prior to cheese manufacture. Salmonellosis outbreaks associated with cheese have occurred in the UK.

Seafood

Seafood (most usually prepared from fresh and seawater fish, molluscs or crustaceans) is a major source of protein, and both toxic and infectious disease can be associated with its consumption. Allergic illness can also result from seafood consumption, however this, together with consumption of non-microbiological toxins such as heavy metals, is beyond the scope of this section. Seafood is highly perishable because psychrotrophic bacteria often constitute a high proportion of the microflora: spoilage can therefore occur rapidly at refrigeration temperatures. In addition, seafood naturally contains high concentrations of non-protein nitrogenous compounds that can be rapidly converted to off flavours and taints. Hence, for fresh seafood products, there is often a much quicker food chain between catching, harvesting and retail (sometimes including live animals) than that for meat and poultry, which are consequently treated differently. Partly due to the

faster spoilage rate, a higher proportion of seafood is preserved as frozen, canned, bottled, pickled or smoked than for meat and poultry. Because of the prevention of spoilage, the ice used for chilling on board fishing vessels should be of good microbiological quality, or clean refrigerated seawater may be used on board ships. If water quality is suspect, chlorinated or otherwise treated water should be used. On fishing vessels, holds and container boxes should be cleaned properly between catches to prevent build-up of contamination. Potential reservoirs for food poisoning from seafood are outlined in Table 5.8.

Seafood may be contaminated with food poisoning agents prior to harvest. These include the algal toxins diarrhoetic shellfish poisoning (DSP), paralytic shellfish poisoning (PSP), amnesic shellfish poisoning (ASP) and ciguatera toxin. All of these groups of toxin are highly stable and survive normal cooking processes. DSP and PSP result from particular environmental conditions that produce blooms of some species of marine dinoflagellates that synthesize a toxin during growth. Molluscs ingest these organisms and concentrate the toxin, which affects humans and other warm-blooded animals. The toxins are not denatured by cooking or eliminated by cleansing of shellfish in purification tanks. Hence the only available control measure is to prohibit collection of shellfish when, during periods of dinoflagellate blooms, the toxins in the shellfish approach dangerous concentrations. Ciguatera toxins are also associated with accumulation of algal toxins, but in this instance, occur in tropical reef fish. As with DSP and PSP, control of ciguatera toxin relies on the quality of the raw materials.

Fish are parasitized by various eukaryotes, and the nematode *Anisakis* spp. and cestode *Diphyllobothrium* spp. are also pathogenic to humans. As these pathogens are killed by cooking and freezing, infections are more common in parts of the world where fish is eaten raw. However, with the increase in consumption of raw fish in the UK, as well as the possibility of survival during smoking and other curing processes, these rather rare infections may occur more often in the future.

Shellfish caught or harvested close inshore (such as crabs, lobsters, shrimps and prawns) as well as shallow water sea-fish are prone to surface terrestrial pollution from micro-organisms derived from the faeces of both humans (via sewage) and other

Table 5.8 *Food poisoning agents associated with seafood*

Stage in food chain	Agents	Notes
Pre-harvest contamination	DSP, PSP	Algal toxin most usually accumulated in filter feeding shellfish. Toxin survives cooking
	Ciguatera	Algal toxin accumulated in tropical carnivorous reef fish. Toxin survives cooking
	Hepatitis A and norovirus	Viral contamination of filter feeding shellfish via sewage. Especially associated with oysters, mussels, cockles and clams consumed raw or lightly cooked
	Giardia and *Cryptosporidium*	Protozoan parasite contamination of filter feeding shellfish via sewage. As above, may be associated with consumption of raw or lightly cooked product
	Anisakis and *Diphyllobothrium*	Nematode worm and cestode which naturally occurs in marine fish. Will not survive cooking or freezing, consequently associated with raw fish consumption
Pre- or post harvest contamination which may require growth	Scombrotoxin	Toxin resulting from the conversion of histidine to histamine especially in scombrid fish (tuna, mackerel and bonito). Toxin can be produced any time from catching to final preparation and will survive cooking
	Botulism	Toxin resulting from growth of *Clostridium botulinum* during processing. Mostly type E, which is common in marine muds and sediments. Will not survive thorough cooking
	Vibrio cholerae, *V. parahaemolyticus*, *V. vulnificus*	Contamination from marine and estuarine bacteria. May grow very rapidly on seafood. Will not survive thorough cooking
	Salmonella and *Campylobacter*	Human or animal faecal contamination. Will not survive thorough cooking
	Listeria monocytogenes and *Staphylococcus aureus*	Bacterial contamination from factory sites (*L. monocytogenes*) and food handlers (*S. aureus*)
	Clostridium perfringens	Bacterial contamination from spores present in foods or kitchen areas which will survive cooking. The bacterium can grow rapidly when temperature and time control is poor

DSP, diarrhoetic shellfish poisoning; PSP, paralytic shellfish poisoning.

animals, especially livestock. These can be actively concentrated by filter-feeding bivalve molluscs as part of their normal feeding process. Seafood harvested from coastal waters in many parts of the world, are usually captured by fishing from boats or hand netted from the shore. Fish and shellfish are also grown on commercial fish farms (**aquaculture**). Depending on where they are caught they may be contaminated with a variety of microbial pathogens originating from untreated sewage, such as norovirus and hepatitis virus, *Salmonella* and *Shigella*, *Vibrio parahaemolyticus*, *V. cholerae* or other *Vibrio* spp., and the protozoan parasites *Cryptosporidium* and *Giardia*. Crustaceans should ideally be harvested from unpolluted water and legislation covering classification of shellfish is discussed in Chapter 4, p. 75. Fortunately, these organisms are on the surfaces of fish and shellfish and are usually destroyed during cooking, (although these can cause problems with raw and lightly cooked seafood), but may survive freezing.

Bacterial growth during processing and storage of seafood can also lead to food poisoning. This can be associated with both toxins and the growth of infectious agents. Probably the most common toxin associated with seafood consumption is scombrotoxin, largely because of the high concentrations of histidine occurring in scombrid fish (see Chapters 1 and 4). Bacterial spoilage by the natural microflora of scombrid fish due to poor temperature and time control results in the conversion of histidine to histamine. This process can occur after the fish are caught (especially where the holds of the boats are not refrigerated), in the factory prior to canning, and in restaurants and kitchens with both canned and fresh product. Other bacterial toxins are also important in seafood and this includes staphylococcal toxins (especially with cooked crustaceans) and botulism. *C. botulinum* spores are common in marine muds and sediments and will readily grow in anaerobic environments which may occur in decaying fish as well as improperly processed canned product, both of which have led to outbreaks of botulism (see Chapter 6, p. 139).

Seafood such as fish, shrimps and prawns are sun dried in some countries and contamination by bird droppings or the faeces of other animals can lead to contamination from a variety of pathogens including *Salmonella* spp. Contamination by other food poisoning bacteria can occur after cooking or preserving in factories (e.g. *L. monocytogenes*, a particular problem for smoked fish and shellfish) or in the kitchen (e.g. spores of *C. perfringens*). The growth of both *L. monocytogenes* and *C. perfringens* in seafood via these routes has been associated with outbreaks of food poisoning (see Chapter 6, p. 139).

Table 5.9 summarizes data on 148 general outbreaks associated with seafood consumption in England and Wales between 1992 and 1999. These outbreaks constituted 10 per cent of all outbreaks reported during this period and affected over 2000 people. The most common agents were scombrotoxin, norovirus and *Salmonella* and showed peaks of incidence in the winter (norovirus) and summer (scombrotoxin), suggesting the major problems were contaminated raw product and temperature control.

Foods derived from plants

Foods derived from plants (vegetables, fruits, nuts, grains, salads, herbs, spices, and seaweed) are an essential part of the diet of people around the world. These products are commonly consumed raw as well as processed (including into oils and beverages), and can involve freezing, cooking, pickling, salting, drying, canning and preserving by other means. In developed countries, the health- and nutrition-conscious demand for all-year-round availability of a wide variety of raw product (particularly fruits, salads and vegetables) has resulted in both domestic and worldwide sourcing of fresh products. However, the same practices present additional potential public health problems with these products particularly where faecal wastes from both humans and animals are used as fertilizer or contaminate water for irrigation.

Plant-based foods and food components, as with most other food commodities, can become contaminated with microbiological hazards during their growth in the fields and orchards, harvesting, and post-harvesting handling, storage and distribution. These microbiological hazards originate from their natural food microflora or from organisms present in the soil, air or dust or contamination from animal or irrigation water sources. The latter reservoirs can result from food handlers or via either direct or indirect faecal contamination. Direct faecal contamination can result from wild animals (including birds) which naturally defecate in the places where the food is grown, harvested, processed (particularly for drying) or stored, as well as from livestock. Outbreaks due to various agents (i.e. VTEC, *Salmonella*, and *Cryptosporidium*) have resulted from the collection of fruit, seeds or vegetables from the ground where livestock have been allowed to graze (see Chapter 6, p. 142). Indirect faecal contamination can also result via contaminated water used for

Table 5.9 *General outbreaks of food poisoning associated with seafood in England and Wales 1992–99**

Agents responsible	Number of outbreaks	Seafood type			
		Fish	Molluscan	Crustacean	Other, mixed or not known
Scombrotoxin	47	47	0	0	0
Norovirus	24	0	19	3	2
Salmonella spp.	14	7	1	4	2
Campylobacter spp.	3	1	0	1	1
Clostridium perfringens	3	1	0	1	1
Diarrhoetic shellfish poisoning	1	0	1	0	0
Other and unknown	56	13	33	8	2

*Data adapted from Gillespie *et al.* (2001).

irrigation, washing, or spraying with insecticides or fungicides (see Chapter 6, p. 141). The occurrence of pathogens in faeces has been discussed in earlier sections of this chapter, and for a more detailed consideration of the role of water see Chapter 7.

The natural microflora of plant material as well as the soil, dust and air represents reservoirs not previously discussed; these are predominantly fungal and bacterial (Table 5.10). These potential pathogens will inevitably contaminate plants and plant materials and their control and prevention of food poisoning is predominantly by the quality of raw materials and by proper storage under conditions which do not allow their growth.

Production of mycotoxins in cereals, grains, nuts, fruits and seeds results from the growth of fungi which naturally occur on plants and in the soil. These toxins can occur in spoiled raw materials and where poor storage conditions have been employed. The exclusion of damaged and mouldy products (including fruit used in processed foods and beverages) with control of temperature and humidity during storage is important for preventing mycotoxins entering the food chain; these are further discussed in Chapters 4 and 18.

Bacteria resident in the soil (e.g. *L. monocytogenes*) also represent a potential hazard, and because of the resistance of endospores to dry conditions, members of the genera *Bacillus* and *Clostridium* will also be present in air and dust as well as that from soil. To cause food poisoning, *L. monocytogenes*, *Bacillus* spp. *and Clostridium* spp. all require a period for growth. *L. monocytogenes* has been implicated with outbreaks of preserved vegetables, including a large outbreak in Nova Scotia in 1981 in which contaminated cabbage was used for the preparation of coleslaw. Small numbers of *C. botulinum* spores will naturally be present in vegetable products and these may

survive cooking and other preservation processes. When conditions occur that allow growth, toxin is produced, and this can cause outbreaks of botulism. Vegetable products associated with botulism have included poorly pickled olives, baked potatoes wrapped in foil and cooked vegetables in airtight containers. The last two were inappropriately stored at room temperature for several days. Botulism has also been associated with vegetables preserved in oil and with vegetables sold in modified atmosphere packages. Spores of *B. cereus* and other *Bacillus* spp. will also occur on grains and vegetables and, as with *C. botulinum*, will survive many normal cooking processes. The subsequent growth and toxin production by *Bacillus* spp. in cooked rice and bread (also causing spoilage known as ropy bread) are further described in Chapters 1 and 4.

Among the 1518 food poisoning outbreaks of intestinal infectious disease occurring in England and Wales between 1992 and 2000, 83 (5.5%) were due to salad vegetables or fruit (Long *et al.*, 2002). A total of 3438 people were affected in these 83 outbreaks and the list of agents is given in Table 5.11. Infected food handlers (especially for norovirus) and cross-contamination (*Salmonella*, VTEC and *Campylobacter*) were considered the principal contributory factors in these outbreaks. Among the outbreaks due to *Shigella*, one occurred during this period due to *S. sonnei* in which at least 100 people (with cases in at least six other European countries) consumed iceberg lettuce grown in southern Europe where sewage contaminated water was likely to have been used for irrigation.

Table 5.10 *Food poisoning agents associated with soil, air and dust*

Environmental source	Agents
Soil	*Bacillus cereus* and *Bacillus* spp. *Clostridium perfringens* and *C. botulinum* *Listeria monocytogenes* Fungi including *Aspergillus* spp., *Penicillium* spp., *Byssochlamys*
Air and dust	*Bacillus cereus* and *Bacillus* spp. *C. perfringens* and *C. botulinum*

Table 5.11 *Outbreaks of infectious intestinal diseases associated with salad vegetables or fruit in England and Wales 1992–2000*

Pathogen	Number of outbreaks
Salmonella Enteritidis	24
Norovirus	13
Salmonella Typhimurium	7
Campylobacter spp.	5
Shigella spp.	4
Other *Salmonella*	3
VTEC* O157	2
Clostridium perfringens	1
Other and unknown	24

Adapted from Long *et al.* (2002).
*VTEC, vero cytotoxin producing *Escherichia coli*.

Other foods and beverages

Clearly the above description is not exhaustive of all food types, and other food types such as honey act as additional reservoirs of infection. Honey should not be fed to young babies because it is a potential source of spores of *C. botulinum* and its consumption has been associated with infant botulism. In addition, some foods contain multiple components (such as sandwiches) and their potential to act as reservoirs of food poisoning agents and vehicles of food poisoning will be influenced by the individual components and degree of handling. However the general principles of maintaining good and wholesome ingredients, preventing cross-contamination and inhibiting microbial growth (often by temperature and time control) equally apply to these food types. The same general principles apply to beverages including milk and can include a wide range of ingredients, many originating from plants. The reservoirs and sources of contamination are similar to those previously described earlier in this chapter, although it is important to remember the role of water (including ice) (see Chapter 7).

Summary

Transfer of micro-organisms or toxins resulting in food poisoning can occur at various stages during the food chain, including in raw products prior to harvesting, during slaughter or processing, from factory sites, and from cross-contamination in the kitchen. This transfer occurs from

- person to person
- animal to animal
- animal to human
- human to animal
- or by direct contact with the environment.

An understanding of these reservoirs and routes of infections is essential for the prevention of foodborne illness.

SOURCES OF INFORMATION AND FURTHER READING

Bowen AB, Braden CR (2006) Invasive *Enterobacter sakazakii* disease in infants. *Emerg Infect Dis* **12**: 1185–9.

Doyle MP, Beuchat LR, Montville TJ, eds (1997) *Food Microbiology: Fundamentals and Frontiers.* Washington: American Society for Microbiology.

Gillespie IA, Adak GK, O'Brien SJ, Brett MM, Bolton FJ (2001) General outbreaks of infectious intestinal disease associated with fish and shellfish, England and Wales, 1992–1999. *Commun Dis Public Health* **4**: 117–23.

Gillespie IA, Adak GK, O'Brien SJ, Bolton FJ (2003) Milkborne general outbreaks of infectious intestinal disease, England and Wales, 1992–2000. *Epidemiol Infect* **130**: 461–8.

Jay JM (2003) *Modern Food Microbiology*, 6th edn. Kluwer, New York: Plenum Publishers.

Kessel AS, Gillespie IA, O'Brien SJ, *et al.* (2001) General outbreaks of infectious intestinal disease linked with poultry, England and Wales, 1992–1999. *Commun Dis Public Health* **4**: 171–7.

Little CL, Surman-Lee S, Greenwood M, *et al.* (2007) Public health investigations of *Salmonella* Enteritidis in catering raw shell eggs, 2002–2004. *Lett Appl Microbiol* (In press).

Long SM, Adak GK, O'Brien SJ, Gillespie IA (2002) General outbreaks of infectious intestinal disease linked with salad vegetables and fruit, England and Wales, 1992–2000. *Commun Dis Public Health* **5**: 101–5.

Mattick K, Durham K, Hendrix M, *et al.* (2003) The microbiological quality of washing-up water and the environments of domestic and commercial kitchens. *J Appl Microbiol* **94**: 842–8.

Smerdon WJ, Adak GK, O'Brien SJ, Gillespie IA, Reacher M (2001) General outbreaks of infectious intestinal disease linked with red meat, England and Wales, 1992–1999. *Commun Dis Public Health* **4**: 259–67.

6

Epidemiology

Jim McLauchlin, Christine Little, Gordon Nichols, Richard Elson, Iain Gillespie

Surveillance and epidemiology	114	Policy development	131
Surveillance systems	115	Burden of illness	132
Field investigations and descriptive studies	124	Factors contributing to outbreaks of food poisoning	133
Analytical studies	125	Examples of outbreaks and incidents	133
Attribution	129	Summary	143
Evaluation	131	Sources of information and further reading	143

Compiling an evidence base for the control of food poisoning and application of good food hygiene practices requires collection, analysis and interpretation of data on the occurrence of foodborne disease. Therefore it is essential to have an understanding of how data are collected, how food poisoning agents are identified and how this information is translated into interventions to prevent more cases occurring.

Epidemiology The study of the patterns and causes of health-related events (disease, hospital admission, etc.) in defined populations, including the control of health problems. Health-related events are often referred to as **outcomes** and the factors which lead to them as **exposures**.

Surveillance The ongoing systematic collection, analysis and interpretation of outcome-specific data, closely integrated with the timely dissemination of these data to those responsible for control and prevention. Surveillance has also been described as '**information for action**'.

Outbreaks The recognition of two or more linked cases, or when the observed number of cases exceeds that expected.

Sporadic cases Single cases of disease which are not recognized as being part of an outbreak.

Burden of disease Estimates of the true scale of disease, for example in terms of the total morbidity, mortality and economic costs.

Intervention Action taken to prevent infections.

SURVEILLANCE AND EPIDEMIOLOGY

Monitoring trends and investigating the causes and effects of foodborne diseases entails communication between a wide range of professional groups including clinical and food microbiologists, epidemiologists, medical doctors, veterinarians, environmental health officers, food and/or public health regulators, food manufacturers, wholesalers, retailers, statisticians and mathematical modellers, as well as the ultimate consumer, the general public. Surveillance and epidemiology therefore involve multidisciplinary teams which rely on close co-operation locally, nationally and sometimes internationally. Mechanisms must therefore be developed for establishing and maintaining working relationships, information exchange and successful co-operation. Coherent networks, often between multiple groups, are vital for successful epidemiological investigations, and involve both written and oral communication on multiple levels between a wide range of partners and stakeholders. The roles of the various professional groups in the investigation of food poisoning are outlined in greater detail in Chapters 20 to 32. The core functions and activities of these multidisciplinary teams and the methods used for the investigation of foodborne illness are shown in Box 6.1.

Box 6.1 Investigation of food poisoning: core methods

- **Routine surveillance:** The ongoing systematic collection, analysis, interpretation and dissemination of data including outbreak data
- **Field investigations and descriptive studies:** Initial responses and data collection with observations from routine surveillance and generation of hypotheses about possible sources of infection and routes of transmission
- **Analytical studies:** Application of methods (based on statistical probabilities) to evaluate causes and modes of transmission and the credibility of hypotheses generated by routine surveillance and field investigations
- **Attribution:** The process of ascribing a food poisoning agent to causing disease
- **Evaluation:** Systematic determination and communication of the effectiveness and efficiency of any specific activity with respect to predefined goals. For example, the effect of interventions to prevent a foodborne pathogen entering the food chain, such as the vaccination of laying flocks to prevent carriage of *Salmonella*
- **Policy development:** Development and dissemination of foodborne disease control strategies and healthcare policy to food and public health regulators at national and international levels.

Each of the categories in Box 6.1 will be considered in more detail later in this chapter. A key role of epidemiological investigations is determining the cause of incidents of food poisoning and ensuring that the correct interventions are implemented so that further cases of disease are prevented. Causes of food poisoning are determined by a chain of factors and usually derived from three sources:

- Microbiological factors: This includes identification of the agent (usually the detection of a micro-organism or toxin in a laboratory) in clinical and/or food specimens. The identification process is usually, but not always, straightforward and also includes information on the food poisoning agent's distribution and concentration in the specific food. Details of some of these micro-biological factors are given in Chapters 2–5, but further information is considered in the following section.

- Environmental factors and transmission routes: These are the factors which lead to sufficient numbers in food of the agent which causes disease, when an individual is exposed to it. These have been discussed in Chapters 3 and 5.
- Host factors: These include the presentation and symptoms in affected individuals (see Chapter 4) and the behavioural, genetic and social factors are discussed briefly in this chapter.

SURVEILLANCE SYSTEMS

Methods of surveillance are similar for all infectious diseases and include the collection and analysis of mortality data (causes of death), statutory notification, laboratory reports, general practice reports, hospital data and surrogate reports. Routine surveillance data for food poisoning in England and Wales are most usually derived from three sources:

- statutory food poisoning notifications
- national surveillance of laboratory confirmed infections and intoxications
- national surveillance for general outbreaks.

Reports of food poisoning for England and Wales from 1982 to 2005 derived from these three data sources are shown in Figure 6.1.

Sources of data for routine surveillance of food poisoning

Statutory food poisoning notifications
Under the Public Health (Control of Disease) Act 1984, all doctors in clinical practice (general practitioners [GPs]) have a statutory duty to notify the proper officer of cases of food poisoning. (In England and Wales the proper officer is usually the Consultant in Communicable Disease Control [CCDC] who is also called a Consultant in Health Protection and who works for the Health Protection Agency [HPA]). Food poisoning was not defined in the 1984 Act but was subsequently defined as 'any disease of an infectious or toxic nature caused by or thought to be caused by the consumption of food or water'. This includes all food and waterborne infections and intoxications (including those due to toxic chemicals) but not illness due to allergies or food intolerances. The Public Health (Infectious

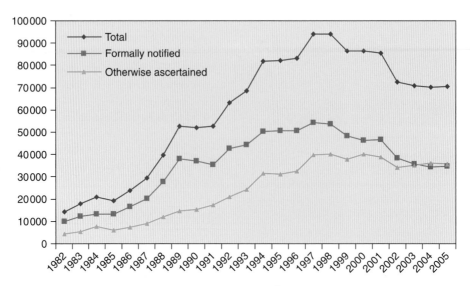

Figure 6.1   *Food poisoning reported in England and Wales. (Source: Health Protection Agency [www.hpa.org.uk/infections/topics_az/noids/food_poisoning.htm])*

Disease Regulations) 1988 requires collection of data on the name, age and sex of affected patients. This should be submitted in a timely manner to enable CCDCs and environmental health practitioners (EHPs) to investigate possible incidents which might pose a continued risk to public health. Notifi cations are based on clinical diagnoses and do not depend on laboratory confirmation of infection or intoxication. In addition to formal notifications, cases may be ascertained by other means such as those discovered during investigation of outbreaks, as a result of complaints by members of the public, from hospital admissions or from laboratory notifications. All notifications are collated locally and, following anonymization, sent weekly to the Registrar General at the Office for National Statistics (ONS). National data are published in the *Health Protection Report* (previously known as the *Communicable Disease Report*; available at www.hpa.org.uk/publications/ PublicationDisplay.asp?PublicationID=89). These data are also available from the HPA website in tabulated form (www.hpa.org.uk/infections/topics_ az/noids/food_poisoning.htm) and can be amended by local teams via quarterly returns to the ONS, if, for example, person-to-person spread or if animal contact has been demonstrated. Statutory notifications provide a crude estimate of the burden of disease because only a proportion of cases are notified. In addition, there is under-reporting because not

all people who are ill seek medical attention, or patients are notified as infected, and some seek medical attention via telephone consultations to NHS Direct. This reporting pyramid is illustrated in Figure 6.2, and has been discussed for different pathogens in Chapter 4.

There is another category of statutory notification, some of which are foodborne, and these are known as **notifiable diseases**. Food poisoning due to cholera, typhoid and paratyphoid are notifiable diseases under the provisions of the Public Health (Control of Disease) Act 1984. Although not generally considered to be 'food poisoning', typhoid and paratyphoid can be transmitted via food from a patient or carrier to other patients or in water soiled by urine or faeces. Cholera is also spread by contaminated water and food. The disease generally occurs in regions of the world where there is limited availability of clean water and inadequate sewage disposal. Sudden large outbreaks are usually caused by a contaminated water supply rather than by direct person-to-person contact.

National surveillance of laboratory confirmed cases

Data on laboratory confirmed cases of foodborne illness, for example by detection of a potential pathogen in a sample of faeces, have been produced in England and Wales by the HPA (previously the

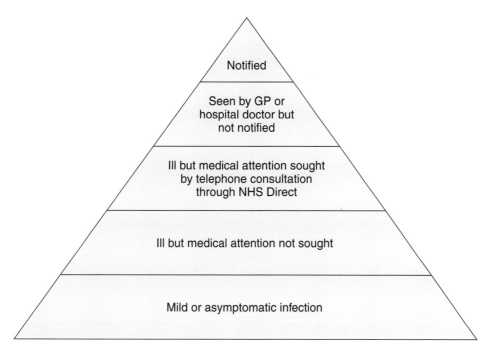

Figure 6.2   *Disease reporting pyramid for food poisoning. GP, general practitioner; NHS, National Health Service*

Public Health Laboratory Service [PHLS]) for over 50 years. These laboratory data, together with statutory notifications, are also published in the *Health Protection Report* and on the HPA website (see address on p. 116). Reports are compiled via electronic reporting to a central database (LabBase) at the **HPA Centre for Infections (CfI)** in London. Data on the laboratory which initially detected the pathogen together with age, sex, data of birth, date of onset, specimen type, clinical and epidemiological features, name of pathogen or toxin detected, if the infection contributed to the patient's death (if appropriate), and laboratory and anonymized patient identifiers are included. These data are also augmented for a subset of specific pathogens with characterization (typing) data from reference laboratories (most of which are also at the CfI in London). Additional data are also collected for specific pathogens when further efforts are required (because of the extreme seriousness of the infection or if there is a specific problem) – these are known as **active surveillance data**. Laboratory confirmed reports represent only a true fraction of the actual numbers of cases, again due to a reporting pyramid (Figure 6.3). This laboratory reporting pyramid is also affected by laboratory test protocols, which may change over time either due to improvements in testing technologies or due to laboratory resources being re-allocated to address different problems.

The absolute numbers of notifications from both statutory and laboratory reports rose after 1982 (probably due to greater awareness of the requirement for reporting), and peaked in 1997 and 1998 with over 90 000. The numbers of cases reported have now declined to about 80 000 (Figure 6.1), probably because of reduced numbers of reports of *Salmonella* and *Campylobacter* infections (see Chapter 4 and Figure 4.1, p. 61). The recent reduction in the numbers of statutory notifications to a greater extent than the laboratory confirmed data is probably due to telephone consultations through NHS Direct, which would previously have involved a GP consultation.

Syndromic surveillance and surrogate surveillance

Syndromic surveillance is the collection of data on single disease presentations (such as the numbers of patients with diarrhoea or vomiting) regardless of their cause. **Surrogate surveillance** is the collection

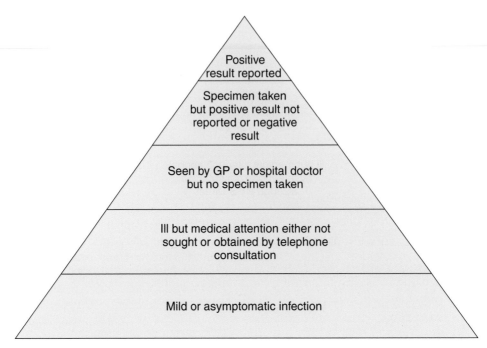

Figure 6.3   *Laboratory reporting pyramid to the Health Protection Agency Centre for Infections (CfI) for food poisoning. GP, general practitioner*

of data based on behaviours that act as a substitute for a medical consultation or laboratory examination (such as the purchase of anti-diarrhoeal medication from pharmacies). Both these surveillance methods are heavily reliant on electronic capture of data, for example from GPs, by telephone enquiries to NHS Direct, from retail pharmacies or from employee self-sickness absence returns. With greater IT connectivity, together with the availability of reliable near-patient testing and self-testing products, these types of surveillance system are likely to become much more widely used in the future.

Use of surveillance data

The provision of surveillance data allows key descriptive information to be gathered systematically and is equivalent to 'monitoring the pulse' of a population. In addition to data collection, the provision of routine surveillance includes data management, mapping and methods of analysis, interpretation, and data presentation. One of the first tasks for any surveillance system is to decide what to count. Therefore it is essential to establish a **case definition** (a set of criteria for classifying

individuals) at the outset for all epidemiological studies. The case definition can include, for example, individuals with a particular disease syndrome, sets of symptoms, other health conditions, infected by a specific species or type of pathogen, resident in a specific area, or with an onset during a specific time period. Some case definitions are nationally or even internationally recognized, and these are invaluable in allowing comparisons with other data including those which have been historically collected or are from other regions or countries.

The main purposes of surveillance are:

- Systematic collection of data including the early description of changes in disease pattern, which will enable rapid investigation and application of appropriate control measures.
- Analysis of these data to produce statistics (including the determination of the **prevalence** of infection within a population) and provide a timely distribution of the information in a readily understandable form to those required to take action.

- Interpretation of the statistics, for example to provide information to:
  - monitor long-term trends
  - assess the needs for interventions
  - predict future trends
  - collate data on newly recognized or rare infections.
- Continued monitoring to evaluate the effects of any action and provide evidence to evaluate disease control measures and prevention programmes.
- Planning and costing of public health services for prevention and control.

Routine surveillance systems can sometimes point to possible sources of foodborne infection, but are unlikely to provide detailed answers to specific questions necessary for control. However, routine surveillance data are useful for the **generation of hypotheses** (a provisional theory about the reservoir, vehicle of infection, route of transmission, which is consistent with all or the majority of the observations), which can be tested by more detailed investigation. Routine surveillance systems provide ongoing collection of data and consequently may provide only a minimal dataset which will, at any given time, be to a greater or lesser extent incomplete. However, valuable information on seasonal changes in disease, information about age distribution and evidence of recent unusual exposures (e.g. travel) can often be gleaned from routine surveillance systems. Where more formal investigation is warranted a descriptive 'trawling' questionnaire can be used to gather information on a wide range of exposures for a small subset of patients to come up with hypotheses for what the source of infection might be.

Human or computer-based **exceptional reporting algorithms** (reporting systems that identify unusual reporting patterns above what would be expected in comparison to historical patterns) can identify when there is temporal or geographic increases or clustering of cases over short or long time periods so that further investigation can be instituted. Mapping is also used to supply descriptive information about distribution. The extension of surveillance internationally through national and international surveillance networks has allowed the detection of outbreaks linked to individual products causing food poisoning across different countries or even continents that would not have been detected previously.

Routine surveillance provides information on the seasonal patterns of infection for gastrointestinal pathogens (see Chapter 4). For example, with *Salmonella* infections, the summer occurrence is thought to be related to the increase in seasonal temperature and is not particularly useful in source tracking, although it is possible to detect outbreaks by reference to the seasonal occurrence in disease through an exceptional reporting system algorithm. For *Cryptosporidium* infections, spring and autumn peaks are thought to be more associated with animal infections around lambing and calving (spring) and travel and swimming pool-related transmission (late summer). Norovirus and rotavirus infections are more common over the winter. Listeriosis shows a strong late summer to early autumn peak, although the reason for this is not understood. *Campylobacter* infection shows a strong increase in the late spring/early summer and this seasonality does not appear to be explicable by rainfall, temperature or other obvious physical factors. Flies have been put forward as a potential vector for transmission (Nichols 2005), but additional research is required to confirm or refute this hypothesis.

The routine surveillance and public health infrastructures differ among countries, with the biggest differences being between developing and developed countries. In addition, there are usually lower levels of morbidity and mortality in infants and children, less acquired immunity in adults and a more restricted range of pathogens in developed than in developing countries (see Chapter 18). Within the European Union (EU) there are differences between the results generated from different routine surveillance systems for many different pathogens, for food poisoning and for rates (this is a product of clinical and/or microbiological practice and surveillance) of gastrointestinal illness, although the documentation of these differences is poor. Initiatives are currently underway to improve pan-European surveillance. For example, zoonoses surveillance is performed for all member states on 16 of the zoonotic diseases of infections in humans (in 2005, 197 363 *Campylobacter*, 176 395 *Salmonella*, 9630 *Yersinia*, 3314 verocytotoxin producing *Escherichia coli* [VTEC], 1439 *Listeria*, 1218 *Brucella* infections were reported) together with antimicrobial resistance, incidences in animals and in feed across Europe. This is performed for the EU by the European Food Safety Authority (EFSA, see http://www.efsa.europa.eu/en/science/monitoring_zoonoses/reports/zoonoses_report_2005.html) and it is envisaged that this will improve the identification of meaningful national differences within the EU. Data are also produced by the European Centre for Disease Prevention and Control (ECDC, http://ec.europa.eu/health/index_en.htm) and the World Health Organization (WHO, www.emro.who.int/tdr/index.asp).

Outbreak surveillance

Sources of data

A **general outbreak** is defined as that 'affecting members of more than one private residence or residents of an institution' and is distinct from family outbreaks which affect members of a single residence. Surveillance of general outbreaks was introduced in England and Wales by the PHLS in 1992. A standardized structured questionnaire is sent to the appropriate CCDC to be completed by the lead investigator when an outbreak investigation has been completed. This questionnaire seeks to collect data on the setting in which the outbreak occurred, the mode of transmission, causative organism, and details of laboratory and epidemiological investigations. A similar questionnaire is also designed specifically designed for waterborne infections. Completion of these questionnaires and participation in this surveillance scheme is purely voluntary (**passive surveillance**). Data on general outbreaks obtained in this way have already been used in the discussion of food types, reservoirs and vehicles of infection in Chapter 5. A more detailed consideration of the use of questionnaires is given in the following section.

Use of outbreak data

The objectives of outbreak surveillance are to:

- identify routes of transmission
- identify trends in pathogens
- identify trends in food vehicles
- detect new pathogens and/or vehicles
- identify the impact of outbreaks in different settings
- assess the impact of specific interventions.

The retrospective examination of outbreaks, particularly where good outbreak investigations have

been undertaken and comprehensive outbreak reports have been produced, can be instructive in providing evidence for the causes of foodborne diseases (see Chapter 32). Much of the public health activity is focused on the detection, examination and prevention of outbreaks, and this is one of the most useful ways of examining transmission routes. However, there may be variation in the quality and strength of evidence for the mode of transmission and vehicle of infection, which can be an area of considerable uncertainty in any individual outbreak (O'Brien et al. 2002). Information on the identification of routes of transmission is inevitably influenced by those outbreaks which are investigated and confirmed through microbiological and epidemiological analysis. This information is more likely to be obtained from large rather than small outbreaks, or those with unusual vehicles or agents. In addition, outbreaks tend to occur at social functions affecting a defined cohort and are more likely to be associated with contaminated products from restaurants, wholesale or retail outlets. However, outbreaks occurring in these settings are more likely to be identified than, for example, diffuse community outbreaks. Outbreaks are uncommonly identified for some organisms (e.g. *Campylobacter* infections and listeriosis) where the majority of cases are probably sporadic. This means that the opportunity to examine risk factors from outbreaks is more limited than for other foodborne pathogens. Finally, general outbreaks account for only a small proportion of the total laboratory (and formally notified) cases of foodborne disease. Reports not linked to general outbreaks may be genuine sporadic cases, arise from family outbreaks, or be associated with unrecognized (or unreported) general outbreaks.

Microbiological food surveillance and microbiological typing

Additional sources of data for epidemiological investigations are microbiological surveillance and typing. Microbiological food surveillance involves the compilation of data from laboratory analyses of food (see Chapter 30). This source of information can be used not only for identification of specific problems or as part of wider investigations, but also to establish the types and numbers of organisms derived from a particular source. This can include the monitoring of pathogens in raw meats to estimate the amount of contamination, for example, by *Salmonella*, *Campylobacter* and VTEC.

Use of microbiological data

Monitoring ready-to-eat products can occasionally yield a pathogen that is implicated in human disease or an outbreak, but detection levels are usually low. Data from surveillance of food, as well as that from water or the environment, can contribute to detection in source foods, particularly through timely focused surveys. Veterinary surveillance data of disease incidence and distribution in animals can also be useful in determining likely sources of infection.

The characterization or typing in microbiology reference laboratories of specific species of foodborne pathogens has been invaluable in elucidating their epidemiology (Box 6.2) and has been briefly discussed in Chapter 2.

Box 6.2 Advantages of typing

- Allows the identification of routes of infection and sources of contamination
- Confirms reservoirs of infection
- Distinguishes between pathogenic, and less and non-pathogenic variants
- Provides evidence for the effectiveness of interventions
- Identifies long-term trends and changes including the emergence of new pathogens

---

Along with detecting an organism in a source product, it is particularly useful to identify microbiological contamination associated with an outbreak so that the route of transmission can be identified as well as the source. For example, in outbreaks associated with *Salmonella* Enteritidis infection transmitted by hens' eggs, it is essential to demonstrate that the eggs were either contaminated (the source), that the egg was used in a food product, and that this was as a result of contamination within the kitchen environment or undercooking of the product (the transmission route).

It can also be useful for any pathogens isolated from process quality control to be submitted to reference laboratories for typing because these can occasionally coincide with, or be relevant to, an outbreak.

Terminology used in epidemiology

Epidemiology has a vocabulary all of its own for describing disease and its causes (Box 6.3).

Box 6.3 Common epidemiological terms

- **Case:** A person in the population or study group identified as having the particular disease, health disorder, etc. under investigation
- **Control:** In certain epidemiological studies (see case–control studies p. 127) there is a comparison group consisting of people who differ from cases in disease experience (e.g. well subjects)
- **Population at risk:** A group of people, healthy or sick, who would be considered cases if they had the outcome under investigation
- **Outcome:** All the possible results (e.g. infection with a micro-organism, hospital admission, death) that may stem from exposure to a causal factor
- **Exposure:** A supposed cause of the health effect of interest. Exposures are often described in terms of time, place and person (see the next section)

Furthermore, epidemiological analysis most usually considers infections in terms of time, place and person.

Time

The distribution of cases over time (the epidemic curve) is probably the most common immediate means of assessing outbreaks. The onset of a specific disease with an epidemic curve and consideration of the environment of the cases often provides much information on the possible source of infection. In point source outbreaks (where all cases are exposed at the same time to a single source), all primary cases (those cases exposed to the single source) will occur within the range of incubation periods for that food poisoning agent. An example of a point source outbreak is a *Clostridium perfringens* outbreak at a wedding where all (primary) cases are exposed to a single heavily contaminated food on the afternoon of the reception. In some outbreaks however, point source infection is followed by person-to-person spread to secondary cases; such outbreaks have more complex epidemic curves. An example of an outbreak with a more complex epidemic curve is a foodborne VTEC outbreak occurring in school which presents with a single initial peak, followed by further waves of infection as secondary cases occur when the disease is transmitted to siblings through contact outside school and who were not exposed to the primary source.

Place

The geographical distribution of cases can provide evidence for the source and spread. Obtaining information on the attendance at a specific function or restaurant, or the location from where foods were obtained, remains of vital importance in investigating food poisoning outbreaks. Mapping has been invaluable for suggesting exposures. Clearly locally, nationally and internationally distributed foods are likely to cause outbreaks with very different distributions of cases. Mapping has been particularly useful for environmental or waterborne outbreaks, as demonstrated by the control of an outbreak of cholera by John Snow in 1854 (see Chapter 1, p. 7).

Person

Data on the affected people's age, sex, occupation, travel, ethnic background, leisure activities, etc. are often the first set of information available. For example, because food consumption patterns of babies and young children differ markedly from that of adults, a brief consideration of the age distribution of cases in a food poisoning outbreak can reduce rapidly the foods under consideration as suspect vehicles.

Measurements used in epidemiology

Incidence rate (more often called just incidence) is the number of new cases of a disease that develop within a specified population during a defined time period. Incidence is commonly expressed as the number of cases per 100 000 population in any given year. Prevalence is the number of people who have a particular disease at a specific time.

Attack rate (AR) is the proportion of the total population exposed to an infectious agent that becomes ill, i.e. the number of people who are ill divided by the total number of people, exposed or unexposed. A simple attack rate calculation is shown in Table 6.1. The similar attack rates between exposure to eating chocolate suggest that this is not a risk factor for becoming ill in this example. Mortality is the proportion of a defined population that die each year from a disease.

Table 6.1 *An example of calculation of attack rate*

Eaten chocolate	Not ill	Ill	Total
No	69 (A)	77 (B)	146
Yes	6 (C)	6 (D)	12
Total	75	83	158

AR, attack rate.
$AR_{Exposed} = D/(C+D) = 6/12 = 0.50$ (or 50.0%)
$AR_{Unexposed} = B/(A+B) = 77/146 = 0.53$ (or 52.7%)

Relative risk (RR), also known as the risk ratio, is the risk of illness in those exposed to a factor divided by the risk of illness in those unexposed to the factor. This is the ratio of the attack rates and provides a measure for their comparison. If the relative risk is:

- less than 1, the exposure is **protective**, i.e. there is decreased risk among the exposed group
- approximately equal to 1 (attack rates are equal) there is no association between the exposure and the disease
- greater than 1, the association is **positive**, i.e. there is increased risk among the exposed group.

Using the example in Table 6.1:

$$RR = AR_{Exposed}/AR_{Unexposed} = 0.50/0.53 = 0.95.$$

So although there is a decreased risk among the exposed group, this difference is small and this confirms that the risk of eating chocolate is unlikely to be causing the illness.

Odds of exposure is the number of people exposed to a factor divided by the number of people not exposed to the factor. **Odds ratio (OR)** is the ratio of the odds of exposure in those with the outcome of interest to the odds of exposure in those without. The odds ratio is calculated from the number with the disease divided by the number without. Using the example in Table 6.1:

$$OR = (D/C)/(B/A) = (6/6)/(77/69) = 0.90.$$

In well-designed studies of rare diseases, odds ratios are approximately similar to relative risks in that values of greater than 1 indicate increased exposure.

Generally, attack rates and relative risk are used in cohort studies and odds ratios in case–control studies (see pp. 125–7). Tables compiled from epidemiological studies of illness and exposures are known as **contingency tables**.

Statistical association

A number of different analytical techniques are available, and these involve mathematical (statistical) comparisons of groups to quantify measures of association. These statistical tests are used to investigate if differences between the proportions of specific groups are greater than those which would be obtained by chance, i.e. they are statistically significant. For example, in a food poisoning outbreak, the relationship between those who were or were not ill and those who did or did not eat a suspect food vehicle is tested for statistical significance. If the analysis shows that there is a statistical association between eating the suspect food and illness, it supports the theory that the food was contaminated and provides evidence that this was the cause of the outbreak. It is beyond the scope of this chapter to describe in detail these statistical tests, and at the start of any epidemiological investigation, it is essential to obtain advice from a qualified statistician who specializes in epidemiological investigations.

The commonly used statistical tests include the **chi-square (χ^2)** and **Fisher's exact** tests; the latter is more applicable to smaller samples. The level of significance required to demonstrate that a difference is not merely the result of chance (i.e. not due to any cause) is specified beforehand. The commonest significance level used is 95 per cent (**p** or **probability values** of 0.05), that is, there is a 1 in 20 (5 per cent) likelihood that chance alone would account for the difference between the two groups. A further measure of the accuracy of estimations is provided by the **confidence interval (CI)**. A 95 per cent CI is usually used and this denotes that one can be 95 per cent confident that the true value of the estimate lies within this range. The wider the CI the less accurate the estimate. Simple-to-use statistical software packages are widely available and provide some of these requirements, for example Epi Info™ (www.cdc.gov/epiinfo). However, expertise is required for designing statistical analyses and interpreting epidemiological studies. The reader here

should be aware of two further effects, confounding factors and bias.

Confounding factors are those factors which offer an alternative explanation for an observed association. They are associated with the exposure under investigation and independently associated with the outcome of interest. For example, in the investigation of a *Salmonella* outbreak an association between the consumption of both fish and hollandaise sauce was observed. The hollandaise sauce was made with contaminated eggs and was the source of the outbreak, but both foods appeared to be risk factors for disease, as most people who ate the fish also ate hollandaise sauce. The association between fish and disease is therefore confounded by the effect of hollandaise sauce. Consideration of these may be important in investigation of food poisoning outbreaks because dietary exposures can be linked. The effects of confounders can be minimized by careful study design (often based on prior experience of investigating similar incidents) and the analysis of strengths of association by single and multiple variables (**single variable** and **multivariable statistical models**) to assess the independent effects of individual risk factors. Finally, there is an effect of **bias** (the introduction of spurious effects by systematic selections or deviations resulting in incorrect conclusions). Bias can result in both the incorrect presence of an association as well as the absence of an effect. Examples of the possible effects of bias are:

- unintentional selection of cases (e.g. inclusion only of those who are most acutely ill)
- intentional prompting of cases by investigators to respond with the 'correct answers' as they perceive them
- cases and controls responding differently because the former has a different recall (because they were ill) than the latter
- cases responding unintentionally (as well as intentionally) with specific answers because they have learnt the 'correct answer' from a national media campaign and are likely to benefit with some form of compensation.

Types of investigations

The objectives of outbreak investigation are to:

- determine the cause by identifying the vehicle, pathogen (if any) and mode of transmission
- prevent further cases by removing the source of contamination or infection, isolating or treating cases
- provide evidence to support conclusions
- monitor the effectiveness of control measures
- prevent future outbreaks by identifying novel pathogens, vehicles or modes of transmission and reporting these.

When used in outbreak investigation, the primary purpose of analytical epidemiology is to contribute to the first and third of these objectives.

In any foodborne disease outbreak, people may become ill after consuming food that has been contaminated with pathogens. The food is known as an **exposure** and the illness is known as an **outcome**. The ill people are usually part of a larger group of people known as the **population at risk**. The population at risk may be a tightly defined group such as wedding guests or may be less defined such as inhabitants of a town, region or country. The population at risk, however, may have been exposed but does not become ill. This may be due to several reasons including a resistance to disease, consumption of a part of the food that was not contaminated, or they did not eat the same foods as the ill people. The aim of epidemiology in outbreak investigations is to examine the effects of different exposures (foods consumed) on the outcomes (ill or not ill) within the population at risk. Before epidemiological studies can be used, **hypotheses** must be developed. Epidemiological studies are used to test these hypotheses to identify the cause and routes of infection. The main hypothesis may become apparent early on in the investigation. For example, if the majority of cases reported eating cooked meat purchased from one butcher's shop but did not share any other exposures, then the cooked meat or something else in the butcher's shop would be a hypothesized vehicle of infection. Epidemiological studies are therefore used to investigate associations (relationships between two or more sets of observations without an indication of the underlying path between them) and identify **risks** or **risk factors** (relationships between two or more sets of observations where there is, or is suspected to be, an underlying pattern). For example, when investigating an outbreak of food

poisoning at a wedding, there was an association between a group of individuals who became ill after attending this event, and the risk was in consuming a dish containing cooked salmon.

Questionnaires

To ensure accurate and comparable records of all patient interviews, data should be obtained by using carefully designed standardized forms or questionnaires. Wherever possible, questionnaires should be either initially piloted on a small group of cases and amended as necessary, or be based on a form which has been previously used successfully. Examples of questionnaires used by the HPA to obtain data from cases of food poisoning can be obtained from the website (www.hpa.org.uk/infections/topics_az/gastro/menu.htm). Questionnaires must be administered in as unbiased way as possible and in the same way to all individuals regardless of their health status. Questionnaires are often administered as face-to-face interviews or by telephone: the latter can be useful for rapid capture of data. Self-administrated questionnaires where the respondents submit completed forms by post or electronically have also been used since they are cheap and quick to administer. However self-administration can suffer from reduced response rates and greater variation in the accuracy of data in interpreting the questions posed. It has previously been noted that there may also be limitations with accuracy of recall which decreases with increased time after an event. Problems may also occur with accuracy of recall depending on the outcome of the event. People who became ill with food poisoning after attending a particular event have a different (and often more accurate) recall of what foods they ate than those who remained well – this effect is known as **differential recall bias**.

FIELD INVESTIGATIONS AND DESCRIPTIVE STUDIES

Field investigations

Field investigations can involve a variety of actions from a simply telephone enquiry to clarify an anecdotal report of a case of infection, to co-ordinating the efforts of a team to characterize the extent of an outbreak. These were often previously described as 'shoe leather epidemiology'. The objectives of such investigations may differ but often lead to the identification of additional otherwise unreported or unrecognized cases (also known as **case finding**). Such investigation of a food poisoning outbreak may rapidly identify hypotheses for likely sources of infection and routes of transmission which can be tested more formally with analytical methods. However, this is certainly not always the case. A common problem can be the length of time between the start of illness and the interview with the patient resulting from delays in attendance at a GP, laboratory detection and reporting to surveillance. People can readily forget what they ate a few days ago and find it very difficult to recall the details of meals eaten over a month ago.

Descriptive studies

Descriptive studies are usually based on distributions or proportions of cases which fall into categories or rates of occurrence within subgroups of the population. Analysis of routine surveillance data described previously is part of this category of data analysis. Descriptive studies include those used to measure what proportion of a given population can be classified as being in a diseased state at a given point in time – these are known as **cross-sectional** or **point prevalence** studies. Where these are applied on multiple occasions, data on both the size of the population and numbers of diseased individuals is necessary – these are known as **incidence** or **longitudinal** studies. It is often important to compare the rate at which a disease occurs over time, for example longitudinal studies are necessary to investigate if there has been a change in the rate of listeriosis cases over time despite the increase in the population of those over 60 years of age (one of the 'risk groups' for contracting this disease). Data for descriptive studies are usually fixed or **discrete**, e.g. age, sex, symptoms, date and time of onset, and severity and duration of illness, occupation and nationality.

ANALYTICAL STUDIES

Although routine surveillance, field investigation and descriptive approaches may be sufficient to identify a cause, more rigorous methods are often required in the investigation of both sporadic cases and outbreaks of foodborne disease. **Analytical studies** are those which use specific techniques to answer an individual question or test a hypothesis. Analytical techniques rely on comparison of affected and unaffected groups. They are complementary to microbiological studies because when a specific pathogen is detected in the food supply, this alone does not identify the source of infection in affected individuals. Analytical epidemiological evidence is necessary to demonstrate an association between exposure and disease. Analytical studies investigate both outcome and exposure in contrast with descriptive studies, which investigate either exposure or outcome. The usual requirements of analytical studies are given in Box 6.4.

> **Box 6.4 Some requirements of analytical studies**
> - **Design** – determining the appropriate strategy, writing justifications and protocols, developing case and control definitions, calculating appropriate sample sizes, designing questionnaires and data acquisition methods
> - **Conduct** – securing appropriate permission, co-operation and ethical clearance, extracting records, locating and interviewing subjects, collecting and handling specimens and managing data
> - **Analysis** – calculating rates, creating comparison tables, measures of association (risk or odds ratios), tests for significance and confidence intervals
> - **Interpretation** – evaluating the strengths and weaknesses of the study, putting study findings into perspective, identifying key messages and making sound recommendations
> - **Communication** – producing a report with an abstract, publication of scientific paper and report, informing interested parties and identifying interventions

There are a number of different study designs for analytical epidemiological studies and it is beyond the scope of this chapter to describe all of these in detail. However, the cohort and case–control types both have a role in the investigation of foodborne disease and will be described briefly here.

Cohort studies

Cohort studies are used to investigate defined groups or **cohorts** (named after the group of soldiers who constituted one tenth of a Roman Legion). Used retrospectively for outbreak investigation, this approach applies epidemiological techniques to 'natural experiments' in which the cohort is (or has been) exposed to a risk factor and a proportion of the cohort becomes ill. Cohort studies are probably the most common analytical method used for the investigation of local, point source food poisoning outbreaks and are suitable where the entire population at risk:

- is known
- was known to be disease-free prior to being exposed to the hypothesized source of infection
- is expected to be relatively easy to follow up.

Cohort studies are, for example, suitable to investigate a group of people who have eaten together, with illness becoming recognized relatively soon afterwards, for example at a wedding function. The cohort is all of the group who attended the wedding, and so were potentially exposed to the foods being investigated. The food consumed by each member of the group, and if possible the amount, is collected. The statistical analysis is similar to that for case–control studies and food-specific attack rates can be calculated.

The cohort method has the advantage over case–control studies in that there is no need to identify and select controls, so the possibility of bias is reduced. However bias can be introduced by misclassification. This can occur when cases and 'non-cases' cannot be identified accurately. For example, in a *Salmonella* outbreak, if only the faeces from patients with diarrhoea is examined, those 'cases' who have mild or no symptoms but who have been exposed to the contaminated food and have the bacterium present in their faeces will be misclassified as non-cases. A second problem with cohort studies is bias due to loss to follow-up. Here an inability to interview non-cases (who are less likely to respond since they were not ill) can invalidate the results of this type of study. Hence it is desirable to treat all cases and non-cases in exactly the same way, including the microbiological investigations used and efforts to locate subjects after an event.

If follow-up of an entire cohort is poor, or is likely to be problematic (e.g. delegates at an international conference), or the cohort is so large that following up all cases would represent a waste of resources, exposure data from ill people can still be compared with that of well people to study disease. This is known as a **nested case–control study**, so called as it is a case–control study nested within a cohort study.

Examples

Examples of two cohort studies on outbreaks with data from food poisoning outbreaks are given in Tables 6.2 and 6.3. Thirty cases of *Salmonella* food poisoning were reported in a staff canteen serving 241 employees. Food-specific attack rates for the meal preceding the outbreak (see Table 6.2) showed that 30 of 161 who ate egg mayonnaise were ill, giving an attack rate of 19 per cent compared with none of 51 who did not eat it. There was a choice of egg mayonnaise or steak, so that eating steak was significantly associated with not being ill and the egg mayonnaise was the likely vehicle of infection. Microbiological evidence is now needed to confirm that the strain of *Salmonella* in the egg mayonnaise (as well as that from the supplier of the eggs or from other items in the kitchen where cross-contamination could have occurred) was isolated from the affected employees

Table 6.2 *Food-specific attack rates for the meal preceding an outbreak of food poisoning in staff canteen*

Food type consumed	Ate			Did not eat			Difference in attack rates P*
	Ill	Not ill	Attack rate (%)	Ill	Not ill	Attack rate (%)	
Egg mayonnaise	30	131	19	0	51	0	<0.0005
Steak	0	27	0	30	154	16	<0.05
Potato	8	49	14	21	125	14	NS
Pears	21	95	18	9	84	10	NS
Sandwiches	8	69	10	22	107	17	NS
Orange juice	13	60	18	17	121	12	NS

*Chi-square 1 d.f. = chi squared test with 1 degree of freedom. Chi-square test is used to test whether the observed frequencies of individuals with given characteristics (e.g. they were ill/ate a particular food) are significantly different from the expected frequencies from some specific hypothesis.
NS, not significant.

Table 6.3 *Attack rates of illness for all food items from a school picnic lunch*

Food type consumed	Ate			Did not eat			Difference in attack rates *P* *
	Ill	Not ill	Attack rate (%)	Ill	Not ill	Attack rate (%)	
Meat sandwiches	41	24	59	35	8	23	0.002
Egg sandwiches	19	16	84	57	16	28	0.00002
Cheese sandwiches	31	12	39	45	21	47	0.3
Biscuits	49	20	41	27	12	44	0.5
Muffin	36	18	50	40	14	35	0.1
Apple	45	21	47	31	10	32	0.2
Orange juice	65	32	49	11	0	0	

*Exact probability using Fisher's equations. Fishers exact test is used to analyse 2 by 2 tables where any of the cells has an expected value of <1.

No., number of individuals.

and was the vehicle of infection. In a second food-poisoning outbreak, staphylococcal intoxication occurred amongst 30 children and three adults after a school picnic. Attack rates were calculated from the food eaten by 83 of the 85 picnickers. Results showed that the illness was confined to those who ate the school packed lunch with 32 of 76 (42 per cent) affected compared with none of the 7 who did not eat the sandwiches. A more detailed analysis of the 76 who ate the packed lunch showed that meat sandwiches and egg sandwiches produced the highest differential attack rates (Table 6.3). From the analysis distinguishing those who ate both types of sandwich, only one type or neither, it was confirmed that illness was associated with both the egg and the meat sandwiches. The picnic lunch was prepared too far ahead and not kept refrigerated.

Case-control studies

Case–control studies begin with the identification of individuals with and without a particular outcome (e.g. disease, hospital admission, etc.) and retrospectively attempts to identify **risk factors** associated with the diseased group. This technique is useful for comparing dispersed cases with a control population selected by a variety of routes and is used where:

- the total population at risk is not known, or so large in relation to the number of people ill that it is not possible to include them all in a study
- follow-up of all cases is expected to be difficult, or when the population is so large in proportion to the number who are ill that it is not cost effective to include them all in the study.

An example of where a case–control study is used is when a nationally distributed food is thought to be responsible for an outbreak such as a sudden rise in the reporting of an uncommon serotype of *Salmonella* with cases spread over a wide area. Although it may be clear that there is an outbreak, there may not be a single meal in common. Interviews with cases may suggest several foods distributed throughout the affected area that could be contaminated. By showing that cases are significantly more likely than unaffected controls to have eaten one of the foods under investigation, the most likely food can be determined. The diet of 'other people' is discovered by asking a sample of well people to be 'controls' by providing details of the foods that they have eaten.

In a case–control study, there should be a specific hypothesis that consumption of a single, or small number of foods is associated with disease. Controls should be people who have had similar opportunities to eat the suspect foods. Consideration needs to be given to whether controls should be matched. For instance, if the suspect food is a chocolate bar and most of the cases are children, matched controls would be children of similar age living in the same area. Adults selected here as controls would be inappropriate since, in general, they are less likely to eat chocolate. Controls can be chosen from neighbours and friends of the cases or from various registers and lists, such as people who are registered with the same GP as the case. Each case will usually have one, or preferably more than one, control. Data from a case–control study are analysed by standard statistical methods.

Using a Geographic Information System (GIS) it

is possible to link datasets and conduct a case–control study based on geographic data rather than information from a questionnaire. While this is not likely to be particularly useful for the investigation of *Salmonella* infections, which are usually linked to contaminated food, it can be more valuable with *Cryptosporidium* infections, in which transmission from animals through water is more likely.

Example

An example of a case–control study is provided in Table 6.4. In a national outbreak of *Salmonella* Typhimurium DT104 infection in the summer of 2000, consumption of salad vegetables prepared away from home was one of the primary hypotheses as a risk factor for illness. This hypothesis was tested using a case–control study. Single variable analysis found a strong association

between lettuce eaten away from home and illness. This food item was consumed by 15/22 cases and 12/52 controls. Multivariable analysis confirmed this association to be independent (odds ratio 7.28, 95 per cent CI 2.25, 23.57) and highly significant ($P<0.001$).

Communication

The findings from surveillance and outbreak investigations together with the methods for their control must be communicated. This communication can be part of the management of an individual outbreak to ensure that the correct interventions have been implemented. This will prevent further illness by eliminating any continuing hazards as well as reducing the likelihood of further primary or secondary cases occurring. However, communication should extend wider than this to allow general

Table 6.4 *Example of a case–control study*
(A) Single variable analysis of foods eaten away from home*

Variable		Cases	Controls	Odds ratio	95% confidence interval	P value[†]
Eat any food prepared away from home?	Yes	18	24	5.25	1.38, 21.67	0.01
	No	4	28			
Chicken sandwich away from home	Yes	4	2	5.88	0.80, 52.39	0.05[F]
	No	17	50			
Chicken from Indian restaurants	Yes	5	1	15.00	1.48, 370.98	0.01[F]
	No	17	51			
Lettuce	Yes	15	12	7.14	2.07, 25.64	<0.001
	No	7	40			
Tomatoes	Yes	11	8	6.05	1.67, 22.66	0.003
	No	10	44			
Cucumber	Yes	9	6	7.67	1.85, 33.42	0.002
	No	9	46			
Carrots	Yes	2	2	2.58	0.23, 28.70	0.57[F]
	No	19	49			
Mayonnaise	Yes	6	9	1.91	0.49, 7.36	0.34[F]
	No	15	43			

(B) Full multivariable model

Explanatory variable	Odds ratio	95% confidence limits	P value
Chicken from Indian restaurants eaten away from home	8.3	0.77, 89.88	0.05
Lettuce eaten away from home	7.28	2.25, 23.57	0.0006

*Adapted from Hortby *et al.* (2003).
[†]Chi-square test except [F] where Fisher's exact test was used.

lessons to be learnt by all of those involved with the food chain. This communication extends to all levels of education, as well as to the production of written reports including outbreak control reports, advice in trade journals, peer review publications and advice to the general public. Finally, information from surveillance and outbreak investigations must feed into policy at both a national and international level (see p. 131) for the improvement of foodborne disease control strategies.

ATTRIBUTION

Microbiological factors have already been previously discussed in Chapters 2–5 and it is important to reiterate here that food poisoning agents are diverse in nature, and that foodborne disease manifests in different ways. However, a microbiological factor which has not been considered is the process of ascribing a food poisoning agent to causing disease: this process is known as **attribution**.

While investigating the transmission of tuberculosis and anthrax in the nineteenth century, the pioneering work of Robert Koch in Germany established a series of conditions for attributing a microorganism as the cause of a specific disease. Although Koch did not state these criteria exactly in the form given in Box 6.5, these became known as **Koch's postulates**.

Box 6.5 Koch's postulates

- The disease agent must be found in all cases of the disease and its distribution must correspond to the anatomical sites of the lesions of the disease
- The agent must be able to be grown in pure culture outside the body of the host for several generations
- The process of re-introduction (inoculation) of the pure culture into a susceptible host, usually an experimental animal (although this can also be a human volunteer) must reproduce the disease
- The agent itself must also be recovered from the experimentally inoculated subject

---

These postulates have proved invaluable for understanding many infectious diseases, including those which are transmitted through food. Indeed, Dr Betty Hobbs' work in the 1950s in human volunteer feeding experiments (which included

herself) fulfilled Koch's postulates and firmly established *Clostridium perfringens* (then named *Clostridium welchii*) as a cause of diarrhoea (Hobbs *et al.* 1953). Although Koch's postulates provide a **gold standard** (the condition of greatest certainty against which other observations and experiments should be compared) for agent attribution, it has subsequently proved difficult or impossible to fulfil these criteria for many microbial diseases, including some which are foodborne (see Box 6.6).

Box 6.6 Reasons why Koch's postulates cannot always be applied during agent attribution

- Not all micro-organisms can be cultured outside their host
- Some diseases are caused by toxins
- As a result of host responses, a disease may only manifest a considerable time after the agent is no longer present in the host
- Diseases may be due to the interactions between multiple agents, or to additional risk factors, this is especially true in the gastrointestinal tract which is a not a sterile anatomical site
- In the absence of any suitable animal model, it may be unethical to reproduce the disease using human volunteer experiments because a specific disease may have severe consequences or be untreatable

---

Partly because of difficulties in applying Koch's postulates, the problem of attribution has been addressed in a somewhat modified form known as the **Bradford Hill criteria** (Table 6.5), named after the English epidemiologist and statistician Austin Bradford Hill. Key to this approach is, in addition to the considerable amount of information already available in the scientific literature, the concept that similar organisms will behave in a similar way. This may have to be modified in some instances because not all similar organisms of the same species have specific virulence factors, e.g. only some *E. coli* are able to induce haemolytic uraemic syndrome (see Chapter 4). However, this reservation is now becoming less important with improved understanding of the pathogenicity mechanisms of many species of micro-organisms and the more widespread availability of methods (particularly based on molecular biology) to routinely detect virulence factors. These techniques allow organisms which are sometimes quite diverse in nature but use similar

Table 6.5 *Modification of the Bradford Hill criteria for causality in relation to foodborne disease*

Criteria	Description	Examples in relation to food
Analogy	Are there other similar illnesses that behave in a similar way?	Do organisms with similar characteristics cause disease related to food consumption under similar conditions?
Biological gradient	Is the disease more common in those people with most exposure to the risk factor?	Is the occurrence of disease related to the amount of food consumed?
Coherence	Do the epidemiological data conflict with other biological and clinical data suggesting causality?	Does information on food quality conflict with epidemiological evidence?
Consistency	Do the results from different researchers all suggest an association?	Have there been previous reports of disease associated with consumption of this or a similar food?
Experiment	Is it possible to design experimental interventions to demonstrate causality?	Do attempts to improve the quality of food (including withdrawal of contaminated product) reduce the occurrence of disease?
Plausibility	From what is already known of the biology of the potential pathogen, is it plausible that the exposure causes disease?	Is the implicated organism likely to survive the food process?
Specificity	Is the disease specific to contact with the risk factor or are there other known causes?	Are other sources responsible for any of the disease such as person-to-person or zoonotic transmission?
Strength of association	Is any association between disease and the risk factor, as demonstrated in epidemiological study, statistically significant?	Are the numbers of people with and without disease sufficient to prove an association with food consumption?
Temporality	Does the disease follow exposure to the proposed risk factor (rather than precede it)?	Does the occurrence of disease correspond with known incubation periods, delays in reporting, seasonal increases etc.?

mechanisms to produce diseases to be identified much more readily. Much of the useful information on individual food poisoning agents has derived from descriptive information on sporadic cases and from outbreaks. At an early stage this involves preliminary descriptions of the pathogen, its isolation and association with patients and sources. Assessing the overall public health problem of a newly recognized pathogen is dependent on more general replication of results in multiple episodes of disease. The Bradford Hill criteria also include non-microbiological factors that could be used in investigating the causality of possible food-poisoning agents in relation to foodborne disease, and these are further considered elsewhere in this chapter.

Attribution of illness can also be used to ascribe, in a quantitative way, the contribution of different food and food types. This process can be performed using different methods as well as different information sources which do not necessarily always give the same answers. These types of study can include information from one or more of the following sources: the species of pathogen or types of agent which have defined reservoirs; data from all cases of food poisoning as well as from sporadic cases and outbreaks; and estimates of food consumption. This type of approach works much more successfully for some pathogens and in certain countries. In a recent study (Adak *et al.*, 2005) the contribution of different food groups to all cases of food poisoning in the UK between 1996 to 2000 was estimated (Table 6.6). It was estimated that almost three-quarters of the foodborne illness was due to poultry, red meat, eggs and complex food (those containing ingredients of various food types in which the precise source of infection could not be established). These types of study are very much part of a developing field and similar mathematical approaches, particularly for national and international food policy, will be discussed later.

Table 6.6 *Estimated impact of different food types on the numbers of cases of foodborne diseases in England and Wales*.

Food type	Cases (%)	Deaths (%)
Poultry	502 634 (29)	191 (28)
Eggs	103 740 (6)	46 (7)
Red meat	287 485 (17)	164 (24)
Seafood	116 603 (7)	30 (4)
Milk	108 043 (6)	37 (5)
Other dairy products	8794 (<1)	5 (<1)
Vegetables and fruit	49 642 (<1)	14 (2)
Rice	26 981 (2)	5 (<1)
Complex foods	453 237 (26)	181 (26)
Infected food handlers	67 157 (4)	14 (2)
Total	1 724 316	687

*Based on Adak *et al.* (2005).

EVALUATION

Epidemiological techniques have an important role in the systematic determination of the **effectiveness** (the ability to produce intended or expected results) and **efficiency** (the ability to produce intended results within a minimum time and resource) of any specific activity with respect to pre-agreed goals. This type of activity could be driven locally, but is more likely to be at a national or international level through national public health (such as the HPA) or regulatory (e.g. the Food Standards Agency [FSA]) organizations. This type of activity is outside the scope of this book but could include the effect of interventions to prevent a foodborne pathogen entering the food chain, such as the vaccination of laying flocks to prevent carriage of *Salmonella*.

POLICY DEVELOPMENT

As the study of epidemiology has already been defined to include the 'control of health problems' at the start of this chapter, it is worth a brief discussion of this topic with respect to strategies for controlling foodborne disease and healthcare policy. This activity is carried out by national (e.g. the FSA) and international food regulators such as the EFSA, ECDC, Food and Agriculture Organization of the United Nations (FAO) and the World Health Organization (WHO). Although much of this is outside the scope of this book, it is important to briefly consider one aspect – mathematical modelling including **microbiological risk assessment (MRA)**. A further refinement of an MRA is where models provide a numerical estimate of risk in the form of a probability distribution – a **quantitative microbiological risk assessment (QMRA)**. A brief description of the MRA process is given below and further details of the process can be obtained from the FAO's website (www.fao.org). This is an emerging science which enables mathematically models to be constructed, which characterize **hazards** (biological, chemical or physical agents in food that may have an adverse health effect) to obtain a measure of **risk** (the probability of an adverse affect and the magnitude of that effect consequential to a hazard in food). To generate an MRA, a risk analysis is performed which comprises:

- **Risk assessment:** The evaluation of known or potential health effects resulting from exposure to foodborne hazards. This process is further subdivided into:
  - hazard identification (the identification of known or potential health effects associated with a particular agent)
  - **hazard characterization**, the quantitative or qualitative evaluation of the nature of the adverse health effects, including a dose response (the determination of the relationship between the magnitude of the exposure and the frequency of adverse effects)
  - **exposure assessment**, the qualitative or quantitative evaluation of the degree of intake
  - **risk characterization**, integration of the hazard identification, hazard characterization and exposure assessment into an estimation of the adverse effects including attendant uncertainties.
- **Risk management:** The process of weighing policy alternatives to accept, minimize or reduce assessed risks and select appropriate options.
- **Risk communication:** A process of exchange of information and opinion among risk assessors, risk managers and other interested parties.

QMRAs have had considerable use in formulating policy for food additives, chemical contaminants, pesticide and other residues. However, these have presented considerably more problems when applied to microbial hazards. This is partly because micro-organisms are heterogeneous in their ability to cause disease, even within a species, and can clearly change in concentration within different parts of the food chain because of their ability to grow as well as die. Key to conducting MRAs is the attribution of pathogens to sources and understanding the pathways associated with transmission from source to people. Epidemiological data are important in suggesting which pathogens may be associated with which foods as well as the levels of microbial contamination of the food product at the time of consumption, and the amount of the product consumed at each meal by different members of the population. Epidemiological data are also important in providing information on dose–response relationships especially because, in the absence of animal models, it is often unethical to obtain this by any other route.

MRAs are important to those involved with food regulation in that not only does this process allow an estimation of risk to humans, but this also provides a framework for organization of data and allocating responsibilities for action in dealing with such risks. In addition, MRAs can be used to assess the effects of any interventions, and provide a **cost–benefit analysis** of such interventions. These types of analyses have proved extremely useful for the management of bovine spongiform encephalopathy (BSE) and the consequent variant Creutzfeldt–Jakob disease (vCJD) epidemic, and will be increasingly used for the more common foodborne pathogens.

BURDEN OF ILLNESS

The burden of foodborne illness has been remarkably difficult to estimate and is subject to the degrees of under-reporting discussed previously and illustrated in Figures 6.2 and 6.3 (pp. 117 and 118). The infectious intestinal disease study (IID study) conducted in England between 1993 and 1996 compared cases of gastroenteritis with matched controls (Anon 2000). From this study it was estimated that gastrointestinal infections affected 20 per cent of the population in England each year, comprising 9.5 million cases at a cost of £750 million. The laboratory-based methodology used in the IID study failed to identify a potential aetiological agent or toxin in 49 per cent of the cases. This study provided a valuable benchmark from which to calculate, for example the overall number of days ill, the number of days in hospital and the number of deaths due to different food poisoning agents. An example of such an estimate is given in Table 6.7. From these data it can be estimated that 91 per cent of the hospital bed days and 76 per cent of the total deaths are accounted for by *Salmonella*, *C. perfringens*, *Campylobacter* and *L. monocytogenes*. As with disease attributions and QMRAs, these types of study are very much part of a developing field, however similar approaches have been taken in North American and European countries (Flint *et al.*, 2005), and are also being developed for use in national and international food policy.

Table 6.7 *Estimate of cases of indigenous foodborne diseases in England in 2000 by causes of death*.

Agent	Total (%)	Admissions to hospital (%)	Hospital bed days (%)	Deaths (%)
Salmonella	41 616 (3)	1516 (7)	8 793 (10)	119 (25)
Clostridium perfringens	84 081 (6)	354 (2)	5240 (6)	89 (19)
Campylobacter	359 466 (27)	16 946 (82)	62 701 (71)	86 (18)
Listeria monocytogenes	194 (<1)	194 (1)	3473 (4)	68 (14)
Unknown agents	642 043 (48)	488 (2)	1465 (2)	65 (14)
Escherichia coli O157 (VTEC)	995 (<1)	377 (2)	2149 (2)	22 (5)
Other	152 596 (11)	847 (4)	4581 (5)	22 (5)
Norovirus	57 781 (4)	37 (<1)	143 (<1)	9 (2)
Total	1 338 772	20 759	88 545	480

*Based on Adak *et al.* (2002).

FACTORS CONTRIBUTING TO OUTBREAKS OF FOOD POISONING

In previous chapters, the causes of food poisoning, characteristics of the agents responsible together with their sources or reservoirs and the conditions which allow survival and growth have been considered. It is instructive to consider further what lessons can be learnt from data collected by the HPA from 1900 general outbreaks of food poisoning reported in England and Wales between 1992 and 2005. The outbreaks occurred in a wide variety of settings, the most common being restaurants (26 per cent) and hotels (11 per cent). Table 6.8 shows that 76 per cent of these outbreaks were of bacterial origin, 7 per cent were due to viruses, 3 per cent due to toxin (scombrotoxin), <1 per cent due to parasites (*Cryptosporidium*) and the remaining 14 per cent were either of mixed aetiology, due to other agents or where the food poisoning agent was not known. Half of these outbreaks were due to *Salmonella*: 28 per cent *S.* Enteritidis PT4, 12 per cent other *S.* Enteritidis phage types, 6 per cent *S.* Typhimurium and 5 per cent to other salmonella

Table 6.8 *Food poisoning agents in 1900 general outbreaks of food poisoning in England and Wales, 1992–2005*

Pathogen/toxin	Total (%)
S. Enteritidis PT4	525 (28)
S. Enteritidis Non-PT4	231 (12)
Clostridium perfringens	229 (12)
Norovirus	134 (7)
S. Typhimurium	121 (6)
Other salmonellas	100 (5)
Campylobacter	77 (4)
Scombrotoxin	61 (3)
Verocytotoxin producing *E. coli* O157	49 (3)
B. cereus	45 (2)
S. aureus	34 (2)
B. subtilis	17 (1)
Other or mixed aetiology*	26 (1)
Unknown	251 (13)
Total	1900

* Five or fewer outbreaks including those due to: *Shigella sonnei*, astrovirus, *Cryptosporidium*, *Shigella flexneri*, rotavirus, enteropathogenic *Escherichia coli* other than vero cytotoxin producing *E. coli* O157, *Bacillus* spp. and diarrhoetic shellfish poison (DSP).
Health Protection Agency, unpublished data.

types. Outbreaks can be due to a number of different factors which include:

- infected food handler
- inadequate heat treatment
- cross-contamination
- inappropriate storage including freezing, thawing, refrigeration, warm handling or cooling as well as preparation too far in advance
- and other faults including contaminated raw products, inadequate hygiene and a lack of food safety training.

One or more of these contributory factors was reported in 578 outbreaks (30 per cent) and for more than a third of outbreaks (638; 34 per cent) information on contributing faults was not reported.

The distribution of the contributory factors for the most common pathogens is shown in Table 6.9. Consumption of raw foods such as shell eggs and poultry were mainly associated with *S.* Enteritidis PT4 and in these outbreaks inadequate heat treatment, cross-contamination and inappropriate storage were most often reported. A similar pattern was seen with all other salmonella infections. In outbreaks due to *C. perfringens* multiple factors were frequently recorded with inadequate cooling and reheating playing the most important roles. In norovirus outbreaks, infected food handlers, contamination of raw products (in 'other faults') together with cross-contamination were the most common contributory factors. For *Campylobacter* and VTEC (both low-dose infections), cross-contamination was the most important fault. Inappropriate (refrigerated) storage was the most common fault for scombrotoxin outbreaks. Examples of outbreaks in different settings and food groups as well as for various food poisoning agents are given below.

EXAMPLES OF OUTBREAKS AND INCIDENTS

The final section of this chapter briefly describes outbreaks of food poisoning in a variety of settings where problems occurred at various stages along the food chain. Most of the examples described occurred in the UK. These outbreaks provide examples for a range of the food poisoning agents transmitted via the major food groups together with measures used

Table 6.9 *Contributory factors for the most common food poisoning agents in 1262 general outbreaks of food poisoning in England and Wales, 1992–2005.*

Pathogen/toxin	Fault*				
	Infected food handler (%)	Inadequate heat treatment (%)	Cross-contamination (%)	Inappropriate storage (%)	Other faults (%)
S. Enteritidis PT4	71 (14)	217 (41)	191 (36)	163 (31)	48 (9)
S. Enteritidis Non-PT4	24 (10)	87 (38)	97 (42)	64 (28)	50 (22)
C. perfringens	1 (<1)	81 (35)	14 (6)	100 (44)	18 (8)
Norovirus	48 (36)	10 (7)	18 (13)	6 (4)	23 (17)
S. Typhimurium	18 (15)	30 (25)	53 (44)	32 (26)	15 (12)
Other salmonellas	16 (15)	27 (32)	51 (51)	39 (38)	16 (16)
Campylobacter	1 (1)	21 (27)	37 (48)	9 (12)	10 (13)
Scombrotoxin	0	0	5 (8)	30 (49)	11 (18)
E. coli O157 VTEC	3 (6)	11 (22)	23 (47)	4 (8)	8 (16)
Other and mixed	11 (16)	10 (14)	15 (21)	34 (49)	9 (13)
Unknown	29 (12)	29 (12)	30 (12)	43 (17)	29 (12)

*In 30 per cent of outbreaks more than one fault was identified, therefore each row adds up to more than 100 per cent.
Health Protection Agency, unpublished data.
VTEC, verocytotoxin producing E. coli.

to control the outbreaks and lessons learnt. Some of these outbreaks occurred over 30 years ago and were particularly serious or unusual, but in some the scenarios were typical of deficiencies which were described in the first edition of this book in 1953. Where possible, references for the original descriptions are given for those wishing to obtain further information for each outbreak. Readers may find it helpful to cross-reference with the sections on each of the agents in Chapter 4.

Human reservoir

Contamination from a food handler
In 1996 there was a wedding reception in North Yorkshire where 47 of 111 guests reported illness (predominantly vomiting) within 20–65 hours of attendance (Patterson *et al.* 1997). Laboratory and epidemiological investigations were consistent with **norovirus** infection and the source of the outbreak was traced to a kitchen assistant who vomited into a sink on the day before the wedding which was then used for preparing vegetables. The sink was disinfected with a chlorine-based disinfectant and used for preparation of a potato salad on the following day. This outbreak illustrates the extremely high transmissibility of norovirus together with its survival in the kitchen environment. Vomiting in a food preparation area is an extremely serious incident, indeed transmission may also occur via person-to-person spread as well as airborne transmis-

sion, and any such incidents (as well as any gastro-intestinal illness) should be reported to the manager or proprietor as soon as possible.

Meat products

Contamination of raw product
In 2004, six cases of **trichinellosis** were detected in southern France after a meal of wild boar meat (Gari-Toussaint *et al.* 2005). The meat had been locally hunted, killed and dressed without veterinary control, frozen at −35 °C for 7 days, thawed, cooked and then eaten semi-rare. Samples of frozen meat from the same carcass were subsequently examined and encapsulated *Trichinella britovi* was detected. Given local hunting practices, the risk of trichinellosis from consumption of wild boar is likely to continue in this region of France (wild boar is consumed infrequently in the UK). However, controls for prevention include the recommendation to cook the meat to an internal temperature of 65 °C and to freeze sufficiently to kill this nematode parasite (at least 10 days at −25 °C or 4 weeks at −20 °C).

Contamination of a cooked product from factory sites
Between 1977 and 1989 there was a near doubling in the numbers of cases of **listeriosis** in the whole of the UK (McLauchlin *et al.* 1991). This upsurge consisted of over 355 cases (94 deaths), and was

due to two strains of *L. monocytogenes*. Sampling of pâté during 1989 showed that product from one Belgian manufacturer was much more heavily contaminated with *L. monocytogenes* than similar products from other manufacturers. The isolates from the people affected in this epidemic and from the majority of the contaminated Belgian pâté were indistinguishable. Patients infected by the epidemic types were more likely to have eaten pâté than those infected by other strains. As the epidemic strains of *L. monocytogenes* were recovered from multiple batches of pâté collected nationwide, the most likely source of contamination was from sites within the manufacturing environment, probably after cooking. In June 1989 the manufacturer voluntarily withdrew this product from sale, and this was followed by a rapid decline in the numbers of reported cases and thus the outbreak was controlled. Following outbreaks of listeriosis in Switzerland and the USA associated with the consumption of soft cheese, in 1989 the UK Department of Health issued warnings to the general public advising pregnant women and the immunocompromised not to consume mould-ripened soft cheese. As a result of the outbreak described above, similar warnings were issued to the same groups not to eat pâté. This outbreak highlights the problems of a large public health emergency resulting from the contamination of an internationally produced food product from a food manufacturing environment.

Cross-contamination between raw and cooked product

One of the largest outbreaks of VTEC O157 in the UK was that around Wishaw in Lanarkshire, Scotland, during 1996 (Pennington 2000). Initially a single case of bloody diarrhoea in a 5-year-old child was recognized, which was followed by the recognition of an unusual cluster of a small number of cases in a single laboratory. However it rapidly became clear that a highly unusual occurrence was taking place, in that during November and December a total of 503 cases of infection were recognized with 21 deaths: 279 were microbiologically confirmed as due to the same strain of VTEC O157. Epidemiological and microbiological evidence linked cases with consumption of meat products from a local butcher who both produced and sold these products. The cases were linked not only to retail sales, but also to a lunch in the church hall, a

birthday party in a public house and a nursing home, which were supplied with meat products from this same manufacturer. Following legal proceedings against the manufacturer failures were found in:

- training to employees, including management and supervision to enforce food safety measures
- use of temperature probes to monitor the cooking process and ensuring that meat was cooked to the correct temperatures to eliminate VTEC
- enforcing cleaning schedules in both the shop and factory to prevent cross-contamination
- separating raw and cooked meat products by providing separate knives, tables, scales, vacuum packers, etc.
- provision of a complete list of the places supplied by the butcher to those investigating the outbreak
- local authority inspections.

The outbreak was controlled locally by closure of this manufacturer, recall of product and advice to the public not to consume these products. This outbreak also led to a wider review of food safety policy including legislation, guidance and practices in dealing with food poisoning outbreaks. The review's recommendations included practices and hygiene in premises handling raw and cooked meats that were not subject to approval under the then Meat Products (Hygiene) Regulations 1994. This led to a selective licensing scheme for these premises which came in to force in 2000 where licensing conditions included documentation of Hazard Analysis and Critical Control Points (HACCP), food hygiene training of staff, physical separation of raw meat and unwrapped cooked meat or other food products and (wherever possible) the use of separate staff as requirements to ensure food safety. The new European hygiene legislation in force since 2006 (see Chapter 15) has introduced documentation of HACCP across all food sectors or industries; therefore the licensing scheme for butchers was withdrawn in 2006.

Eggs

Contamination of raw product which was processed frozen

In 2004, 16 guests at a wedding (including the groom) developed **salmonellosis** (Holtby *et al.*,

2006). No problems were identified in the kitchen where the food was prepared and a cohort study established an association between illness and the consumption of 'sesame prawn toast'. None of the food product was available for examination but *S.* Enteritidis PT14b was recovered from the faeces of infected patients. Further typing (plasmid and pulsed-field gel electrophoresis [PFGE] analysis) showed that this bacterium was indistinguishable from isolates from imported Spanish eggs. The sesame prawn toasts were prepared from another manufacturer using raw shell egg, frozen and sold with advice for cooking at 180 °C for 4 minutes from frozen.

Egg and egg products were previously strongly associated with *S.* Enteritidis PT4, but these declined following vaccination of chickens and improvement in the way eggs were sold (Gillespie *et al.*, 2005). The most likely source of *Salmonella* contamination in this outbreak was from imported eggs: this bacterium is likely to survive the freezing process and was probably not destroyed by the insufficient cooking. There was subsequent epidemiological evidence for another outbreak due to this product. Control was by training of kitchen staff in the adequate cooking of this product (together with re-issuing of guidance by the FSA to caterers on proper cooking of egg products) and modification of the process by the manufacturer. In Europe, *Salmonella* is now controlled in the egg production chain under Regulation (EC) No. 1168/2006. Every Member State will have to work towards reducing the number of laying hen holdings contaminated with *Salmonella* by a specific minimum percentage each year, with steeper targets for Member States with higher levels of *Salmonella*. The first target deadline is set for 2008. It is also planned under this Regulation that from January 2010, eggs from *Salmonella*-infected flocks will be treated in a manner that guarantees the elimination of *Salmonella*, e.g. the heat treatment of contaminated eggs. Contaminated eggs will therefore be required to be sent for processing into egg products.

Dairy products

Contamination of raw product

In 1995, 48 of 260 junior school children became ill with diarrhoea, **Cryptosporidium** was detected in the faeces of 16 of 20 children where specimens were available for analysis (Gelletlie *et al.* 1997).

The initial hypothesis for the route of transmission for this outbreak was by more usual routes for this pathogen of contamination of drinking water or swimming pool use. A cohort study was conducted among the children and the only exposure which was significantly associated with illness was drinking school milk. During the period of the outbreak, the school received milk from a small-scale local producer. On inspection there was evidence that the pasteurization plant had not been working correctly prior to this event. This outbreak illustrates the need to consider all possible routes of transmission during outbreak investigations. Microbiological evidence was not available for the aetiological agent for over half of the cases, and this parasite was not detected in the faeces of cows associated with this dairy or from samples of milk, albeit that these were collected after the outbreak was over. The outbreak itself was the result of a point source exposure and therefore ceased without further control measures. However, there was sufficient evidence to prevent repetition of this outbreak by cancelling the contract for supply of milk from this producer.

Toxin produced in an ingredient prior to food manufacture

Yoghurt has a low pH, and hence is a very unusual vehicle for food poisoning. An outbreak of **botulism** occurred in northwest England in 1989, the largest outbreak of this disease recorded in the UK (O'Mahony *et al.* 1990). A 47-year-old woman was admitted to a hospital in northwest England with suspect botulism. Her son had been admitted to a second hospital with suspect Guillain–Barré syndrome where a third patient was suspected to have the same syndrome. During the next day, two more patients were admitted to hospital together with another two children to a third hospital. Four of the patients required ventilation to assist with their respiration. On 10 June a diagnosis of suspect botulism was made in a third child in the third hospital. Preliminary investigations showed that seven of the eight patients had eaten a single brand of hazelnut yoghurt in the week before onset of symptoms: the remaining patient was too ill to be interviewed. On the basis of this information a decision was made to stop the production of all of this producer's yoghurt, to withdraw all products from sale and to advise the general public to avoid this brand of hazelnut yoghurt. Eventually a total of

27 patients were identified aged between 14 months and 74 years, one of which died: none of these had onset of infection after the day following the implementation of control measures. *Clostridium botulinum* toxin type B was detected in:

- a blown can of hazelnut conserve (Figure 6.4)
- opened and unopened cartons of yoghurt
- a specimen of faeces from one of the patient.

The hazelnut conserve was prepared by heating hazelnuts, water, starch and other ingredients to 90 °C for 10 minutes, and then pumping the mixture into cans which were sealed and heated in boiling water for 20 minutes. The cans were stored at room temperature and added to yoghurt mixtures prior to dispensing into cartons.

This outbreak illustrates the result of successful communication between clinical and microbiological colleagues together with implementation by food regulators of appropriate interventions for the control of a public health emergency. The appropriate interventions were made on the basis of brief descriptive information and resulted in the prompt withdrawal of implicated food. It also illustrates the potential for an unusual food to act as a vehicle of infection. Failures in the processes of preparing the hazelnut conserve were: insufficient heat treatment to kill *C. botulinum* spores and inadequate preservation to prevent the subsequent growth of this bacterium. This was combined with a failure to recognize a faulty product indicated by the blowing of the can: the production of gas in canned products is usually due to microbial growth which should be

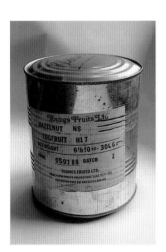

Figure 6.4 *Blown can of hazelnut conserve associated with an outbreak of botulism in 1989*

easily recognized by this yoghurt manufacturer as unsatisfactory and potentially hazardous.

Contamination during a manufacturing process

There was an unusual increase in the numbers of *Salmonella* Ealing infections recognized in the national reference laboratory during 1985 (Rowe et al. 1987). Forty-one cases were reported during November and December: the annual totals had been between 23 and 52 over the previous four years. Among the 76 cases detected between January 1985 and January 1986, there were a high proportion of infants. A case–control study was performed among the infants and there was a highly significant association between consumption of infant formula dried milk from a single manufacturer and illness. S. Ealing was isolated in low numbers from 4 of 267 sealed packets and the product was withdrawn from sale. Production at the factory ceased and the source of contamination was traced to a hole in the inner lining of the spray dryer allowing escape of powder and its return from contaminated insulation material. Although the source of contamination was never established, the top of the dryer was constructed from interlocking steel plates which could allow liquid to contaminate the insulation material. It is possible that water from a partly covered water-tank or bird dropping on the roof of the building contaminated this equipment. The factory was not able to eradicate this Salmonella contamination and did not resume commercial production. This outbreak highlights the result of a single problem in a food manufacturing process. It also demonstrates the need to obtain basic details of the affected patients, in this instance, and for analysis of a centrally held national database on typing data. This is vitally important since considerations of the diet of this patient group dramatically reduced the food types considered for investigation.

Cross-contamination between unpasteurized and pasteurized products

Outbreaks in hospitals can be particularly problematic because of the large groups of patients in close contact with each other as well as with staff and visitors in an enclosed environment. These patients are often highly susceptible to infection as well as already being acutely ill, and the risk of cross-contamination and secondary spread is higher than in many community settings. In May 1997, three elderly in-patients in a 557-bed district general hospital in Scotland were identified who became unwell with mild gastroenteritis. VTEC O157 was detected in their stools (O'Brien *et al.* 2001). Infection control measures were immediately instituted and an outbreak control team (OCT) meeting was convened on the day of diagnosis. A total of 886 stool samples were collected from staff, patients and community contacts and screened for the bacterium. Thirty-seven individuals were found to be excreting the bacterium (these were the same rare phage type 8 and VT1+ VT2+), and 12 individuals had enteric symptoms: overall 16 were in-patients, 11 were staff and 10 cases occurred in the community. Except for two of the community carriers, all individuals with the VTEC in their stool had attended a concert in the hospital. There was a strong relationship between the occurrence of infection and the consumption of home-baked cream-filled cakes prepared in a domestic kitchen, which had been brought to the party. Pasteurized cream and milk were used in the preparation of the fresh cream, but the owner of the kitchen also obtained unpasteurized milk from a farm where the same type of VTEC was detected in the faeces of dairy cattle. Although the exact route of contamination could not be determined, the most likely scenario was cross-contamination in the kitchen. Despite the age of the patients (mean 82 years) there were no deaths, and no secondary infections were detected within the hospital. This outbreak highlights the need for rapid investigation of outbreaks to prevent secondary spread as well as problems with the introduction of domestically prepared food into hospitals.

Fish and shellfish

Contamination with a toxin prior to harvest
In 1997, 49 people presented with acute-onset (within 30 minutes) nausea, vomiting and abdominal pain, together with feeling feverish for more that 8 hours. All patients had eaten mussels in two London restaurants (Scoging and Bahl 1998). Diarrhoetic shellfish poisoning (DSP) toxin was detected at 25–37 µg/100 g of mussel flesh collected from the restaurants. The mussels were produced in the UK. As normal cooking does not inactivate these types of toxins, the critical control point is the quality of the raw food component and

the waters of shellfish beds. Control of the DSP intoxications involved withdrawal of batches of contaminated product (which had already been consumed by the time this outbreak had occurred) as well as by the monitoring of shellfish and shellfish harvesting beds with their closure when contamination occurs. No more cases of intoxication were identified with subsequent shellfish harvested from the implicated beds when they were re-opened.

Contamination of raw product which is eaten without cooking
In January 2004, 22 adults reported vomiting and/or diarrhoea, 6–36 hours after consumption of raw oysters (Gallimore *et al.* 2005). Norovirus was detected in the faeces of the affected patients, however no oysters were available for microbiological testing. No other sources of infection were identified. The oysters were produced in Northern Ireland in grade A beds (i.e. live bivalve molluscs collected from these beds must meet the health standards laid down in Regulation [EC] No. 853/2004 and can therefore be collected for direct human consumption) and had been depurated for 42 hours prior to shipping on ice. Prior to shipping, the oysters had passed the standard bacteriological tests for *Listeria*, *Salmonella*, *E. coli*, *Vibrio*, total coliforms and total viable count. This outbreak highlights the problem with a product that is eaten raw and was contaminated with virus despite the absence of a bacteriological indication of faecal contamination. The critical control point for such products is the point of production, and all reasonable steps must be taken to prevent faecal contamination.

Incomplete cooking, cross-contamination, and poor temperature and time control
In 1997, a cluster of a rare *Salmonella* type (*S. Enteritidis* phage type 19) was isolated from the stools of four patients in the Poole Public Health Laboratory. Eventually eight people were recognized, who became ill with severe diarrhoea and vomiting (one was admitted to hospital) within 24 hours after consumption of cooked cockles (Greenwood *et al.* 1998). All of the patients obtained their cockles from a fish and chip shop (three of the cases were the owner of the shop, and her son and daughter) where some of the shellfish were displayed at room temperature. *S. Enteritidis* phage type 19 was isolated from the faeces of all patients and another case was identified but from

which no further information could be obtained. No cockles were available for microbiological examination by the time the outbreak was investigated. The supplier reported collecting a large batch of cockles from an unclassified bed in a large harbour and these were boiled in several batches using a large domestic saucepan. It was not possible for the manufacturer to specify the time or temperature of cooking. Hence the heat treatment of some of these batches may have been inadequate and cross-contamination between batches may have occurred. As this type of S. Enteritidis is unusual in the UK, the most likely source of contamination was sewage discharge from a ship in the harbour. However, this bacterium was not recovered from the harbour sea water, albeit that this was collected 10–21 days after the outbreak. As illness occurred in one case after having only 'tasted' the cockles, these may have been heavily contaminated, and this is consistent with growth of the bacterium resulting from poor temperature control after cooking. This outbreak would not have been recognized if it had been due to a common S. Enteritidis type. Control measures for the outbreak were to provide advice on safe cooking and handling of shellfish through a press release and local radio broadcast. In addition, written advice was sent to all local restaurants, pubs, clubs, takeaways, hotels and guest houses about the hazards of buying shellfish from casual traders.

Contamination during processing and toxin production prior to consumption

In 1978 four elderly people in the UK developed botulism after consuming Alaskan-produced tinned salmon. Despite treatment with antitoxin, two of the patients died. The diagnosis of botulism was confirmed by the detection of C. botulinum type E toxin in the serum of all four patients. Gram-positive rods and spores were detected in stained preparations of the remnants of the tinned salmon, and C. botulinum type E as well as type E toxin were detected. There was no evidence of under-processing (heating) at the factory. The implicated tin of salmon had been produced about a year before consumption and contained a defect which resulted in a small hole in the seam (Figure 6.5). This hole allowed contamination of the contents, probably from the factory because C. botulinum type E is common in marine environments. This bacterium had clearly grown in the contents of the can, and being non-proteolytic (unable to break down proteins) did not produce gas or visible taints to make the product unpalatable. There was only a single defective can identified in the batch produced, and no other cases of botulism were detected. This outbreak highlights the potential for fatal food poisoning from a single defect in an otherwise safe manufacturing process.

Poor temperature and time control after cooking

In 1975, 56 of 219 guests at a dinner became ill after 9–12 hours with a diarrhoeal illness for 1–3 days (Hewitt et al. 1986). At the dinner, cold salmon salad, roast beef in gravy and lemon meringue pie with cream had been served. Food remnants were available for analysis and no potential bacterial pathogens were detected except for high numbers of C. perfringens in the samples of salmon. High

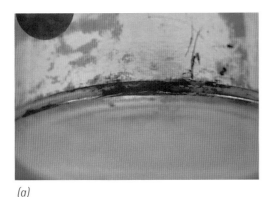

(a)

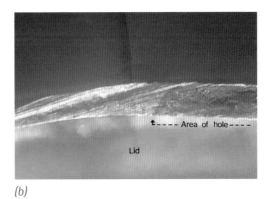

(b)

Figure 6.5   Can which contained salmon associated with an outbreak of botulism in 1978. (a) Outside of can showing defect in seam. (b) Cut section through seam showing hole which allowed material to enter and contaminate the can

levels of *C. perfringens* were also detected in the faeces of eight of the ill patients: no other pathogens were detected. The salmon were prepared by wrapping them in foil, placing them in boiling water for 30 minutes, leaving them to cool overnight at ambient temperature and served the next day at lunch time following skinning and portioning. The evidence for the aetiological agent comes from samples submitted from a small proportion of all those affected, however this diagnosis is consistent with the incubation period for *C. perfringens* food poisoning. This bacterium is most often associated with poor temperature and time control of meat and poultry dishes, however, this outbreak serves as a reminder that other food types can be associated with transmission. The route of transmission was obtained by a descriptive study alone. Catering for large functions (weddings, institutional meals etc.) can be problematic, and good catering practices are essential to prevent outbreaks. As the outbreak was already over by the time the investigation was started, control was not possible in this instance. However, this highlights the importance of identifying poor catering practices and communicating this information to those involved in the production and serving of food at these types of events.

Poor temperature and time control

Two examples illustrate that poor temperature control can occur throughout the food chain and result in scombrotoxin food poisoning. In these examples, problems occurred either at the point of production in the food factory or where the food was prepared. The first example occurred in London in three outbreaks occurred at restaurants in 1995 (McLauchlin *et al.* 2006). In the first outbreak four people became ill, and developed a rash and dizziness within an hour of eating a meal including cooked tuna steaks. The histamine in fresh tuna steaks collected from the restaurant was found to be greater than 331 mg/100 g (which is toxic). In the second outbreak, 16 people were ill with headache and rash 1 hour after consuming cooked fresh tuna steaks which were found to contain 595 mg of histamine per 100 g. In the final outbreak two people were ill with a rash, vomiting and burning mouth after 2 hours: histamine in fresh tuna steaks was detected at 170 mg/100 g. All three outbreaks were associated with the same batch of vacuum-packed tuna which was produced and frozen at a

factory in Sri Lanka. All tuna from this factory was withdrawn. Spoilage occurred at the factory which was closed prior to institution of better processing (refrigeration) procedures.

The second (unrelated) example also occurred in London, in 1997 when seven office workers reported headache, rash and diarrhoea, 1 hour after eating tuna sandwiches bought from a sandwich bar at about 1 pm. The sandwiches were prepared at 6 am and tuna remnants from a can, tuna/mayonnaise mix as well as sandwich on display all contained more than 245 mg/100 g histamine. However, because unopened cans from the same batch all contained less than 3.9 mg/100 g of histamine, spoilage resulting from poor temperature control had occurred in the sandwich bar. Prevention of subsequent outbreaks was by improved temperature and time control procedures.

Vegetables, salads, fruit and grain products

Contamination during harvest

In 1983 a banquet was held for 10 people in a hotel in Scotland. Raspberry mousse was served at the banquet, and six of eight people who consumed this developed jaundice 24–38 days later, which was subsequently confirmed as due to hepatitis A virus (Reid and Robinson 1987). The two exposed individuals who did not develop illness were shown to have antibodies against the virus and were therefore immune. Fifteen members of the hotel staff also became ill, two of whom denied eating the mousse. Nine secondary cases were identified including four members of the public, who dined at the hotel approximately a month after the mousse had been served when the outbreak among the staff was at its height. Additional cases arose in a waitress and four family members of one of the primary cases. The supplier of the raspberries had purchased frozen berries from the producer, and this product had been implicated in a previous outbreak. Fruit was picked by itinerant workers who lived on caravan sites which had poor toilet facilities. At peak fruit picking times, outbreaks of hepatitis A among the workers were common. This outbreak illustrates the survival of a foodborne pathogen when the product is frozen and the importance of eliminating contaminated product identified as a problem in the first outbreak to prevent further cases of infection. It also illustrates the long incubation period of some pathogens, and the need to control secondary spread from primary cases infected from food. The outbreak was controlled by exclusion of affected staff from work when ill, and training of the food handlers (including the fruit pickers) in hygienic practices when dealing with food.

Contamination prior to harvest

Soft fruit (in this instances raspberries) was also involved with a series of large outbreaks of cyclosporiasis in the USA and Canada during the mid-1990s. During 1996, 1465 cases of cyclosporiasis were detected in 20 states in the USA and in Canada (Herwald *et al.* 1997). *Cyclospora cayetanensis* is a protozoan parasite which is specific to humans, and, in northern Europe and North America, is particularly associated with recent foreign travel to the Indian subcontinent, the Far East, Central and South America. However, among the large numbers of cases, foreign travel was not identified as a risk factor. Illness was associated with consumption of raspberries grown in Guatemala from as few as five farms. This outbreak illustrates the effect of global sourcing of food where contamination of a food product in one country resulted in the 'export' of food poisoning over very large geographical areas. The outbreak was initially controlled by an import ban on soft fruit to the USA from Guatemala. Although the exact source of contamination was not totally explained, the use of sewage-contaminated water for irrigation as well as for preparation of insecticide and fungicide sprays was suspected as the contamination route. Longer-term control was achieved by the improvement of water quality used in these agricultural environments.

Contamination prior to harvest

Salad products have also been involved with foodborne outbreaks. In 2000, 361 cases of **Salmonella** Typhimurium phage type 104 were detected in England and Wales (Hortby *et al.* 2003). Although the cases were distributed over most of the country, a third of the cases occurred in the Midlands. The *S.* Typhimurium was unusual in that it was resistant to six different antibiotics. A case–control study was performed and 22 cases and 52 controls were interviewed by telephone (see Table 6.4, p. 128). Several food items eaten away from the home were initially significantly associated with illness:

following a final multivariable analysis, chicken in Indian restaurants ($P = 0.05$) and lettuce ($P = 0.0006$) eaten outside the home in fast-food restaurants were significantly associated with illness.

This investigation therefore identified lettuce as the most likely vehicle for infection, however because of the short shelf-life of salad products it was not possible to acquire any salad products for microbiological analysis. In addition, because of complexities in the food supply chain, no individual farm was identified with producing the salad. The numbers of cases due to this *S.* Typhimurium type peaked between August and September after which there was a rapid decline in their number. Although the exact mechanism for contamination was not identified, the following were considered possible routes:

- use of contaminated water for irrigation
- use of contaminated water to apply pesticides or other dressings
- use of human or animal sewage as a fertilizer
- use of contaminated water to wash crops once harvested
- transport of harvested crops in a contaminated vehicle or storage system.

This outbreak illustrates that microbiological and epidemiological evidence for the exact source of infection and vehicle is often not obtained and that outbreaks can end without any specific preventive action being taken. However, it is extremely important that these are investigated and any lessons learnt are communicated so that they might prevent the future occurrence of similar episodes.

Contamination during manufacture and production of toxin

In Italy in 1984, a family outbreak of acute **staphylococcal food poisoning** was reported (Woolaway *et al.* 1986). This was followed shortly by cases in Luxembourg and France and 47 cases were identified in at least 10 sites in England and Wales. As the largest cluster (30 cases) occurred in a girls' boarding school, a cohort study was conducted at this single site. The cases presented with nausea, abdominal pain, vomiting, loss of appetite, headache, diarrhoea and fever within 4 hours of an evening meal, and there were significant associations between illness and consumption of pasta ($P<0.0006$) and 'chipsteak' ($P = 0.05$). Microbiological analysis of samples of the implicated dried pasta found the pasta to be contaminated with staphylococcal enterotoxin type A as well as high levels of *Staphylococcus aureus*. These outbreaks were therefore likely to be due to pasta contaminated at the factory. Pasta is an unusual food vehicle for food poisoning, although, as demonstrated here, heat stable toxins are likely to survive normal cooking of this product. The ingredients of the pasta included wheat, water, egg, and it was dried slowly at 'warm temperatures' when presumably the *S. aureus* (most likely introduced from a food handler) was able to grow. On subsequent storage of the pasta, the toxin remained (and presumably biologically active) while the bacterium no longer remained viable. The implicated batches of pasta were withdrawn from sale across different European countries. Following improved hygiene and processes in the factory there was no recurrence of this problem. This outbreak illustrates the potential for food poisoning incidents to occur across national borders and the need for international surveillance and alerts.

Poor handling after cooking

In Finland in 1975, 18 people became ill within 2 hours of consuming a warm meal of meat, rice and vegetables (Raevuori *et al.* 1976). The warm portions had been packaged in cardboard boxes two days previously and stored in a refrigerator prior to regeneration by microwave cooking. In the food samples from the central kitchen, high levels of **Bacillus cereus** were detected in the rice ($>10^8$ CFU/g) and in the meat (10^6 CFU/g). No other pathogens were detected. The short incubation period here suggest a microbiological toxin, and *B. cereus* seems the most likely agent since this bacterium was present in high numbers and no other pathogens (particularly *S. aureus*) were detected in samples of the food. For unequivocal attribution of the infective agent, *B. cereus* emetic toxin should have been detected in a sample of the implicated food.

Cooked rice was first recognized as a cause of food poisoning through contamination with *B. cereus* in 1971. *B. cereus* can give rise to two distinct forms of foodborne disease, the emetic and diarrhoeal syndromes. Evidence from England and Wales and other countries indicates that food poisoning attributed to enterotoxigenic *B. cereus* continues to occur in association with the con-

sumption of cooked rice, particularly from Chinese or Indian take-away restaurants. In this outbreak, refrigeration was likely to have been poor because the warm rice was packaged in cardboard boxes: refrigeration will not inactivate the *B. cereus* emetic toxin. Control of this outbreak was not possible as all cases had resolved by the time of investigation. However, the use of rice of good microbiological quality and improved temperature and time control of the cooked product should prevent recurrences.

Beverages

Contamination of raw product

Contamination of beverages represents similar hazards to those of contaminated food. Two examples are given here of contamination of raw product of beverages.

In 1991 in Massachusetts, USA, 23 cases of **VTEC O157** infection occurred: 22 had diarrhoea (16 bloody diarrhoea, and four haemolytic uraemic syndrome) (Besser *et al.* 1993). Six patients were hospitalized. A case–control study was performed and a significant association was found between the disease and consumption of fresh pressed apple juice (known as cider in Massachusetts). VTEC was not detected in any sample of apple juice. Ninety per cent of the apples were 'drops' (collected from the ground) and were not washed prior to milling. The most likely source of contamination was from cattle which also lived on the same farm where the juice was produced. Recommendations were given to prevent further occurrence by improved hygiene (including washing applies prior to pressing), pasteurization of the pressed juice, and addition of sodium benzoate.

In 1974, a total of 2467 hospitalized cases and 48 deaths due to **cholera** occurred in the Lisbon area of Portugal (Blake *et al.* 1977). A case–control study showed that there was a strong association with consumption of a single manufacturer's bottled water: the cases were found to have either consumed bottled water, visited the spa or worked at the spa within 5 days of symptoms. The source of contamination was suspected to be at the source through the limestone aquifer, either from surface rainwater or via a nearby river. The outbreak was controlled by ceasing production from the spring, by drilling a new spring at higher altitude and using ultraviolet irradiation prior to bottling the water.

Summary

Epidemiology provides the evidence base for the control of food poisoning and the application of good food hygiene practices by the collection, analysis and interpretation of data on the occurrence of foodborne disease. This process includes co-ordination and communication between a wide range of professions involved with the safety of food, including clinical and food microbiologists, epidemiologists, medical doctors, veterinarians, environmental health officers, food and public health regulators, food manufacturers, wholesalers, retailers, statisticians, mathematical modellers, etc., as well as the final consumer, i.e. members of the public. The roles of epidemiological investigations in preventing food poisoning are:

- providing and interpreting surveillance data
- determining the causes of food poisoning
- ensuring that the correct interventions are implemented for individual outbreaks and incidents and assessing the effect of these interventions
- ensuring that information is available to food regulators at national and international levels to influence control strategies and healthcare policy.

All websites cited in this chapter and given below were accessed in March 2007.

SOURCES OF INFORMATION AND FURTHER READING

Adak GK, Long SM, O'Brien SJ (2002) Trends in indigenous foodborne diseases and deaths in England and Wales: 1992 to 2000. *Gut* **51**: 832–41.

Adak GK, Meakins SM, Yip H, *et al.* (2005) Disease risks from foods, England and Wales, 1996–2000. *Emerg Infect Dis* **11**: 365–72.

Anon (2000) *A Report of the Study of Infectious Intestinal Diseases in England*. London: The Stationery Office.

Ball AP, Hopkinson RB, Farrell ID, *et al.* (1979) Human botulism caused by *Clostridium botulinum* type E: the Birmingham outbreak. Q *J Med* **191**: 473–91.

Besser RE, Lett SM, Weber JT, *et al.* (1993) An outbreak of diarrhea and hemolytic uremic syndrome from *Escherichia coli* O157:H7 in fresh pressed apple cider. *JAMA* **269**: 2217–20.

Blake PA, Rosenberg ML, Florencia J, *et al.* (1977) Cholera in Portugal, 1974. *Am J Epidemiol* **105**: 344–8.

Bradford Hill A (1965) The environment and disease: association or causation? *Proc R Soc Med* **58**: 295–300.

Flint JA, van Duynhoven YT, Angulo FJ, *et al.* (2005) Estimating the burden of acute gastroenteritis, foodborne diseases and pathogens commonly transmitted by food: an international review. *Clin Infect Dis* **41**: 698–704.

Gallimore CI, Cheesebrough JS, Lamden K, *et al.* (2005) Multiple norovirus genotypes characterised from an oyster-associated outbreak of gastroenteritis. *Int J Food Microbiol* **103**: 323–30.

Gari-Toussaint M, Tieulié N, Baldin JL, *et al.* (2005) Human trichinellosis due to *Trichinella britovi* in southern France after consumption of frozen wild boar meat. *Eurosurveillance* **10**: 117–18.

Gelletlie R, Stuart J, Soltanpoor N, *et al.* (1997) Cryptosporidiosis associated with school milk. *Lancet* **350**:1005–6.

Gillespie IA, O'Brien SJ, Adak GK, *et al.* (2005) Foodborne general outbreaks of *Salmonella* Enteritidis phage type 4 infection, England and Wales 1992–2002: where are the risks. *Epidemiol Infect* **133**: 795–801.

Greenwood M, Winnard G, Bagot B (1998) An outbreak of *Salmonella enteritidis* phage type 19 infection associated with cockles. *Commun Dis Public Health* **1**: 35–7.

Herwald BL, Ackers ML, the *Cyclospora* Working Group (1997) An outbreak in 1996 of cyclosporiasis associated with imported raspberries. *N Engl J Med* **336**: 1548–56.

Hewitt JH, Begg N, Hewish J, *et al.* (1986) Large outbreaks of *Clostridium perfringens* food poisoning associated with consumption of boiled salmon. *Epidemiol Infect* **97**: 71–80.

Hobbs BC, Smith ME, Oakley CL, *et al.* (1953) *Clostridium welchii* food poisoning. *J Hyg* **51**: 75–101.

Holtby I, Tebbutt GM, Anwar S, *et al.* (2006) Two separate outbreaks of *Salmonella enteritidis* phage type 14b food poisoning linked to the consumption of the same type of frozen food. *Public Health* **120**: 817–23.

Hortby PW, O'Brien SJ, Adak GK, *et al.* (2003) A national outbreak of multi-resistant *Salmonella enterica* serovar Typhimurium definitive phage type (DT) 104 associated with consumption of lettuce. *Epidemiol Infect* **130**: 169–78.

Last JM (ed.) (2001) *A Dictionary of Epidemiology*, 4th edition. New York: Oxford University Press.

McLauchlin J, Hall SM, Velani S, Gilbert RJ (1991) Human listeriosis and pâté: a possible association. *BMJ* **303**: 773–5.

McLauchlin J, Little CL, Grant KA, Mithani V (2006) Scombrotoxic fish poisoning. *J Public Health* **28**: 61–2.

Nichols GL (2005) Fly transmission of *Campylobacter. Emerg Infect Dis* **11**: 361–4.

O'Brien SJ, Murdoch PS, Riley AH, *et al.* (2001) A foodborne outbreak of Vero cytotoxin-producing *Escherichia coli* O157:H-phage type 8 in hospital. *J Hosp Infect* **49**: 167–72.

O'Brien SJ, Elson R, Gillespie IA, *et al.* (2002) Surveillance of foodborne outbreaks of infectious intestinal disease in England and Wales 1992–1999: contribution to evidence-based food policy? *Public Health* **116**: 75–80.

O'Mahony M, Mitchell E, Gilbert RJ, *et al.* (1990) An outbreak of foodborne botulism associated with contaminated hazelnut yoghurt. *Epidemiol Infect* **104**: 389–95.

Patterson W, Haswell P, Fryers PT, Green J (1997) Outbreak of small round structured virus gastrointenteritis arose after kitchen assistant vomited. *Commun Dis Rep* **7**: R101–3.

Pennington TH (2000) VTEC: lessons learned from British outbreaks. *J Appl Bacteriol* **88**: 90S–8S.

Raevuori M, Kiutamo T, Niskanen A, Salmenen K (1976) An outbreak of *Bacillus cereus* food-poisoning in Finland associated with boiled rice. *J Hyg* **76**: 319–27.

Reid TMS, Robinson HG (1987) Frozen raspberries and hepatitis A. *Epidemiol Infect* pp. 109–12.

Rowe B, Begg NT, Hutchinson DN, *et al.* (1987) *Salmonella Ealing* infections associated with consumption of infant dried milk. *Lancet* **ii**: 900–3.

Scoging A, Bahl M (1998) Diarrhetic shellfish poisoning in the UK. *Lancet* **352**: 117.

US Department of Health and Human Services. Principles of Epidemiology in Public Health Practice: An introduction to applied epidemiology and biostatistics, 3rd edn. Self Study Course SS1000 (available from: http://www.cdc.gov/mmwr/preview/mmwrhtml/mm5542a5.htm).

Woolaway MC, Bartlett CLR, Wieneke AA, *et al.* (1986) International outbreak of staphylococcal food poisoning caused by contaminated lasagne. *J Hyg* **96**: 67–73.

Wall PG, de Louvois J, Gilbert RJ, Rowe B (1996) Food poisoning: notifications, laboratory reports and outbreaks – where do the statistics come from and what do they mean? *Commun Dis Public Health* **7**: R93–100.

7

Water supply, waterborne infection and sewage/sludge disposal

Gordon Nichols

Water as the most important food resource	146	Standards and legislation	155
Worldwide burden of disease related to water for drinking and agricultural use	148	Sewage, animal waste and risk	160
		Problems with *Cryptosporidium*	162
Disease emergence related to water, food and food animals	149	Water use in food production, retail and households	164
Infections transmitted through water	149	Summary	165
Contamination of foods by water	153	Sources of information and further reading	165

Water is a universal requirement for organic life and is essential for survival. Water is also used in the removal of waste and its treatment. The treatment of sewage and other wastes is important in ensuring drinking water supplies are not a source of diarrhoeal diseases. In developed countries water treatment has resulted in supplies being relatively safe from contamination but cryptosporidiosis is still an important infection in these countries. Where chlorination or other disinfection is not used there is a risk of infection. Contaminated drinking water and poor levels of sanitation are still an important cause of morbidity and mortality, particularly among young children.

Drinking water Water used for drinking and other purposes.

Private water supply Water coming from sources other than a water company or utility, often small scale and usually not from an extensive supply distribution network.

Sewage Waste matter from domestic or industrial establishments which is carried away in a sewer.

WATER AS THE MOST IMPORTANT FOOD RESOURCE

Water is required for life and, besides **drinking water**, it is used for cleaning and preparing food, bathing, washing clothes and equipment, flushing waste, irrigating crops, extinguishing fires, swimming, transporting goods and people, and in manufacturing goods and generating energy. The quality and quantity of the water provided by **utilities** (the supply services for water) can strongly influence the economic and physical health of communities. This is a key reason why most towns and cities are located close to rivers. Because water is so important to human life there are strong environmental laws to ensure contamination of natural environments and surface and underground water reserves are controlled.

People require water on a daily basis and can survive extended starvation but not sustained lack of water (Ukety 1993). There are a variety of water-related diseases associated with infections and toxins, and these are summarized in Table 7.1. There is a direct effect of wastewaters on drinking water, thus this chapter examines the water we drink and the waste we produce. Disease related to recreational and other water use will only be discussed as it relates to food contamination.

Table 7.1 *Types of water-related problems and disease associated with infectious agents and microbial toxins*

Type of water-related problem	Nature of disease	Example of agents or diseases
Waterborne	Water passively transmitting the agent	Cholera, typhoid, cryptosporidiosis
Water washed	Diseases due to insufficient water	Trachoma, scabies, shigella dysentery
Water based	Diseases where the pathogen completes its lifecycle in water	Dracontiasis, schistosomiasis, diphyllobothriasis, gnathostomiasis
Water vectored	Diseases transmitted by insects which breed in water	Yellow fever, dengue, filariasis, malaria, onchocerciasis, sleeping sickness
Fish- or shellfish-related infections	Diseases where the agent is consumed in or acquired from seafood	*Vibrio parahaemolyticus, Vibrio vulnificus,* viral gastroenteritis
Wound contamination	Contamination of damaged skin or wounds from water or aquatic organisms	*Aeromonas hydrophila, Mycobacterium marinum*
Foods containing water	Diseases where food or drinks are made from contaminated water	Cryptosporidiosis, cyclosporiasis
Foods contaminated by water	Diseases where food or milk is contaminated by infected irrigation or processing water	Typhoid, dysentery, salmonellosis
Airborne infection	Diseases where a waterborne agent is transmitted by aerosol	Legionnaire's disease
Airborne toxicosis	Disease where exposure is due to an aerosolized microbial toxin	Dinoflagellate blooms
Cyanobacterial disease	Diseases associated with consumption of or contact with cyanobacteria or their toxins	*Microcystis aeruginosa, Schizothrix calcicola, Anabaena flos-aquae*
Dinoflagellate- and diatom-related diseases	Diseases resulting from the accumulation of dinoflagellate toxins in shellfish and fish	Ciguatera poisoning, diarrhoetic shellfish poisoning, neurotoxic shellfish poisoning, paralytic shellfish poisoning
Recreationally acquired infection	Diseases associated with immersion in water	Pseudomonas dermatitis, fish tank granuloma, amoebic meningoencephalitis, leptospirosis, legionnaire's disease
Opportunistic waterborne infections	Infections acquired from water which affects people with impaired immunity	*Mycobacterium* spp.
Drowning related infections	Respiratory infections following near-drowning incidents	Aeromonas respiratory tract infection
Occupationally acquired infection	Diseases associated with particular occupations	Leptospirosis, schistosomiasis
Contamination of water for injection	Diseases associated with the injection of non-sterile water	*Clostridium botulinum, Clostridium novyi*
Water contamination of devices	Infections acquired from the use of dialysis machines, contact lenses, syringes, respirators etc.	Dialysis related cyanobacterial toxicosis, *Mycobacterium* spp., Enterobacteriaceae, acanthamoeba
Water excess	Diseases due to too much water, as in a flood	*Vibrio cholerae,* Enterotoxigenic *E. coli*
Damp conditions	Diseases due to living in conditions where it is damp	*Stachybotrys chartarum*
Food stored damp	Storage of food in damp conditions	Mycotoxins (e.g. aflatoxin, patulin, ochratoxin)

WORLDWIDE BURDEN OF DISEASE RELATED TO WATER FOR DRINKING AND AGRICULTURAL USE

Water has been a prominent source of human infectious disease throughout history, causing large outbreaks of diarrhoeal disease and all too frequently death. The pathogens implicated in waterborne outbreaks over the past century have changed in response to:

- changes in human activity
- improved sewerage and drinking water systems
- increased recreational water activity
- improved diagnostic techniques
- a greater understanding of waterborne disease.

A review of the burden of disease attributable to selected environmental factors and injury among children and adolescents in European countries in 2001 found that in young children, diarrhoea attributable to inadequate water and sanitation accounted for 5.3 per cent of deaths and 3.5 per cent of **disability-adjusted life years (DALYs;** Valent *et al.* 2004). In developing countries morbidity and mortality can be high and the outcome of infection is worse when children have underlying malnutrition. In addition, there is a substantial worm burden derived from food, water and poor hygiene in many developing countries, and these infections can impair both physical and mental development as well as reduce the ability to work in adults. Pruss *et al.* (2002) estimated the worldwide disease burden from water, sanitation and hygiene to be 4.0 per cent of all deaths and 5.7 per cent of the total disease burden (in DALYs) worldwide, taking into account diarrhoeal diseases, schistosomiasis, trachoma, ascariasis, trichuriasis and hookworm disease.

The pandemics of cholera in the nineteenth and twentieth centuries (Table 7.2) were not exclusively as a result of contaminated drinking water, but water has played a major part, along with contaminated seafood, in the epidemiology of this disease. Epidemic cholera in India and Bangladesh in 1992 was caused by a new strain of toxigenic *Vibrio cholerae* O139 Bengal. This has spread throughout Southern Asia but is not yet a pandemic. Similarly, typhoid outbreaks that result from contaminated water are uncommon in all developed countries, but remain a serious problem in some developing countries.

A large burden of illness and death in the world today derives from agents that cause diarrhoea, even though diarrhoeal infections are now much less common in developed countries because of improved drinking water treatment, sewage disposal systems and public health infrastructure. However, they still cause significant morbidity and mortality in developing countries, particularly in association with war, flooding and population movements. The lack of adequate drinking water facilities in both urban and rural communities, together with high level of diarrhoeal infections, poor systems of waste

Table 7.2 *The seven pandemics of cholera*

First pandemic	1817–1823 Asiatic Cholera originated near Calcutta and spread to south-east Asia, China and Japan but did not reach Europe
Second pandemic	1826–1837, began in Bengal and spread through India. Cholera entered UK in 1831 (31 000 died)
Third pandemic	1846–1863, reached Europe and the USA in 1848. John Snow observed during the 1848 London epidemic that the disease was spread by contaminated water
Fourth pandemic	1863–1866, spread first to the Middle East, then to the Mediterranean and on to New York. Tens of thousands died, but public health reforms moderated the death toll
Fifth pandemic	1881–1896, improved sanitation, diagnosis and quarantine kept it from reaching many European cities and the USA. Robert Koch discovered that *Vibrio cholerae* caused the disease
Sixth pandemic	1899–1923, also affecting Asia but failing to reach western European cities or the USA, again due to developments in water treatment and sanitation
Seventh pandemic	1961–present, began in Indonesia and reached Peru and neighbouring countries. It continues with periodic outbreaks in many areas of the world. The outbreak in Peru partly resulted from a halt in drinking water chlorination

disposal and poor standards of hygiene, contribute to high rates of diarrhoeal disease in young children. Deaths following infection among infants and young children are usually due to dehydration or anaemia resulting from worm burden. Adults usually get infected through contaminated water and food, although there is a substantial degree of immunity to the commoner intestinal infections, along with a higher rate of asymptomatic carriage of enteric pathogens where waste disposal is poor.

In developed countries, although the classic waterborne pathogens have become less important, new concerns have arisen. During the past 30 years a range of new pathogens, such as *Campylobacter* and *Legionella* (the cause of Legionnaire's disease), have been identified as waterborne. The protozoan *Cryptosporidium* is increasingly being recognized as a problem, with a number of large outbreaks identified throughout the world. An increase in the numbers of immunocompromised individuals in developed countries has also changed our perception of risks from waterborne micro-organisms that were previously considered harmless. *Mycobacterium* spp. and microsporidia can cause debilitating illness in people with untreated human immunodeficiency virus (HIV) infection.

In the UK, the microbiological quality of drinking water from public supplies is now better than ever before. Private water supplies that are not provided by a statutory water company are generally of poorer microbiological quality than public supplies. Although it is estimated that less than 1 per cent of the UK population is served by a private domestic supply, many more people are exposed to this water through its use in food production and in commercial residential establishments.

Water is also vital for the production of both arable crops and livestock. Without water, crops cannot grow and animals die. Land can be irrigated with potable ground water, untreated surface water or other contaminated water in addition to precipitation. Control measures need to be in place to ensure that the contamination of crops and the exposure of animals to contamination are minimized.

DISEASE EMERGENCE RELATED TO WATER, FOOD AND FOOD ANIMALS

Emergence of agents causing diarrhoeal diseases, particularly the new types of *Salmonella*, frequently occurs within a small group of animals. Infection then spreads from within farm environments to a wider range of animal species and subsequently to humans. Emergence involves not only expansion of a single strain of *Salmonella* within a host species, but also gradual genetic variation over time to produce new types, with mutation and recombination contributing to the change.

Examples of this emergence are not particularly well documented at the farm level because human pathogens do not necessarily cause ill health to animals, and hence monitoring is patchy. However, emergence over years of strains can be observed in human disease surveillance data, and the contribution of different food animals to human disease has been documented. In particular, individual clones can emerge as a result of special affinity for the host species (e.g. *S.* Enteritidis in chickens) or spread within and between herds as a result of particular animal management practices. Because animals defecate on fields and consume the grass that is in close proximity to the faeces, there are good reasons why transmission within herds or flocks is common. The use of untreated water may add to this recycling of pathogens within farms, as does the common occurrence of small mammals, birds and insects in these settings. Indigenous and imported animal feed can contribute to the seeding of new strains within agricultural animals. The movement of animals between farms and through markets can similarly contribute to the acquisition of new organisms by individual animals.

INFECTIONS TRANSMITTED THROUGH WATER

The range of pathogens causing waterborne diseases have been reviewed recently (Percival *et al.* 2004). The range continues to expand because of ongoing technological advances in microbial detection.

Bacterial diseases

In developing countries, a large range of bacterial pathogens can cause human diseases. Most of these are spread via contaminated food, flies and poor hygiene as well as through drinking water. Contamination of water is predominantly from human and animal faeces. *Vibrio cholerae*, the causative agent of cholera, gives rise to acute and life-threatening diarrhoea and dehydration, and remains the classic waterborne disease in developing countries (Table 7.2) although foodborne transmission and general hygiene are also important. *V. cholerae* is thought to be able to survive in plankton in a **viable but non-culturable state** and numbers increase as the temperatures change (Colwell 1996).

Many large waterborne outbreaks of typhoid and paratyphoid fever occurred in the UK before the 1930s, caused by *S.* Typhi and *S.* Paratyphi B, respectively, both of which are associated with a low infectious dose. These outbreaks were the result of contamination of drinking water with faecal material from infected patients or carriers. The last major outbreak of typhoid via mains water occurred in Croydon, London, in 1937 and was caused by a typhoid carrier working with an untreated water supply (Galbraith *et al.* 1987). As a result of improvements in water sanitation, particularly the subsequent widespread use of chlorine, only two more small outbreaks of mains water associated typhoid have occurred in the UK. Between 300–400 cases of typhoid and paratyphoid fever are detected per year in England and Wales; most of these are contracted abroad. Substantial waterborne outbreaks still occur in developing countries, and there are problems with antibiotic resistance.

Besides *S.* Typhi and *S.* Paratyphi B, other salmonellas are well recognized as waterborne pathogens. Although chlorination has reduced their frequency, outbreaks can still occur when there is gross faecal contamination of treated drinking water. Most salmonellas have a high infectious dose and require nutrient-rich environments for proliferation, so *Salmonella* infections are much more commonly associated with food than water.

Shigella spp. cause dysentery, and have been associated with outbreaks around the world that have involved the ingestion of contaminated drinking water. Outbreaks of waterborne *Shigella* dysentery are usually the result of inadequate treatment. In the UK, such infections have not occurred in recent years.

Despite being the most common bacterial cause of gastroenteritis in the UK, the epidemiology of *Campylobacter* remains somewhat unclear. Outbreaks of waterborne infection have usually involved the consumption of non-chlorinated water. *Campylobacter* spp. cannot multiply in water, although they can survive for extended periods; this and the low infectious dose make these pathogens well adapted to spread via water. *Campylobacter* is the most common pathogen associated with outbreaks in UK linked to private drinking water supplies occurring, for example, in campsites, hospitals and schools. *Campylobacter* isolated from natural waters may not always be pathogenic to humans; *Campylobacter* isolated from untreated water supplies in France comprised 14 types in 891 samples: all except one were considered non-pathogenic (Megraud and Serceau 1990).

Although most strains of *Escherichia coli* are non-pathogenic, several types are known to cause enteric illness in humans. The strains are classified based on the possession of distinct virulence factors, and include enteropathogenic (EPEC), enterotoxigenic (ETEC), enteroinvasive (EIEC), verocytotoxin producing (VTEC) and enteroaggregative (EAggEC) *E. coli* (see Chapter 4). In developing countries, contaminated water is a principal vehicle for transmission of *E. coli* infections, either by direct consumption or by contamination of foods during preparation or crop irrigation. It is less common in developed countries with higher standards of general hygiene. However, drinking water contaminated by sewage or animal waste has been implicated in outbreaks.

VTEC *E. coli* O157 can cause severe bloody diarrhoea and renal failure (haemolytic uraemic syndrome), and infection can be fatal. *E. coli* O157 and other VTEC strains have become an important public health problem in recent years, with more than 20 000 cases of infection and up to 250 deaths per year in the USA. Transmission of infection has been linked to the consumption of undercooked ground beef, unpasteurized milk and a variety of other foods. Contaminated drinking water and recreational water can also be a significant routes of infection. Water was first associated with *E. coli* O157 infection in two isolated cases in 1985, both of which were the result of ingestion of untreated water. A large outbreak in USA, affecting 243 people, of whom 4 died, followed the installation of 45 water meters after the repair of two ruptured mains in an non-chlorinated supply. Drinking water was also implicated in an outbreak affecting children in Czechoslovakia. Due to the low infective dose of *E. coli* O157, waterborne transmission will continue to occur. However, chlorinated mains drinking water supplies present little risk as a source of infection in the UK. Chlorination is equally effective in eliminating *E. coli* O157 and non-pathogenic *E. coli* strains from water. Private water supplies, however, are frequently untreated and have high rates of faecal contamination. Thus, these have been identified as an area of concern.

Viral diseases

Viral outbreaks associated with drinking water are generally from non-chlorinated supplies or those in which chlorination has failed. These outbreaks are more common in countries where chlorination of mains supplies is not universal. The organisms include: adenovirus (Kukkula *et al.* 1997), coxsackievirus B1, enteric cytopathogenic human orphan (ECHO) virus, hepatitis A virus, hepatitis E virus, norovirus and rotavirus.

Enterovirus infections are among the most common causes of aseptic meningitis. Worldwide there are reports of recurring outbreaks, especially during the summer, favoured by conditions of poor hygiene and contaminated water. Transmission is predominantly through the faeco-oral route or by droplet infection. The most commonly implicated species are coxsackie B and ECHO virus. ECHO viruses have a worldwide distribution and usually occur as 'summer flu' or aseptic meningitis and meningoencephalitis in toddlers and infants. Hepatitis A virus causes infectious hepatitis and is spread from person to person by the faecal–oral route. Infection causes illness in adults but is often asymptomatic in children. A vaccine is available and recommended for travellers to developing countries. Hepatitis A virus can spread through faecal contamination of water and food. Hepatitis E virus is also spread by faecal contamination of water and food and is predominantly found in travellers returning from Asia, China and Africa. The infection is similar to hepatitis A virus, but can be severe and life-threatening in pregnant women. Person-to-person spread is uncommon and large scale waterborne outbreaks have been reported in developing countries (for further details of hepatitis viruses, see Chapter 4, p. 80).

Norovirus is the most common cause of viral gastroenteritis in adults with a higher incidence in the winter. It causes projectile vomiting in all age groups. Outbreaks commonly occur in semi-closed environments such as residential institutions, hospitals, schools and cruise ships, and are easily spread from one person to another. Waterborne and foodborne outbreaks also occur, these are particularly associated with consumption of raw shellfish. Sapovirus is a calicivirus and a relatively uncommon cause of mild and self-limiting diarrhoea in babies. There are no reports of transmission by drinking water or recreational water. Rotavirus is the major viral cause of gastroenteritis in childhood both in the UK and worldwide. Most children have been infected by the age of 5 years. In the UK it occurs as a mild self-limiting illness, but causes large numbers of deaths in developing countries. The primary infection produces lasting immunity and symptomatic re-infection is uncommon. Only a few incidents of waterborne rotavirus transmission have been reported and these often involve other pathogens.

Adenoviruses can cause acute respiratory disease and conjunctivitis and serotypes 40/41 may cause acute diarrhoea in young children. These viruses replicate in the intestinal tract and may be present in sewage and natural waters. Outbreaks linked to drinking water are rare, more commonly they are related to swimming pools. For further details of viral gastroenteritis, see Chapter 4, p. 73.

Parasitic infections

Parasitic infections can be acquired from food or water used in its production. The responsible parasites include protozoa (microparasites) and helminths (macroparasites). Many parasites have a very specific life cycle and a number are transmitted through drinking water. Foods deriving from aquaculture (Anon 1999) can be a particular problem, and many parasitic diseases are linked to irrigation associated with particular types of food production.

Helminth diseases

The cycle of human helminthic diseases usually involves food, water or wastewater, and the implicated organisms include trematodes (e.g. *Fasciola* spp. and *Schistosoma* spp), cestodes (e.g. *Echinococcus* spp. and *Taenia*) and nematodes (e.g. *Anisakis* and *Ascaris*). Prevention of these diseases in both developing and developed countries usually involves breaking the disease transmission cycle and reducing exposure of people to these parasites. They are sensitive to freezing and cooking so these methods can be used for preventing disease. Macroparasites have different disease kinetics from microparasites (which besides protozoa include viruses and bacteria) in that not only do they grow and go through the reproductive cycle within their human hosts but do not increase in numbers. Unless there is **autoinfection** (infection transmitted from one's own gastrointestinal infection, see Chapters 2 and 4), the number of parasites present is usually related to the number of infected stages (e.g. ova) passing into the body.

Protozoan diseases

A range of protozoan parasites have been associated with drinking water and food. Pathogenic protozoa are common in developing countries and much of the disease diagnosed in developed countries is in people returning from abroad. *Toxoplasma, Cryptosporidium* and *Giardia* are the main protozoa of concern in developed countries and can cause problems in immunocompromised people. *Cyclospora cayetanensis* has emerged as a foodborne and waterborne pathogen in developing countries and has been a particular problem in fruits and vegetables imported into North America from Central and South America. *Entamoeba histolytica* and *Sarcocystis* can cause water or foodborne diseases in developing countries. Microsporidia may be transmitted through water and food but are usually only associated with disease in immunocompromised people.

Cryptosporidium can cause large outbreaks of waterborne or foodborne gastroenteritis. Most people have diarrhoea for a few days to a couple of weeks followed by the remission of symptoms. Chronic infection can occur in people with compromised T cell conditions such as acquired immune deficiency syndrome (AIDS) or severe combined immunodeficiency (SCID) in which prolonged periods of watery diarrhoea are life-threatening. *C. cayetanensis* causes watery diarrhoea that can last for many weeks. It occurs worldwide but is more common in developing countries. Person-to-person spread does not occur because the oocysts need to mature within the environment for 1–2 weeks before they become infectious. In developing countries transmission is possibly through sewage-contaminated water, and contamination of fruit and vegetables with sewage-contaminated water used for irrigation or pesticide application (see Chapter 6, p. 141).

The lifecycle of *Toxoplasma gondii* involves a sexual cycle with oocyst production in cats and other felines and an asexual lifecycle in other mammals and birds. The parasites form cysts within the secondary host's tissues and the lifecycle is completed when the carnivorous primary host consumes the secondary host. Humans get infected after eating inadequately cooked meat from infected secondary host species such as agricultural animals or from oocysts contaminating food or water. Toxoplasmosis is common in most countries of the world and is usually a sub-clinical condition.

Toxoplasmosis in pregnant women can lead to mental retardation and loss of vision in congenitally infected infants. Intestinal and hepatic toxoplasmosis, pneumonia, disseminated infection, cerebral and ocular infection and death can occur in immunosuppressed or immunocompromised patients. Outbreaks of infection have been associated with food, milk, water and environmental contamination with oocysts from feline faeces. Waterborne infections arise when oocysts excreted with the faeces by infected felines entering drinking water. Demonstrating outbreaks is difficult because diagnosis is by detection of antibodies in serum samples and most infections are not serious enough to cause a visit to the doctor. However, outbreaks have been reported in both developing and developed countries.

Sarcocystis is a genus of protozoans containing more than 100 species with an obligatory two-host lifecycle involving a definitive host (usually a carnivore) and an intermediate host (usually a herbivore). Hosts can be avian, mammalian and reptilian. Human infections are more common in developing countries than developed ones. The sexual generations occur in the small intestine of definitive hosts which shed infective sporocysts in their stools and present with intestinal sarcocystosis. Asexual multiplication occurs in the skeletal and cardiac muscles of intermediate hosts which harbour cysts (sarcocysts) in their muscles and present with muscular sarcocystosis. Sarcocysts are long sinuous cylindrical objects, classified by their three-dimensional appearance. Humans can get intestinal sarcocystosis through the consumption of raw meat containing sarcocysts and muscular sarcocystosis after drinking water or eating food contaminated with sporocysts. The main species are *S. hominis* (acquired from infected beef) and *S. suihominis* (from pork). Waterborne infection in humans has not been reported but is likely to occur in the same way as waterborne toxoplasmosis (i.e. through sporocysts contaminating drinking water). Clinical sarcocystosis is less commonly diagnosed than toxoplasmosis and is not usually associated with fetal infection or abortion in humans and only occasionally in animals.

Giardia spp. are flagellated protozoans that parasitize the small intestines of mammals, birds, reptiles and amphibians. Giardiasis is a common cause of diarrhoea worldwide. The symptoms of giardiasis range from asymptomatic to a transient or persistent acute stage, with steatorrhoea, inter-mittent diarrhoea, and weight loss, or to a sub-acute or chronic stage that can mimic gall bladder or peptic ulcer disease. Sources of infection in addition to humans are thought to include wild and domestic animals. Experimental inoculation of animals and human volunteers indicates that *Giardia* has a low infective dose (10–25 cysts). Outbreaks of infection related to drinking water, recreational water and food have been described. The cysts of *G. duodenalis* are relatively resistant to chlorine, although less resistant than *Cryptosporidium* oocysts. Outbreaks related to drinking water can occur, although they have mostly been associated with recreational water use. The cysts can remain viable in cold water for months. For further details on pathogenic protozoa, see Chapter 4.

Diatom and dinoflagellate diseases

These are protozoan organisms that can produce a range of potent toxins. They occur predominantly in saltwater and, under the right conditions, can produce blooms that result in 'red tides'. These have toxic effects on fish and other sea-life. The toxins accumulate within shellfish (causing diarrhoetic shellfish poisoning and paralytic shellfish poisoning in humans) or pass up the food chain and make some carnivorous fish toxic to eat, causing ciguatera poisoning (see Chapter 4, p. 81).

Fungal diseases

Fungi cause spoilage in foods that become wet or are stored before proper drying. They can also cause chronic diseases through the production of a range of carcinogenic and toxic metabolites known as **mycotoxins**. Other similar but non-toxic fungi are used in food production. In addition a large range of mushrooms and toadstools are toxic and can cause severe acute illness and death.

Alternaria spp., *Cladosporium* spp., *Fusarium* spp. and *Mucor* spp. have been implicated in a rare disease called **alimentary toxic aleukia** (an often fatal disease – characteristics include skin inflammation, vomiting, diarrhoea, and fatal bleeding). This disease has been associated with mouldy grain crops that are allowed to remain in the fields during the winter. The syndrome is thought to result from the toxic metabolites fusariogenin, epicladosporic acid and fagicladosporic acid. It does not occur in the UK.

Aspergillus spp. spores are common but can occasionally cause respiratory illnesses when inhaled. *Aspergillus* spp. grow on foods and produce mycotoxins that have carcinogenic potential, particularly aflatoxins. The aflatoxin-producing species include *A. flavus*, *A. parasiticus* and *A. nomius*. *A. ochraeus* can produce ochratoxin A that is postulated as a cause of Balkan endemic nephropathy (a non-inflammatory, chronic, slow progressing kidney disease, frequently associated with urinary tract tumours). *Penicillium verrucosum* can also occur as a contaminant of cereal crops and produces ochratoxin A. *A. versicolor* can produce sterigmatocystin. *A. versicolor*, *A. flavus* and *A. tamarii* can produce cyclopiazonic acid, which is thought to be responsible for 'kodua poisoning' in India. Some strains of *A. flavus* can produce aflatrem – these are tremorogenic neurotoxins. *A. clavatus* and *P. expansum* produce the mycotoxin patulin and this has become an issue in relation to apples. These fungi have been implicated in alimentary toxic aleukia. For further details on mycotoxins see Chapter 4 (p. 89) and Chapter 18 (p. 326).

CONTAMINATION OF FOODS BY WATER

The contamination of food by water is largely controllable through the implementation of **Hazard Analysis and Critical Control Points (HACCP)** in developed countries, but is a particular problem in developing countries where the processes and infrastructure of food production and retail are less developed, and the burden and range of diarrhoeal diseases in the population is greater. Much of this can be overcome if food is being exported through:

- HACCP control by the companies organizing production
- by paying particular attention to the quality of irrigation water and washing water

- quality assurance
- hygiene and screening of food handlers.

With regard to food produced for indigenous consumption, much of which does not pass through retail, there can be minimal controls on quality or hygiene. Quality is controlled by purchasing behaviours and is strongly influenced by appearance and price.

As development is often led by initiatives to improve water supply there is a need to understand how these changes contribute to improved human health. It is important that development contains sustainable improvements in hygiene and wastewater management as well as drinking water treatment, and that the arrangements for moving from a free new resource to a paid-for service are arranged in a socially non-divisive way. The difficulties in supplying networks of water distribution across widely dispersed rural communities can be substantial and make adequate food hygiene difficult to pass to all.

Feeding infants

Breast-feeding is protective for babies in that it can prevent diarrhoeal and respiratory diseases (*Salmonella*, *Campylobacter* and rotavirus infections). This protection derives from maternal antibodies present in the breast milk, and seems to wane within 2 months of stopping breast-feeding. Infant formula milk is reconstituted with water, and use of boiling water to make up baby milk can be an effective way of reducing risk from contamination if it is rigorously conducted.

Household food and water hygiene

In the home, water is used for drinking, cleaning raw food during its preparation, washing utensils, surfaces and containers during preparation, cleaning hands and washing up. Water from a mains supply should be as good as water treatment and disinfectant residual allow and hand pumps can provide clean water in rural communities (Figure 7.1). However, illegal connections can compromise water quality.

Water storage and treatment

As houses often do not have access to mains water, the way water is stored within the house is important in the extent to which it can become faecally contaminated. Simple point-of-use interventions can be effective in reducing diarrhoeal diseases. Access to substantial water storage and the quality of water available has been shown to be strongly associated with height-for-age and prevalence of diarrhoea.

Harvesting crops

The harvesting of crops uses local and migrant labour, and their cleanliness can depend on the provision of toilet facilities and running water at the site of harvesting. Insecticide or herbicide sprays made up with contaminated water have the potential to cause outbreaks of infection. This could

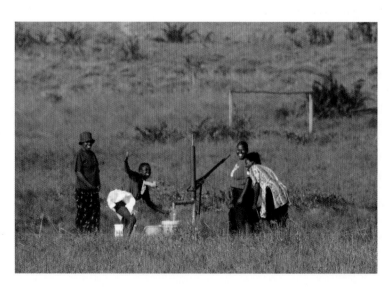

Figure 7.1 *Hand pumps can provide clean water in rural communities*

also explain the outbreaks associated with C. *cayetanensis* infected produce imported into the USA (see Chapter 6, p. 141).

Markets

Markets provide an additional opportunity for the contamination of foods because here foods are exposed to people, flies and environmental contamination. There is also the problem of food getting contaminated via the hands of the people selling these products, as markets may not have adequate toilet or washing facilities.

STANDARDS AND LEGISLATION

Purpose of standards and regulations

The standards for drinking water have evolved over the years and have traditionally been based on the use of the following microbiological indicators:

- coliforms
- thermophilic coliforms (*E. coli*)
- faecal streptococci (enterococci)
- sulphite reducing clostridia (*Clostridium perfringens*).

E. coli (the non-pathogenic majority of isolates) requires rich nutrient conditions and relatively high temperature for growth and thus will not normally grow in water in temperate regions. This and the fact that *E. coli* is abundant in the gastrointestinal tract of animals, has made it a useful indicator of faecal contamination and regulatory standard for many years. Enterococci are additional faecal indicator organisms that have been shown to correlate with risk of waterborne infection in health studies. Sulphite-reducing clostridia are used as indicators of past faecal contamination because the spores persist for longer than *E. coli* and enterococci in water. More recently the presence of *Cryptosporidium* oocysts has been used to indicate failure of filtration to remove faecal contamination (The Water Supply [Water Quality] [Amendment] Regulations 1999 SI 1524, www.opsi.gov.uk/SI/si1999/19991524.htm). The heterotrophic plate counts at 22 °C and 37 °C have value in showing changes in the contamination of water over time but are not thought to be linked to ill health (World Health Organization [WHO]

2003). These indicators are used to monitor both the contamination of waters that are used as sources for drinking water and as an indication that treatment has been effective. The processes for water production are moving to Water Safety Plans (WSPs), which are analogous to the HACCP principles used in food production, and involve catchment protection as well as effective treatment.

World Health Organization guidelines

The WHO first published guidelines for drinking water quality in 1984/85 and these, together with updated versions, are the basis of much of world legislation. These guidelines include considerations of the distinct and complementary roles of the water supplier and the surveillance agency, the problems with private water supplies, the central role of microbiological monitoring and the need to link surveillance information to engineering improvements and remedial measures. More recently the WHO has initiated WSPs as an improved approach to water safety, but this approach adds to and does not invalidate the original recommendations.

The WHO WSPs provides the most effective means of consistently ensuring the safety of a drinking-water supply by the use of a comprehensive risk assessment and risk management approach that encompasses all steps in water supply from catchment to consumer. WSPs use a systematic assessment, effective operational monitoring, and management plans that describe what should be done during normal operation and in emergency situations.

Water framework directive and other European Union regulations

The quality of water in European Member States is a source of concern to people and the Water Framework Directive (http://ec.europa.eu/environment/water/water-framework/index_en.html) was designed to tackle pollution on a European basis. Other pieces of legislation that contribute to this are:

- the Urban Waste Water Treatment Directive (http://ec.europa.eu/environment/water/water-urbanwaste/index_en.html)
- the Nitrates Directive (www.defra.gov.uk/Environment/water/quality/nitrate/directive.htm)

- the Drinking Water Directive
  (http://ec.europa.eu/environment/water/
  water-drink/index_en.html)
- the Bathing Water Directive
  (http://ec.europa.eu/water/
  water-bathing/directiv.html)
- the Directive for Integrated Pollution and
  Prevention Control (IPPC)
  (http://europa.eu/scadplus/leg/en/lvb/
  l28045.htm).

Drinking Water Directive

The European Union (EU) Drinking Water Directive is the basis of most drinking water regulations in Europe. The objective of this legislation is:

> to protect human health from the adverse effects of any contamination of water intended for human consumption by ensuring that it is wholesome and clean.

Governments must ensure compliance with these regulations and any national changes are additional to these. In relation to infections, the Directive stipulates that drinking water must not contain *E. coli* or enterococci in 100 mL as a parametric value. There are also indicator parameters for *C. perfringens* (0/100 mL) and colony count at 22 °C (no abnormal change over the levels normally detected). Similarly water offered for sale in bottles or containers (except natural mineral waters and medicinal waters) must not have *E. coli*, enterococci or *Pseudomonas aeruginosa* in 250 mL and must have colony counts at 22 °C and 37 °C of less than 100/mL and 20/mL, respectively, as parametric values. There are also indicator parameters for bottled waters that include *C. perfringens* (0/100 mL), coliforms (0/250 mL) and colony count at 22 °C (no abnormal change). This legislation covers water used in the food industry unless it can be established that the use of such water does not affect the wholesomeness of the finished product. It covers water for cooking, drinking, food preparation and washing and other domestic purposes as well as to premises for food production, processing and preservation purposes. It applies to water from a distribution network, tanker or in bottles or containers. The general obligations of the Directive state that:

> water intended for human consumption shall be wholesome if it is free from any microorganisms and parasites and from any substances which, in numbers or concentrations, constitute a potential danger to health and which meet minimum requirements for check and audit monitoring.

This Drinking Water Directive pre-dates the *Cryptosporidium* Regulations (1999) and does not make any specific recommendations in relation to *Cryptosporidium* apart from testing waters that are positive for *C. perfringens*. Because the general obligations state that wholesome water should be free from parasites, it might be assumed that some supplies in England and Wales that have oocyst counts of 1 or 2 per 1000 L are not considered as wholesome. However, it is usually difficult to demonstrate that such oocysts are of a *Cryptosporidium* species that is able to infect humans and occur in sufficient numbers that are likely to cause human disease.

UK legislation

Implementation of the EU Drinking Water Directive into UK law was through the Water Supply (Water Quality) Regulations 2000 (www.opsi.gov.uk/SI/si2000/20003184.htm). These regulations use the same microbiological parameters but include coliforms as an additional national parameter for service reservoirs and water treatment works.

Cryptosporidium contamination has been a problem in water supplies, contributing to waterborne outbreaks. Regulation of this problem is through the Water Supply (Water Quality) (Amendment) Regulations 1999 SI No.1524. This requires water providers to assess the risks of treated water being contaminated with *Cryptosporidium* oocysts. If the risk assessment indicates there may be a risk then water companies are required to conduct continuous monitoring of *Cryptosporidium* contamination by filtration of 1000 L of water over 24 hours for every day of the year. The *Cryptosporidium* regulations have had an impact on the occurrence of cryptosporidiosis in the population in England and Wales through pressure on water providers to improve treatment standards and increased investment in water treatment.

Natural mineral waters and bottled water

Regulation of bottled water is through the Natural Mineral Water, Spring Water and Bottled Drinking

Water (Amendment)(England) Regulations 2003 (SI No 666, www.opsi.gov.uk/sr/sr2003/20030182.htm), which are based on the Natural Mineral Water, Spring Water and Bottled Drinking Water Regulations 1999 (SI No 1540, www.opsi.gov.uk/SI/si1999/19991540.htm). The microbiological parameters should be measured within 12 hours of monitoring and the Regulations state that water must not contain *E. coli*, enterococci or *Pseudomonas* in 250 mL and the colony counts at 22 °C and 37 °C must be less than 100/mL and 20/mL, respectively.

The safe sludge matrix

There is general agreement that the best way of managing sewage sludge is by its application to agricultural land as a fertilizer and soil conditioner. However, such application needs to be controlled in a way that does not allow pathogens to recycle and affect human and animal health. The Sludge (Use in Agriculture) Regulations 1989 SI 1263 (www.opsi.gov.uk/si/si1989/Uksi_19891263_en_1.htm) have been designed to protect both the environment and human and animal health where sewage sludge is used on agricultural land.

The 'Safe Sludge Matrix' (www.adas.co.uk/media_files/Publications/SSM.pdf) consists of a table of crop types, together with clear guidance on the minimum acceptable level of treatment for any sewage sludge (often referred to as **biosolids**) based product which may be applied to that crop or rotation (Table 7.3). The agreement between Water UK and the British Retail Consortium, organized by ADAS, was reached in September 1998 and included inputs from the Environment Agency, the Department of Environment Transport and Regions and the Ministry of Agriculture Fisheries and Food (MAFF, now Defra), the National Farmers Union, Country Landowners Association, food manufacturers and food processors. The agreement provides a framework which gives the retailers and food industry confidence that sludge re-use on agricultural land is safe and was driven by the desire to ensure the highest possible standards of food safety. The Matrix enables farmers and growers to continue to use the beneficial properties of sewage sludge as a valuable and cost-effective source of nutrients and organic matter.

The main impact of the Matrix has been the phasing out of raw (untreated) sewage sludge use on agricultural land for food production from 31 December 1999. The use of untreated sewage sludge on agricultural land meant for non-food crops was banned from 31 December 2005. The use of conventionally treated sludge on grazed grassland was banned from 31 December 1998. Conventionally treated sludge can be applied to grazed grassland only where it is deep injected into the soil. The regulations require that there will be no grazing or harvesting within 3 weeks of application. Where grassland is reseeded, sludge must be ploughed down or deep injected into the soil. Conventionally treated sewage sludge can be applied to the surface of grassland or for forage crops such as maize, which will subsequently be harvested, but there can be no grazing of that land within the season of application.

The requirements are more stringent where sludge is applied to land meant for vegetable crops, particularly those eaten raw (e.g. salad crops). Conventionally treated sludge can be applied to agricultural land which is used to grow vegetables in the rotation, provided that at least 12 months have elapsed between application and harvest of the following vegetable crop. Where the crop is a salad which might be eaten raw, the harvest interval must be at least 30 months. Where enhanced treated sludges are used, a 10-month harvest interval applies.

Water for irrigation and washing vegetables on farms

River water can get polluted from a variety of sources (Table 7.4) and can be composed of a high proportion of treated sewage effluent as well as inputs from animal sources. Water used for irrigating crops should ideally be free from faecal organisms. Groundwater sources are useful because they are generally less contaminated than surface ones. Strategies to reduce the risks of contaminating fruit and vegetables include:

- improving the microbiological quality of irrigation water
- restricting poor quality water to products that are unlikely to be eaten raw
- drip or surface irrigation
- washing of the fruit and vegetables in water containing chlorine.

Table 7.3 *The ADAS Safe Sludge Matrix: used to decide what sewage sludge is safe to use in soil for the fertilization of different crops**

Crop group	Untreated sludges	Conventionally treated sludges	Enhanced treated sludges
Fruit Apples, pears, plums, cherries, currants, berries, vines, hops, nuts	✗	✗	✓ 10-month harvest interval applies
Salad Lettuce, radish, onions, beans (runner, broad, dwarf French), vining peas, mange tout, cabbage, cauliflower, broccoli, calabrese, courgettes, celery, red beet, carrots, herbs, asparagus, garlic, shallot, spinach, chicory, celeriac	✗	✗ 30-month harvest interval applies	✓ 10-month harvest interval applies
Vegetables Potatoes, leaks, sweetcorn, Brussels sprouts, parsnips, Swedes, turnips, marrows, pumpkins, squashes, rhubarb, artichokes	✗	✗ 12-month harvest interval applies	✓ 10-month harvest interval applies
Horticulture Soil-based glasshouse or polythene tunnel production (tomatoes, cucumbers, peppers etc.), mushrooms, nursery stock and bulbs for export, basic nursery stock, seed potatoes for export, basic seed potatoes, basic seed production	✗	✗	✓ 10-month harvest interval applies
Combinable and animal feed crops Wheat, barley, oats, rye, triticale, field peas, field beans, linseed, flax, oilseed rape, sugar beet, sunflower, borage	✗	✓	✓
Harvested grassland and forage Maize silage, grass silage, haylage, hay, herbage, seeds	✗	✓ No grazing in season of application – 3 week no grazing and harvesting interval applies	✓ 3 week no grazing and harvesting interval applies
Grazed grassland and forage Grass, forage, turnips, sweeds, kale, fodder mangolds, beet, forage rye, forage triticale, turf production	✗	✗ Deep injected or ploughed down only – 3 week no grazing and harvesting interval applies	✓ 3 week no grazing and harvesting interval applies

✗ = Not allowed.
✓ = Allowed.
*Source: www.adas.co.uk/media_files/Publications/SSM.pdf. Reproduced by kind permission.

Land contaminated with manure or water containing *E. coli* O157 can remain contaminated for many weeks.

Water for animal watering and washing carcasses

Faecal contamination of animal carcasses can some- times amount to kilos of dried faecal mass. Washing animals before euthanizing them can reduce contamination problems in the abattoir. Use of clean and uncontaminated water for watering and washing animals is important in reducing the risks of contamination to the food chain. This is particularly true of washing udders before milking cows.

Table 7.4 *Sources of pollution**

Sources of pollution	Point source or diffuse	Potential pollutant
Effluent discharges from sewage treatment works	Point source	Nitrogen (N) and phosphorus (P), persistent organic pollutants, pathogens, solids, litter
Industrial effluent discharges treatment	Point source	N, oxygen-depleting substances and a broad spectrum of chemicals
Industrial processes	Point source	Broad spectrum of chemicals released to air and water
Oil storage facilities	Point source	Hydrocarbons
Urban storm water discharges	Point source – arising from storm water runoff (from paved areas and roofs in towns and cities) entering the sewer network	N, P, oxygen-depleting substances, heavy metals, hydrocarbons, pathogens, persistent organic pollutants, suspended solids, settleable solids, litter
Landfill sites	Point source	N, ammonia, oxygen-depleting substances, broad spectrum of chemicals
Fish farming	Point source	N, P, oxygen-depleting substances, pathogens
Pesticide use	Diffuse	Broad spectrum of chemicals
Organic waste recycling to land	Diffuse	N, P, pathogens
Agricultural fertilisers	Diffuse	N, P
Soil cultivation	Diffuse	Soil, N, P
Power generation facilities	Diffuse	N, sulphur
Farm wastes and silage	Point/diffuse	N, P, oxygen-depleting substances, pathogens
Contaminated land	Point/diffuse	Hydrocarbons, organic chemicals, heavy metals, oxygen-depleting substances
Mining	Point/diffuse	Heavy metals, acid mine drainage
Leaking pipelines	Point/diffuse	Oil, sewage, pathogens

*Source: Foundation for Water Research (2005) Information Note FWR – WFD16 (www.euwfd.com/FWR-WFD16-0.pdf). Reproduced by kind permission.

Shellfish depuration

Bivalve molluscs are grown in estuarine and coastal areas with differing levels of faecal pollution. Live bivalve molluscs can only be harvested from production areas with fixed locations and boundaries that the local (competent) authority has classified as A, B or C in accordance with Regulation (EC) No 854/2004 (http://europa.eu.int/eur-lex/pri/en/oj/dat/2004/l_226/l_22620040625en00830127.pdf). Molluscs from class A can be sold directly while those from class B require depuration (allowing them to filter feed in a clean water supply for a suitable period of time). For class C supplies the molluscs need relaying before they can be sold for consumption. The main purpose of depuration is to allow bacterial contamination to be naturally eliminated from the molluscs. Purification for the removal of viral contamination is a less efficient and more prolonged process rather than the one day usually needed for bacterial de-contamination. For further details on shellfish classification see Chapter 4, p. 75.

HACCP and drinking water safety plans

In the same way that HACCP has been used in the food industry to control contamination of food and protect public health, the Water Industry and regulators are using WSPs to look at the sources of contamination from catchment to consumer's tap. The approach is designed to systematize the normal practices of water management (Davison *et al.* 2005).

Multiple barriers

Methods for preventing contamination of water that is the source of drinking water can include simple measures such as fencing fields to prevent animals getting to areas where animal faeces can pass into the water (catchment management). There is usually a flocculation stage that facilitates the removal of much of the particulate material from the water followed by filtration, disinfection and the incorporation of a residual disinfectant into distribution. The multiple barrier approach is designed to deal with the differing qualities of source waters and the main pathogens that are likely to be present. Within drinking water supplies several things can go wrong and can lead to outbreaks. Heavy rainfall can cause temporary increases in the levels of contamination from animal and human faeces. Poor management of filter operation and backwashing can cause breakthrough of pathogens although outbreaks will usually be prevented by the disinfection. This is not the case with cryptosporidiosis where disinfection with chlorine has little impact on oocyst viability.

Private water supplies

Private water supplies are those that are not supplied by a mains drinking water supply company and are regulated by specific legislation (Private Water Supplies Regulations 1991, www.opsi.gov.uk/SI/si1991/Uksi_19912790_en_1.htm) and enforced by local authorities. In Scotland there is the Private Water Supplies (Scotland) Regulations 2006 (www.opsi.gov.uk/legislation/scotland/ssi2006/ssi_20060209_en.pdf)

Private water supplies have been classified into a number of categories (Table 7.5), with the larger supplies deriving from deep boreholes and the smaller ones from springs and wells that are strongly influenced by surface waters. Category 2 supplies are those allowed for commercial use in food premises.

SEWAGE, ANIMAL WASTE AND RISK

There is a cycle of pathogenic and non-pathogenic micro-organisms within the environment and passing between humans, domestic and wild animals. This is exemplified by the tapeworms *Taenia saginata*

Table 7.5 *Classification of private water supplies*

Class	Number of people supplied with the water	Average daily volume of water supply (m³/day)
Category 1*		
A	>5000	>1000
B	501–5000	101–1000
C	101–500	21–100
D	25–100	5–20
E	<25	<5
F	Single dwelling	–
Category 2†		
1	N/A	>1000
2	N/A	101–1000
3	N/A	21–100
4	N/A	2–20
5	N/A	<2

*Category 1 supplies domestic properties.
†Category 2 supplies commercial premises, food production, schools and other institutions.
N/A not applicable

and *T. solium*, whose life cycles have evolved over millions of years to require both human and animal infection for the organisms to be maintained. Other pathogens can pass from animals to humans and vice versa in a less cyclical way and then emerge in a particular niche. This can lead to a pathogen entering an animal population, becoming endemic in the population and causing human disease. The cycling of human pathogens back to agricultural animals has been reduced over the years by improvements in the treatment of sewage, but the effluents from sewage treatment works still pass into rivers and can reach both wild and agricultural populations. Similarly, agricultural animal waste is an important source of river water contamination. Costal waters therefore get contaminated by rivers, and this contamination is at its greatest following periods of heavy rain. This in turn can result in the contamination of shellfish beds with both human and animal pathogens.

In addition to the cycling of pathogenic organisms, there is also a dynamic cycling of the organisms that represent the microbial flora of people and animals, but there is little evidence that this cycling has a major impact on human or animal health. There are clear examples of human pathogens that are present in animals and birds as a constituent of the normal flora (e.g. *Campylobacter*).

Management of human waste

To reduce the transmission of food-poisoning organisms from faeces to food, over the past two centuries, many approaches have been adopted for the disposal of human waste. The general principle is that raw faeces is known to be a plentiful source of the agents of diarrhoeal diseases and should be disposed of through sewers (the pipework system that transports sewage to a waste processing plant). Raw sewage, if left to compost (termed nightsoil) can be a significant source of worm eggs, such as those of *Ascaris lumbricoides*, which require time in the environment to become infectious. These sources can also contribute to widespread environmental contamination following periods of flooding. Sewage should be treated using one of a variety of treatment regimens in a three-stage process:

- Primary stage – removal of insoluble particulate material by screening, the addition of coagulants, followed by settlement.
- Secondary treatment – removal of dissolved organic matter as measured by the **biological oxygen demand (BOD)**. This treatment is achieved through secondary aerobic treatment by activated sludge, trickling filters, lagoons and extended aeration and other processes and results in a substantial reduction in BOD.
- Tertiary treatment – physical, chemical and biological removal of inorganic molecules and viruses.

Most sewage treatment works are designed to deal with the changes in flow rate associated with normal rainfall, but where there is a particularly heavy downpour the storm drains open up and large amounts of sewage (and animal waste) can be washed into natural water bodies, particularly rivers. This is the main reason why people should avoid the recreational use of rivers after heavy rain. The contamination during heavy rainfall is not uniform – sewers sometimes get washed out at the start of the rainfall with its subsequent dilution with large amounts of relatively clean rainwater. Outbreaks of waterborne disease are more common during the period after heavy rain.

The effluent from sewage treatment is commonly disposed off in rivers and can make up a substantial percentage of river water, particularly during periods of drought. Sludge can be further treated to reduce the numbers of pathogens present through mesophilic-anaerobic-digestion, dewatering (removing water from the solids), composting etc., and may be used on agricultural land under certain defined conditions (see Table 7.3, p. 158). Sewage effluent can also be burned.

Septic tanks that take the waste from one or a few houses can contribute to the contamination of groundwater or private water supplies if they are not managed properly.

Management of animal waste

The volume of faeces from agricultural animals exceeds that from humans by a factor of about 10. During the summer much of this waste is deposited on the land where animals are grazing and decomposes on the fields. During winter periods when animals are kept indoors, the waste is collected as slurry and allowed to settle in tanks. This material is often re-applied to the land in a muckspreading process at particular times of the year. The use of animal faecal matter as a source for 'improving' the soil makes this a useful resource for farmers but its application to land can cause problems with contamination of river water. This is controlled by the Environment Agency and farmers can be fined for applications or accidents that lead to contamination of natural waters.

Shellfish can be particularly affected by contaminated water. The classification of shellfish beds is designed to reduce the exposure of shellfish to high levels of organic pollution (see p. 159). While depuration can reduce the levels of bacterial contamination of shellfish from estuaries contaminated with sewage or slurry it is ineffective at reducing viral contamination.

Management of wildlife

A large variety of zoonotic infectious diseases are derived from wild animals and have the potential to infect people through the food chain. This includes transmission of:

- *Mycobacterium bovis* from badgers to cattle in the UK
- trichinellosis to humans from wild pig and fox populations in continental Europe
- foot and mouth disease from wild herbivores to domestic livestock in some parts of Asia.

Transmission cycles

Transmission pathways for many parasitic infections can be delimited by a clear understanding of the life cycle through primary and intermediate hosts. However, bacterial transmission cycles can be complicated and, although it can be relatively easy to trace the source of a *Salmonella* outbreak to a particular host animal or bird species, it is often difficult to determine how the source of infection infected this host. Wildlife can act as reservoirs of infection for domestic animals and birds and transmission from one to the other can occur through water, food or the environment.

Insects and disease transmission

Insects can transfer food-poisoning organisms from animal faeces to other animals and to humans. The larvae of many fly species grow in faeces or rotting vegetation. Flies may transmit *Campylobacter* from animal faeces into chicken houses through ventilation ducts. Indeed, flies may also transmit material from animal faeces to human food and could contribute to human *Campylobacter*-related disease (Nichols 2005). There are practical difficulties in providing epidemiological evidence that fly transmission is occurring because disease is likely to be sporadic and the route of transmission from a contaminated source different for each fly. An hypothesis for an association derives from the particular seasonal distribution of *Campylobacter* cases that appears to follow increase in fly numbers in Spring. Where human faeces are exposed to flies there is also the potential for flies to transmit *Shigella* spp. and other enteropathogenic organisms. Because the flies that are most likely to be involved are houseflies (*Musca domestica* and *Fannia canicularis*) and blowflies (*Calliphora* spp., *Lucilia* spp.) that can grow in rotting domestic waste as well as faeces, the risks of foodborne transmission are likely to be greater where kitchen waste is not managed efficiently. Flyborne transmission is likely to be more common when eating outdoors rather than inside and in the countryside rather than in cities.

PROBLEMS WITH *CRYPTOSPORIDIUM*

Specific difficulties with *Cryptosporidium*

Cryptosporidiosis is a common cause of gastro-intestinal infection, with drinking water outbreaks contributing significantly to the total cases per year. The Water Supply (Water Quality) (Amendment) Regulations 1999 SI 1524, have had an important effect on drinking water production through the introduction of risk assessment and continuous monitoring. This, together with increased investment in water treatment, appears to have resulted in a reduction in cryptosporidiosis. Outbreaks highlight some problems for food producers in preventing contamination of foods either through water being a constituent of the product, or through irrigation or washing.

Outbreaks of cryptosporidiosis generally result from the parasite's resistance to disinfection coupled with inadequacies in filtration of both drinking water and swimming pool water. There were 149 outbreaks of cryptosporidiosis in the UK between 1983 and 2005 (Table 7.6) and although food was implicated in four of these, two involved a possible food vehicle followed by community spread and another was at an adult training centre where a specific food associated with the outbreak was not identified. The final outbreak was associated with inadequately pasteurized milk and is described in Chapter 6, p. 136. The scientific literature has many reports of other food-related outbreaks of cryptosporidiosis. One outbreak was associated with the consumption of fresh-pressed apple juice at an agricultural fair in the USA and appeared to result from collecting apples from the ground which became contaminated with calf faeces. Other outbreaks have been associated with the contamination of foods by kitchen staff. Detection of outbreaks can be difficult because it is difficult to detect oocysts in food, and there are difficulties in routinely typing isolates from both faeces and environmental sources where the number of detected oocysts is low.

In addition to outbreaks, disease can be transmitted in small clusters where there is no evidence of a common source. About a third of cases occur in clusters or outbreaks and two-thirds as sporadic disease. There is comparatively little evidence about what causes sporadic cryptosporidiosis. A case–control study of sporadic disease identified differences in the epidemiology of cryptosporidiosis between *Cryptosporidium hominis* and C. *parvum* in that ice cream and raw vegetables (particularly tomatoes) were both strongly negatively associated with C. *parvum*-related illness. The reasons for this negative association are not clear.

Table 7.6 *Summary of* Cryptosporidium *outbreaks in the UK by transmission route: 1983–2005**

Outbreak source/transmission route	Total number of outbreaks	Total number of cases (laboratory confirmed)
Public drinking water supply	55	7097 (5821)
Private drinking water supply	6	176 (30)
Swimming pool	43	799 (490)
Interactive water features	3	189 (70)
Paddling pools	2	13 (6)
Other recreational water	2	27 (12)
Animal contact	16	936 (294)
Farm (transmission route unknown)	3	25 (19)
Foodborne	4	140 (81)
Person-to-person	10	279 (116)
Unknown	5	148 (141)
Total	149	9829 (7080)

Source: Based on Nichols *et al.* (2006).

Effects of treatment processes on oocyst viability

A study of the survival of both *C. hominis* and *C. parvum* (the two species most often associated with disease) reported oocysts remaining viable for up to 14 days following most chemical treatments in different osmotic solutions at different pHs of food; treatments with one or more of the following significantly increased inactivation:

- high salt
- glycerol
- sucrose
- ethanol.

Such treatments can therefore contribute to prevention but should not be relied on as the sole critical control factor. *Cryptosporidium* oocysts are inactivated by drying (Anderson 1986) and by heating to pasteurization temperatures. They can also be inactivated by ultraviolet irradiation.

'At risk' foods

Cryptosporidiosis can cause human disease through the contamination of fruit used to produce unpasteurized fruit juices. Salad and soft fruit remain vulnerable to *Cryptosporidium* (as well as to *Giardia*, *Cyclospora* and helminth ova) via contaminated irrigation water or from the water used for washing. In developing countries there are similar risks from *Cyclospora* oocysts. Studies have demonstrated contamination of salad products with enteric protozoa, mostly in developing countries.

Detecting contamination

Raw food ingredients may be contaminated as is the water used for food processing, particularly in developing countries and also from irrigation water in developed countries. *Cryptosporidium* oocysts are sensitive to hot water and it has been suggested that this can be a suitable way of cleaning and decontaminating carcasses. Outbreaks of cryptosporidiosis may occur in tourist resorts where they are unlikely to be detected through normal surveillance processes.

What to do in a waterborne outbreak

The drinking water supply can, despite the best efforts of water providers, become contaminated with *Cryptosporidium*. Outbreaks can be effectively managed by following the advice set out in expert committee reports (Bouchier 1998). When an outbreak occurs, many food-related problems can arise. Food producers who use drinking water as a component of the final product need to ensure that any contamination will not result in viable oocysts in the final product. Premises that use drinking water for food preparation purposes need to ensure that water is boiled before use. The owners of vending machines need to be confident that there is an effective means of removing or inactivating oocysts if water is used in these machines.

Because some contamination events and outbreaks are not recognized, a 'belt and braces' approach to ensuring that *Cryptosporidium* oocysts do not contaminate food products should be considered. This may involve a heating or a filtration stage in production.

Detecting outbreaks through surveillance

Outbreaks are generally detected through laboratories or local public health teams noticing a greater than normal number of cases over a short timescale. Action at an early stage can contribute to a reduction in further cases. Early in an outbreak, an **outbreak control team** (OCT) is established with representatives from the laboratories, local authority, health authority and, if the water is suspected, the water company covering the area of the outbreak. The OCT has to assess the situation, with a close examination of new cases and compilation of descriptive epidemiology (e.g. age, sex, geographic and temporal distribution). The OCT must ensure that an appropriate epidemiological investigation is undertaken, including:

- conducting a trawling questionnaire on a small number of affected patients to establish hypotheses for what risk factors might have caused the outbreak
- determination of any changes in food or water supply that might have contributed to an increased risk of exposure
- conducting of an analytical case–control or cohort study to provide statistical evidence for disease associations.

Along with this process goes determining possible interventions and communicating the information to other professionals and the public. Further details about the detection and management of outbreaks are given in Chapters 6 and 32.

WATER USE IN FOOD PRODUCTION, RETAIL AND HOUSEHOLDS

Water is an essential requirement in food processing plants, catering and retail premises.

Hand washing is essential for food handlers producing ready-to-eat products and this should be accompanied by a biocidal wash (see Chapter 8). Food handlers working in such production areas may come from developing countries with higher rates of carriage of intestinal pathogens, thus it is important to ensure that staff wash their hands thoroughly after visits to the toilet. The production area needs to be regularly cleaned to reduce the possibility of areas of contamination that can be transferred to the production line. This includes drains, surfaces and equipment. Care needs to be taken to prevent splashing and spraying during washing which can create aerosols. Washing of raw produce prior to processing should preferably be done in a separate room or site from ready-to-eat food production areas.

Washing hands during food preparation is an effective way of preventing foodborne disease (see Chapter 8). In particular, thorough washing of hands, equipment and surfaces after handling raw poultry and other raw meats is essential. It is also important to ensure that towels used to dry hands are not contaminated with foodborne pathogens and regular cleaning of cloth towels or use of single-use paper ones is advisable. Similarly, because dish-cloths often remain damp for extended periods, they can harbour pathogens, which are then easily transferred to ready-to-eat foods from contaminated surfaces or hands. Taps and surfaces can become contaminated as a result of washing raw meat (e.g. chicken) prior to cooking, as can sinks that are used for washing poultry and subsequently used for washing salads.

Hot water temperature needs to be kept above 50 °C to prevent *Legionella* contamination, particularly where aerosols may be created. In relation to food the risk relates more to the food workers than to contaminated food.

When examining supply security and safety, it is important to remember that if there is a failure in drinking water supply quality, as when *Cryptosporidium* contaminates potable supplies, then the safety of the food may be compromised. For foods or beverages with a high percentage of drinking water in the final product (e.g. soft drinks), there may be value in using additional controls and membrane filtration to the treated mains water. In the event of drought or flooding, water storage may assist in securing production.

Summary

Microbiological contamination of food with water can occur at many stages between the farm and the dinner plate. These potential risks can be eliminated through HACCP, provided that the risks are fully understood, the critical control points are examined and measures are taken to prevent contamination.

All websites cited in the text and below were accessed in December 2006.

SOURCES OF INFORMATION AND FURTHER READING

Anderson BC (1986) Effect of drying on the infectivity of cryptosporidia-laden calf feces for 3- to 7-day-old mice. *Am J Vet Res* **47**: 2272–3.

Anon (1999) *Food Safety Associated with Products from Aquaculture – Report of a Joint FAO/NACA/WHO Study Group*. Technical Report Series, No 883. Geneva: World Health Organization, pp. 1–62.

Bouchier I. (1998) *Cryptosporidium* in water supplies; Third report of the group of experts. London: Department of the Environment, Transport and the Regions, Department of Health, pp. 1–171.

Colwell RR. (1996) Global climate and infectious disease: the cholera paradigm. *Science* **274**: 2025–31.

Davison A, Howard G, Stevens M, *et al.* (2005) *Water Safety Plans – Managing Drinking-water Quality From Catchment to Consumer*. Geneva: World Health Organization, pp. 1–244.

Galbraith NS, Barrett NJ, Stanwell-Smith R (1987) Water and disease after Croydon: A review of water-borne and water-associated disease in the UK 1937–86. *J Institution Water Environ Manage* **1**: 7–21.

Kukkula M, Arstila P, Klossner ML, *et al.* (1997) Waterborne outbreak of viral gastroenteritis. *Scand J Infect Dis* **29**: 415–18.

Megraud F, Serceau R (1990) Search for *Campylobacter* species in the public water supply of a large urban community. *Zentralbl Hyg Umweltmed* **189**: 536–42.

Nichols GL (2005) Fly transmission of *Campylobacter*. *Emerg Infect Dis* **11**: 361–4.

Nichols GL, Chalmers RM, Sopwith W, *et al.* (2006) *Cryptosporidiosis*: A report on the surveillance and epidemiology of *Cryptosporidium* infection in England and Wales. Drinking Water Directorate Contract Number DWI 70/2/201.London: Drinking Water Inspectorate.

Percival SL, Chalmers RM, Embrey M, *et al.* (2004) *Microbiology of Waterborne Diseases*. Edinburgh: Elsevier, pp. 1–480.

Pruss A , Kay D, Fewtrell L, *et al.* (2002) Estimating the burden of disease from water, sanitation, and hygiene at a global level. *Environ. Health Perspect* **110**: 537–42.

Ukety OT (1993) Trachoma in northeastern Zaire: a study of 22 cases. *Ann Soc Belg Med Trop* **73**: 61–6.

Valent F, Little D, Bertollini R, *et al.* (2004) Burden of disease attributable to selected environmental factors and injury among children and adolescents in Europe. *Lancet* **363**: 2032–9.

World Health Organization (2003) *Heterotrophic Plate Counts and Drinking-Water Safety: the Significance of HPCs for Water Quality and Human Health*. London: IWA Publishing (available at: www.who.int/water_sanitation_health/dwq/HPCFull.pdf).

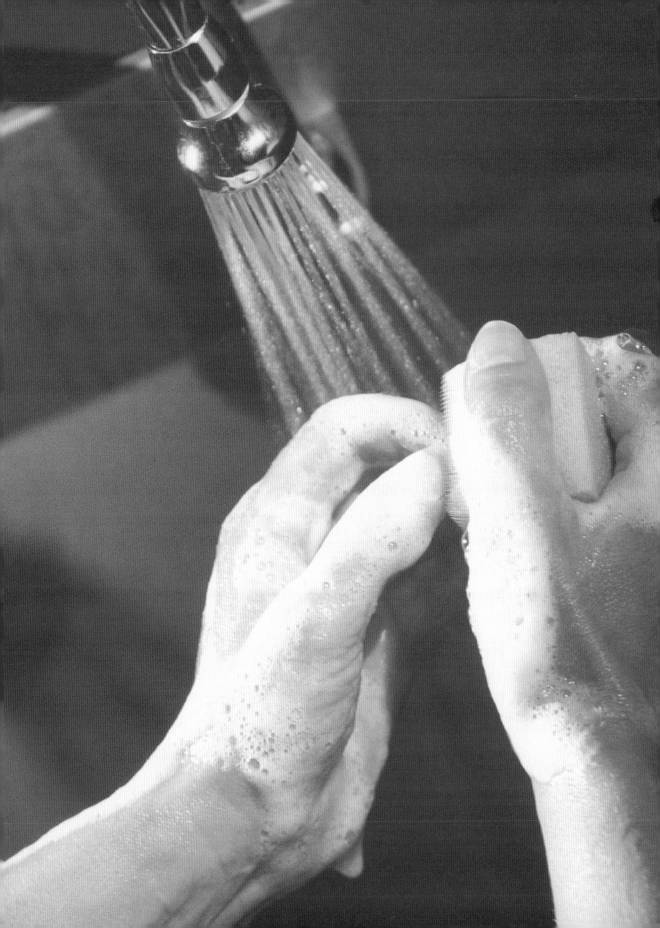

FOOD HYGIENE IN THE PREVENTION OF FOOD POISONING

In Part 2 the chapters include details of effective preventive measures. Consideration is given to care of the hands and other points of personal hygiene, to storage, preparation and cooking methods, retail sale and factory practices. Coverage for the kitchen includes cleaning methods, design of premises and equipment, sterilization and disinfection. Microbiological specifications, legislation and education are necessary corollaries to control the incidence of disease from food. There is also a chapter on food hygiene outside the developed world, as well as consideration to survival in the wilderness.

Personal hygiene of the food handler

Richard Elson

Food handlers as a source of contamination	169	Personal cleanliness and protective clothing	173
Hands	169	Food handlers' fitness to work	175
Nose and throat	170	Training	178
Gastrointestinal tract	170	Summary	179
Prevention of food contamination by food handlers	171	Sources of information and further reading	179

Food handlers can be a source of food contamination and facilitators of cross-contamination. Personal hygiene of food handlers is extremely important in the prevention of food poisoning, which is principally associated with cleanliness of the hands. Identification of ways in which food handlers may contaminate food can help develop appropriate interventions to reduce or eliminate the risk of contamination.

Personal hygiene This is the maintenance of personal health, particularly by cleanliness. Personal hygiene is often principally limited to the care of the hands.

Food handler A worker in the food industry whose hands come in direct contact with food.

FOOD HANDLERS AS A SOURCE OF CONTAMINATION

All living organisms have commensal organisms living on or in them. Humans are no exception and micro-organisms can be found on the hands, hair and skin, in the nose and throat and in the gastrointestinal tract. Humans may occasionally harbour pathogenic organisms, either as carriers or subclinical infection. Mary Mallon (Typhoid Mary) is a famous example of a cook who, either unwittingly or deliberately, infected more than 1300 people with typhoid in the USA in the early 1900s. Food handlers can also contaminate food with unwanted objects such as hair, skin, nails and jewellery, which in turn can be contaminated with micro-organisms.

HANDS

The very nature of preparing and serving food means that the food handler's hands frequently come into contact with foods, thus providing an opportunity for hands to contaminate and become contaminated. Food handlers whose work involves touching unwrapped foods to be consumed raw or without further cooking or other forms of treatment belong to the **high-risk food handler group**.

Bacterial flora of the hands

The flora of the human hand is complex and comprises bacteria, viruses and fungi, and can be described as **resident** or **transient**. Resident flora live on the skin, are the normal permanent microflora, and are not easily removed by hand washing. Resident flora do not, however, usually pose a threat of infectious disease. The bacterium *Staphylococcus aureus* is the only resident micro-organism that poses concern with regard to food safety. Transient flora can be any pathogenic micro-organism including bacteria (e.g. *Escherichia coli*) and viruses (e.g. norovirus), and are picked up accidentally. This flora resides on the skin for a short period of time only. Transient flora are of concern to the food industry because they attach only loosely to the skin surface and are easily transmitted by hands to food and surfaces unless removed by, for instance, adequate washing of hands. Transient flora can be picked up from food preparation or kitchen areas including raw foods, surfaces, equipment and refuse or the toilet. Hands must be kept clean and washed as frequently as necessary (Box 8.1).

Box 8.1 When to wash hands
- Always before starting/recommencing work
- After using the toilet
- Before handling cooked or ready-to-eat foods
- After handling or preparing raw food
- Before gloving and after glove removal
- After any non-food contact such as touching skin/face/hair, sneezing or blowing the nose

---

Damage to skin on the hand, such as wounds and cuts, presents a greater risk of infection and contamination because there will be many more organisms. Cuts, burns and other raw surfaces, however small, are particularly a problem as a reservoir of staphylococci. Food handlers should ensure that infected lesions and cuts on exposed areas of the skin (hands, arms, face, neck, scalp) are totally covered with a distinctive coloured waterproof dressing.

Waterproof dressings help to prevent the passage of bacteria outwards from serous fluid and inwards from fluids in the environment. People with inflamed or obviously infected lesions or sores on hands, or other parts of their body, should not handle foods. Dermatitis is a widespread cause of occupational ill health and the food and catering industries account for about 10 per cent of this. Dermatitis can be caused by water, foods, detergents, foods and cleaning chemicals. Skin affected by conditions such as dermatitis or eczema can be preferentially colonized by staphylococci and care should be taken to avoid touching irritant substances or to expose broken skin to very hot water. Food handlers developing these conditions through their work should report to the manager of the food business who should then take appropriate action. Employers are under a legal obligation to prevent occupational dermatitis by removing or replacing materials that may cause these conditions or providing appropriate gloves or other materials.

NOSE AND THROAT

It is estimated that about 25 per cent of the UK population harbours staphylococci in their nasal passages. Staphylococci are found in the nasal mucosa as well as on hands and other skin surfaces, particularly in damaged areas (such as cuts, burns, abrasions) and pustular lesions (such as boils, carbuncles, whitlows and styes). Due to legal temperature control requirements for the storage of food, the observed frequency of foodborne staphylococcal outbreaks has declined in the past 20 years.

Streptococci may also be found in the nose and throat and can cause a wide range of infections in humans. However, foodborne infection is infrequent. The infection may not present with classic food poisoning symptoms, and the sequelae can be serious, particularly in vulnerable groups. Zoonotic infections with *Streptococcus equi* subsp. *zooepidemicus* have been reported in association with the consumption of cheese, however, these incidents have been attributed to inadequate pasteurization of the milk used in cheese making rather than contamination by food handlers. Outbreaks of group A streptococci infection associated with food handlers having cuts on their hands have also been reported. As well as being aesthetically unpleasing to customers, food handlers who touch their nose, spots or cuts may increase the risk of passing staphylococci from hands to foods: these practices should be strongly discouraged.

GASTROINTESTINAL TRACT

The human gastrointestinal tract contains millions of microbes that are essential to the digestive process. Most of the gut microflora are harmless. However, pathogenic viruses, bacteria or parasites can be present in the intestinal tract and faeces of people with gastrointestinal illness, even after symptoms have resolved. People with diarrhoea or other symptoms of gastrointestinal disease should not work in areas where food is handled while they are symptomatic, whatever job they are doing. Intestinal pathogens are more likely to spread from the fluid stool of diarrhoea than from a well-formed stool. Explosive vomiting and diarrhoea commonly occur as a result of viral gastroenteritis and can cause widespread contamination of the immediate environment and directly infect other people.

Cross-contamination can also occur when areas are incorrectly cleaned or sanitized. Virus particles can survive for some time on hard surfaces, but more so on soft surfaces, which are harder to clean effectively. Aerosol sprays are formed when toilets are flushed, and general toilet cleanliness is more difficult with fluid excreta. Where vomiting occurs in a food handling area, any exposed food should be disposed of. The area should be cleaned and subsequently disinfected with a freshly prepared hypochlorite-based cleaner that releases 1000 ppm of available chlorine (according to the manufacturer's instructions). It is the responsibility of the food handler to inform their manager if they are ill. For some infections, medical clearance must be sought from an appropriate medical professional (see section on Food handlers' fitness to work, p. 175).

PREVENTION OF FOOD CONTAMINATION BY FOOD HANDLERS

Hand washing

Effective hand washing is one of the cornerstones of personal hygiene and preventing food poisoning. Its importance was first demonstrated by Dr Ignaz Semmelweiss in 1847 who suspected that infections causing childbed (puerperal) fever in an Austrian maternity hospital were being transmitted by clinicians who were not washing their hands between consultations. Semmelweiss instigated a personal hygiene regimen for doctors between seeing patients; this resulted in a drop in mortality from over 12 per cent to less than 3 per cent.

Investigations of the bacterial flora of the hands before and after washing with soap and water alone, or with antiseptic, have shown that the soap and water wash is effective for removal, or at least reduction in numbers, of coliforms and other Gram-negative intestinal organisms on the hands. Jewellery may interfere with the effectiveness of hand washing and should not be worn by those handling ready-to-eat foods. The resident population of staphylococci, although usually reduced, can still be cultured from the hands after washing. Occasionally it can become more profuse than before because of their dislodging from hair follicles and cracks in the skin surface. Due to the difficulty in altering the resident flora on the hands, washed

hands do not necessarily mean safe hands. Thus, foods which readily support the growth of staphylococci, such as heat-treated dairy products, should not be touched with the hands. Such foods must be refrigerated after preparation and before consumption. Figure 8.1 shows the growth of bacteria from a hand impression following various exposures and treatments.

Alcohol hand disinfectants may also be used and act as a convenient disinfectant after hand washing. These disinfectants are only effective when used on physically clean hands as they are inactivated completely by any organic matter. Their convenience and importance are emphasized by their use in healthcare settings to prevent nosocomial infections (infections acquired in hospital). However, they are not a legal requirement in food premises and may be a cause of occupational dermatitis.

It is a legal requirement to provide adequate washbasins in food premises, exclusively for washing hands. These basins must be provided with hot and cold (or mixed) water. Materials for cleaning hands and for hygienic hand drying should be available. It is good practice that the temperature of a mixed water supply, if provided, should be about 50 °C. Where a mixed supply is not available, a plug or stopper can be used to enable mixing of water to a suitable temperature which also reduces the possibility of re-contaminating clean hands when turning taps off. Ideally, taps should be non-hand operable and should be considered when refurbishing premises. Washing facilities should be kept clean and in good order. Drying facilities can be in the form of paper towels, roller towels in cabinets or hot air dryers. The number and location of the washbasins will depend on the size and type of the business. However, they should always be readily available and there should be a sign stating that these are for hand washing only. A suitable set-up for hand washing is shown in Figure 8.2.

Washbasins should be well maintained, located close to toilet facilities and easily accessible to encourage use – for example, at the entrance to a food preparation area. Areas where high-risk open foods are routinely handled should have dedicated hand wash basins. Soap or detergent must be available. It is good practice to have a bactericidal detergent in a dispenser or provide disinfectant wipes for use after hand washing, particularly in areas where high-risk foods are handled.

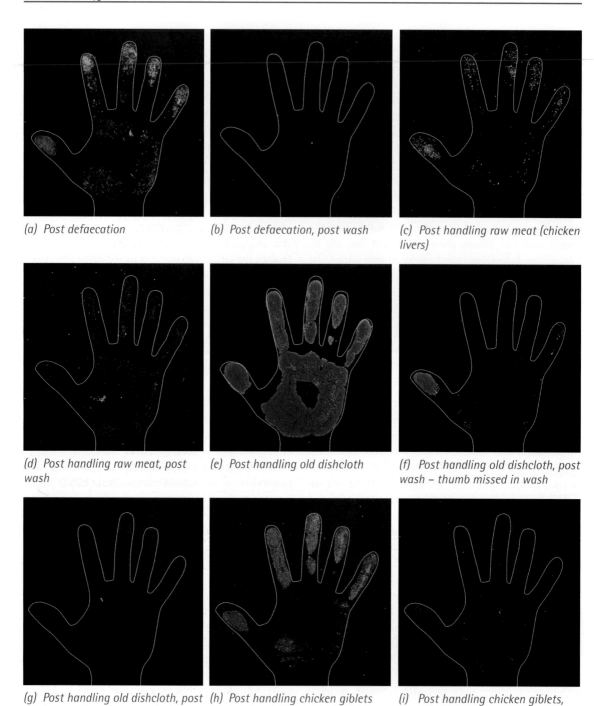

(a) *Post defaecation*   (b) *Post defaecation, post wash*   (c) *Post handling raw meat (chicken livers)*

(d) *Post handling raw meat, post wash*   (e) *Post handling old dishcloth*   (f) *Post handling old dishcloth, post wash – thumb missed in wash*

(g) *Post handling old dishcloth, post wash*   (h) *Post handling chicken giblets*   (i) *Post handling chicken giblets, post wash*

Figure 8.1   *Colonies of bacteria growing on agar following a hand impression (outlined) (photographs courtesy of Peter Hoffman)*

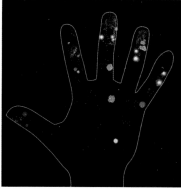
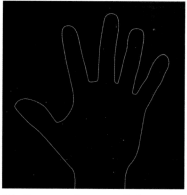
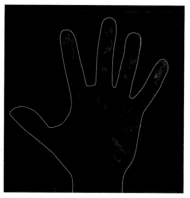

(j) Post mopping-up spill from raw meat

(k) Post mopping-up spill from raw meat, post wash

(l) Clean hands wiped on damp, used towel

Figure 8.1   *(continued) Colonies of bacteria growing on agar following a hand impression (outlined) (photographs courtesy of Peter Hoffman)*

Signs, strategically placed at the entrance to food preparation rooms, in toilets and around wash hand basins will remind staff of the need to wash hands regularly. Suitable pictures (e.g. Figure 8.2) may also encourage effective hand washing. Effective hand washing involves six steps and these are illustrated in Figure 8.3. The minimum washing time should be 20 seconds. Some food establishments dispense creams and lotions for the hands.

These serve as a barrier and/or keep the hands soft and supple, thus reducing roughness and cracks which can harbour bacteria. Such creams may also incorporate a disinfectant to prevent the growth of contaminants in the cream itself. Perfumed hand creams should not be used when handling open food.

PERSONAL CLEANLINESS AND PROTECTIVE CLOTHING

Regulation [EC] No. 853/2004 states that every person working in a food handling area shall:

- maintain a high degree of personal cleanliness
- wear suitable, clean and, where appropriate, protective clothing.

These requirements should be regarded in the context of the working environment and the degree to which a person has contact with food. For example, a warehouse worker who does not handle open food would not be expected to comply stringently with the first requirement.

Personal cleanliness covers washing and drying hands on a regular basis, not wearing jewellery or false nails that could contaminate foodstuffs, and dressing any wounds appropriately. Smoking, spitting, eating and drinking are prohibited in food handling areas, and **food handlers** are under a general obligation to keep fingernails short and

Figure 8.2   *A suitable hand washing station*

(a) Step 1: Wet hands thoroughly under warm running water and squirt liquid soap onto the palm of one hand

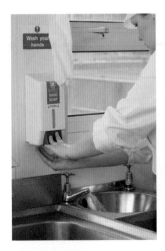

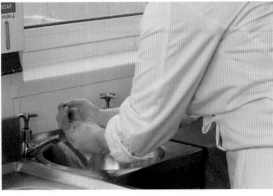

(b) Step 2: Rub hands together to make a good lather

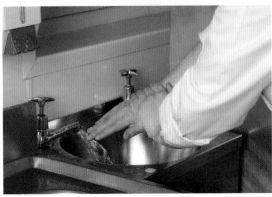

(c) Step 3: Rub the palm of one hand along the back of the other and along the fingers. Then repeat with the other hand

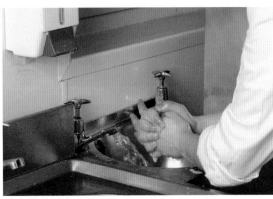

(d) Step 4: Rub in between each finger on both hands and around thumbs, fingertips and nails

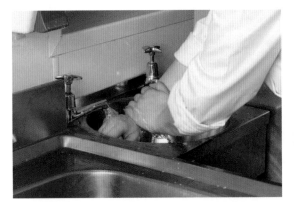

(e) Step 5: Rinse off the soap thoroughly with clean running water

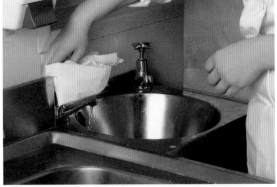

(f) Step 6: Dry hands thoroughly (using a paper towel, hand dryer or cabinet roller towel). Turn off the tap with the towel and dispose of towel, or by elbow/knee (non-hand) operated lever action

Figure 8.3 *The six steps of hand washing (courtesy of the Food Standards Agency)*

clean, and behave in a manner that will not spread bacteria – for example, by licking fingers, biting nails, or touching the nose, etc.

Protective clothing protects food from the food handler rather than vice versa and must be worn in areas where open, high-risk food is being handled. It should be clean, durable and light coloured. Protective clothing can be a source of bacterial contamination and should therefore be kept clean. However, clothes can be a source of physical contamination by shedding fibres, and because of buttons and other fasteners. Best practice guidelines promote the wearing of suitable, clean and appropriate outer clothing by food handlers. Visitors and contractors should also be subject to the same standards of personal hygiene as employees. Hair should be kept neat and tidy. Although it is not a legal requirement, it is good practice for food handlers to wear hats, hair coverings or nets as well as snoods (for beards and moustaches). Hair restraints also discourage the touching of hair.

In some high-risk environments, such as ready-to-eat food processing environments, clothing becomes particularly important in the prevention of contamination. Many modern food processing environments have 'dirty' or low-care areas (where raw ingredients are received or foods are prepared to a minimal level by washing or grading) and 'clean' or high-care areas (where handling or processing of a product to its finished state is carried out). Staff are usually segregated to work in either of these areas to prevent cross-contamination. Colour coding of protective hats, clothing or parts of clothing, for example collars, can be used to distinguish staff in the two areas. Staff entering or working in high-care environments must not travel to work in protective clothing and suitable changing facilities should be provided at the place of work. Staff working in these areas should also enter through a specially designated area and must follow specified procedures for changing into visually distinctive clean overalls and footwear.

Gloves and other barriers

Gloves act as a physical barrier between hands and food, yet may become contaminated if they are not washed as often as hands or changed regularly. In addition, latex gloves may contaminate food with latex, to which some consumers are allergic. Gloves are often worn for the handling and assembly of salads, sandwiches and other foods that will not be subject to further cooking. The aim is to restrict the passage of staphylococci from hands to foods. Where gloves are worn, these should be disposable and 'single use'.

Other barriers to contamination include utensils, film wraps, food grade paper and reversed food bags. Gloves or other barrier techniques must not be used as a substitute for good hand hygiene. However, combining the use of clean suitable gloves with other barrier techniques ensures lower contamination risks.

FOOD HANDLERS' FITNESS TO WORK

Health

Chapter VIII of Regulation [EC] No. 853/200 contains a specific requirement relating to the health of food handlers, which is applicable to all member states of the European Union. This legislation states:

> No person suffering from, or being a carrier of a disease likely to be transmitted through food or afflicted, for example, with infected wounds, skin infections, sores or diarrhoea is to be permitted to handle food or enter any food-handling area in any capacity if there is any likelihood of direct or indirect contamination. Any person so affected and employed in a food business and who is likely to come into contact with foods to report immediately the illness or symptoms, and if possible their causes to the food business operator.

The 1996 UK Department of Health guidelines for food business managers state:

> Anyone suffering from diarrhoea and/or vomiting should report this to their manager and leave food handling areas immediately. If there is only one episode of diarrhoea and/or vomiting in a 24 hour period and no fever, then the person can return to work. If the symptoms persist, then they should only return to work only when vomiting has ceased for 48 hours and/or the bowel habit has returned to normal for 48 hours.

The UK Health Protection Agency (HPA) also produced guidelines in 2004 designed to prevent

Table 8.1 *Recommended control measures* for high-risk food handlers[†]*

Causative agent/illness	Exclusion beyond clinical recovery	Recommended control measures for food handlers	
		Microbiological clearance	If food handler is a contact of a case
Aeromonas spp. *Bacillus* spp. *Campylobacter* spp. *Clostridium perfringens* *Cryptosporidium* spp. *Cyclospora cayetanensis* *Escherichia coli* (not VTEC) *Salmonella* spp. (not typhoid and paratyphoid) Viral gastroenteritis Yersiniosis	48 hours after first normal stool	No	Reinforce hygiene advice
Amoebic dysentery (*Entamoeba histolytica*)	Until microbiological clearance obtained	One stool, obtained at least 1 week after the *end* of treatment examined for *E. histolytica* cysts	Screen to detect if cyst excreter (careful assessment needed to evaluate significance as many cysts non-pathogenic)
Cholera (*Vibrio cholerae* O1 or O139)	48 hours after first normal stool	When indicated (suspect hygiene/poor sanitation), two consecutive negative stools taken at intervals of at least 24 hours	Reinforce hygiene advice
Clostridium botulinum	Not appropriate	No	Treatment of those at risk. Examination of faecal and serum specimens may be indicated
Escherichia coli (VTEC)	Until microbiological clearance obtained	Two stool specimens not less than 48 hours apart are negative	Exclude until microbiological clearance obtained
Giardiasis (*Giardia duodenalis*	48 hours after first normal stool	No	Screening may identify those who need treatment
Hepatitis A	Seven days after onset of jaundice and/or symptoms	Not relevant	Consider for prophylaxis Asymptomatic contacts of a case of hepatitis A can continue to handle food providing good hygienic practice is adhered to
Listeriosis (*Listeria monocytogenes*)	No	No	Reinforce hygiene advice
Marine biotoxins Scombrotoxin poisoning Ciguatera poisoning	No	No	Reinforce hygiene advice
Non-cholera *Vibrio* spp.	No	No	Reinforce hygiene advice

Table 8.1 *Recommended control measures* for high-risk food handlers[†]*

Causative agent/illness	Recommended control measures for food handlers		
	Exclusion beyond clinical recovery	Microbiological clearance	If food handler is a contact of a case
Staphylococcus aureus	48 hours after first normal stool Skin: septic lesion treated and healed	No Lesions healed	Reinforce hygiene advice
Shigellosis	*Shigella sonnei*: 48 hours after first normal stool *S. dysenteriae, S. flexneri, S. boydii*: until microbiological clearance obtained	*S. dysenteriae, S. flexneri, S. boydii*: (two negative stool samples taken at intervals of not less than 48 hours)	Contacts of *S. dysenteriae, S. flexneri, S. boydii*: exclude until microbiological clearance obtained
Enteric fever (typhoid and paratyphoid)	Until microbiological clearance obtained	Six consecutive negative stool specimens at weekly intervals starting 3 weeks after completion of treatment	Exclude until two consecutive stools obtained 48 hours apart are negative after treatment commenced
Taenia solium	Until microbiological clearance obtained	Two negative stools at 1 and 2 weeks post treatment	Screen serologically for evidence of cysticercosis
Thread worm	Until treated	Until treated	Treat all contacts

*Recommendations of the Health Protection Agency ad hoc Working Group of the former PHLS Advisory Committee on Gastrointestinal Infections (2004).
[†]High-risk food handler: a person who handles unwrapped food meant to be consumed raw or without further cooking or other forms of treatment.
VTEC, verocytotoxin producing *E. coli*.

person-to-person spread of gastrointestinal infection. The HPA guidelines complement and supplement the Department of Health's guidance. Both pieces of guidance apply to food handlers whose work involves handling unwrapped food to be consumed raw or without further cooking or other forms of treatment, i.e. the high-risk food handler group. The requirements of both pieces of guidance are only effective when supported by good hygiene practice.

Screening and stool testing

UK and EC legislation place the responsibility on the food business operator to satisfy themselves that food handlers do not pose a hygiene risk to their product. However, food handlers are also obliged to inform their supervisor if they are suffering from any illness likely to affect the safety of food. Large companies may assess the health of their staff before they start work and may not allow them to resume handling food if the employee:

- has been ill in the past 7 days
- has been in contact with some one with enteric fever in the past 21 days
- is a suspect typhoid or paratyphoid carrier.

If a carrier state is suspected, it should be confirmed by microbiological examination. This is also relevant to employees returning from a holiday abroad

with symptoms of illness. Food businesses may also consider including the requirement to report illness as a condition of employment. Table 8.1 summarizes these requirements, along with exclusion criteria for people with, or contacts of, the more common gastrointestinal infections. Pre-employment stool testing or testing of an employee recovering from a diarrhoeal illness are not strict requirements. However, some micro-organisms/ infections require special consideration: enteric fever (typhoid and paratyphoid); verocytotoxin producing *E. coli* (VTEC); bacillary dysentery/ shigellosis; amoebic dysentery; pork tapeworm; hepatitis A.

TRAINING

The ability to maintain high standards of hygiene is a critical element in preventing contamination of food by food handlers. Food handlers should be not only adequately supervised but also have ongoing training and instruction in the importance of personal hygiene and hand washing. Use of appropriate language or translated material, where necessary, is a fundamental element of training. The knowledge and practice of food handlers should be regularly assessed. Further information on types of food hygiene training courses is provided in Chapter 17.

Summary

Good hygiene practice, a critical factor in preventing spread of infection, is essential for all food handlers to protect consumer health and ensure a safe food supply. The primary concern is the avoidance of microbiological contamination of food by infected food handlers, whether by direct contact with open food, or by indirect contact, such as from surfaces in production and processing areas. Food handlers with gastrointestinal infections are especially likely to contaminate food and the environment. Managers in the food industry have an important role in minimizing the risk of contamination of food by ensuring that all staff understand the importance of good personal hygiene and receive training in the safe handling of food. All training should be appropriately targeted, with particular emphasis on the high-risk food handler. The main considerations in prevention of food contamination by food handlers are:

- a good work environment with clean, hygienic work premises and adequate toilet, hand washing and changing facilities
- training and/or instruction, and supervising staff in the safe handling of food
- good personal hygiene practice by food handlers
- the reporting by food handlers to management of relevant infectious or potentially infectious conditions so that appropriate action (including exclusion) can be considered.

Food handlers are under a legal obligation to maintain a high degree of personal cleanliness as well as informing their manager when they are ill. Owners of food businesses must ensure that management systems, including HACCP, exclude food handlers when they report ill health and ensure that they receive regular training in food hygiene issues. These measures are only one step in the complex chain of events that ensure the food provided to the consumer is safe and personal hygiene should always be seen in this context.

All websites cited below were accessed in November 2006.

SOURCES OF INFORMATION AND FURTHER READING

Health Protection Agency (2004) Preventing person to person spread following gastrointestinal infections. A Guide for Public Health Physicians and Environmental Health Practitioners. An ad hoc Working Group of the former PHLS Advisory Committee on Gastrointestinal Infections. *Commun Dis Public Health* 7: 362–84.

Department of Health (1995) *Food Handlers: Fitness to Work* and *Food Handlers: Fitness to Work Guidance for Food Business Managers*. London: The Stationery Office.

Food Standards Agency (2006) *Safer Food Better Business*. London: Food Standards Agency (available at: www.food.gov.uk/foodindustry/regulation/hygleg/hyglegresources/sfbb/).

Foodlink. Your complete guide to food safety (available at: www.foodlink.org.uk).

9

Food preparation, cooking, cooling and storage

Paul A Gibbs

Introduction	180	Storage	196
Preparation	180	Summary	199
Cooking	181	Sources of information and further reading	200
Cooling	194		

Food preparation is the act of converting raw food material (whether cereal, fruit, vegetable, fish or meat) into a form ready for consumption or further processing. The Hazard Analysis Critical Control Point (HACCP) system is a structured, systematic approach to ensuring food safety. Hazard analysis identifies and assesses potential hazards in food processing, and Critical Control Points (CCPs) are identified where effective control measures can be defined, applied and monitored. The HACCP system is now internationally recognized and incorporated into legislation.

Cooking Heating food to make it more acceptable to a consumer or easily digestible, and/or to eliminate or reduce the levels of spoilage and pathogenic organisms. Only heating to temperatures >100 °C eliminates all micro-organisms (e.g. sterilization at 121 °C for 15 minutes).

Storage Holding of food under appropriate conditions, e.g. dry storage for powders, chill storage for raw meats, fish, fruit and vegetables.

Cool storage Treatment to temperatures below ambient. **Refrigeration** at 4 °C reduces or prevents growth of most micro-organisms. **Psychrotrophic** micro-organisms are those which continue to grow slowly at refrigeration temperatures, and include some pathogens and spoilage organisms. **Freezing** to −18 °C inhibits all microbial growth and many physico-chemical changes that cause deterioration. However, some chemical/enzymatic changes may lead to slow deterioration at these temperatures.

INTRODUCTION

The principles of HACCP can be applied to commercial (and domestic) catering and food preparation of a wide variety of raw materials, processes, and combinations of ingredients used. Qualitative risk assessments are also often done for the prevention of food poisoning in both domestic and commercial settings. Quantitative risk assessment can be difficult to apply because data on human infections, dose responses, etc. are limited, even in the UK, where good data on food poisoning and infections are otherwise available.

PREPARATION

Raw materials are frequently contaminated with many pathogenic and spoilage microbes, including bacteria, yeasts and moulds. General removal of gross 'soil', e.g. by washing with potable water, will reduce the level of contamination but not eliminate it. Even using dilute solutions of chlorine (bleach), as is often recommended, will reduce the surface contamination by only about 1–2.5 log colony forming unit (CFU)/g or mL. Most plant materials have a hydrophobic (waxy) surface that resists washing and protects adherent micro-organisms. In some salad items it has been clearly demonstrated that plant tissues can accumulate specific pathogens through the root system. No amount of washing or treatment with a disinfectant will kill these contaminants. However, a recent observation suggests that exposure to dilute peroxide and ultraviolet (UV) light, can kill pathogens within plant tissue by generation of short-lived free radicals. But such a process is only suitable for commercial treatment of ready-to-eat vegetables.

In addition to cleaning the raw food material, it is most important to maintain hygienic conditions in food preparation areas, i.e. clean hands, working surfaces and implements, and frequent washing with appropriate detergents and/or sanitizers. Many micro-organisms can quickly colonize surfaces and form an adherent film (biofilm). Such biofilms allowed to develop on surfaces can be difficult to remove and become a continuous source of spoilage and pathogenic organisms. Most of the organisms in biofilms are in the stationary phase of growth and generally more resistant to high temperatures, cleaning agents, physical removal, etc. Stationary phase organisms may also exhibit enhanced virulence traits, e.g. toxin production, invasive enzymes, etc. through a phenomenon called quorum sensing or cell–cell signalling. In commercial food preparation, it is now quite common to use plastic conveyor belts impregnated with a highly effective antimicrobial, triclosan. This has been shown to reduce considerably the number of viable microbes on the surface and biofilm formation.

In the preparation of rolled joints of meat, contamination from the surface of the meat or from the working surface can reach the centre of the joint during rolling. The centre reaches the cooking temperature more slowly and later than the rest of the joint, is heated for the shortest time, and also cools the slowest. Thus food poisoning caused by *Clostridium perfringens* occurs by these means. There has been considerable controversy about the hygienic status of chopping (cutting) boards, i.e. plastic versus wood. Plastic is generally recommended since wood is porous and swells when wet and so may trap organisms within the crevices. However, the surface of plastic is readily cut, increasing the sites where microbes can adhere strongly and avoid the action of cleaning agents. It has also been shown that the natural oils in some woods may be bactericidal, i.e. killing bacteria throughout the life of the chopping board. However, cleaning plastic with strong sanitizers, e.g. alkali, caustic or chlorine solutions, in combination with high temperatures, is highly effective. Such cleaning methods are not recommended for wood. Nevertheless, plastic chopping boards can get stained by vegetable juices and this is extremely difficult to remove. A common method of assessing the efficacy of removal of food material and microbes is by measurement of residual adenosine triphosphate (ATP) as a marker of microbial contamination. It has been shown that even after bacteria have been removed from or killed on plastic chopping boards by the normal operation of a commercial washing machine, only when much more rigorous cleaning was applied, did the stains disappear together with residual ATP. Although the consensus of opinion is still in favour of plastic cutting boards in commercial and domestic catering, these should be colour coded for separate use for raw vegetables, raw meats and cooked items, and cleaned effectively and dried before storage.

COOKING

Food is cooked via heating by many and various means. Heating is the most common method of preparing food for consumption. Cooked food is more appetizing, in most cases is easier to digest, and heating to temperatures above about 60 °C for several minutes (e.g. pasteurization) destroys many food spoilage and food poisoning micro-organisms. Nevertheless, heat-resistant spores resist cooking, and if the food is held warm, these will germinate and grow rapidly, potentially leading to food poisoning. Elimination of all viable microbes (sterilization), including spore-forming foodborne pathogens, can only be achieved at temperatures exceeding 100 °C (see Chapter 3). The physicochemical parameters of a food matrix can have a marked effect on the heat resistance of micro-organisms. In general, low pH values will reduce the D value, whereas low water activity (a_w) produced by high sugar content will increase the D value, often to a surprising degree. For example, in cocoa liquor or chocolate (water content about 0.5–1.0% w/w, a_w about 0.60), salmonellae can survive heating to 100 °C for several minutes even though they are normally killed by pasteurization (e.g. 72 °C for 15 seconds). For further discussion of D, a_w and resistance to heat see Chapter 3.

When microbial growth that results in production of foodborne toxins, occurs in a food, some of these toxins may be difficult or impossible to destroy by cooking, e.g. *Staphylococcus aureus* (enterotoxin), *Bacillus cereus* (emetic toxin; cerulide), some mycotoxins, or the shellfish toxins. Cerulide, for example, will resist temperatures of 121 °C for several hours. However, other toxins, e.g. botulinum neurotoxin, are destroyed by boiling for about 5–10 minutes.

Food that is eaten immediately after cooking, while still hot, should not give rise to food poisoning or infections. However, under-cooking has given rise to some serious cases or outbreaks of foodborne infections. Under-cooking of poultry, such as at a barbecue, causes salmonellosis, whereas under-cooking of hamburgers has led to infections and deaths from vero cytotoxin-producing strains of *Escherichia coli*.

Cooking, rapid cooling and adequate reheating of foods, if done carefully and with prevention of re-contamination after cooking, is a safe and useful method of mass catering (see 'cook–chill', 'cook–freeze' and '*sous vide*' processes described later in this chapter). However, cases of botulism have resulted from holding cooked foods at ambient temperatures and then reheating, e.g. foil-wrapped baked potatoes.

Developments in mass preparation, cooking, packaging, refrigeration and distribution of food have led to considerable changes in eating habits. These include preparation of meals cooked from raw materials in the home (**scratch cooking**), to reheating pre-cooked meals (**convenience cooking**) at any time of the day (or night), leading to 'eating-on-the-go' or 'grazing'. The wide availability and variety of such pre-prepared meals, together with an increase and variety in the hours spent away from home by family members, has also led to a decrease in the time a family spends together eating and socializing, with each family member being able to choose what and when they eat.

Methods of cooking

Heat is transferred to food items by several means. The least effective way is by hot dry air (since that medium has a low specific heat), such as used in domestic ovens, whether convection only or fan-assisted. Until a food item has much of the water removed by heat, the temperature of the food will not exceed about 100 °C, even though the oven temperature may be above 200 °C. Some domestic fan-assisted ovens have the facility of injecting steam into the air stream.

Heating of liquids for pasteurization or temperatures at or above 100 °C, e.g. for sterilization, can be achieved by indirect means: through a heat exchanger with steam or hot water; by direct injection of steam into the flowing product, or by spraying the liquid product into a vessel maintained at the required temperature and pressure with steam. Each of these methods has particular advantages and disadvantages for different products.

Cooking in steam under pressure raises the temperature and reduces the cooking time considerably. Thus a pressure of 1 bar (10^5 Pa) raises the temperature to 121 °C and reduces cooking time to minutes. At this temperature, sterilization is achieved in 15 minutes, as in a laboratory or hospital autoclave. In these times of rising fuel prices, pressure cooking has much to recommend it to domestic and commercial caterers alike. Frying in oil at high temperatures serves to rapidly heat, brown and dehydrate foods, e.g. potato chips, meat, or fish. Until the food is dehydrated, the temperature will not exceed 100 °C, even though the oil may be at 200 °C. Grilling or toasting is achieved by infra-red radiation from a hot surface, and the brown surface coloration is the result of dehydration and high-temperature chemical reactions between the food constituents. Cooking with microwaves relies on transfer of energy to water molecules by high-frequency radiowaves, and is in effect a type of boiling. The speed of heating by microwaves (not requiring preheating of an oven) is particularly suitable for reheating of pre-prepared meals.

Pasteurization of liquids, especially of milk and raw liquid egg, has, over many years, proved to result in safer products insofar as vegetative food-borne pathogens are destroyed (e.g. salmonellae). However, chilled storage and a limited shelf-life are necessary to minimize the growth of the surviving spores and some other heat-resistant microbes. The benefits of pasteurization of milk are reversed by re-contamination.

During production of evaporated, condensed or powdered milk, there is considerable heating, and as the milk becomes more concentrated, the heat resistance of any vegetative organisms present also increases. Thus milk must be pasteurized before any concentration begins. For example, it has been clearly demonstrated that salmonellae can survive the concentration of milk to 40 per cent solids and then spray drying. Boiling is similar to pasteurization, but at the higher temperatures (about 100 °C) all foodborne vegetative cells are killed rapidly. Poaching of fish in water, either on a hob or in a low oven, is designed to retain the flavours of the fish without causing hardening of the flesh. At the lowest temperatures used, about 50–55 °C, there is a probability that certain vegetative foodborne pathogens will survive, e.g. *Listeria monocytogenes* or vero cytotoxin producing *E. coli*.

Pressure cooking and steaming enable food to be cooked within minutes and, in conjunction with steam-heated pans they can replace the boiling top and its battery of pans. Domestic pressure cookers – specially designed, securely closed, heavy saucepans with some form of pressure relief valve – are commonly used for rapid cooking or reheating foods or meals, at pressures of up to 1 bar and achieve 121 °C (Figure 9.1). Raising the temperature by 10 °C approximately doubles the rate of chemical reactions and halves the cooking time: about 20 minutes boiling can be reduced to less than 5 minutes pressure cooking at 1 bar.

Modern commercial pressure cookers/steamers are of two types:

- **dynamic or high pressure**, where steam jets will rapidly defrost and cook frozen food at 0.8–1.0 bar;
- **low pressure**, operating at about 0.4 bar when there is greater flexibility and control of the cooking process.

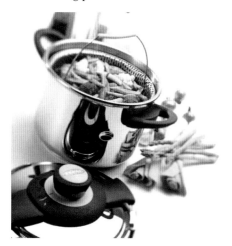

Figure 9.1 *A domestic pressure cooker. Photo courtesy of Tefal Ltd.*

In a pressure cooker, as in a laboratory or hospital autoclave, sterilization occurs if the conditions are hot enough for sufficient time. At a pressure of 1 bar, the temperature will probably reach 121 °C and sterilization will be achieved in 15 minutes. At pressures below 1 bar, sterilization cannot be assured although most bacteria and many spores will be destroyed.

Convection ovens rely on dry hot air from the heating source (gas flame or electric element), and conduction of the supplied heat from the heated surface to the interior of the food. A temperature gradient is established from the surface to the centre: the surface of the food will dry and become brown (oxidized and caramelized) while the interior retains most of the original moisture. Internal temperatures will rarely exceed 100 °C until all water is boiled away, but as the internal temperature exceeds 65–70 °C for several minutes, vegetative cells will be killed, although spores will survive. Even on removal from the heat source, there will still be a temperature gradient that results in further heating of the interior of the food.

Most electrically heated ovens used to be pure convection ovens, i.e. the heat was transferred around the food by movement of the hot air rising from the heat source (electric elements at the sides of the oven), cooling slightly and transferring heat to the food. This is a relatively slow method of cooking, but is convenient as the top of the oven will be several degrees hotter than lower, thus allowing foods to be cooked together at different temperatures. Gas-heated ovens are pure convection ovens.

It is now more common to have a fan in an oven (**forced air convection oven**) that re-circulates the hot air in the oven, improving heat transfer considerably, and cooks faster, more evenly, and more effectively. The oven shelves can be filled with food and given there are sufficient gaps for circulation of air, cooking is achieved throughout the oven without affecting efficiency. Similar articles of food will be equally cooked almost regardless of their position in the oven. Cooking times generally can be reduced by about a third compared with those of the conventional oven, or, alternatively, the temperature can be reduced by about 20–30 °C. Forced air convection ovens are available in three types according to the speed of air movement and the input of heat. Care is needed to select the correct oven. As with conventional ovens, vegetative cells of bacteria are killed but not all spores. Some fan ovens have a facility for injecting hot water/steam into a fast-moving hot air stream thus increasing the humidity, decreasing the surface drying effect, but increasing considerably the rate of heat transfer due to the latent heat of condensation of steam onto the food.

Infra-red cooking (grilling or toasting) relies on radiant heat (infra-red rays) from an open fire, charcoal barbecue, hot electric element or gas-heated grill, and will cook food relatively slowly, requiring a temperature gradient to be established from the surface inwards. Only observing the intense browning on the surface and not measuring the internal temperature of foods, especially meat and fish, can lead to under-cooking. Such poor cooking practice, especially with barbecues, has led to outbreaks of food poisoning. Generally, the causative organisms are salmonellae, although occasionally *Campylobacter* spp. from poultry are responsible. However, poor hygiene may also be a contributory cause, because there are no means of readily washing utensils used for handling raw foods before manipulating the cooked foods. Under-cooked hamburgers have been associated with vero cytotoxin-producing *E. coli* infections, especially in the USA. This organism appears to be a commensal in bovine animals and does not cause disease in them. In humans the infection, thought to result from ingesting very few bacteria, is extremely serious; the verocytotoxin causes severe kidney and liver damage, and is sometimes fatal. (See Chapter 4, p. 67.)

Steam ovens cook food by direct contact with steam in the cooking chamber, and the cooking is much faster than in hot air ovens (due to the latent heat of condensation of steam). Generally, these ovens are commercial or catering-type cookers, although there are a few domestic steam ovens on the market. Steam enters the chamber or compartment at 0.4 bar (low pressure) or 1 bar (high pressure) and may be connected directly to a steam line or have a steam generator built-in (as in the domestic steam cookers). Some cookers use heated containers of water within the cooker (convection generators) to produce the steam. The appropriate steam temperature within the cooking space is 100 °C. Steam cookers fed with high-pressure steam usually have a capacity of only one to two pans as they cook the food faster than a low-pressure or convection generator-type of cooker. A drain in the bottom of the cooker removes the condensate, and preheating leads to even shorter cooking times. Some models have a thermostat that adjusts to the size of compartment load and original product temperature. Steam cookers are especially good for dense root products such as potatoes and carrots, as well as fragile vegetables (broccoli and asparagus), rice, shrimp and eggs in their shells. Commercially, chickens or turkeys may be rapidly cooked whole, but because the surface is not browned as in a hot air oven, a spicy or flavoured browning paste is applied to the surfaces before cooking. The carcasses may be packed in heat-resistant plastic bags under a vacuum, but not as highly evacuated as in *sous vide* packaging. Covering food in steam ovens, as in all ovens, increases the cooking time.

Microwave ovens heat food rapidly via high frequency radiowaves. These ovens use little electricity and reheat cooked food quickly; food may be covered during cooking or reheating as the microwaves easily penetrate through glass or plastic but not metal. Microwave ovens are used in conjunction with a deep freeze for fast food service, both in commercial catering and in the home. Microwaves heat food by the transfer of energy to molecules, especially water molecules. The waves penetrate into the food, the distance depending on the type of food, as they gradually lose energy. This energy is absorbed and converted into heat which then spreads inwards by conduction. Most foods need to be stirred during heating or left to stand at the end of the cooking process to allow the centre to reach the same temperature as that near the surface of the food. As the surface of foods encounters the microwave energy first, there is a strong tendency for the water molecules to be 'boiled-off', thus cooling the food surface: steam or water vapour absorbs microwave energy poorly. If the effect is sufficiently marked, some vegetative microbial cells survive on the surface. Covering or wrapping a food item minimizes water vapour loss and hence cooling effects, as well as allowing cooking by steam. However, foods high in fat and sugar, and low in water, have a tendency to become extremely hot. Christmas puddings and rich fruit cakes can burst into flames in microwave ovens!

Metal containers impede microwave cooking by reflection and may even cause a breakdown in the microwave generating system – sometimes seen as sparks or heard as crackling within the oven. Even a metal decorative design on a plate or cup, e.g. of gold or silver, can cause damage. There is a tendency towards uneven cooking in microwave ovens, which can be checked by covering the cooking plate with a flour paste and cooking until dark areas become visible. Uneven cooking is partially overcome by the inclusion of a turntable which rotates the food during cooking, and also mode or wave stirrers, e.g. rotating antennae, deflect the waves off the metal walls of the oven to give a more even power distribution. Turning solid foods and stirring liquids or semi-solid foods at intervals during the cooking period will distribute the heat. As the microwaves heat only the food and not the container, care must be taken to keep the oven and the containers clean. It has been shown that organisms can survive in dried films on the microwave oven walls.

The drawbacks of microwave cooking are irregular heat penetration and lack of browning; these can be overcome by incorporating hot air streams (as in a conventional oven), e.g. the **Mealstream Micro-Aire** ovens are designed for fast-food menus. These cook by continuous or 7-second pulsed microwave energy, in combination with forced air convection, making use of the adjacent infra-red wave band as the source of heat. They can be used to roast, bake, fry, grill, braise and boil, and save labour, food, power, space and time compared with traditional cooking methods. There is less dirt and the hygiene is thereby improved. Ventilation requirements are also reduced. Nevertheless, microwave ovens must be kept clean as only a small gap because of a food particle in the door seal can result in leakage of microwave energy into the kitchen with exposure of workers; microwaves cook humans just as well as food!

Ohmic heating is an industrial process requiring special equipment and control systems. Heating of liquid food flowing in a pipe is achieved by passing an alternating electric current through the liquid along the length of the pipe. The conductivity of the food must be carefully controlled and also any particles must be as uniform as possible and have conductivity similar to that of the fluid part. The process is therefore only suitable for large batches, e.g. of soup mixes, which can be pasteurized or sterilized followed by rapid cooling and aseptic filling into sterile cartons.

Slow cooking dates back to ancient times when stone pots were first used for this purpose. This cooking process became popular in the 1970s and 1980s with the increasing costs of fuel and food: maximum tenderness can be obtained from less expensive cuts of meat when they are cooked slowly at low temperatures. With the current steep rises in costs of fuel (2005–06) there has been renewed interest in electric slow cookers or crock pots in both the USA and Britain as a means of economy, and for 'cash-rich, time-poor' households. A typical slow cooking vessel consists of a glazed earthenware bowl and lid with an outer aluminium casing containing an electrical heating element. The heat used is approximately 60 W on low and 120 W on the high setting – which is equivalent to that of a light bulb. Most slow cookers have a timer or thermostat that starts the cooking process on high power and switches to low power after a pre-set time or at a pre-set temperature. Others require manual re-setting to low power.

Some concern has been expressed about the possible bacteriological hazards of cooking food at low temperatures for long periods of time. Survival of organisms (especially C. *perfringens*) can occur in the centre of meat and poultry during slow, low-temperature cooking, and that growth may occur during the prolonged holding period. However, the hazards of using slow cookers are no greater than those of conventional cooking methods provided that the manufacturer's instructions are followed. Although the heating rate may be slower than by more conventional means, the time spent in the temperature zone permitting microbial growth is short and any increase in the numbers of vegetative cells is negated as higher temperatures are reached. Bacterial spores will survive, but if the holding temperature is correct, there is no outgrowth of spores of food poisoning organisms during the holding cycle. Outbreaks of C. *perfringens* food poisoning have occurred with holding temperatures of about 45–50 °C: the spores germinate at about 50 °C and multiply rapidly on further cooling with doubling times of about 12 minutes at 45–48 °C in meat. However, as with other methods of cooking, it is important that the food be eaten immediately when hot or removed from the casserole, cooled rapidly and refrigerated.

When a dish containing red kidney beans is to be cooked in a slow cooking vessel, the beans should be pre-cooked by boiling for at least 10 minutes before they are added to the other ingredients. The red kidney bean **haemagglutinins** have been known to cause food poisoning when the beans are cooked from the raw state in an electric casserole. The temperatures are sufficient to cook food and kill vegetative cells of bacteria, but not to inactivate the toxic component of the bean.

Electronic catering-size slow cookers and ovens are also available. They cook meats at low temperatures to a predetermined centre (of the food) temperature detected by means of a probe. When the required temperature is reached in the centre, the oven switches to a non-cooking cycle which holds the food at 63 °C for several hours, even overnight, until required. It is claimed that shrinkage is minimal and that natural enzyme action during the holding cycle makes the meat more tender. However, most meat enzymes will have been destroyed by the higher temperatures of the cooking cycle, and it is more likely that tenderization occurs because of slow hydrolysis of the tendon structures by the elevated temperature of the holding period.

Cook-chill is a catering system in which cooking of food is followed by fast chilling, storage under controlled low temperatures just above freezing point, 0–3 °C, and subsequent reheating immediately before consumption. The many advantages of the cook-chill system include: centralization of stores, saving on staff, better portion control, and a better balance of the day's work, thus avoiding the traditional peaks of production around mealtimes. From a microbiological point of view, it is more difficult to achieve good control over temperatures and times for cooking and cooling of larger batches of foods than it is for small amounts of food cooked individually. The dangers of cross-contamination between raw materials and other foods can be reduced by the preparation of single items at a time when equipment is not being used for other foods. If necessary, samples taken from large batches can be checked bacteriologically before they are eaten.

Abuse of temperature control in the preparation, storage, distribution or reheating of food is more likely to result in hazards to health in a cook-chill system than by the cook-freeze method. Cross-contamination during cooling with psychrotrophic food poisoning bacteria such as *L. monocytogenes*, or survival of spores of psychrotrophic strains of *Clostridium botulinum*, and subsequent moderate temperature abuse (5–7 °C), would allow growth to potentially hazardous levels. The chilling process should commence within 30 minutes of the food leaving the cooker and be complete within a further period of 1.5 hours. Chilled foods should be distributed under controlled conditions and the temperature must not exceed 10 °C. Experimentally, it has been shown that botulinum toxin production can occur within 10 days at 8 °C. Cooked foods should be reheated to at least 70 °C before consumption. The maximum life of the cooked products when held at or below 3 °C should not exceed 5 days, including both the day of cooking and the day of consumption. This is a rather short shelf-life, but does allow freedom to prepare meal items in bulk throughout the working day, without the time constraints inevitable in traditional catering operations. If the storage temperature exceeds 5 °C, but does not rise above 10 °C, the food should be consumed within 12 hours; if 10 °C is exceeded the food should be regarded as unsuitable for use, since there would have been time sufficient for microbial growth. There is still some controversy regarding shelf-life, because the industry code indicates 10 days at <5 °C and 5 days at <10 °C.

A Code of Practice issued by the Department of Health for both the cook-freeze and the cook-chill systems (Department of Health 1989) does not apply to chilled foods prepared under special conditions of processing and packaging that provide a product with an expected shelf-life of more than 5 days, for example *sous vide*. In the basic *sous vide* process, raw or par-cooked food is put in high-barrier plastic bags or pouches and hermetically sealed under vacuum. The food is then cooked at low temperatures, either in hot water baths or steam-heated ovens, often only at pasteurization temperatures (65–75 °C). The food may be served immediately, or more usually, chilled to 0–3 °C, stored for up to 21 days, reheated and the bag opened for service of the meal. The microbiological advantages of the process are largely concerned with the lack of opportunity for cross-contamination between cooking, chilling and reheating before serving, unlike cook-chill or cook-freeze where foods may be only lightly covered during cooling and storage.

The *sous vide* process does not kill all food poisoning organisms, some spores will survive, so the chilling process must be rapid – usually cold showering of the bags while still in the cooker – and the chill holding temperature must be very carefully controlled. The system improves both the nutritional value and the palatability of foods through minimizing oxidative changes (e.g. of unsaturated oils), and the longer potential storage life gives greater flexibility in catering and retail operations. However, there are drawbacks to the system that include a greater risk of spoilage or even food poisoning if production controls are not carefully applied. Storage under vacuum may mask signs of spoilage, and surviving facultative or anaerobic organisms may multiply and produce toxins. Of particular concern are the spores of psychrotrophic *C. botulinum* (types B, E and F). Recommendations have been made for reduction of these spores by 6 log by cooking times and temperatures equivalent to 90 °C for 10 minutes. Careful selection of raw materials and hygienic preparation all help to minimize problems with these organisms, but they cannot be eliminated. It is not a process recommended for domestic catering, although there have been attempts to market 'vacuum packaging kits' for *sous vide* food processing in the home. Similarly, although there have been attempts to market *sous vide* products at retail, this is now rarely done as the temperature controls necessary to assure safe shelf-life cannot be guaranteed either at retail or in the home. A general guide to *sous-vide* processing with

particular emphasis on the microbiological safety of the technology, is available (CCFRA 1992).

Cook-freeze is a system whereby high-quality food is prepared and cooked in economic quantities, retained in a state of 'suspended freshness' by rapid freezing and freezer storage, and served when and where required from finishing kitchens with low capital investment and minimal staffing. Food is prepared, cooked, and frozen centrally and distributed frozen to service areas for final heating and service (Figure 9.2). Rapid freezing may be done in blast freezers or by spraying with liquid nitrogen in special cabinets or tunnels.

The many advantages of the cook-freeze system are similar to cook-chill systems described above, but there is less emphasis on careful control of temperatures since below about −5 °C there is no significant microbial growth, although there will be physico-chemical degradation of foods by ice crystal formation and possibly some very slow enzymic activity. From a microbiological point of view, there is more time available for samples taken from large batches to be checked bacteriologically before they are eaten. However, mistakes in batch preparation can lead to larger outbreaks of food poisoning than small-scale cooking on a day-to-day basis. In dealing with large quantities of food, there is an increased hazard because of greater difficulty in ensuring adequate heat penetration and rapid

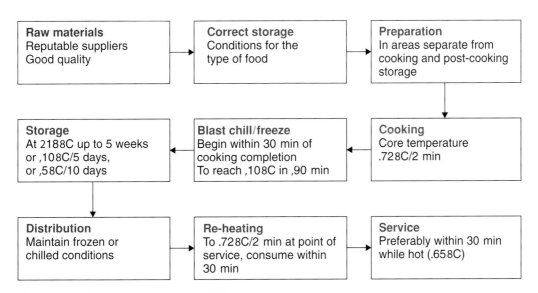

Figure 9.2 *Flow diagram for cook-chill/freeze process*

cooling after cooking. The main emphasis in cook-freeze, as in any other catering system is correct storage between cooking and service to prevent multiplication of organisms that may have survived the heat process or reached the food after cooking.

Cooking frozen food – the common use of home freezers and the marketing of both raw frozen food and ready meals has led to much discussion on the hazards of cooking from the frozen state, particularly joints of meat and poultry. It has been a long accepted practice to cook small items such as vegetables, fish fingers, beefburgers, pies, chops and ready meals, without preliminary thawing. Individually, these items are relatively small so there is little delay in heat penetration and adequate cooking is ensured in fairly short periods of time, whether by grilling, frying, oven or microwave heating. With the changes in eating habits – individual meals in the home, eating on the go, 'grazing' – cooking foods from frozen, especially by microwaves, is on the increase.

The main difficulty arises in the cooking of joints of meat and poultry from frozen. Although some frozen food companies and authors of books on home freezers and cookery advocate cooking meat from the frozen state and give times and temperatures to use, it is safer to thaw frozen meats before cooking. However, when a frozen joint or poultry carcass is cooked, the outside may appear to be well done while the centre remains quite raw. As stated in the beginning of this chapter, vegetative organisms present in the centre of a rolled joint or in the cavity of poultry, may survive and if the cooked food is stored incorrectly, they can multiply to numbers able to cause food poisoning. Even if recommendations for cooking times and temperatures are laid down, there will be occasions when rules are forgotten. 'Doneness' is usually judged by the external appearance of meat and by probing with a sharp implement: meat thermometers, unfortunately, are rarely used.

Small meat joints or poultry carcasses will be consumed quickly, possibly at one meal. The number of organisms surviving cooking will probably be too small to cause illness. However, catering-size joints are a much greater hazard as they are more likely to be cooked in advance of need and improperly stored before use because of lack of adequate cooling facilities. The cooking of large joints from the frozen state requires much longer times and hence more fuel. Proper cooling is also much more difficult and the cooking and cooling of large joints should be strongly discouraged.

Food poisoning outbreaks have been attributed to the large 'banqueting' size frozen turkeys, often 14–18 kg in weight. Problems with handling this size of carcass occur at all stages of preparation, cooking and storage. The time needed to thaw the meat may be several days; thorough cooking to the centre without over-cooking the exterior is difficult and cooling prior to refrigerated storage needs several hours in the absence of mechanical coolers such as cold rooms with fans or blast chillers. Thus there are multiple opportunities for survival and growth of food poisoning organisms, in particular, salmonellae and *C. perfringens*. In recognition of these difficulties, a predictive modelling program for estimating the growth of *C. perfringens* during cooling has been developed and is freely available on the internet. Other similar predictive models are there for the survival of other organisms during heating (see http://www.ifr.ac.uk/safety/growthpredictor).

Cooking of specific food items

Meat and poultry dishes

Heat penetrates slowly into joints, poultry carcasses, and made-up dishes such as pies, and adequate cooking times and temperatures should be allowed for the centre to reach almost 100 °C. For instance, a 3 kg meat pie requires an oven temperature of 177–204 °C for 2.5–3 hours for the centre to approach boiling point. An outbreak of salmonellosis from several pies of two smaller sizes has been reported. The minced meat, probably already contaminated with salmonellae, was hand-filled raw into the pastry cases and it was thought that the cooking, at 232–246 °C for 25–30 minutes, was either inadequate to destroy the contaminants or that there were temperature fluctuations. It has been pointed out that pies made with raw meat should be cooked to the point where the centre achieves close to 100 °C, even though the pastry may become a little over-brown in the process. It is worthwhile to note that for the red muscle colouring of meat to change to the familiar grey cooked colour, the temperature must be at least 73 °C. Heat penetrates meat slowly and English rare roast beef which remains red inside, has not reached an internal temperature of more than 63–65 °C.

Slowly cooked rare beef used for sandwiches has caused *C. perfringens* food poisoning.

Comment has already been made about under-cooking of hamburgers (beef patties), which has caused infections (including deaths) from infection with verocytotoxin-producing *E. coli* O157:H7, particularly in the USA. Several studies have made recommendations regarding cooking temperatures and times, but essentially, the centre of burgers should be cooked to a minimum temperature of 70 °C for 2 minutes or equivalent. Browning – lack of pink colour – of the centre of the burger is now not an appropriate method of determining that the safe cooking temperature and time have been reached. Some ground (minced) beef can turn brown before being fully cooked, whereas some fully cooked minced beef can still retain some pink colour. Advice on equivalent core cooking time/temperature combinations is provided in the Department of Health (1992) guidelines that cover the safe cooking of meat.

Pre-cooked meat is often used for making pies and pasties so that the final cooking time is sufficient only to bake the pastry. The temperature reached in the centre of the mass of meat – sometimes mixed with vegetables – would not necessarily destroy sporing or even non-sporing organisms, which would multiply actively while the meat was still warm. Between 1988 and 1991, 146 of 611 (24%) general outbreaks of food poisoning in England and Wales in which the vehicle of infection was traced were due to *C. perfringens;* the foods most commonly implicated were cold and reheated meat and poultry, and stews, casseroles, curries and minced meat dishes. Thus a change in cooking methods and a greater awareness of the necessity for rapid cooling and cold storage will help to eliminate this type of food poisoning. The numbers of *C. perfringens* cases has decreased in the past decade, probably due to the intelligent use of cooling and refrigeration in the home and in catering outlets – but only to be overtaken by cases of salmonellosis and campylobacteriosis, mainly from poultry sources and generally due to cross-contamination of cooked items!

Part cooking of meat in hot weather or at any other time, is poor catering practice. Some organisms will be killed but others may be encouraged to multiply. The final cooking may be too light either to kill bacteria or to destroy toxins. It is safer to keep meat in the raw state overnight, preferably in the cold, and to cook it thoroughly on the day when it is required. If, from motives of economy or for some other reason, it is essential to cook meat the day before it is eaten, it should be cooked thoroughly, cooled rapidly and refrigerated overnight. When there is insufficient refrigerator space, there should be a strict rule that all dishes of stewed or boiled meat, whether stews pies, or joints, must be cooked and eaten the same day, preferably with no delay between cooking and eating and certainly no more than 1–2 hours. The danger of eating meat and poultry cooked a day or two earlier seems to be far greater in the communal canteen dealing with larger masses of meat than in the home, although in no instance should cooked meat be allowed to stand at a warm temperature for several hours.

Well-roasted solid meats should be safe, but the roast rolled joint frequently gives trouble because the contaminated outside is folded into the centre, where the joint is the slowest to heat and cool. The size and shape of joints of meat are important in relation to heat penetration and heat loss. Temperature recordings from thermocouples during cooking have shown that the temperature at any point within the meat depends on the distance of the point from the outer surface of the meat. The centre of large, bulky cuts of meat will, therefore, take longer to heat and cool than that of long, slim portions of similar weight. It has also been shown experimentally that the centre of large portions of meat are slower to heat-up in a hot-air oven than in a moist-air or steam oven (see p. 182).

The use of pressure cookers for quick, high-temperature cooking solves many of the difficulties associated with the preparation of foodstuffs on the day they need to be eaten hot. Even heat-resistant spores are killed by this method of cooking, given the correct time and temperature (see p. 183). Canteen-prepared tongue has been a frequent vehicle of *C. perfringens* and staphylococcal food poisoning, although this item of food is now less commonly eaten. *C. perfringens* from the organisms already present in the raw tongue, and staphylococci from the hands of the cook, multiply in the cooked product as a result of handling after cooking. Outbreaks of food poisoning are often associated with cold or warmed poultry meat. Salmonellae and *C. perfringens* are commonly present in frozen or chilled birds. The spores of C.

perfringens may not get killed by cooking and can grow later during the long slow cooling and kitchen storage. Salmonellae may survive in under-thawed and under-cooked carcasses, although they are most often picked up after cooking, from traces of the raw product left on surfaces and utensils. If the meat is left unchilled, the organisms will grow in it.

Outbreaks of *Salmonella* food poisoning from spit-roasting can occur. Unless the cook is aware of the dangers, drips can result in contamination between fresh raw carcasses and those that are part cooked. Cross-contamination also occurs when handling both raw and cooked carcasses with the same tools or hands without thorough washing. Careful instructions are needed for thawing, cooking and, most importantly, for handling and storage of cooked poultry. Staphylococci are usually transferred by hands after cooking. Cooked carcasses may be cut and torn apart while still warm and the portions piled high on trays, so that the rate of cooling is slow, even if these are refrigerated. When the meat is removed from the refrigerator or cold room the next day, organisms continue to grow and produce toxin. Any meat that must be handled while still warm after cooking, and which is not refrigerated promptly, is a potential source of food poisoning. Cooked ham is similarly readily contaminated with staphylococci from hands or slicing machines improperly cleaned and sanitized, and although the growth of many organisms is inhibited by the curing salts present, staphylococci are very tolerant of these preservatives.

Dairy foods

The hazards associated with the preparation of food a day or so ahead of consumption also apply to custards, trifles, blancmange and other milk puddings; these dishes should be freshly cooked unless they can be chilled quickly and stored in a refrigerator.

Gentle heating of milk, as in pasteurization, destroys vegetative cells of hazardous organisms so that the milk is made safe unless re-contaminated. However, it should be remembered that spores will survive pasteurization and efficient chilling and continuing refrigeration is essential to minimize their germination and growth. *B. cereus* is the most common spore-former to survive. If refrigeration is insufficient, there will be growth of this bacterium, resulting in the phenomenon of 'bitty cream'. This

occurs because the natural detergent-like activity of lecithin, which maintains the cream in small droplets, is destroyed by lecithinase produced by *B. cereus*. As a result the droplets coalesce to form large particles, with the appearance of an oily layer on hot drinks such as tea.

Food poisoning from the growth of *B. cereus* in milk is rare because growth of this bacterium is preceded by obvious spoilage. However, in the mid-1960s, when milk was mixed with other ingredients, such as starch products, heated to make blancmange (varieties of vanilla-flavoured puddings) and stored at ambient temperatures for a few hours, *B. cereus* emetic food poisoning was very common (Becker *et al.*, 1994). Growth of the organism in the presence of starch (as in cooked rice – see p. 193) seems to favour production of emetic toxin.

'Sterilized milk' means that a temperature is reached at which almost all bacteria are destroyed, and the milk will be close to sterile for an indefinite period as long as it is kept in the sealed container. **Ultra heat treated (UHT) milk** is subjected to high temperatures by indirect or direct application of steam, cooled rapidly and packaged aseptically; not all spores are destroyed, but the chilled shelf-life of the milk in unopened cartons may be as long as 3 months. However, if the raw milk has been held on the farm or in silos at the dairy in chilled conditions for too long, there may be considerable growth of pseudomonads. Pseudomonads do not cause acidic spoilage of milk (like lactic acid bacteria), but many of this group of organisms release lipolytic and proteolytic enzymes that are more heat resistant in UHT conditions than spores. These enzymes are destroyed by pasteurization but not completely so by the short times (<3 s) at 141 °C used for UHT milk. Sealed cartons of UHT milk may spoil enzymically over a period of 1–3 months, generating a soft clot (proteolysis) and/or rancid flavours (lipolysis).

There have been some noteworthy episodes of food poisoning from powdered (spray-dried) milk. Several outbreaks have been described in the UK (due to staphylococcal enterotoxin and *Salmonella enterica* subsp. Ealing) (see Chapter 6, p. 137) and in the USA (due to *S. enterica* subsp. New Brunswick) (see Chapter 6). Milk must be pasteurized before concentrating (to 40 per cent solids) by heating under vacuum and spray drying. Vegetative cells in concentrated milk are much more heat resistant than those in normal milk and can survive spray drying, even though the air temperature in the drier may be >240 °C. Cross-contamination of the dried milk (e.g. during cooling of the hot powder with filtered external air from handling machinery), although rare, has occurred. During 1985, in the UK, a powdered baby milk formula that came from a contaminated site in a spray-drying tower led to several cases of salmonellosis in babies (Rowe *et al.* 1987).

Confectionery creams are susceptible to bacterial contamination, and they should be prepared and stored under strict hygiene conditions. All ingredients should be free from pathogens and gross bacterial contamination. Equipment should be scrupulously clean and disinfected frequently, preferably by heat. Savoy bags for dispensing cream and other toppings (and also mashed potato) should be made of materials which can be washed and boiled after use, such as cotton, linen or nylon or other suitable materials. After boiling they should be dried thoroughly and stored in a special place protected from dust or other sources of contamination. Disposable paper bags may be better for this purpose.

Although it is considered necessary to ensure that people handling cream and milk are free of salmonellae, the presence of these organisms in the cow is probably of even greater importance. In some parts of the world, *Brucella abortus* is still found in cows and *Brucella melitensis* in goats. However, *Brucella* and others such as the tubercle bacilli are pathogenic for these domesticated animals, and are a hazard for those who drink raw milk in countries without eradication schemes and without pasteurization. The abolition of the sale of raw milk in Scotland has reduced the occurrence of outbreaks of salmonellosis and *Campylobacter* infection attributable to milk.

Infant bottle feeds

Careful precautions are necessary during the preparation and storage of bottle feeds for infants. Bacteria may be introduced into prepared feeds from the constituents as well as from bottles, teats, utensils and hands during preparation. High bacterial counts may be due to growth during cooling and storage at ambient temperatures. Feeds contaminated with pathogenic bacteria including *B. cereus* and other aerobic spore-forming bacilli, may be given to infants unless care is taken at every stage of preparation. Considerable hazards are associated with the use of breast milk substitutes in developing countries, including over-dilution of the powder, preparation with unboiled, contaminated water, and inadequate washing and disinfection of bottles and teats.

There is a continuing interest in the procedures of hospital kitchens and in the preparation of milk and safe infant feeds. Hospitals in the UK, USA and in some other countries, use **terminal sterilization techniques**, e.g. terminal heat treatment of complete feeds in feeding bottles, in a pressure cooker or steamer. The incidence of *E. coli* enteritis in infants has been markedly reduced by these procedures. Cooked feed is poured into sterilized bottles; a sterilized or disinfected teat is placed on each bottle and covered with a paper cap; the complete bottled feeds with teats are placed in small crates, ready for feeding each child for a day, and given a terminal heat treatment in a pressure cooker or steamer. Special equipment is available for cleaning and disinfecting bottles and teats. Much care, attention and legislation have been given to the hygienic production of milk, both in liquid and dried form, for the general public; similar care is needed to ensure a safe clean product for infants.

An organism that has more recently been of considerable concern in infant feeds, including its presence in dried milk, is the bacterium *Enterobacter sakazakii*. Premature infants and those with underlying medical conditions may be at high risk for developing *E. sakazakii* infection. Several outbreaks have occurred in neonatal intensive care units worldwide. However, an apparently healthy full term newborn infant in Iceland also became ill prior to hospital discharge and had permanent neurological sequelae. The growing number of outbreaks of infection among newborns strongly suggests that milk-based powdered infant formulas have served as the source of infection. Notably, the results of one investigation suggest that even low levels of *E. sakazakii* in milk-based powdered infant formula (i.e. levels within the currently accepted limit for the presence of coliforms in milk-based powdered infant formula in a 1994 Codex Alimentarius document), can lead to development of infection. There have been reports of infection due to *E. sakazakii* resulting in meningitis in a neonatal intensive care unit in the USA. In subsequent investigations, a cluster of newborns with *E. sakazakii* infection or colonization were identified in association with a powdered infant formula containing these bacteria.

Nasogastric tubes used for babies unable to suck because they are premature or ill may become contaminated. The small capsule through which the milk or other fluid is injected into the small-bore plastic tube must be handled; the liquid may overflow and the lumen of the tube coated in coagulated milk affording a good medium for bacterial growth during the time (24–48 h) that it may be in place. Bacteria from the hands of nurses, the nasopharynx of the baby, the environment of the cot and even from the mother, may multiply in the tube. Various pathogens have been isolated in large numbers from tube washings, including *S. aureus*, enteropathogenic *E. coli*, salmonellae, *Pseudomonas* and *Klebsiella*. Little is known of the effect on the infant, although with a poorly developed immune system, the infant must be at increased risk of infection. However, so far no alternative method of feeding has been suggested. Nasal feeding in adults carries the same risks. It is important that there is strict microbiological quality control of the ingredients and stringent hygienic precautions are taken during the preparation and handling of all enteral feeds. It has been shown that bacteria can survive and multiply in feeds with low pH and high osmolarity as well as in isotonic feeds of neutral pH. Likewise, care must be taken in the administration of all enteral and nasogastric feeds. Although the complete feed is supplied in a sterile sealed pack, either home-produced or from commercial sources, it may be given to the patient over a long period of time – 24 hours or more. Ward temperatures are often high and ideal for bacterial multiplication. All associated tubes and attachments must be sterile and care must be taken to avoid contamination while the feeding set is attached to the patient; and the possibility of bacteria from the patient growing back up the tube, should be minimized.

The Parenteral and Enteral Nutrition Group of the British Dietetic Association has produced a guidance document on microbiological control in enteral feeding. It proposes microbiological limits for raw materials used as enteral feed ingredients and the finished product (in the nutrient container prior to administration) and also gives guidance on administration, sources of contamination and sterilization and disinfection. The Group recommends that dried ingredients with an aerobic plate count of greater than 200/g should be rejected and that liquid ingredients should not exceed 10 organisms/mL. The products should be free from *Salmonella*, *Escherichia coli*, *Klebsiella* spp., *Pseudomonas* spp., *Clostridium* spp., *S. aureus* and *B. cereus*. The administration time of non-sterile complete feeds should be limited to 4 hours to ensure that microbial numbers will not exceed 1000/mL at the end of administration.

Other infant feeds

Meat-based and vegetable broths, and fruit purées, are common weaning foods for infants during the second 6 months after birth. Care of these foods, which may be canned, bottled or prepared in large quantities in the home, is important because they are excellent media for the growth of bacteria. The sterile contents of small bottles or cans are intended to be eaten at one meal. Closure methods for bottles have been designed to prevent opening by curious mothers anxious to know the smell of the product before purchase. The preparation in the home of small quantities for individual meals may be uneconomical; large quantities may be either divided into smaller portions and stored after prompt cooling for a few days only in the refrigerator or divided into meal-sized portions and frozen. Contaminants can be introduced from hands or from utensils, and they will grow rapidly in warm weather without refrigeration. Infants are more sensitive than adults to foodborne infections and are more likely to get dehydrated because of diarrhoea and vomiting.

All foods and liquids intended for infants should be stored in covered containers in a refrigerator or, if canned, the portion left in the can should be covered to prevent cross-contamination and refrigerated. Three days should be the maximum time of storage. Supplies prepared for 2 days should be divided into two portions to avoid further contamination by handling. Where there is no refrigeration, the covered container should be stored in the coolest place available, and the food boiled immediately before the meal. When the indoor temperature is greater than 21 °C and there is no refrigeration, meat and vegetable meals must be freshly opened and anything left over should be discarded. All containers and utensils used for the preparation of infant feeds should be boiled after cleansing and allowed to drain dry.

Egg products

Small numbers of salmonellae may be present in unpasteurized egg products, including liquid and dried whole egg, white, and yolk. *S.* Enteritidis was more common in most sources of eggs (and poultry) in the UK market until recently (and still more common in Spanish eggs today), and it has been the major source of foodborne salmonellosis in the past decade. Whole eggs should be cooked until the yolk is solid, and liquid egg mix for commercial catering operations must be pasteurized and rehydrated powders cooked within 2 hours of preparation unless refrigerated in small amounts. Such egg products should only be used in recipes requiring thorough heat treatment. Similarly, scrambled eggs, fried eggs and omelettes should also be cooked until quite hard. Lightly cooked dishes containing eggs (or separated eggs contents, such as egg white for meringues) should be avoided.

An outbreak of food poisoning which occurred in an army camp illustrates a number of these points. Reconstituted spray-dried whole egg was prepared early one morning; part of it was scrambled for breakfast and eaten by 70 men, only one of whom was affected. The portion which remained was allowed to stay in the cookhouse until late afternoon, when the original bacterial population, including salmonella, would have increased enormously. The mixture was lightly scrambled with insufficient heat treatment to kill all the salmonellae, and 16 of the 20 men who ate it were taken ill. However, it has been clearly demonstrated that salmonellae in egg white are eliminated very rapidly when the white is mixed with icing sugar to make 'Royal icing'. But this does not occur so readily when making marzipan with egg yolk.

Mayonnaise prepared from raw egg yolk, vinegar, oil and salt to a traditional recipe and stored at ambient temperature overnight will kill any salmonellae present in the egg. Refrigeration immediately after preparation will permit salmonellae to survive. Reducing the level of vinegar, or full or partial replacement by lemon juice, will not only permit survival of salmonellae, but, at ambient temperature, may allow growth. The level of acetic acid is critical for the safety of mayonnaise, and citric acid is not as effective as vinegar at killing salmonellae.

Cake mixes

Recently, availability and variety of ready-made cakes and other bakery products in retail has greatly increased, mainly through expansion of supermarkets. Packaged mixtures for cakes and sponges are still popular with some consumers, but these have given rise to outbreaks of salmonella food poisoning in the USA and Canada because of the inclusion of salmonella-contaminated egg products. Such mixes should not be used unless there is an assurance that the mix does not include egg products or, if it does, the egg product was subjected to pasteurization before being mixed with the other ingredients of the powder. The centre of some cakes may not reach temperatures sufficient to kill salmonellae. Clostridial spores in flour may germinate in under-cooked cakes, pastry, bread and other baked cereal products where the water activity is sufficiently high to allow growth.

Gelatine

Powdered gelatine is another substance that requires particular care in preparation and addition to foodstuffs because it may contain a large and varied bacterial flora. Melted gelatine in water is used in cooked meat pies and also for other purposes such as for glazing meat loaves, cold meats and pâtés. For preparation, the gelatine should be nearly boiled, and used as rapidly as possible with the temperature maintained above 60 °C. This procedure may involve the use of a higher concentration of gelatine (or gelatine of a higher Bloom strength) than formerly needed at low temperatures to produce an effective gel. Microbiological standards that stipulate the absence of salmonella for the various forms of gelatine used for cooking (and also for feeding animals) will reduce the hazards associated with this product. Gelatine as glaze and as jelly for pies has been responsible for outbreaks of food poisoning when used with poorly designed filling equipment (leading to difficulties in cleaning and sanitizing) or when prepared in bulk with the re-use of glaze that dripped off foods after coating. Similar problems (salmonellosis) have occurred with aspic jelly in which gelatine is the main setting agent.

Coconut

Methods of pasteurization in the production of desiccated coconut are much improved, but contamination with salmonellae, although reduced to a minimum, can occur; in the UK further heat treatment is usually applied. Coconut milk in the shell is sterile unless the outer husk of the nut or seed is damaged and bacteria pass through into the white flesh.

Rice

Dried polished rice has low counts of bacteria but *B. cereus* is frequently present, and its spores can survive cooking. The spores germinate into vegetative bacilli which multiply in non-refrigerated cooked rice (and in other cereal products) with production of emetic toxin. Cooking of rice in bulk at the end of a night's catering in restaurants and leaving to cool in the kitchen overnight, followed by rapid frying of the rice next day, has led to outbreaks of *B. cereus* food poisoning presenting with vomiting within 2–3 hours after consumption. This is sometimes termed 'Chinese restaurant syndrome', because this was the general cooking practice followed in these restaurants. The emetic toxin of *B. cereus* is very heat resistant; autoclaving at 121 °C for 15 minutes, together with frying, destroys only a small fraction of the toxin. Cooked rice if readily cooled, by running cold water through the mass in a sieve, and storing it in the refrigerator, as described above for other cook-chill foods, will prevent the growth of *B. cereus* and consequently toxin production. When rice (or other cereals containing *B. cereus*) is combined with meat ingredients (as in meatballs), the food poisoning syndrome is more often due to the diarrhoeagenic toxin.

Salad vegetables and dessert fruit

In large-scale catering it is recommended that vegetables and fruits with thin skins used for salads and desserts should be washed in water containing a solution of sodium hypochlorite (about 50–100 ppm free chlorine). To facilitate the correct use of hypochlorite, a marked washing container should indicate a known volume of water and a small measure should be used to add the required volume of concentrated solution (60–80 ppm is considered to be satisfactory for this purpose). The household use of hypochlorites for salad vegetables (including watercress) and fruits is also advocated; exposure to solutions should not be less than 30 seconds. However, many experimental studies have shown that the best reduction that may be achieved is about 2.5 log CFU/g of the produce, and generally <1–1.5 log CFU/g, depending on the smoothness and hydrophobicity (waxiness) of the plant surface. This treatment will only affect organisms on the outer surfaces of produce, and it has been clearly shown that outbreaks of salmonellosis and of vero cytotoxin-producing *E. coli* (in sprouting seeds) can occur from these organisms being taken up by the root hairs, and distributed internally through the stems and leaves of the plants.

The poor sanitary conditions and polluted water in some countries, particularly in the developing world, emphasize the need for care of vegetables and fruits purchased in shops and local markets. Similar care should be taken in developed countries that import such produce. As well as the direct transfer of bacilli and protozoa, from product to consumer, cross-contamination from raw to cooked vegetables may occur in the kitchen.

COOLING

Temperatures below the optimal range for growth of mesophilic micro-organisms (about 15–40 °C) results in reduction in the growth rate, or if sufficiently low, cessation of growth. Rate of cooling is important to prevent growth of surviving microbes, particularly through the critical temperature range between 45 °C and 10 °C. Removal of heat from large blocks of food is difficult to achieve rapidly, e.g. blocks or rolled joints of meat for cooking should be only about 2.5 kg (5–6 lb) and cooled in forced chilled air (blast chilling or freezing) or in circulated cold water. In some commercial cooker-coolers for cooking packages of meat joints, the cooking is done in circulated hot water that is replaced at the end of the cooking cycle by circulating chilled water. Similarly, rice cooked in bulk is best cooled by running cold water through the mass of rice before storage in chill. In the current regime of high energy prices, older technologies can be used again, such as cool larders (as in older houses), and evaporative cooling with water from earthenware pots.

Domestic and small–scale catering

Over 99% of homes now have refrigerators that are changed, on average, every 3–5 years. Domestic refrigerators are intended to keep food cold and not to cool hot food, which may overheat the cooling coils, causing moisture to condense on adjacent cold foods and growth of bacteria and moulds. Cooked foods should therefore be cooled before they are placed in the domestic refrigerator. The cooling time should be short – within 2 hours of cooking.

The penetration of heat into large joints of meat and the loss of heat after cooking are slow, so that cuts should be limited in size to 2.7 kg (6 lb) unless special precautions are taken for cooling in a chilled atmosphere with good air circulation. In homes and small catering establishments without cool rooms, hot meat should be left covered in a cool and draughty place for not longer than 1.5 hours before refrigeration.

Large bulks of food should be portioned into smaller lots to accelerate cooling, and liquids decanted into shallow containers for the same reason. Hot foods can be placed directly in large refrigerators with proper ventilation where they will cool more rapidly. For small catering establishments, a simple circulating fan installed in a well-ventilated cooling room or larder situated on the north side of the building will provide a satisfactory cooling system. Cabinets with shelves, containing a fan and air filter can be designed for quick cooling. Shallow rather than deep containers provide a larger cooling area for stews, gravies and other liquid foods prepared in bulk. Household refrigerators can be adapted to provide space for shallow trays stacked one above the other for the cold storage of liquids, and once cool the food can be transferred to clean deep containers.

Proper facilities for the thawing, cooking, cooling and storage of large turkey carcasses are essential. Faults in preparation and storage of turkey meat had led to many outbreaks of salmonellosis and C. perfringens food poisoning. Similarly, large-scale outbreaks of C. perfringens food poisoning were common in mass catering during the late 1940s and 1950s. They still occur when large joints of meat are improperly cooled. Such importance is attached to proper cooling regimens that modelling programs have been developed to predict the growth of C. perfringens during cooling of meats (see page 187). Storage of large cuts of meat cooked by boiling or by other methods not requiring surface temperatures above 100 °C, should be discouraged.

Large-scale catering and food production

The rapid cooling of food cooked in bulk, intended to be eaten hours or even days later, is difficult. Investigations to determine the cooling rate of large cuts of meat have shown that immediate storage in a well-ventilated cold room is the most effective method: 2.3 kg cuts of meat cool from 70 °C to 10 °C in 1.5–2 hours.

In commercial premises, blast chillers may be used to increase the speed of cooling (Figure 9.3). A cooling rate survey in the USA showed that rapid chill refrigeration through 'blast chillers' cooled food at a consistent rate, whereas with walk-in coolers it was impossible to ensure steady cooling rates. In some food factories hot food is initially cooled in wind tunnels (measuring about $1.5 \times 1 \times 24$ m long). Metal trays with food are carried through on conveyor belts and subjected to wind from a fan 1.5–2 m in diameter. Cupboards with descending cold air streams are also used.

For large catering establishments that need to cool masses of food required for frozen or chilled meals, the temperature of the cooling rooms should

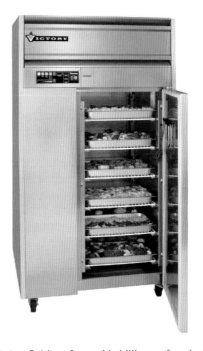

Figure 9.3   *Cabinet for rapid chilling or freezing. Photo courtesy of Victory Refrigeration Ltd.*

be maintained at 10 °C. Although most new kitchens have this facility (e.g. for school canteens), it is desirable that accommodation for efficient cooling be provided in all kitchens cooking for large numbers of people. Some producers of cook–chill or cook–freeze foods use a spray of liquid nitrogen within specially designed cabinets to achieve a rapid reduction of temperature before chill or frozen storage.

Ways in which the food handler can help to prevent food poisoning have been discussed in previous chapters. However, in the absence of facilities to aid rapid cooling and storing foods under cold conditions, bacteria will multiply to dangerous levels and toxins may accumulate.

Improvised cooling

Traditional domestic approaches to cooling involve cool cupboards or larders located on a north wall, fitted with slate, marble or stone slabs and with high and low ventilators protected against flies. Where the air flow is limited, a small fan is helpful. Foods should be covered but all materials must allow an exchange of air, otherwise there will be an increase in humidity, which will encourage mould and bacterial growth. Other older provisions for **cool storage** included boxes, louvered to allow a free flow of air but protect the contents from rain, hung on a wall away from direct sunlight.

Many methods have been devised to keep food cool in the home. Porous earthenware vessels cooled with water help to keep foods such as milk and butter cold by evaporation. Muslin cloth covering a bottle of milk or other container may be kept damp by dipping the four corners in cold water held in an outer receptacle; the container should be placed in a draught and out of the sun. A small louvered cupboard standing in water contained in a large basin or bath may be used for more bulky foods. Milk delivered after a family leaves for work should be placed in an insulated box, such as a polystyrene container, kept by the door in the shade. Some of these methods could be useful even today, given the rise in energy costs.

Frozen packs of food allowed to thaw should be cooked and eaten within a short time; a vacuum flask will keep frozen foods solid for an extra day and delay the growth of bacteria for 3–4 days. Insulated containers designed to keep ice-cream solid are becoming quite common; they will delay the growth of bacteria for at least 24 hours. Frozen meals for elderly and incapacitated people living alone may be stored in either of these containers for 2–3 days after delivery.

A wide variety of insulated containers, cool boxes or bags and cold packs (sealed plastic boxes or envelopes containing a liquid with a high heat capacity to be frozen at home before use) are now available. These can be used to keep food cool during transport, for example, from supermarkets, to picnic sites or while travelling. Such containers are also useful for keeping foods frozen after shopping at supermarkets or freezer centres. Insulated containers may be purchased with a 12 V thermo-electric cooling/heating lid for use in the car or a boat.

STORAGE

Cold storage

In the UK, summer temperatures usually vary between 18 °C and 20 °C; in the occasional heat-wave temperatures rise up to 36 °C. Winter temperatures are usually 1–5 °C with occasional cold spells and warm days when temperatures of 10 °C occur. Kitchen and shop temperatures will be considerably higher. Temperatures across Europe can be much higher and lower than these, and refrigerators must work much harder to maintain low temperatures in summer.

The incidence of food poisoning is highest in the summer, but cases and outbreaks occur throughout the year. C. *perfringens* grows rapidly in food left to cool in the warmth of a kitchen, as do many other foodborne pathogens, and food poisoning will occur in any season. Adequate cold storage facilities in homes, shops and canteens reduce the incidence of food poisoning; no other method can effectively replace cold storage as a preventive measure.

Low temperatures affect micro-organisms in different ways. As the temperature falls, bacterial activity declines. Therefore foods which support bacterial growth should be stored at low temperatures to prolong their life and maintain safety. When foods are 'chilled' or stored at temperatures close to but above freezing point, some bacteria will grow slowly (e.g. the food spoilage group such as pseudomonads, but also psychrotrophic foodborne infectious organisms such as *Yersinia enterocolitica* and *L. monocytogenes*), but in the frozen or solid state, many micro-organisms will be killed directly in the process of freezing – the most lethal temperatures being in the range −5 °C to −10 °C; the remainder will not multiply and their numbers gradually diminish. Hence freezing preserves foods for a long time, whereas chilling merely delays the growth of organisms and extends the shelf life of the food.

Chilled storage

In the refrigeration trade, the term 'chilling' is used to cover any reduction in the normal temperature of the food concerned. For example, the ripening of tropical fruits is delayed during transit by storage at a temperature not far below that of the atmosphere, whereas the decomposition of imported meat is delayed by storage at −3 °C to 1 °C (usually in controlled atmospheres) on ships. In large chill stores, where there is no forced air movement, moisture can be transferred from warmer areas of the store to colder areas; thus the surface of the colder foods, if uncovered, can become moist and allow mould growth. An additional benefit of refrigeration of meat carcasses is that the atmosphere in the chill room has a low humidity, and as a result the surface of the meat dries, further limiting the growth of micro-organisms. Some foods cannot be chilled at too low a temperature because there may be harmful changes. The flesh of apples turns brown if chilled below 3.5 °C, and similarly in bananas, and the resistance of some fruits to moulds may be destroyed by chilling, so that the rate of spoilage by moulds is increased.

With regard to pathogenic organisms, some strains of salmonellae will grow at 10 °C, but not at 5 °C. *S. aureus* will not grow below about 10 °C; between 15 and 20 °C there is growth and toxin production. *C. perfringens* will not grow at temperatures much below 15–20 °C. Most strains of *C. botulinum* will grow very slowly at 10 °C and in some instances toxins may be formed at this temperature. At 5 °C some strains of *C. botulinum* type B (non-proteolytic) and types E and F can grow and produce toxin at 3.5 °C. Predictive models are available, which can be used to assess the risk of botulinal growth and toxin production (see page 187).

Unlike most pathogenic organisms, both *Y. enterocolitica* and *L. monocytogenes* can grow slowly at refrigerator temperatures. Thus there are limits to the storage of foods that may be contaminated with these organisms for prolonged periods at chill temperatures. For lightly preserved foods, such as salted, smoked and cured meats, cold-smoked fish, the chilled shelf-life must be limited to contain the growth of *L. monocytogenes* below 100 CFU/g at the time of consumption. Mathematical models are available to predict the growth of these pathogens (and others).

Bacteria are able to multiply slowly at chill temperatures, and under prolonged domestic refrigeration at 4–5 °C will gradually spoil foods. Domestic refrigerators usually operate at temperatures well above the ideal, often between about 8 °C and 10 °C. Milk, for example, will develop 'off' flavours and odours (soapy, bitter, fruity) from the growth of bacteria better adapted to the cold (psychrotrophic) which differ from those which grow and sour the milk at higher ambient temperatures (the lactic acid bacteria). Foods of good bacteriological quality may be kept in a satisfactory condition at 4 °C for 4–7 days. For example, meat is preferably 'hung' to achieve 'maturity' for up to 10 days in chilled conditions, but surface growth of spoilage organisms is controlled to some extent by drying of the surface. If drying does not occur, spoilage is more rapid. Storage at just below freezing, can lead to excessive surface drying of meat, and growth of specific spoilage moulds – producing 'whiskery beef'.

Food handlers should be instructed in the correct use of refrigerators and cold rooms. In particular, they must be taught that the cleanliness and safety of a refrigerated foodstuff are dependent on the extent of bacterial contamination before refrigeration as well as on the temperature of refrigeration. They must also be made aware that extreme cold merely delays the growth and multiplication of bacteria which immediately renew their activity when the food is transferred to a warm room. This applies to both food spoilage and food poisoning organisms. The rule must be 'first in, first out' for foods.

Deep freeze storage

The freezing of foodstuffs, particularly slow freezing, to approximately −18 °C kills many organisms, and the rate of death of the remainder will depend partly on the temperature of storage and partly on the food substrate. Of the food poisoning organisms, those of the salmonella group are usually killed most rapidly on freezing and generally die in 1 month. Staphylococci on strawberries kept at −18 °C die in 5 months. However, salmonellae have been isolated after years of frozen storage from whole egg products and meat. The spores of C. *perfringens* and C. *botulinum* are not affected by freezing and the toxin of C. *botulinum* has considerable resistance to alternate freeze–thaw cycles at a temperature as low as −50 °C. Staphylococcal enterotoxin (and toxins in general) has been shown to withstand a temperature of −18 °C for several months. Moulds and yeasts endure freezing conditions better than bacteria, thus refrigerators and freezers should be kept thoroughly cleaned and free from fungal and yeast growth.

When highly contaminated foodstuffs are kept frozen, changes occur in the food owing to the slow activity of surviving organisms or enzymes over a long period of time. Thus there may be slow spoilage during storage in the frozen state, although far less, of course, than that which would occur in the unfrozen food. Freezing will not restore the freshness of a food already highly contaminated or spoiled by bacterial action. When a frozen food is thawed, those bacteria which have survived will recommence growth, causing decomposition, so that the keeping time of the food is limited and it must not be left at room temperature too long before being eaten, nor should it be re-frozen. Manufacturers take great care in the preparation of frozen foods and provide instructions on the packet for their correct use. A temporary period of thawing due to power cuts or failure of the freezer cabinet or even during shopping and transport home, does not necessarily mean that the partially thawed food should be discarded. Discretion must be used depending on the length of time, rise in temperature, and general condition of the food. While the central core is still frozen, the outside will be cold enough to stop most bacteria growing. Frozen food should be eaten as the manufacturer intends, freshly thawed from the original frozen state. Cycles of thawing and freezing will lead to quality deterioration as well as bacterial hazards. If a thawed food cannot be used immediately it should either be discarded or thoroughly cooked and re-frozen as a cooked dish.

Cold storage accommodation

Every kitchen should have ample cold storage space that is conveniently available. Where the size of the establishment justifies the extra expense, there should be a walk-in cold room with metal shelves and, in addition, one or more household refrigerators, so that foods with strong odours, such as fish, are kept separate. A well-defined air space or a cold air curtain between the cold room and the kitchen will prevent the warm air from the kitchen reaching the cold room. The temperatures of all domestic refrigerators and cold rooms should be checked regularly with thermometers placed in positions where they can be read easily, and records kept. Cold rooms and domestic refrigerators ideally should be maintained at temperatures of 1–4 °C. Several surveys of refrigeration units in hotels, restaurants and homes have shown that about 20 per cent are set or are running at temperatures above those recommended. The Food Hygiene (England) Regulations 2006 have been tightened with respect to the temperature at which certain foods should be maintained. A two-tier system is in use whereby certain foods must be kept at temperatures not greater than 8 °C and 5 °C for foods in the highest risk group, with shorter and longer shelf-lives – 10 days at 5 °C, 5 days at 10 °C, although there are still debates about refrigerated shelf-life.

The life of food in the refrigerator is limited and the longer it remains there, the shorter its life on removal. It has been shown that when the initial count of bacteria was low, the appearance of slime on refrigerated meat was delayed for 18 days; when counts were high before refrigeration, slime appeared in 8 days. Recommendations for the temporary storage of various foodstuffs have been made by the Food Standards Agency in the UK and similarly in the USA.

Refrigerators and freezers should be defrosted regularly, automatically or according to the manufacturer's instructions. They should not be overcrowded, so that air may circulate freely; it is advisable to check the contents at the time of defrosting and foods exceeding their recommended storage period, should be discarded. Space in the refrigerator ought to be available to store cooked and uncooked foods separately; because there may be cross-contamination from raw to cooked foods, store cooked foods above raw foods. Aluminium foil, greaseproof paper, or polythene or flexible film wrapped around foods, will prevent loss of moisture and minimize the spread of odours and flavours to other foods. Many foodstuffs commonly stored in a refrigerator do not encourage microbial growth and they can be safely kept for a few days in a cool room on a slate or stone slab. Milk can be stored in the cool room during the winter, but in the summer it should be refrigerated whether in bottles or cartons. Open vessels (e.g. jugs) containing milk, should be covered, and the outside cleaned before they are placed in the refrigerator, cold room or larder.

Most unopened canned goods do not require refrigerated storage. However, large cans of ham and similar cured meats which have only undergone a process of pasteurization, should be kept under cold storage (<8 °C – to prevent growth of mesophilic strains of *C. botulinum* that are relatively salt tolerant) until required.

When defrosting, the walls and shelves of refrigerators should be washed with a detergent-sanitizer and warm water (preferably alkaline to leave a surface unfavourable to the growth of moulds) and carefully dried before the food is replaced. If a refrigerator is switched off in holiday times, it must be emptied and carefully dried to prevent mould growth and the door left slightly open. Dust should also be removed from exterior cooling elements (condenser coils) for better heat transfer.

Other food storage

In addition to refrigerated and cool storage, there should be cool, dry, light and airy cupboards or rooms for canned and other packaged goods stacked on shelves and marked for rotation. Dry, powdered and granular foods such as flour, sugar, dried milk, tea, oatmeal, sago, rice, egg powder and coconut are stored in metal bins or metal or glass jars with close-fitting lids. These containers should be at least 450 mm (18 inches) above the floor to allow space for cleaning. Goods packed in cardboard or wooden crates or cases, should be clear of the floor and preferably on higher shelves. Exterior packaging that may have become contaminated during transport or handling, should be removed before entering the store room. Store rooms should be designed to discourage vermin, flies and dust, and they should be easy to clean. Dried fruit, fish or meat should be kept cool and dry. It is important to avoid conditions which could lead to condensation of moisture on the surface.

Summary

- Food preparation prior to cooking cannot eliminate all micro-organisms, but can limit their numbers and growth by good hygienic washing procedures (where appropriate) and strict adherence to conditions of temperature and time.
- The growth of most food-poisoning organisms is limited by chill and dry conditions.
- Cooking by any means of heat transference to achieve internal temperatures above about 70 °C, will eliminate vegetative cells of pathogenic and spoilage organisms, although spores will survive.
- The growth of surviving organisms is limited by rapid chilling (to below 10 °C) and chill storage (≤5 °C), or freezing.
- Commercial systems of cook-chill and cook-freeze permit rapid cooking and cooling.
- In domestic situations, chilled or frozen storage is the most important factor in extending the shelf-life and safety of prepared foods.

All websites cited in this chapter and below were accessed in November 2006.

SOURCES OF INFORMATION AND FURTHER READING

Becker H, Schaller G, von Miese W, *et al.* (1994) *Bacillus cereus* in infant foods and dried milk products. *Int J Food Microbiol* **23**: 1–15.

CCFRA (Campden and Chorleywood Food Research Association) (1992) *Guidelines for* Sous Vide *Processing.* Chipping Campden, UK: CCFRA.

Department of Health (1989) *Chilled and Frozen Guidelines on Cook-Chill and Cook-Freeze Systems.* London: HMSO.

Department of Health (1992) *Safer Cooked Meat Production Guidelines.* A 10 point plan. London: Department of Health.

Food Hygiene Working Group (1997) *Industry Guide to Good Hygiene Practice: Catering Guide.* London: Chadwick House Group Ltd, CIEH.

Food Standards Agency (2006) *Safer Food Better Business.* London: Food Standards Agency (available at: www.food.gov.uk/foodindustry/regulation/hygleg/hyglegresources/sfbb).

Institute of Food Research (2006) Growth Predictor & Perfringens Predictor (available at: www.ifr.ac.uk/safety/growthpredictor). *A predictive modelling program for estimating the growth of food-borne pathogens and for* C. perfringens *during cooling.*

Rowe B, Hutchinson DN, Gilbert RJ, *et al.* (1987) *Salmonella Ealing* infections associated with consumption of dried milk. *Lancet* ii: 900–3.

10

Food hygiene in modern food manufacturing

Robert Mitchell

Introduction	201	HACCP	205
Risk analysis, risk management and HACCP	201	Summary	207
Prerequisite programmes	202	Sources of information and further reading	208

The general principles of food hygiene in terms of hazards and risks for food manufacturing are no different from those of other food handling operations. The hazards are also the same but the risks can be far greater because of the sheer numbers of consumers who could potentially be affected, particularly in large-scale operations.

Hazard A chemical, physical or biological agent that can harm the consumer.

Risk The probability that a hazard will occur. Sometimes the risk will also contain an element of severity.

Hazard Analysis and Critical Control Point (HACCP) system A systematic way of analysing the potential **hazards** in a food operation, identifying the **points** in the operation where the hazards may occur, and deciding which are **critical** to consumer safety – these are the **critical control points (CCPs)**. The CCPs are then monitored and remedial action, specified in advance, is taken if conditions at any CCP are not within the safe limits.

Food hygiene requirements There are almost as many food manufacturing processes as there are food types, encompassing a vast range of raw materials and many different sizes of operation. Consequently, a list of hygiene rules and regulations would be either too long and detailed or too restricted to be applicable in all situations. Recognizing this limitation, bodies such as the Codex Alimentarius Commission Food Hygiene Committee have made efforts to clarify the principles of food hygiene, elucidating the rationale behind these principles and providing examples as to how the principles can be applied.

INTRODUCTION

The Codex Alimentarius Commission is an international body, which was set up under the auspices of the World Health Organization and the Food and Agriculture Organization. Its aims are to protect the health of the consumer and ensure fair practices in the food trade by the development and publication of standards and codes of practice for adoption by governmental and non-governmental organizations worldwide. The World Trade Organization has effectively adopted Codex guidance as the basic standard for all international trade in foods. Indeed, many governmental organizations, including the European Union, use the Codex guidance as the basis for their own legislation.

This chapter will follow a format paraphrasing the Codex General Principles of Food Hygiene (Codex Alimentarius 2001) where appropriate.

RISK ANALYSIS, RISK MANAGEMENT AND HACCP

Modern food manufacturing operations are diverse and complex, having adopted formal, structured, science-based solutions derived from **risk analysis** (Box 10.1) and associated risk management strategies such as **HACCP**.

Box 10.1   Risk analysis

Risk analysis is a scientific system comprising:

- **Risk assessment** – what is the risk, how severe will it be and who will it affect?
- **Risk management** – how can the risk be minimized or eradicated? It is a scientific system for selecting control options based on a risk assessment, e.g. HACCP.
- **Risk communication** – how can it be communicated in context?

HACCP is not a substitute for the Codex general principles of food hygiene. Although it is technically possible to build the Codex principles into the HACCP system, this could overly complicate its application. In practice, it is better to have the hygiene requirements in place *before* beginning the HACCP process. Therefore, Codex recommends that the application of the general principles should be as **prerequisite programmes** that must be in place before the HACCP process can begin.

PREREQUISITE PROGRAMMES

Prerequisite programmes comprise seven areas, each of which will now be considered in turn.

Personnel hygiene

Personnel hygiene applies to anyone involved in any capacity in the manufacture of food. Food safety requires that all personnel are committed to ensuring that the food reaching the consumer is as safe as possible. Commitment focuses the attention of all personnel, from the managing director to those on the factory floor, to the over-riding hygiene objectives of the business. Commitment to good hygiene calls on financial and staff resources and can sometimes conflict with production imperatives such as throughput or the cost/quality of raw materials.

The objective of personnel hygiene is to ensure that those who come directly or indirectly into contact with food are not likely to contaminate it. This is achieved by maintaining an appropriate degree of personnel cleanliness, and behaving and operating in an appropriate manner (Box 10.2). People who do not maintain the appropriate degree of personal cleanliness, or who have certain illnesses or conditions,

or who behave inappropriately can contaminate food and transmit infections to consumers (for further details see Chapter 8).

Box 10.2   Some principles of personnel hygiene for food handlers

- Do not handle food or enter food handling areas if you are suspected to be suffering from or carrying a disease or illness likely to be transmitted through food
- Report any such illnesses to the management
- Wear suitable protective clothing
- Wash hands before handling foods, after using the toilet and between handling raw and cooked food

---

Premises

Premises are any places where food or ingredients are stored, handled or processed. Food premises must be properly designed and easy to clean. The layout of premises can critically affect food safety. For example, to exclude *Listeria monocytogenes* from cooked foods, factories are designed to completely separate 'low risk' (uncooked products) and 'high risk' (cooked product) areas. Attention to good hygiene design and construction, appropriate location, and the provision of adequate facilities, is necessary to control **hazards** effectively (Box 10.3).

Box 10.3   Objectives of good premises design

Equipment and facilities should be located and constructed to ensure that:

- contamination is minimized – premises are located away from environmental pollution, flooding or pest infestation
- high- and low-risk foods, staff and equipment are separated where appropriate design and layout permit
- appropriate maintenance and cleaning to minimize airborne contamination
- surfaces and materials, in particular those in contact with food, are non-toxic, suitably durable, and easy to maintain and clean
- walls and floors made from impervious non-toxic materials
- suitable facilities are available for temperature, humidity and environmental controls
- there is effective protection against pest access and harbourage
- there is an adequate supply of potable water
- there are adequate personnel facilities

Maintenance and sanitation of premises are important to permit continuous effective control of food hazards, pests, and other agents likely to contaminate food. The procedures include ensuring adequate and appropriate maintenance and cleaning; control of pests; management of waste; monitoring of effectiveness of maintenance and sanitation procedures.

Examples of ways in which this can be achieved are:

- The premises and equipment are easy to clean and minimize food contamination.
- Specified cleaning procedures are followed and monitored. The cleaning programmes should ensure that appropriate parts of the premises are sanitized, and pest control procedures to prevent access or infestation are monitored and effective.

Product

Raw materials

It is essential that raw materials are either safe in themselves or that the processing will make them safe. The manufacturer must know the history of each batch of raw material in terms of source, age and storage conditions. Knowledge of its chemical, physical and microbiological status is vital. This can require a range of analyses based on appropriate sampling plans. The results need to be interpreted in time to allow acceptance or rejection of the raw material. For products with a short shelf-life it is not always possible to wait for the results of such tests, so the manufacturer may have to rely on auditing the supplier of the raw material.

Product design

The product must be safe in terms of microbiological, chemical and physical hazards. Most food processes are designed primarily to eliminate or prevent the growth of pathogenic micro-organisms. For example, traditionally preserved foods (cheese; yoghurt; salted and cured meats and fish; dried meats, fish, vegetables and fruit; pickled foods and jams) were designed to prevent the growth of *Clostridium botulinum*, a particularly deadly pathogen. Given the dangerous effects of *C. botulinum* toxin, it is absolutely critical that the correct process is applied every time foods are manufactured otherwise deaths can occur. Current market trends towards foods with low or no additives or preservatives, less processing, and longer shelf-life are, in some products, eroding the margins of product safety.

The factors that control the growth or survival of micro-organisms in food include: time, temperature, water activity, acidity, atmosphere and preservatives. These are discussed in detail elsewhere in this book, particularly Chapters 3 and 4. With a few notable exceptions such as canned or frozen foods, these factors rarely operate individually and combinations of physical and chemical limiting factors are usually responsible for limiting microbial growth. This situation, in which none of the factors are effective in themselves but their combined synergistic effect is, is referred to as the hurdle concept. In other words the combined effect is greater than the effect that would be expected by the sum of each individual component.

When designing minimally processed foods, it is vital to be able to predict how various combinations of factors will affect the growth, death or survival of the organisms of concern. There are two ways to do this:

- Challenge testing – the organisms of concern are inoculated into food with a specific combination of factors and their growth, death or survival is monitored throughout the intended shelf-life of the product. Obviously, this is costly, time-consuming and subject to the vagaries of microbiological sampling and analysis.
- Predictive microbiology – sophisticated modelling and computer programming are combined with traditional microbiology to develop software that can predict how a given organism will react to combinations of chemical and physical limiting factors.

Predictive microbiology programmes are now freely available on the internet (for example see the Institute of Food Research webpage: www.ifr.ac.uk/Safety/GrowthPredictor/default.html; and Combase: www.combase.cc/).

Product design must also take account of the three factors:

- Cost – includes the price of raw materials, packaging, capital equipment, energy and labour. Each of these includes a cost associated with safety, i.e. cheaper might not be safest.

- Quality – the product should comply with the appropriate quality requirements including shelf-life, taste and appearance.
- Legislation – the product must comply with all relevant safety legislation, including labelling requirements.

Process control

Process control renders the raw material safe and fit for human consumption. The opposite is also true in that process control also reduces the risk of manufacture of unsafe food by taking measures to assure the safety and suitability of food at each stage in the operation by controlling food hazards. Process control is achieved by:

- formulating design requirements with respect to raw materials, composition, processing, distribution, and consumer use
- designing, implementing, monitoring and reviewing effective control systems.

Some examples of process controls are: implementation of an appropriate HACCP plan; quality assurance (QA) checks on raw materials and auditing of suppliers; exclusive use of potable water.

Distribution

An efficient distribution system is that which will deliver an uncontaminated product to the customer in time and at the correct temperature. Food may become contaminated or may not reach its destination in a suitable condition for consumption if effective control measures are not in place during transport, even when adequate hygiene control measures have been taken earlier in the food chain. During distribution, measures should be taken to:

- protect food from potential sources of contamination
- protect food from damage likely to render the food unsuitable for consumption
- provide an environment which effectively controls the growth of pathogenic or spoilage micro-organisms and production of toxins in food.

Some examples of effective distribution systems are: separation of food and non-food items during distribution; temperature control maintained at all times; conveyances and containers are kept clean and in good repair.

Retailer

The retailer must handle foods in a way that does not compromise their safety. Manufacturers need to take proper account of the storage and display conditions at the retailer when determining processing conditions and shelf-life.

Consumer

The consumer is the king. Above all else, consumers expect that the foods they buy will be safe. Loss of consumer confidence can lead to loss of repeat sales or product withdrawals. Worse still, if the scare is serious enough then consumers can lose confidence in a whole sector of the industry resulting in loss of business for all the manufacturers of a particular product. The industry can take years to recover, e.g. a typhoid outbreak in the UK in the 1960s associated with canned corned beef resulted in a dramatic decline in the sale of all canned foods that lasted several years.

Consumers are also the last link in the food chain and as such have a responsibility to handle food properly and to follow the instructions on the label. The food manufacturer must label products clearly and correctly and ensure that the consumer is able to comply with them. Insufficient product information, or inadequate knowledge of general food hygiene, can lead to products being mishandled resulting in illness, or products becoming unsuitable even when adequate hygiene control measures have been taken earlier in the food chain.

Products should bear appropriate information for the consumer to enable them to handle, store, and prepare the product safely and correctly. Consumers should have enough knowledge of food hygiene to enable them to:

- understand the importance of product information
- make informed choices appropriate to the individual
- prevent contamination and growth or survival of foodborne pathogens by proper storing, preparing, cooking and use.

HACCP

HACCP is the internationally accepted system for managing hazards in foods (Codex Alimentarius 2001). HACCP has a number of advantages over traditional control methods. These include:

- Control is rapid and proactive, therefore remedial action can be taken before problems occur.
- Control includes features that are easy to monitor such as time, temperature and appearance.
- Control is cheap compared with chemical and microbiological analyses.
- Control is effected by those persons directly involved with the food.
- Many more measurements can be taken for each batch of product because control is focused at critical points in the operation.
- HACCP can be used to predict potential hazards.
- HACCP involves all staff in product safety, including non-technical personnel.
- HACCP focuses resources on controlling those aspects of the operation that are critical to consumer safety.

Practical application of HACCP

The Codex Alimentarius Commission has published useful guidelines for the practical application of HACCP (Codex Alimentarius 2001). These have been further clarified by others (Mitchell 1992, 1998). In addition, guides for the application of HACCP in small- and medium-sized business are also available (WHO 1999).

HACCP may appear to be complex, but closer inspection reveals it consists of several simple steps:

- **Assemble the HACCP team.** HACCP entails a team effort from key personnel involved in the full range of activities associated with the product. A typical multidisciplinary team might include: food technologists; microbiologists; engineers; the production manager; the quality assurance manager; the hygiene manager. The team must be fully trained in the principles and application of HACCP or should include someone with this expertise. The support and commitment

of all staff, including senior executives, are essential to the success of the exercise. These are enhanced by a communication and education programme for all levels of staff, not just those directly involved in the HACCP and its implementation.

- **Describe product.** A full description of the product should be drawn up including information on composition and distribution, and the usual use of the product by the end user or consumer. This step focuses attention on the likely uses or misuses of the product after it leaves the control of the food producer or operator.
- **Construct a flow diagram.** All the steps in an operation, from the raw materials through to the processing, distribution, retail and customer handling stages are defined in a flow diagram. The word 'step' refers not only to operations, processes or procedures, but also to raw materials. Details needed include times and temperatures of cooking, cooling or storage; chemical, physical and microbiological details of ingredients; quality assurance and management systems; shelf-life details; customer handling, especially whether the final product is ready to eat or will be cooked prior to final consumption.
- **Verification of the flow diagram.** All members of the HACCP team then verify that every step in the flow diagram is an accurate representation of the normal running of the food operation by expert knowledge and on-site inspections. The flow diagram must be updated to take into account any deviations from the original version.
- **Listing of all hazards associated with each step and any control measures.** The HACCP team lists all the biological, chemical or physical hazards that may reasonably be expected to occur at each step and describes the **control measures** that can be used to eliminate them or reduce their occurrence to acceptable levels. More than one control measure may be required to control a specific hazard. For example, if the hazard is the survival of *Salmonella* in a cooked, ready-to-eat product, there might be a number of control measures at the cooking stage including the length of time of cooking

coupled with the cooking temperature; temperature of product prior to cooking; temperature distribution within the oven. More than one hazard may be controlled by one control measure, i.e. cooking designed to destroy *Salmonella* will also kill *Listeria*.

- Determine the CCPs. This is the heart of HACCP. The keywords for success are flexibility and common sense. Operations that appear to be similar might not necessarily have the same CCPs because of differences in operating procedures. A decision tree, such as the Codex Decision Tree can help in determining CCPs. The intention is to minimize the number of CCPs and focus control resources at those points and still make a safe product. If a hazard is identified at a step where control is needed for safety but no effective control measures exist, the step, process or product need to be modified to permit control.
- Establish critical limits for each CCP. Critical limits must be specified for each control measure. Characteristics that can be measured quickly and easily are preferred. Examples of these include assessments of temperature, time, moisture level, pH, water activity, available chlorine and organoleptic parameters such as visual appearance and texture.
- Establish a monitoring system for each CCP. Monitoring is measurement or observation at a CCP to detect loss of control in time for corrective actions to be taken to regain control of the process. In addition to identifying the most appropriate monitoring system, the team should address the following issues:
  - WHO will monitor. For example, the job title of the person who will carry out the monitoring. Designated operators must be trained to carry out their monitoring functions properly.
  - WHEN they are to monitor. This should be often enough to detect potential problems and rectify them with corrective actions before they become serious.
  - HOW and WHAT they are to monitor. This is precisely how the monitoring is to be carried out, e.g. the temperature of a joint of meat should be measured in the very centre, which is the slowest point to cook.
  - Establish corrective actions. These are the actions to bring the CCP back under control when monitoring shows that the CCP has deviated from its critical limits, e.g. increase the time or temperature of cooking.
- Establish verification procedures. These are used to verify the HACCP procedure is working correctly. Verification procedures include internal auditing systems, microbiological examination of intermediate and final product, and a review of customer complaints.
- Establish record keeping and documentation. Efficient and accurate record keeping is essential to the successful application of HACCP. The amount of documentation should be appropriate to the nature and size of the operation.
- Review of the HACCP plan. Any alterations to the system, e.g. changes to the raw materials, product, process, or consumer handling should trigger a review of the whole HACCP plan to ensure that it is still relevant and is delivering a safe product. An annual review of the HACCP plan is a good idea even if no alterations are thought to have occurred.

Figure 10.1 illustrates an actual HACCP plan and its implementation.

(A) Parameter associated with the implementation of HACCP in a large-scale factory producing thousands of chicken pies each day. Note how the control options have focused down to only three CCPs

HACCP team	8 members
Time to do HACCP Plan	5 days
Time to fully implement HACCP Plan	2 months
Number of steps	916
Number of potential hazards	82
Number of control points	120
Number of critical control points	3

(D) Simplified flow diagram

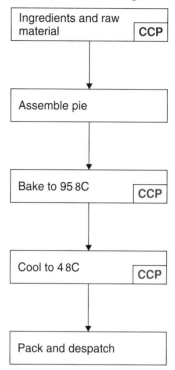

(B) Monitoring details of one CCP (baking)

Control measures	Action	Frequency	Responsible person
Thorough cooking	Record temperature at coldest point	Every batch	Oven operator
Thorough cooking	Determine oven heating profile	Installation/annually	Engineer
Thorough cooking	Check thermometer	Weekly	Quality assurance manager
Thorough cooking	Train oven operator	On appointment	Department manager

(C) Two of the associated corrective actions

Critical limit	Deviation	Corrective action	Person responsible
95 °C	<95 °C	Continue to bake	Oven operator
95 °C	<<95 °C	Dispose of product	Department manager

Figure 10.1   *Hazards Analysis and Critical Control Points (HACCP) – chicken pie manufacture*
CCP, critical control point

Summary

The complexity of food hygiene practices in modern food manufacturing reflects the increasing complexity of food processes, food business and the food chain. More modern, structured scientific approaches now build on well established food hygiene practices to encompass risk analysis, and, in particular, risk management strategies such as HACCP.

All websites cited in this chapter and below were accessed in November 2006.

SOURCES OF INFORMATION AND FURTHER READING

Campden and Chorleywood Food and Drink Research Association (1992) *HACCP: A Practical Guide.* Technical Manual No.38. Campden Food and Drink Research Association, Chipping Campden, Gloucestershire, England.

Joint FAO/WHO Food Standards Programme, Codex Alimentarius Commission (2003) *Codex Alimentarius Food Hygiene Basic Texts.* Rome: Secretariat of the Codex Alimentarius Commission Joint FAO/WHO Food Standards Programme, FAO.

Mitchell RT (1992) *How to HACCP. Br Food J* **94**: 16–20.

Mitchell RT (1998) Simple HACCP. *Meat Hygienist* pp. 21–3.

World Health Organization (1999) *Strategies for Implementing HACCP in Small and/or Less Developed Businesses* (available from: www.who.int/foodsafety/publications/fs_management/haccp_smallbus/en).

11

Food hygiene in the retail trade

Alec Kyriakides

Introduction	209	Delicatessen counters	222
General principles	210	Bakery	225
Transport and distribution	210	Take-away food and in-store restaurants	228
Produce	214	Home delivery	229
Meat	217	Summary	231
Fish	220	Sources of information and further reading	231

Food retailing is the process of selling food products at a range of outlets: from the 'corner shop' to the large supermarket. Throughout the retailing system there is a need for safe management of many food types that require different storage and processing conditions, as well as transport and distribution to the outlet and to the customer. Even though each type of food, process and stage has its own particular food hygiene challenges, the over-riding factors at every stage are that the food sold to the customer should be fit to eat, of good quality and safe. It is the retailer's responsibility to ensure that the food is prepared, stored and presented under conditions which do not introduce food poisoning organisms or encourage their growth and spread. Although food retailing operations can be complex, the process of assuring safety principally involves the understanding of a few key principles (Table 11.1).

Shelf-life The length of time allowed for a product to be eaten, after which unacceptable deterioration may occur such as wilting, drying, microbial spoilage or, less frequently, growth of pathogenic micro-organisms to unacceptable levels. The shelf-life should be clearly labelled as either the **best before date** (after which the food is no longer of appropriate quality, but remains safe to eat) or the **use by date** (after which it is no longer safe to eat).

Cross-contamination The process whereby micro-organisms are transferred to foods either from other foods or from contact with food preparation surfaces, machinery, utensils, hands or airborne contamination.

Clean as you go The process of continuously implementing good hygienic practices in food manufacturing, storage and retailing environments.

INTRODUCTION

Retail food businesses are the principal interface between food products and the consumer. In the UK, the public spends approximately £120 billion per year in over 100 000 grocery stores (IGD 2006). Over 90 per cent of grocery stores have a sales area of less than 280 m^2 (<3000 ft sq) although supermarkets and hypermarkets (280 m^2 to more than 2322 m^2 (25 000 ft sq)) account for over 75 per cent of sales. Regardless of the size of the business, the key responsibility of the retailer is to ensure that food is handled in such a way that it remains safe and of an acceptable quality prior to consumption (Box 11.1). Although many food retail outlets merely operate as a 'vehicle', buying food from manufacturers and selling it to the public, food retail has diversified significantly in recent decades. Nowadays, many businesses, both large and small, undertake some food processing on the premises, which can range from simply slicing and wrapping of a food such as cooked or cured meat to on-site manufacturing, e.g. cooked chicken, pizzas. The boundaries between retail and catering are also becoming less distinct with the development of 'take-away' counters in food retail outlets and in-store restaurants.

Box 11.1 Principles of food safety in the retail trade

- Ensure safety of products and ingredients being purchased
- Safe storage of products on site to avoid contamination or temperature abuse
- Careful preparation or handling of the foods to avoid contamination
- Appropriate cooking and cooling (or hot holding) of foods to destroy contaminants or prevent growth
- Display foods in a manner that avoids contamination and temperature abuse
- Up-to-date management of stock control and safe shelf-life

This chapter will explore the principles outlined in Box 11.1 for each of the areas of a typical food retail outlet while also discussing the challenges faced in retail outlets of differing sizes. The framework of legislation governing the safety of food in the UK is the Food Safety Act 1990 and subsequent amendments together with the Food Hygiene (England) Regulations 2006 (SI No 14) and its equivalent for each country in the UK. This legislation executes and enforces European Union legislation on food hygiene (Regulation [EC] No. 852/2004 of the European Parliament) and of the Council on the hygiene of foodstuffs; and is consistent with Regulation (EC) No. 178/2002 of the European Parliament and of the Council laying down the general principles and requirements of food law, establishing the European Food Safety Authority and laying down procedures in matters of food safety. This is discussed further in Chapter 15.

GENERAL PRINCIPLES

Food safety has to be actively managed in a food business, it does not happen by chance. Currently, accepted best practice to manage food safety is through the use of a Hazard Analysis and Critical Control Point (HACCP) approach. All food retailers have a legal obligation to identify and manage their food safety risks using a hazard analysis approach (Regulation [EC] No.

852/2004). The general principles of managing food hygiene and safety in retail stores are summarized in Table 11.1. The diversity of retail operations in any one store means that implementation of these principles can be complex. The following sections discuss the key risks and controls for different areas of a retail store in further detail. More hazards than those listed may need consideration, but this chapter attempts to prioritize those areas that form the primary focus for food safety management.

TRANSPORT AND DISTRIBUTION

Vehicles and equipment used to transport foods from manufacturers to retail distribution centres or directly to stores, together with the distribution centres themselves, are integral to ensuring the safety of the end product. Products may be transported loose, in open crates, in boxes, using purpose-built racking or in containers. Transportation may be in vehicles at ambient temperatures or as chilled or frozen. Distribution can be regional, national or international: the time in transport consequently varies from hours to days or even weeks. Distribution centres are often used by manufacturers to consolidate their own products (primary consolidation centres) before despatch to a retail or wholesale distribution centre. These centres are used by retailers to consolidate foods of similar types to redistribute them efficiently to individual stores. The chain of transportation and storage can therefore be extensive, and opportunities exist for weaknesses in any one of these operations to compromise the safety of foods throughout the chain. Distribution centres can be very large (23 000–69 700 m^2 or 250 000–750 000 ft sq) and it can be challenging to ensure safety while managing foods on such a scale.

The key food safety areas requiring particular attention during storage and distribution are:

- temperature control
- pest control
- contamination (microbiological and chemical)
- shelf-life.

Temperature control

Transportation of food involves extended periods in vehicles in all types of weather ranging from sub-

Table 11.1 Key hazards and controls in food retail operations

Factor	Hazard	Control
Temperature control		
Cooking	Survival of contaminating pathogens, e.g. Salmonella spp., Escherichia coli, Campylobacter spp., Listeria monocytogenes	Cook to 70 °C for 2 minutes or equivalent
Cooling	Growth of surviving spore-forming bacteria, e.g. Clostridium perfringens, Clostridium botulinum, Bacillus spp.	Cool to <5 °C in 6 hours maximum (see text for bulk meats)
Storage	Growth of surviving spore formers, e.g. C. botulinum and post-process contaminants, e.g. L. monocytogenes	Store chilled foods at 8 °C or less (ideally ≤5 °C) and hot foods held at >63 °C. Transfer cold foods from delivery vehicles to chillers and from chillers to display cabinets quickly, e.g. within 30 minutes
Contamination		
Microbiological	Cross-contamination of pathogens, e.g. Salmonella spp., E. coli, Campylobacter spp., L. monocytogenes from raw to ready-to-eat foods or from unhygienic equipment, utensils and food contact surfaces	Keep raw foods separate from ready-to-eat foods in storage and display Use separate utensils, equipment and surfaces for raw and ready-to-eat foods or wash and disinfect them between use Prevent transfer of contamination from raw to ready-to-eat foods by employees through effective handwashing, use of gloves and clothing changes Control contamination of foods via infected individuals by excluding those with enteric illness and ensuring wounds are covered Regular and effective cleaning and disinfection of food contact surfaces, equipment and utensils and non-contact surfaces, e.g. floors, underneath display cabinets (using separate, dedicated cleaning equipment)
Chemical	Contamination of food with chemicals or chemical taints, e.g. cleaning fluids, disinfectants, perfumes	Store foods and chemicals in separate areas and clearly label any chemicals in use, e.g. sanitizer solutions
Physical	Physical debris falling into open foods, e.g. flaking paint, hair, earrings, wood from pallets, stones, tissue paper	Ensure effective maintenance programme for building, equipment and utensils to avoid physical hazards Personnel policies, e.g. no false nails, no jewellery, covering of hair Suitable protection of open food to prevent contamination Washing of prepared foods to remove stones, e.g. in-store salads Minimizing use of wooden crates Use of coloured paper for drying hands
Allergens	Presence of allergens, e.g. nuts, peanuts, sesame seeds, in foods with incomplete ingredient labelling or inadvertent cross-contamination with foods containing the allergen	Use of dedicated storage trays, serving utensils, slicing machines, etc. for open foods containing allergens/allergen free Declaration of all allergens on ingredient list or on counter ticket for open foods Display notice on counter that food 'may contain' or is 'not suitable for' specified allergens/allergy sufferers if controls not adequate

Table 11.1 *Key hazards and controls in food retail operations* (continued)

Factor	Hazard	Control
Shelf-life	Growth of pathogens in perishable chilled foods, e.g. *L. monocytogenes*, *C. botulinum*, and ambient foods, e.g. *Bacillus* spp., *C. perfringens* in pies and pastries as a result of exceeding shelf-life	Stock rotation in chillers and display cabinets Time and date coding for short life products on counter tickets Routine code checking of products on display
Infestation	Contamination of food with insects and rodent or bird droppings	Proofing of doors, windows and other openings to ensure tight fit to frame with no gaps Automatic shutters on frequently opened doors Immediate removal of food spillages Food storage on racks/pallets and not floor Good waste-handling practices, e.g. regular removal, enclosed containers Use of infestation monitors, e.g. non-toxic bait traps, electric fly killers, pheromone traps, etc.
Training	Poor understanding of the critical food safety controls leading to failure to control any of the above hazards	Training of employees commensurate with the risks associated with their duties, e.g. training of foundation food safety principles for all colleagues working in store; more advanced training for those handling open foods and managers of store departments

zero to over 40 °C (often higher inside the chamber of the vehicle). Regulation (EC) No. 852/2004 requires that conveyances and containers used for transporting foods should, where necessary, maintain the foods at appropriate temperatures and allow the temperature to be monitored. During storage in distribution centres, foods that are capable of supporting the growth of pathogenic bacteria should be kept at temperatures that will not result in a risk to health. In addition, Regulation (EC) No. 853/2004 details specific temperatures for the transportation and storage of certain foods, for example:

- raw offal – ≤3 °C
- minced meat – ≤2 °C
- meat preparations – ≤4 °C
- other meat – ≤7 °C
- fresh fishery products, thawed unprocessed fishery products and cooked and chilled products from molluscs and crustaceans – temperatures approaching that of melting ice.

Foods most at risk from temperature abuse are chilled foods capable of supporting the growth of pathogenic bacteria. However, it should be recognized that thawing of frozen foods and exposure of some ambient foods to higher temperatures can render them unfit for consumption, e.g. melting ice cream or chocolate, or growth of thermophilic spore-forming bacteria in cans stored above 40 °C. Inadequate temperature control will generally render perishable chilled foods unsafe if they are kept at ambient temperatures for more than 6–8 hours. However, even shorter periods of temperature abuse (2–4 hours) may compromise food safety as the total shelf-life of the product is based on an intact chill chain at all stages. Perishable chilled foods should be kept at temperatures not exceeding 8 °C during transportation or storage unless the legislation specifies even lower temperatures (as described earlier).

The lower the temperature of storage the slower the growth of any micro-organisms present. So for both quality and safety reasons, chilled food is often transported and stored at temperatures of 5 °C or less. Vehicles and storage chillers or freezers should be checked at regular intervals to ensure the correct temperature is being maintained. This can be done with the use of integral continuous temperature monitoring devices in the vehicle or by manual temperature monitoring with a hand-held probe.

To ensure the **chill chain** has been kept intact, temperatures should be checked and recorded before the vehicle is loaded and on receipt at the distribution centre or store. Chillers at distribution centres should also be regularly checked, although many are fitted with continuous monitoring systems linked to pre-set temperature alarms. Monitoring is usually done by viewing the digital readout or by taking an air temperature with a manual probe. If there is evidence of lack of temperature control, between-pack temperatures should be checked to establish the actual product temperatures. If these exceed the specified limit (usually 5 °C or 8 °C) the affected consignment or products are rejected. Measures to ensure maintenance of the chill chain during transportation and storage are listed in Box 11.2.

Box 11.2 Key measures that maintain the chill chain

- Use of refrigeration units with sufficient capacity to hold all of the products and to deal with the volumes of product being held, that is, capable of maintaining chill temperatures in summer months and when full to capacity
- Avoidance of excessive breaches of entrances, e.g. Keeping doors closed, or using strip curtains to restrict excessive air movement
- Rapid movement of foods from vehicles to chillers and vice versa to avoid products warming up

---

Pest control

Infestation is a significant risk during transportation and storage. The physical need to constantly open and close entrances to vehicles and distribution centres to accept deliveries and despatch products means that there is considerable potential for rodent, bird and insect access. Pest infestation also represents a foreign body hazard (i.e. insects in foods) and a route for introduction of pathogenic micro-organisms (via faecal depositions from birds and rodents which, for example, contain *Salmonella* spp. as well as other enteric pathogens). In general, the possibility of infestations cannot be totally eliminated but it can be minimized (Box 11.3).

Where there is evidence of active infestation, ensure that advice is taken from the pest contractor on suitable remedial measures: more detail is provided in Chapter 14.

Microbiological and chemical contamination

Contamination of foods during transportation and storage is a significant risk, principally to open foods (Box 11.4). Vehicles, containers, racking and crates are all used to transport or store a variety of products including raw and ready-to-eat foods and chemicals such as household bleach and cleaners. Historically, most foods were transported in closed boxes but it is now common practice to reduce packaging waste by transporting and storing in open crates. This increases the risk of cross-contamination. Foodborne disease is often difficult to trace if contamination occurs during transportation, although poor transportation practices were the cause of an outbreak of salmonellosis from ice cream that affected an estimated 224 000 people across the USA (Hennessey *et al.* 1996). The ice-cream pre-mix had been transported in a vehicle which had previously transported unpasteurized liquid egg.

Cross-contamination can also occur from the outer packing of pre-packed raw meat products, often as a result of leakage, and it is best practice to avoid direct contact between pre-packed ready-to-eat and raw foods, especially meat and chicken.

Shelf-life

Shelf-life is an important factor that must be adequately controlled to ensure safety in distribution. This is achieved through effective stock control with appropriate procedures for stock rotation, ensuring older stock is despatched before new stock. It usually includes routine code checking of products in distribution depots and centres. Procedures conducted later in the supply chain, that is on receipt at a store, should identify any out-of-code product, but poor stock control at the distribution centre could result in out-of-code product ending up on sale. Distribution depots and centres usually have systems in place that allow only that stock into the system which has a minimum shelf-life on receipt. This shelf-life is a proportion of the total shelf-life of the product and ensures not only that out-of-code stock is not received into the depot but also that sufficient time is available for sale once delivered to the store.

PRODUCE

Fruits, salads and vegetables sold at dedicated greengrocers or at a supermarket have historically not been considered to present a significant food poisoning risk to consumers. However, fruits and salad vegetables are occasionally associated with outbreaks largely caused by faecal contamination with *Salmonella* spp., *Shigella* spp., verocytotoxigenic *Escherichia coli* (VTEC) and *Cyclospora* spp. The increase in international sourcing of such products to provide all-year supply of a wide range of commodities clearly offers greater opportunity for spread of pathogenic micro-organisms.

Intact fruit, vegetables and salad do not present a significant risk in the context of retail store practices, because growth of contaminants is minimal. However, the major area of sales growth in recent years has been in sales of convenience food, and this has also extended to fruits and salad vegetables. Pre-packaged fruits, salads and vegetables are usually sold as ready-to-eat, and these are associated with significant risks if not prepared, handled and stored appropriately. Likewise, the open displays at self-service counters in many retail stores, where customers can choose the prepared items they want to purchase, also presents significant food safety challenges. The key areas that require control with regard to produce are temperature, contamination (microbiological, physical and allergens), pests and shelf-life.

Temperature control

Once the flesh of a fruit, salad or vegetable is exposed by peeling or cutting, it becomes vulnerable to growth of contaminating micro-organisms that can be transferred from the outside during cutting. The extent of growth depends on the intrinsic nature of the food, for example, its pH, moisture, nutrients, but one of the key factors affecting growth is the temperature at which the produce is stored. Once cut, most prepared fruits and vegetables will rapidly spoil through yeast or mould growth if they are not stored at low temperatures. Pre-packaged cut fruits and salad vegetables are usually supplied to retailers after having been washed in water containing a decontaminant such as chlorine. However, even washed produce may occasionally harbour organisms such as *Listeria monocytogenes* or, on rare occasions, enteric pathogens. Such organisms can grow on the exposed surfaces of fruits and salad vegetables, and low temperatures are essential to prevent rapid growth to high levels. As well as being supplied pre-packed, cut fruit and vegetables may also be displayed in open salad bars; and the salads are increasingly being sold mixed with cooked pasta, ham, egg and other similar ingredients. Such foods are equally vulnerable to temperature abuse.

Microbiological, physical and allergen contamination

The products subject to microbiological, physical and allergen contamination in the retail environment

> **Box 11.5 Key measures for temperature control of produce**
>
> - Effective temperature control of chillers and display cabinets and counters (maximum 8 °C but ideally 5 °C or less)
> - Minimum delay in movement of products from the vehicle on receipt at store to the chillers and on replenishment of product (i.e. from chiller to display cabinet or counter – ideally no more than 30 minutes for each operation)
> - Monitoring temperature of chiller and display cabinet or counter with automated systems with digital readout or with high temperature alarms or manual temperature probing of air temperature, between-pack temperature or product temperature (open counter products)

are chiefly prepared, open foods displayed on salad bars (Figure 11.1). Pre-packed fruit and salads may be equally vulnerable but, for these, contamination risks occur during manufacture at a factory. As the products are sold pre-packaged, such contamination should not occur at the retail level and therefore it is not considered here.

It is also important to recognize the potential for malicious contamination with any open food counter. Suitable management includes supervision of the counter at all times and this is best achieved by positioning it next to a busy service counter such as a delicatessen counter. Products should be removed from sale if there are long periods when they may be unsupervised during opening hours.

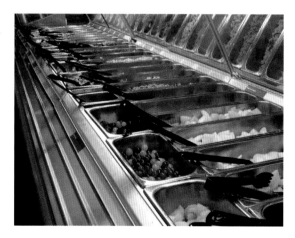

Figure 11.1   *A salad bar*

Box 11.6 Key measures for contamination control of produce

- Produce should be washed with either free-flowing potable water direct from the tap or, if washing in a sink or container, chlorinated water (50–100 ppm free chlorine) or a suitable alternative food grade decontaminant. Produce needs to be washed to remove any microbial contaminant as well as to remove stones and foreign objects that present a physical safety hazard
- Personnel who prepare ready-to-eat foods should be suitably trained in **food hygiene principles**, including prevention of cross-contamination and infectious disease risks. Hands should be washed regularly even if gloves are used, and there should be clear guidelines in place on exclusions and preventive measures for infectious diseases, for example, enteric infections and skin lesions
- Use of 'sneeze screens' at salad bars
- Regular cleaning and disinfection of the containers and equipment, including serving spoons and other utensils on salad bars
- Avoiding the use of allergen-containing ingredients for in-house prepared products on salad bars and providing clear labelling on the display counter and salad bar of the cross-contamination risks, for example, 'May contain allergen x' or 'Not suitable for people with x allergy'

Pest control

Infestation mainly occurs during preparation of produce and also while on display on salad bars. The principal hazard is fly infestation (Box 11.7).

Box 11.7 Key measures for pest control in produce

- Flies should be prevented from accessing the environment by ensuring windows and doors are kept closed and that windows, if open, are suitably screened
- Application of 'clean as you go' principles with frequent cleaning of utensils and storage vessels is important to discourage flies
- Monitor and control fly infestations with appropriately located and managed electric fly killers. These should be positioned close to, but not directly above, open food and should be regularly emptied. Evidence of high levels of insect activity may indicate a broader problem and advice from pest contractors should be sought in such circumstances

---

Shelf-life

Micro-organisms can grow on prepared produce whether they are pre-packaged or on open display. As well as effective temperature control, manage-

ment of stock rotation is essential (Box 11.8) to ensure that the safe shelf-life is not exceeded. This is particularly relevant for products sold on salad bars as they may be subject to routine 'topping up' during the day. So there must be procedures to ensure the shelf-life of the product is not extended through poor management of this practice. In most cases, the product will significantly deteriorate if the shelf-life is too long.

The current shelf-life of pre-packaged products (4–5 days) and open products on the counter (1–2) days offers limited opportunity for excessive growth of microbial pathogens. However, with the use of technologies such as modified or controlled atmosphere packing, it is possible to extend shelf-life to the point at which safety may be compromised in the absence of visual spoilage. *Listeria monocytogenes* is a significant hazard under these circumstances as it can grow under chilled conditions. Indeed, in some pre-packed products, it is not just conventional microbial pathogens that could present a risk, for example, extended shelf-life of pre-packed vegetables often allows anaerobic conditions to develop and thus the potential for growth of *Clostridium botulinum*. Although the current risk associated with this organism appears to be fairly low, future technological advances that extend shelf-life even further may make it more significant.

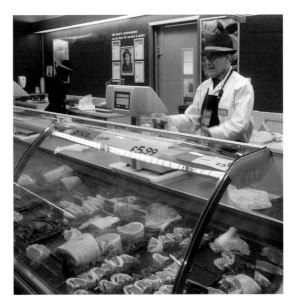

Figure 11.2   *A meat counter*

MEAT

The sale of meat through butchers' shops or from meat counters in supermarkets has always presented significant food safety risks. Meat and poultry can be contaminated with a variety of foodborne pathogens. *Salmonella* spp. contaminates approximately 5 per cent of pork and poultry, *Campylobacter* spp. are present in 50–90 per cent of raw poultry carcasses, and VTEC is an occasional contaminant (<1–3 per cent) of lamb and beef (see Chapters 4 and 5). Their presence represents a significant risk of foodborne disease to the consumer through undercooking and cross-contamination in the home. The same risks exist for food retail businesses selling both raw and cooked meats on the same premises. Until 2006, when the new hygiene regulations were implemented (see Chapter 15), licensing was mandatory for any business selling open raw meat and ready-to-eat foods on the same premises. The risks associated with products bought from butchers' shops and retail meat counters is limited if they handle only raw meat (Figure 11.2) because poor standards of temperature control, hygiene or shelf-life will generally result in product spoilage before it becomes unsafe. However, such outlets also frequently handle ready-to-eat meats and other foods. Practices range from merely slicing pre-packaged meat on a counter to more extensive processing such as preparing, cooking, cooling and storing of bulk meat prior to sale as a commodity to local caterers or as sliced meat on the counter. The key factors requiring control are microbiological contamination, temperature control and shelf-life.

Microbiological contamination

The key food safety control in butchers' shops and retail meat counters is ensuring raw meats do not come into contact with exposed ready-to-eat foods at any stage during storage, preparation and on display (Box 11.9). Raw meats in pre-packaged containers can occasionally be contaminated on the outside of the packaging with pathogens including *Salmonella* spp. and *Campylobacter* spp. (Burgess *et al.* 2005), primarily due to leakage of meat juices.

Cleaning and disinfection of cooked meat counters, utensils and equipment is essential also in the context of preventing contamination with pathogens such as *L. monocytogenes*. This organism can readily gain access to counter tops, serving utensils, slicers (Figure 11.3), etc. and unless regularly removed, levels can significantly increase resulting in extensive cross-contamination of a wide variety of foods using the same equipment. Interim and full clean downs are essential to control such hazards, and cleaning schedules for all utensils, surfaces and equipment should be documented, implemented and recorded. Monitoring the efficacy of cleaning using simple rapid protein, sugar or adenosine triphosphate (ATP) hygiene systems can be useful. Staff should be made aware of cross-contamination risks associated with the use of common cleaning

Box 11.9 Key measures to manage safety hazards while handling meat

- Store raw meat and poultry and cooked meat in separate cold stores and chillers. If this is not possible, ensure they are enclosed in sealed containers or packaging and stored in separate and dedicated areas of the same cold store
- Use separate utensils, equipment, preparation surfaces and, ideally, rooms for raw and cooked meats. If this is not possible, ensure everything is thoroughly cleaned and then disinfected between use. Equipment that is difficult to clean and disinfect (e.g. mincers, grinders, vacuum packers) should never be shared between raw and cooked meats. Colour coded equipment and utensils for raw and cooked products can be helpful to avoid cross-contamination
- Different individuals should handle raw and cooked meats, and ideally meats should be cooked in a double-entry oven so that those preparing the raw meat can place the meat into the oven from one side and those handling cooked meat can remove it from the other. If this is not possible, individuals must change protective clothing and thoroughly wash and disinfect hands between handling raw and cooked meats
- Open raw and cooked meats should never be displayed on the same counter. In the event of a common display counter being used, ensure products are in sealed containers or packaging and that there is a divider between raw and cooked meats
- Staff should serve either raw or cooked meats. If this is not possible, suitable controls should be in place to reduce the possibility of cross-contamination, such as the use of dedicated serving utensils, changing of aprons and thorough washing and disinfection of hands
- Use dedicated equipment, utensils and surfaces for raw and cooked foods including slicers, scales and vacuum packing machinery

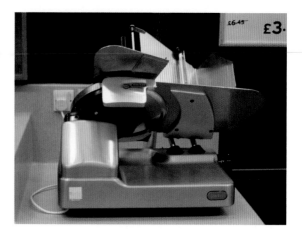

Figure 11.3 *A meat slicer*

Temperature control

Effective temperature control is essential in three key areas with regard to butchers' shops and meat counters.

1 Cooking of raw meat and poultry is a **critical control point**, because this step destroys vegetative bacterial contaminants (as well as other microbial pathogens) present in the raw product. The minimum heat process that must be achieved throughout the meat product to ensure effective destruction is 70 °C for 2 minutes or equivalent (Table 11.2). Cooking processes must be developed to ensure this minimum heat process is achieved. In larger, more sophisticated operations a typical process should be established for the product in the cooking appliance being used under worst case conditions, that is the largest product starting at the lowest in-going temperature, in the coldest part of the oven, with a full oven

Table 11.2 *Time and temperature requirements for destroying vegetative bacterial contaminants on and in food during cooking*

Temperature (°C)	Time
60	45 minutes
65	10 minutes
70	2 minutes
75	30 seconds
80	6 seconds

utensils, for example, cloths and wherever possible dedicated utensils should be used for each. If this is not possible then cleaning utensils should be used for the ready-to-eat areas first, followed by the raw areas and then either disposed off or suitably cleaned and disinfected prior to re-use.

load. Validation will establish the minimum process required to achieve the desired cook and this can then be documented and used as the cooking guideline for all subsequent products. This guideline should be supplemented with routine temperature checks of the product on removal from the oven to ensure the correct temperature has been achieved. Such temperature checks should be conducted with a clean, disinfected temperature probe that is inserted into the thickest part of the meat. The temperatures should be recorded. Validation of cooking processes for meat is not common in small businesses and staff usually rely solely on exit temperature checks using temperature probes. In all cases, temperature probes should be checked to ensure they remain accurate, ideally through external calibration with a reference thermometer or, as a minimum, by checking readouts with iced and then boiling water.

2 Cooling of cooked meats mainly presents a potential problem for bulk meats, when the size of the joint makes rapid cooling difficult. Joints 9 kg or more may be cooked, usually by boiling in cook bags. Extensive periods of warm holding following the cook can present significant risks associated with the growth of surviving spore-forming bacteria such as *Clostridium perfringens*. In general, it is good practice to cool hot foods to 5 °C or less within 4–6 hours of cooking. However, cooling bulk meats according to the criteria given in Table 11.3 achieves a safe product. Large bulk meats, for example, >9 kg can only achieve this cooling profile if they are first cooled for a short period (90 minutes) at

ambient temperatures and then placed in sealed bags into iced water.

3 Storage of cooked bulk meats is an important safety control as such products can be held for long periods prior to slicing and sale. If strict temperature control during storage is not maintained, there is significant opportunity for growth of pathogens. In general, storage temperatures should be as low as possible, that is, 5 °C or less; higher temperatures may be used with associated reduction in shelf-life.

The key measures for effective temperature control are the same as described previously in the Produce section (see Box 11.5, p. 215). Storage temperature is also important for raw meat and poultry although poor temperature control usually results in microbial spoilage well before excessive pathogen growth. Regulation 1906/90/EEC on certain marketing standards for poultry requires fresh raw poultry to be kept and displayed at temperatures not exceeding 4 °C.

Shelf-life

Shelf-life is critical to the safety of cooked meats. Under conditions of effective temperature control (5 °C or less) the principal pathogens capable of growth include *L. monocytogenes* and non-proteolytic strains of *C. botulinum*, which can all grow in food at refrigeration temperatures; *L. monocytogenes* as low as 0 °C and *C. botulinum* down to 3.3 °C. *L. monocytogenes* only presents a risk if it is introduced after cooking – during cooling or slicing. If the meat is cooked and cooled in sealed bags, then the organism is only of concern once the bag is opened, usually when the product is placed on the counter for slicing. The open life of the product should be restricted and, depending on the formulation of the product, a shelf-life of 5 days at 5 °C or less after opening would usually not present a significant risk, even if contaminated with low levels of the organism. The shelf-life of products sliced on the counter is usually much lower than this (1–2 days) because of organoleptic deterioration by drying. *C. botulinum* spores can survive the cooking stage, and, as meat is usually stored in vacuum packs, the anaerobic conditions in the pack and also in the meat itself are ideal for growth. Thus there is great potential for growth of this organism in

Table 11.3 *Cooling conditions for bulk, cooked meat**

Process stage	Uncured meats (maximum cooling time)	Cured meats (maximum cooling time)
Cook to <5 °C	10 hours	12.5 hours
Time between 50 °C and 12 °C	6 hours	7.5 hours

Note: Guidelines assume meat is not contaminated with high levels of spore-forming bacteria.
*Adapted from Gaze *et al.*, 1998.

cooked meats. In the UK, the controls recommended to restrict the growth of *C. botulinum* in chilled food include one or more of the following:

- A maximum chilled shelf-life of 10 days or less after cooking.
- Formulating the product to prevent growth using salt (>3.5 per cent in the aqueous phase).
- Inclusion of other humectants to reduce water activity to 0.97 or less.

Addition of nitrite to cooked cured meats slows down the germination and growth of *C. botulinum* but depending on the levels does not completely prevent it.

FISH

Fishmongers are still a common sight in many high streets. Fish is the most perishable category of food, and is therefore highly vulnerable to growth of contaminating micro-organisms – those that cause spoilage or food poisoning. Historically, the range of fish and shellfish on sale on the fish counter was limited to species caught or farmed in coastal waters. These still represent a high proportion of the fish counter range of products, and include cod, plaice, mackerel, eel, salmon, prawns, crab, mussels and oysters. However, the range has now been significantly extended with exotic varieties being imported from throughout the world and include tiger prawns, clams, tuna, shark and reef fish, such as red snapper and grouper.

Some of these fish present food safety risks that the fishmonger or retailer has limited ability to influence, for example, contamination with natural toxins such as diarrhoetic shellfish poisoning and paralytic shellfish poisoning toxins in filter feeding bivalve molluscs, or ciguatera toxin in reef fish such as red snapper (see Chapter 4, p. 81). Bivalve molluscs such as oysters, mussels and cockles can be contaminated with human enteric viruses that require heat processes to destroy them. A key measure for minimizing exposure to such contaminants is purchasing raw fish and shellfish from reputable supply sources. Outbreaks of foodborne disease have occurred when local retailers and caterers have bought contaminated shellfish from individuals collecting shellfish from local beaches (see Chapter 6, p. 138). The key factors that require management at fishmongers and on fish counters are temperature, microbiological contamination and shelf-life.

Temperature control

Fish counters (Figure 11.4) come in a variety of formats; some simply consist of a bed of ice on which the fish are displayed, others are refrigerated counters with no ice, and yet others use a combination of ice and refrigeration. The purpose of each of these is to keep the fish cold. Fish is highly susceptible to microbial growth and spoilage and this is directly related to the temperature of storage: the lower the temperature the slower the microbial growth and the longer the fish will last. In food safety terms most raw fish will spoil well before the food becomes microbiologically unsafe to eat. However, in some cases, this may not be evident and can itself represent a safety hazard, for example, the microflora of raw scombroid fish (tuna or mackerel), includes species that can decarboxylate the amino acid histidine, present in relatively large quantities in such species, to form histamine (see Chapters 1, p. 10 and 4, p. 88).

Histamine is a very heat stable toxin and it is not destroyed by cooking. Such histamine-producing bacteria can grow at temperatures as low as 4–8 °C and if high levels of histamine is formed (usually >100 ppm) this can result in scombrotoxin poisoning. Legislative levels for maximum amounts of histamine in fish are set between 100 and 200 ppm (Regulation [EC] No. 2073/2005 on the microbiological criteria for foodstuffs). The only effective control is strict management of temperature (in

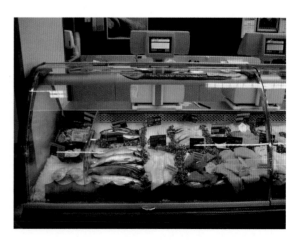

Figure 11.4 *A fish counter*

association with shelf-life control) and temperatures below 3 °C are ideal to prevent growth of histamine-producing bacteria. Fish is usually stored on ice from catch and is received at the fishmongers either on ice or frozen. Procedures that ensure the fish remains near freezing throughout the chill chain are essential for safety and, indeed, quality. Temperature abuse, however mild, is more likely:

● when taking deliveries (at depots or stores)
● when restocking display cabinets or counters
● while on display
● once purchased by the customer.

In general, short periods out of chill i.e. 30–60 minutes will not result in the product temperature increasing significantly if they are in boxes or on ice as the mass of product will maintain good chill temperatures. However, pre-packed products may be delivered in crates or loose and are more susceptible to external temperature fluctuation. Clearly, the prevailing ambient temperature is a critical factor as even short periods out of chill in summer months when temperatures can exceed 30 °C could result in significant temperature elevation. If this occurs during stock replenishment, it can take many hours to bring the product back down to chill temperatures as retail cabinets and counters are designed only to maintain chill temperature. Key measures to prevent temperature abuse include those previously described in the Produce section (Box 11.5, p. 215). In addition, there is a tendency to overfill fish counters as this creates a more strikingly visual display to the customer; displaying all product within the maximum load lines of the cabinet or counter is essential for effective temperature control. Fish are usually placed directly on ice in counters and low temperatures are maintained through contact between the fish and the ice. Over-stacking results in some fish not being in contact with ice and less effective temperature holding. In fish counters that have dual ice and refrigeration units, this is only a problem if fish are stacked so high that they exceed the 'air curtain' or block the air vent. However, with counters that are just ice beds, over-stacking makes the product more vulnerable to temperature abuse.

Some fishmongers cook fish and shellfish on site and the controls specified for cooking of raw meat are equally applicable to fish and shellfish with one notable exception. To ensure safety, bivalve molluscs such as cockles and mussels should be cooked to 90 °C for 90 seconds in the flesh to ensure destruction of enteric viruses such as norovirus; the legal requirement applies to class B and C shellfish only (Regulation [EC] No. 853/2004) (see Chapter 4, p. 75).

Microbiological contamination

Both raw and ready-to-eat fish are usually displayed on the same counter. The presence of enteric pathogens on fish is usually less likely than on red or white meat, but organisms such as *Salmonella* spp. and pathogenic *Vibrio* spp. can occasionally occur. Fish are often contaminated with *L. monocytogenes*. Therefore it is important that the raw and ready-to-eat fish are kept separate to avoid cross-contamination. Traditional fishmongers undertake considerable preparation and handling of fish, such as gutting, filleting and de-skinning, although this is less common on large retail store counters. Preparation presents many opportunities for cross-contamination from raw to ready-to-eat fish and the key measures as previously described in the Meat section should be applied (see Box 11.9). In addition:

● Serve raw and ready-to-eat fish separately using separate serving utensils such as tongs or spoons. Use separate scales or ensure raw and ready-to-eat fish do not come into contact with the scales by using greaseproof paper or plastic bags. Care must be taken to avoid secondary cross-contamination by staff touching the buttons on the scales, tills, etc. and then handling ready-to-eat products with the same hands.
● Cleaning and disinfection of utensils, equipment and surfaces together with separate cleaning of non-contact surfaces, such as floors, under cabinets or counters, is essential to avoid build-up of microbial contaminants. Indeed, it is often poor cleaning and disinfection that result in bad fish odours on fish counters or displays.

Shelf–life

Excessive shelf-life usually results in fish spoilage far earlier than they would become unsafe, with the possible exception of scombrotoxin poisoning as indicated previously. In general, in comparison with other ways of selling, the fish on counters succumbs more rapidly to spoilage because of increased microbial loading through handling and exposure to air. Oxygen in air allows rapid growth of aerobic spoilage micro-organisms such as *Pseudomonas* spp. Fresh fish sold on counters is usually allocated a very short shelf-life from opening, for example, 1–2 days.

Shelf-life is usually of more importance for prepackaged fish, particularly for fish for which vacuum or modified atmosphere packaging is used as this allows shelf-life to be extended. Raw fish packaged in this way will generally achieve a shelf-life of 6–10 days and, if destined to be properly cooked, represents little additional concern other than scombrotoxin poisoning. As already indicated, effective temperature control (<5 °C) will prevent development of bacteria capable of scombrotoxin production even with a longer shelf-life. However, cooked or smoked pre-packed ready-to-eat fish represents more of a concern as a much longer shelf-life is achieved before spoilage becomes evident. If these products are intended to be eaten without further cooking, considerable opportunities exist for growth of any contaminant that survives processing or recontaminates after processing. The principal hazards include *L. monocytogenes* and the non-proteolytic strains of *C. botulinum*, both of which are capable of growth at temperatures below 5 °C, temperatures usually employed for many chilled foods. Cooked and smoked fish and shellfish have been implicated in outbreaks of both botulism and listeriosis, and extending the shelf-life of these products has been a contributing factor.

For many fishmongers, the shelf-life of most of the products is not under their direct control. This is specified by the manufacturer of the incoming material with the retailer merely selling the product either as a pre-pack or loose on the counter after opening the bulk pack. Many fishmongers are not in a position to judge whether the shelf-life is safe or not, and the best means of ensuring safety is to purchase the product from reputable suppliers. When selling previously cooked material, especially if it is received in a bulk pre-pack and then opened and sold loose on the counter, it is essential to ensure the specified maximum shelf-life is not exceeded. Therefore, procedures must be in place to ensure the shelf-life of the original material is transferred to the counter ticket or that procedures are in place to prevent exceeding the total specified shelf-life, for example, if the counter-life is 2 days

and the customer-life is 2 days then product must not be placed on the counter beyond 4 days from its specified use-by date. Unless fish is removed and thrown away every day from the counter, some form of ticketing will be required to ensure old stock does not remain on the counter.

Certain maximum shelf lives of vacuum and modified atmosphere packed products are recommended to control *C. botulinum*: 10 days at 8 °C or less unless other controlling factors are present in the product, that is, pH 5.0 or less, water activity 0.97 or less or aqueous salt content >3.5 per cent. Likewise, if the product is likely to be contaminated with *L. monocytogenes*, growth to levels considered hazardous (>100 CFU per gram) can occur in as few as 5–8 days at refrigeration temperatures (5–8 °C); a shelf-life beyond this needs to be justified. This is now a legislative requirement (Regulation [EC] No. 2073/2005).

DELICATESSEN COUNTERS

Delicatessen counters (Figure 11.5) are present in most medium and large food retail stores and differ quite markedly from delicatessen shops. The mainstay of delicatessen counters and shops are loose, fresh foods of virtually any description, the common factor being that they are usually highly perishable and sold ready to eat. Cheese, pâté, sliced cooked meat, raw dried and fermented meats, olives, dressed salads, pickles, sauces and dips are all commonplace on delicatessen counters. Delicatessen shops tend also to sell a variety of specialist

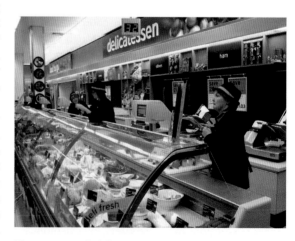

Figure 11.5 *A delicatessen counter*

ambient foods including flavoured oils, dressings, pickles and fruit preserves. In recent years, it has also become common for hot food to be sold from delicatessen counters, such as cooked rotisserie chicken, hot pies, and take-home versions of pre-packaged foods such as ready meals and 'make your own' pizza offers. The average delicatessen counter and shop is replete with what many would tradi-tionally consider to represent 'high-risk' foods. This is because such foods are:

- particularly vulnerable to contamination because they are usually displayed open
- are ready-to-eat
- often extensively handled
- offer significant opportunities for growth of any contaminating micro-organism.

The key areas that require attention are contamin-ation (microbiological, physical and allergens), temperature control and storage, and shelf-life.

Microbiological, physical and allergen contamination

It is unusual for delicatessen counters to display raw meats and ready-to-eat foods on the same counter, although it had been historical practice for stores to co-display open raw foods such as bacon and sausages on the same counter as ready-to-eat foods. This was prohibited in the UK following a large outbreak of *E. coli* O157 infection and the introduction of licensing of those premises handling open raw and ready-to-eat foods. When displaying raw meats together with ready-to-eat foods on delicatessen counters, cross-contamination risks are managed as described above in the Meat section (see Box 11.9). In the absence of raw meats on delicatessen counters, the most significant microbial risk comes from contamination with pathogens from infected food handlers and from cross-contamination via contaminated surfaces, equip-ment and utensils with *L. monocytogenes*.

Many foods on the delicatessen counter are sold open and are subject to extensive handling, especially during slicing. Faecal pathogens from food handlers having, or having recently had, infectious intestinal disease (e.g. caused by *Salmon-ella* spp., *Shigella* spp., noroviruses) or *Staphylo-coccus aureus* from open, infected wounds or lesions are potential hazards. Indeed, perhaps the most

famous example of failure to control such hazards was that of 'Typhoid Mary' who, having contracted enteric fever in the early 1900s, was implicated as the source of over 1000 cases of typhoid in America. Control of these hazards is relatively simple (Box 11.10).

Box 11.10 Key measures to control contamination due to handling

- Have in place an infectious disease policy to manage risks from food handlers returning to work after sickness, overseas holiday or close contact with infected individuals. The general principle would be to exclude those who have had diarrhoea and/or vomiting for a period of 48 hours after they become symptom free. Certain infectious diseases require stool testing and microbiological clearance, for example, typhoid (see Chapter 8).
- Train employees in basic food hygiene principles: handwashing, cross-contamination, covering infected wounds, etc.

Pathogenic bacteria such as *L. monocytogenes* can readily colonize equipment, surfaces and utensils used in food environments and, indeed, can colonize the environment itself. The organism can readily build-up on equipment where food residues are not removed and where the conditions remain moist. This bacterium can then contaminate any foods coming into contact with such equipment or surfaces. Indeed, poor cleaning was considered a significant contributory factor in a major outbreak of listeriosis in France that resulted in 279 cases of listeriosis, 63 deaths and 22 abortions (Goulet *et al.* 1993). Equipment such as slicers for cheese or cooked meats, display cabinets, cracks and scratches in serving dishes and cutting boards all provide an excellent environment for the organism to colonize and multiply. Removal of food residues by cleaning followed by effective disinfection with chlorine or other disinfectants is the only way to ensure *L. monocytogenes* remains under control. It is not possible to eliminate the organism completely from these environments, but the short shelf-life allo-cated to delicatessen foods after cutting or slicing (1–2 days) ensures that the occasional presence of the organism at low levels should not present a significant risk. It is good practice to document cleaning schedules and record that cleaning has been undertaken. It is also common for cleaning to be supplemented with some form of simple indicator of cleaning efficacy such as ATP, protein or sugar tests. All of these assays determine whether residues of food have been left after cleaning, thereby providing conditions that could allow proliferation of residual microbial contaminants.

Any open food is also subject to physical contamination during preparation, slicing or even from customers while on display. Contamination from slicers and loose equipment, for example, screws, broken blades on knives, plastic from packaging, can be minimized through very simple good retail practices including 'clean as you go', regular maintenance and regular checking of equipment after use, for example, for broken or missing pieces.

Allergen cross-contamination is a significant potential hazard due to the wide variety of foods sold open on the delicatessen counter. It is not a legislative requirement to label loose foods with allergen declarations, whether they occur as intentional ingredients of the formulation or as cross-contaminants. However, allergens can present significant hazards to consumers who have particular allergies and can even cause anaphylactic reactions resulting in death. Box 11.11 lists the key measures for good allergen management.

Box 11.11 Key measures for managing allergy risks from foods sold on the delicatessen counter

- Avoid the use of allergens wherever possible, for example, formulations containing peanuts, nuts, sesame, fish and shellfish
- Use separate equipment, utensils and surfaces to handle products that contain allergens and those that do not contain allergens, or wash them thoroughly between use. It is good practice to prepare products that do not contain allergens before those that contain allergens
- Provide clear labelling of foods containing allergens. Where labelling is not possible, maintain readily available and up-to-date lists of product ingredients behind the counter to refer to when asked by a customer
- Display point-of-sale messages if allergen cross-contamination risks cannot be managed to alert customers to any risks, for example, 'May contain allergen x' or 'Not suitable for people with x allergy '

See the section on Bakery products on p. 225 for further information on allergens.

Temperature control

Most delicatessen products are **perishable foods** because they have few intrinsic factors that prevent growth of contaminating microorganisms. Most have neutral pH (e.g. 6–7), high moisture and contain few if any preservatives. Alongside effective **shelf-life management** (see below), management of the chill–chain is a key component of food safety. Perishable foods must be kept at low temperatures right from manufacture through distribution and when in the retail store. Key areas where temperature abuse can occur are when taking delivery of chilled foods prior to storage in chillers, and when replenishing foods due to delays between removal from the chiller and placement in the display unit. In smaller delicatessen operations, these challenges are usually less problematic as deliveries and stock movement for replenishment will be on a smaller scale and opportunities for temperature abuse will be minimal. However, in large retail stores, this presents significant challenges and systems must be in place to ensure movement of stock takes place within periods of time that ensure temperatures do not become elevated. The key measures for effective temperature control such as minimizing delay in movement of product on receipt and during replenishment of display cabinets, and monitoring the temperatures of chiller and retail display cabinets have been described previously in the produce section (see Box 11.5, p. 215).

Shelf–life

As mentioned above, delicatessen products are highly vulnerable to growth of micro-organisms that may be capable of spoilage or food poisoning. The presence of spore-forming bacterial pathogens such as *C. perfringens*, *Bacillus* spp. and *C. botulinum* is inevitable, albeit at low initial levels in many of the foods. The latter two are capable of growth under refrigeration conditions (5–8 °C). Likewise, organisms such as *L. monocytogenes* can be present in delicatessen products due to cross-contamination during preparation, handling, slicing or while on display. Temperature control is important in ensuring that such organisms, if present, cannot grow to unsafe levels. However, as growth can occur even under effective temperature control, this is chiefly prevented by adequate shelf-life control. Most open delicatessen products do not last very long on the counter due to drying and other organoleptic deterioration, and the open counter life for perishable foods is usually just a few days. Restricting chilled shelf-life to 5 days or less will ensure that low levels of contaminating bacteria do not grow to harmful levels over the life of the product. However, many of the foods destined for the delicatessen counter are received in bulk from a producing factory, e.g. cheese, meats, etc., often with very long shelf lives prior to opening. It is essential that appropriate consideration is given to the control of bacterial pathogens in these materials prior to receipt. For example, bulk meats to be sliced on a delicatessen counter may be cooked at a producing factory in sealed containers, cooled, removed from the containers and then finally repackaged. Clearly, opportunities for post-process contamination with pathogens such as *L. monocytogenes* exist at the factory, and although the safe shelf-life of the product is principally the responsibility of the producer, it is essential that this is clearly specified on the product and is adhered to by the retailer. The open retail life that is given to the customer should never exceed the maximum shelf-life allocated to the ingredients, unless it is to be fully re-cooked prior to sale. Adequate management of shelf-life is essential for delicatessen products and procedures to ensure this occurs effectively (Box 11.12).

Delicatessen foods that are not stored in a refrigerator, e.g. baked pies, vegetables in oil, etc. may also require shelf-life restrictions as opportunities exist for growth of a wide variety of food poisoning organisms, all of which will grow much faster when the food is stored under non-refrigerated conditions. Acidified or dry ingredients are not usually subject to any safety restrictions as most pathogenic micro-organisms will not grow if the pH is suitably low (4.5 or less), they are sufficiently dry (<15 per cent moisture) or have a water activity of <0.85. Other foods require shelf-life restrictions. For example, pies that are destined to be eaten warm should be sold within a maximum of 4 hours (see Bakery section). A special mention needs to be made of ambient displayed flavoured oils containing particulates of vegetables, herbs, cheese or other materials. These products are now

---

Box 11.12 Key measures for shelf-life control of delicatessen products

- Stock rotation of material in storage chillers
- Labelling of counter tickets (usually on the reverse) with durability codes, i.e. **use by** or **display until**. This must take into account the maximum life of the ingredient and the customer life, i.e. if the shelf-life when purchased by the customer is 2 days and the maximum life of the open product is 2 days, a counter ticket for that item should be marked to be sold no later than 4 days before the maximum shelf-life of the unopened product
- Stock rotation on open display. Care should be taken to ensure that products are removed from sale when they reach their maximum shelf-life
- Where products are 'topped' up during the day it is important that this is taken into account when marking the maximum shelf-life on the counter ticket, e.g. mark the use by or display until dates of the shortest shelf-life product
- Labelling of the price ticket with a durability code, i.e. use by or **eat within** dates. There is no legal requirement to label products that are loose but it is good practice to ensure the customer is aware of the maximum safe shelf-life of the food and its storage requirements, i.e. chilled etc.

---

commonplace in delicatessen shops. Vegetables in oil such as chilli in oil, garlic in oil, etc. are usually made by simply placing the whole or sliced vegetable into the oil with or without some form of mild cooking process. The cooking at best involves subjecting the product to temperatures that will destroy vegetative food poisoning organisms but will not be sufficient to destroy spores. The combined conditions of high nutrient and moisture content, storage at ambient temperature under an anaerobic environment, i.e. in oil, and with long shelf-lives provide spore forming bacteria like *C. botulinum* ideal opportunities for growth. Indeed, such products have caused outbreaks of botulism in the past. Safety of these products can be achieved if the ingredients used are either dried or acidified prior to use to levels indicated above.

BAKERY

The baker's shop still remains a significant fixture on most high streets and in local shopping areas despite the growth in major retailers with in-house baking facilities. The traditional role of the baker in making bread has been supplemented with the introduction of added-value products, such as cream cakes, pies, doughnuts and a wide variety of cakes, pastries, etc. Indeed, most local bakers now also cater for the lunchtime trade with preparation and sale of sandwiches, salads and other more processed dishes. With the exception of sandwiches, cream cakes and perhaps some of the filled pies and tarts, most foods produced in a bakery are essentially ambient stable and traditional bakery products are usually not associated with foodborne disease. Outbreaks have, however, implicated bakery products mostly through cross-contamination e.g. salmonellosis, hepatitis, etc., although *Bacillus* spp. have also caused illness. The key factors therefore that need control include microbiological, physical and allergen contamination, shelf-life and pest control.

Microbiological, physical and allergen contamination

The vast majority of bakers and in store bakeries make bread through 'scratch' baking, i.e. from raw materials, although some bakeries may simply bake-off previously frozen products. Although this is a relatively simple process of mixing flour, salt, water and yeast, the use of open, automated mixing equipment, the extensively handled and worked product and the open baking tins provide ample opportunity for contamination with foreign objects. Pieces of broken mixing blades, paper or string from dough sacks and mixing utensils and scrapers are a few of the many objects that could fall into and be incorporated and concealed in the dough prior to baking. Such items will only become evident once eaten by the consumer. Control of these hazards is relatively simple (Box 11.13).

Box 11.13 Key measures to control physical contamination in bakeries

- Maintenance of equipment to ensure there are no loose screws, damaged blades, damaged sieves, etc.
- Inspect equipment once used
- Define storage areas for portable equipment and utensils
- 'Clean as you go' processes to ensure loose, open and empty packaging is disposed of in suitable bins

---

Microbiological contamination is mainly a risk for bakery products that are filled or topped after baking, e.g. cream cakes, sandwiches, iced cakes. Outbreaks of salmonellosis due to cross-contamination with raw bakery ingredients, e.g. eggs and an outbreak of hepatitis A virus from a frosted (iced) bakery item contaminated by an infected food handler demonstrate that such simple hazards need to be effectively controlled. The key controlling factors to prevent cross-contamination from raw to cooked foods have already been outlined in the section on meat (see Box 11.9, p. 218) and the same principles apply in bakeries. The main areas for concern in a bakery are hygienic practices of employees and a separate area of the bakery where cooked and ready-to-eat foods are prepared to ensure the products and the surfaces or utensils used to prepared them will not be contaminated from raw ingredients such as eggs or meat.

Staff handling ready-to-eat foods present significant risk to foods when making up and filling cream cakes, icing or when preparing sandwiches. As the vast majority of this is done by manual handling and filling, control of the spread of pathogenic micro-organisms from the food handler to the food is essential. Food hygiene training is essential for such employees with emphasis on reporting infectious disease and personal hygiene controls, i.e. hand washing. To prevent contamination from raw ingredients such as eggs or meat to ready-to-eat foods, it is common for bakeries to have cream rooms where pre-baked cakes are garnished and filled with cream either manually or using automated machinery. Cleaning is essential to ensure safety of perishable bakery products such as cream cakes and particular attention should be paid to the small cream machines. Cream machines usually consist of a chamber with a paddle that whips cream to incorporate air. The cream is drawn through a tube by a screw auger device, leaving through a nozzle and being deposited in or on the baked base. Significant opportunities exist for build up of contaminants such as *L. monocytogenes* in the intricate components of cream machines as they are intrinsically difficult to clean effectively. Full dismantling is usually required to clean cream debris from the machines with periods of soaking prior to reassembly and chemical or hot water sterilization. A useful tip to assess the hygienic status of a cream machine is to lift the lid and smell it before it is to be used, as cream residues in poorly cleaned machines will have a rancid smell.

Allergens are a particular problem for bakeries and bakery counters as many use raw ingredients that are allergens in their own right, e.g. nuts, peanuts, wheat, egg, etc. Many foods can cause allergies and, in the EU, the allergens that require specific controls are nuts, peanuts, sesame, fish, shellfish, milk, egg, gluten, celery, soya, sulphur dioxide and mustard (Directive 2003/89/EC as regards indication of the ingredients present in foodstuffs). If these ingredients are present in a pre-packaged food they must be specified on the label to ensure avoidance by individuals who have specific allergies to them.

In the UK, there is also voluntary labelling of foods in which the allergenic ingredient is not present as a formulated ingredient but from which it may cross-contaminate other food during production. Customers are advised of possible risks by the labelling which indicates that the food may contain the allergen or that it has been made in an environment where allergenic ingredients are also handled. Foods that are sold loose (including most of the foods in a bakery or bakery counter), are exempt from the legislative labelling requirements.

In a bakery environment, the principal risk comes from gluten, nuts, peanuts and egg and the risk is primarily that of inadvertent cross-contamination. The use of common mixing, baking, slicing, packing and display equipment makes the control of allergenic ingredients extremely difficult. In individuals who are extremely sensitive to allergens and where anaphylaxis may result following consumption, levels as low as 0.5 mg (total consumption) of an allergen can trigger a reaction. With the obvious exception of wheat gluten, procedures can be implemented in bakeries to minimize the risk of cross-contamination of allergens but given the low levels of allergen that can trigger a reaction, and difficulties in effectively cleaning equipment where dough is used, most bakeries handling allergens such as nuts, peanuts, etc. are not capable of reducing cross-contamination risks to an acceptable level. In such circumstances, customers to the bakery or bakery counter should be made aware of the potential for allergens that may be present in products using notices on display at the counter or in the bakers shop (Figure 11.6).

Notwithstanding this, it is possible to reduce the risk of cross-contamination through simple measures (Box 11.14).

Box 11.14 Key measures for preventing allergen cross-contamination of bakery products

- Produce, bake and finish, i.e. decorate products containing allergens (nuts and peanuts, etc.) at the end of production in dedicated areas or using dedicated equipment
- Display allergen-containing products in a dedicated area or in separate baskets or containers
- Handle allergen-containing products with dedicated utensils

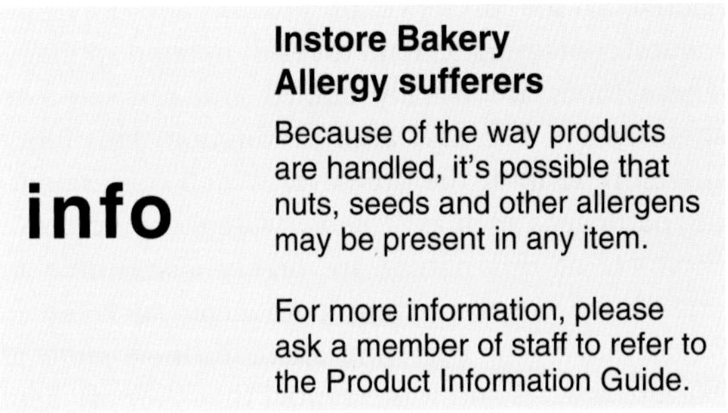

---

info

Instore Bakery Allergy sufferers

Because of the way products are handled, it's possible that nuts, seeds and other allergens may be present in any item.

For more information, please ask a member of staff to refer to the Product Information Guide.

Figure 11.6 *Point of display message in a bakery*

Shelf-life

The majority of bakery products are generally considered ambient stable. However, some products such as custard tarts, sausage rolls, savoury pies are all susceptible to the growth of pathogenic microorganisms capable of surviving the baking process involved in their production. This essentially means spore-forming organisms such as *Bacillus* spp., *C. perfringens* and *C. botulinum*. The speed at which the organisms will grow and render the products unsafe will depend on the products themselves and how dry they become during baking; the lower the moisture the slower organisms will grow. It is generally the filling that provides the conditions to support growth and, under favourable conditions, organisms such as *C. perfringens* and *Bacillus* spp. can grow to unsafe levels within 6–8 hours at warm temperatures in bakeries. It is good practice, if selling foods of this nature at ambient temperature, to display them for no more than 4 hours although certain exemptions have historically applied allowing specified foods (e.g. custard tarts, cooked pies, sausage rolls) to be kept at ambient for up to 24 hours or the entire day on which they are made (The

Food Hygiene Regulations 2006). The scientific basis for this is not clear, and although traditional low moisture and high salt-containing foods may be safe, certain formulations of these products that have higher moisture fillings may be susceptible to growth of pathogens. As already indicated, it is good practice to hold products capable of supporting the growth of pathogenic micro-organisms for no more than 4 hours at ambient temperature, after which time they should be removed from sale and disposed.

For perishable foods such as cream cakes and sandwiches, the shelf-life is usually significantly restricted as the presence of post-process environmental contaminants tend to result in rapid spoilage. These foods are usually chilled and restricted to shelf-lives of 1–2 days after production. This tends therefore to limit the time over which contaminating pathogens such as *L. monocytogenes* could grow. Products of this nature are highly susceptible to growth of contaminating pathogens such as *L. monocytogenes* or surviving spore formers such as *Bacillus* species and it is essential that they are kept refrigerated for the duration of their shelf-life.

Pest control

Infestation is a major issue in bakeries. The need to store large quantities of flour and the difficulty in effectively cleaning bakery environments such as floors with dry cleaning methods means that rodents have ready access to foods. Infestation problems also extend to include insects such as flies, moths and grain weevils (psocids) that can cause considerable contamination of flour. Storing raw materials off the floor and preventing access to rodents by effective proofing of doors to flies by screening of windows are essential. In addition, operating **clean as you go** processes especially for spillages, is an essential way to minimize infestation in bakeries. Pest activity should be monitored using insect and rodent traps and where there is evidence of active infestation ensure the pest contractor issues advice on suitable remedial measures. This is discussed in more detail in Chapter 4.

TAKE-AWAY FOOD AND IN-STORE RESTAURANTS

Many retail food businesses sell hot or warm food for immediate consumption either as the main part of the business (take-away shops) or as part of a larger retail store (supermarket hot-food counters, in-store restaurants, etc.). Such businesses combine many of the risks that are inherent in both food manufacture and catering with the added pressure of periods of high demand e.g. lunch time, pub closing time, etc. The key issues here are temperature control, microbiological and allergen cross-contamination and shelf-life.

Temperature control

Most foods sold at these retail outlets and counters are cooked foods including cooked eggs, meat, chicken, etc., and therefore significant hazards are present on the raw materials that are later cooked. To ensure adequate destruction of vegetative bacterial contaminants, cook products to 70 °C for 2 minutes or a suitable equivalent (Table 11.2). It is essential that the cooking method and appliance used, which can be a domestic appliance in small businesses, delivers the correct cook. It is good practice to use temperature probes for occasional checks, which is a simple and reliable means of ensuring safety in a catering operation. Records of such checks should be kept. Food that is kept hot for extended periods before serving must be kept at a temperature of 63 °C or above and should also have some form of temperature monitoring either of the cabinet or the product. Clearly, it is important when monitoring temperature of ready-to-eat products that the probe itself is properly cleaned and disinfected before and after use. Impregnated alcohol wipes are useful for this purpose.

Microbiological and allergen contamination

Any operation handling raw and cooked foods predisposes itself to the risk of cross-contamination. As take-away shops and in-store restaurants are essentially catering operations, they fall into the class of businesses most often implicated in foodborne disease outbreaks. Environments making take-away or restaurant foods provide ample opportunity for cross-contamination as they are often cramped and with limited resources. However, the key measures to prevent cross-contamination are relatively straightforward (Box 11.15).

Box 11.15 Key measures to minimize the risk of cross-contamination in take-aways and restaurants

- Store raw food separate from cooked foods or, if this is not possible, then in sealed containers or covered and kept below ready-to-eat foods and separated by shelving
- Use different kitchen utensils for handling raw and cooked foods unless the utensil is likely to be 'cooked' itself e.g. ladle, fish slice, etc.
- Do not let ready-to-eat food come into contact with raw foods. This is usually achieved by preparing raw and ready-to-eat foods in separate areas or by cleaning and disinfecting between use

Further details of procedures to avoid cross-contamination is given in the Meat section (see Box 11.9).

Another hazard in such environments for cross-contamination is that of allergens. The best means to avoid cross-contamination is to avoid the use of the allergen, or, if this is not possible, to handle, prepare, cook and serve allergen-containing foods separately. In most environments of this nature, it would not be possible to use such methods to avoid cross-contamination and it is usual practice to alert customers to the risk that allergens may be present in foods that are not designed to contain the allergen (See Bakery section).

Cleaning and disinfection are essential components to ensure food safety in these operations and the principles have already been discussed extensively in the delicatessen section. The use of dishwashers is a useful consideration for many of the utensils used in these types of operations as more aggressive cleaning is often needed to remove cooked-on food (see Chapter 12, p. 235).

Shelf-life

Most take-away and in-store restaurant foods are designed to be eaten immediately after purchase either in the store or restaurant or at home. The expectation is that most food of this nature will be consumed within 1–2 hours at most. Properly cooked food may be contaminated with surviving spore forming bacteria or environmental cross-contaminants such as *L. monocytogenes*. To prevent growth of these foodborne pathogens, hot food should be kept at above 63 °C prior to sale. This is

usually readily achieved as the food is cooked to order. The shelf-life of ingredients is an important factor in the safety of the finished product and it is essential that the recommended shelf-life and storage conditions applied to raw ingredients are adhered to. In some cases, hot food may be designed for either direct consumption or consumption at a later date, e.g. rotisserie chickens. If it is likely that customers will store the product for later consumption or indeed, where leftovers are likely, it is good practice to provide on-pack advice to eat immediately or cool within 2 hours and then refrigerate (IGD, 2000b). Foods cooled in such a way should ideally be fully re-cooked prior to consumption.

Some foods such as pies and pasties, etc., are cooked and intended to be eaten warm, i.e. they are not stored hot but allowed to cool and sold at ambient temperatures. Significant opportunities exist for the growth of surviving spore-forming bacteria in particular, and great care must be exercised when selling such food. The degree to which surviving spore formers will grow to unsafe levels will depend on the factors inherent in the actual pie but organisms such as *C. perfringens* can increase from 10 to 10 000 within 6–8 hours in a high water activity, neutral pH product stored in a warm environment. In the UK, legislation allows such pies to be held for up to a day (The Food Hygiene [England] Regulations 2006) which is regarded as safe for traditional lower water activity pies. However, with a move to reducing salt and the taste benefits of higher moisture and thus higher water activities, it is good practice to sell such products within 4 hours from bake. As most of these types of products are designed for lunchtime or evening trade, they do tend to be consumed within such time periods.

HOME DELIVERY

In the past, home delivery consisted of the local greengrocers' son cycling down with a small amount of groceries in the front basket of his bicycle to the customer's home, usually within a distance that would take no more than a few minutes. Home delivery has expanded significantly in recent years, with large quantities of groceries being delivered over a wide area from a local store or distribution centre. Groceries may be either picked by the store staff, by a dedicated home shopping team or indeed, may be purchased by the customer and left for the store to deliver.

Products are placed in carrier bags and held in the appropriate storage areas prior to loading the delivery vehicle. Bags are placed into dedicated crates and delivery vehicles have any combination of ambient, chilled and frozen compartments. In order to maximize efficiency, vehicles are loaded with groceries for multiple customers, taking into account the likely time for delivery. Deliveries are scheduled within an agreed time slot with the customer. Distances covered by home delivery vehicles can be 22–44 km from the store or distribution centre. The key food hygiene challenges for home delivery are temperature control and chemical contamination.

Temperature control

Vehicles can be scheduled to be out on the road for several hours and this may be further extended due to unforeseen delays in traffic. Temperature control of chilled and frozen foods is critical to ensure food safety. The provisions of Regulation (EC) No. 852/2004 apply to chilled and frozen food in that they must not be kept at temperatures that could result in the growth of pathogenic micro-organisms where such growth would result in a risk to health. The Food Hygiene (England) Regulations 2006 require products that are likely to support growth of pathogenic micro-organisms to be kept at a temperature of 8 °C or less. Mail-order foods are exempt from this requirement but must not be kept at a temperature likely to have a risk for health. For home delivery, this means in practice ensuring food

temperatures do not exceed 8 °C although for durability and quality reasons limits may be set much lower, e.g. 5 °C or less, by individual food businesses depending on the criteria used to establish the maximum shelf-life of their products. Therefore, the use of vehicles with chilled or frozen compartments is often necessary. This allows them to operate for extended periods without affecting the safety of the products. In the absence of this, time restrictions are usually limited by the potential for frozen food to defrost but this is subject to quality effects rather than safety. Like any refrigeration unit, chilled vehicles should have regular checks to ensure the correct temperature is maintained. This issue has been covered extensively in the Transport and distribution section (see p. 210), and checks should be conducted, as a minimum, before the vehicle is loaded with groceries and ideally at several times during the day. Temperatures should be recorded and any deviations investigated.

Chemical contamination

A potential risk exists of spillage of household chemicals (bleach, oven cleaners, toiletries, etc.) which will contaminate foodstuffs during transport. The principal check is to ensure products are not damaged and are placed upright in dedicated carrier bags which are separate from foods. This usually forms part of the training of those picking the shopping. Ideally crates used for transportation of home delivery should have solid bases and sides to contain any spillages and bags holding 'non-foods' should be in separate crates, although this is often not practical for space reasons.

Summary

The low number of foodborne disease outbreaks attributed to food retail premises is a testimony to the effective systems in place in many businesses to manage food safety. However, their size and the large number of customers who purchase food from retailers make any failures at this stage likely to cause large-scale outbreaks. Retail food safety is essentially managed through the application of the similar controls in different combinations for different parts of the retail outlet. These simple principles when operated consistently and effectively will ensure food is not made unsafe or of an unacceptable quality by the retail stage in the food chain. These are:

- temperature control (intake, storage and display)
- cooking and cooling controls
- contamination controls (microbiological, physical, chemical, allergens)
- shelf-life management (stock rotation)
- cleaning and pest control
- personnel hygiene and training.

All websites cited in this chapter and below were accessed in February 2007.

SOURCES OF INFORMATION AND FURTHER READING

Anon (1995) *Industry Guide to Good Hygiene Practice: Retail Guide.* London: Chadwick House Group (available at: http://archive.food.gov.uk/dept_health/pdf/retsec.pdf) Note: 2007 revision in press (see http://www.brc.org.uk and foodstandards.gov.uk).

Anon (1997) *Industry Guide to Good Hygiene Practice: Baking Guide.* London: Chadwick House Group (available at: http://archive.food.gov.uk/dept_health/pdf/complete.pdf).

Burgess F, Little CL, Allen G, *et al.* (2005) The prevalence of *Campylobacter, Salmonella* and *E. coli* on the external packaging of raw meat. *J Food Protection* **68**: 469–75.

Department of Health (1992) *Safer Cooked Meat Production Guidelines. A 10-point Plan.* London: Department of Health (available at http://archive.food.gov.uk/maff/archive/food/bulletin/1996/no80/lanark.htm).

Directive 2003/89/EC of the European Parliament and of the Council of 10 November 2003 amending Directive 2000/13/EC as regards indication of the ingredients present in foodstuffs. *Official Journal of the European Union* L308/15 25.11.2003 (available at www.europa.eu.int/eur-lex/).

Food Standards Agency (2006) *Guidance on Allergen Management and Consumer Information.* London: Food Standards Agency (also available at www.food.gov.uk).

Gaze JE, Shaw R, Archer J (1998) Identification and prevention of hazards associated with slow cooling of hams and other large cooked meats and meat products. Review No. 8. Chipping Campden: Campden and Chorleywood Food Research Association.

Goulet V, Lepoutre A, Rocourt J, *et al.* (1993) Epidémie de listériose en France – Bilan final et résultats de l'enquête épidémiologique. *Bull Epidémiol Hebdomaire* **4**: 13–14.

Hennessey TW, Hedberg CW, Slutsker L, *et al.* (1996) A national outbreak of *Salmonella enteritidis* infections in ice cream. *N Engl J Med* **334**: 1281–6.

IGD (2000a) *Voluntary Labelling Guidelines for Food Allergens and Gluten* (see www.igd.org.uk).

IGD (2000b) *Voluntary Guidelines for the Provision of Food Safety Advice on Product Labels.* London: IGD (see www.igd.org.uk).

IGD (2005) *UK Grocery Retailing.* London: IGD (see www.igd.com).

12

Disinfection and cleaning

Peter Hoffman

Purpose of disinfection and cleaning	233	The practice of cleaning	239
Disinfection	233	Stages in cleaning	241
Sterilization	236	Summary	243
Cleaning	236	Sources of information and further reading	244

Disinfection is the killing or removal of microbes down to safe levels. Disinfection is achieved by using heat or chemicals to kill the microbes, or possibly through the removal of microbes during cleaning.

Effective disinfection can interrupt routes of transmission of infection, but it must be accurately targeted. Random or sporadic disinfection is unlikely to achieve food hygiene.

Cleaning Any process of physical removal of 'soil' (any matter present that should not be part of an item). This matter can contain microbes that are responsible for food poisoning or spoilage and acts as a source of their nutrients.

Disinfectant A chemical that has lethal action on microbes.

Sanitizer A term for disinfectants often used in food industry.

Sterilization The total elimination of all microbes (whether harmful or not).

PURPOSE OF DISINFECTION AND CLEANING

The purpose of **disinfection, cleaning and sterilization** in food hygiene is to prevent both food poisoning and spoilage. Each of these methods has a part to play in controlling the presence and spread of microbes. It is not intended that food handling premises be turned into true sterile zones, but there is a need to identify those areas where harmful microbes exist and, if there is a pathway microbes can use to cause illness, to block such pathways. This can be achieved by good practice, which includes cleaning, disinfection, sterilization or a combination of these. Such an informed approach is essential to the practice of food hygiene. A random approach of sporadic or haphazard cleaning, disinfection or sterilization will not result in food hygiene.

Beware of placing too great an emphasis on cleanliness for its own sake to the possible exclusion of other factors such as good-quality raw materials, separation and handling aspects, thorough cooking, cooling or reheating and proper storage. A clean food preparation area by itself is no guarantee for safe food.

DISINFECTION

Disinfection has a flexible definition. In essence it means the elimination of sufficient disease-producing microbes such that safety is ensured. So the definition of successful disinfection will depend on the situation, taking into account the likelihood of disease transmission in a particular context. If an object does not present a risk of infection, then disinfection of that object is irrelevant. Most people think of specific use of disinfectants as the only means to achieve disinfection, yet this is neither the most common nor the most efficient way to do this. A good working definition of disinfection is elimination of all bacteria, viruses and fungi other than bacterial spores.

Bacterial spores are hardy, heat-resistant life forms produced by the genera *Bacillus* and *Clostridium*. Both have definite roles to play in food poisoning, but this is more related to short- and long-term storage of foodstuffs rather than shortcomings in food hygiene during catering (see Chapters 4 and 5 for details of the roles of these organisms in food poisoning).

Methods of disinfection

There are three methods of disinfection:

- cleaning
- heat
- chemicals.

Cleaning eliminates micro-organisms by their physical removal. This will be discussed in detail later in this chapter. Cleaning must be considered along with other, perhaps more obvious, methods of disinfection when making decisions about food hygiene. Cleaning can be done on its own, or in combination with heat and/or chemicals.

Heat disinfection occupies a fundamental position in food hygiene. Cooking is used to make foods palatable, and at the same time, safe. Many raw foods, primarily meats and meat products, have an unacceptable probability of containing pathogenic micro-organisms. When food is thoroughly cooked, all pathogens except for bacterial spores are killed. Heat, as a more calculated method of disinfection, is one of the oldest processes in microbiology, and is also known as pasteurization (introduced by and named after Louis Pasteur, the nineteenth century microbiologist). This is still used to eliminate pathogenic micro-organisms from milk. In pasteurization, the milk is heated to a variety of temperatures for a corresponding variety of times (the higher the temperature, the shorter the time), for example, 72 ° for at least 15 seconds, kills the bacteria responsible for tuberculosis and other milk-associated pathogens (for further details, see Chapter 3, p. 45).

The method of heat disinfection can also be used for utensils, crockery, cutlery, chopping boards etc. If one or more parts of a dishwasher cycle involves heat of around 80 °C, all the contents will be free from microbes other than bacterial spores. It is usual to include this heat stage in the final rinse in mechanical dishwashing as it facilitates drying. Water at these high temperatures causes serious burns on skin, and it would therefore be hazardous to attempt heat disinfection during hand dishwashing. Hygiene in hand dishwashing is achieved by physical removal of contamination rather than by killing. Thus hand dishwashing is more dependent on training and diligence than mechanical dishwashing and, as such, is more fallible. Dishwashing sinks and handwash basins should be kept separate rather than attempting to use the same facility for both. It can be a disincentive for washing hands if someone else is using the sink for dishwashing.

Chemical disinfection has a limited role in food hygiene. It is far less reliable than heat and usually requires thoughtfully chosen disinfectants; careful controlled application allowing sufficient exposure time; an assessment of the need for pre-cleaning; and rinsing after disinfection.

Some factors that need to be considered when choosing an appropriate disinfectant are:

- The microbicidal range of the disinfectant. All disinfectants do not kill all micro-organisms. It is necessary to know what microbes may be present and whether a particular disinfectant is capable of killing them.
- The ability of a disinfectant to withstand inactivation by a variety of organic matter. Most disinfectants will be inactivated, to varying extents, by organic matter such as dirt and food residues. One can choose a disinfectant that will withstand inactivation or a higher concentration can be used to compensate for inactivation, or one can consider pre-cleaning to remove excess organic matter or a combination of these methods. Detergents and disinfectants can inactivate each other. Never add disinfectants to each other or add detergents to disinfectants unless their compatibility is known. Other causes of disinfectant inactivation are: hard water, contact with a variety of plastics, rubber and cellulose and non-cellulose fibres.
- Disinfectants must be able to reach and make contact with their target micro-organisms. This will not happen if target microbes are protected within layers of dirt which, if present, should be removed by cleaning prior to disinfection. Some

disinfectants claim to have detergent properties in addition to disinfection action – in which case their capacity for disinfection is likely to be exhausted by penetration of organic matter layers.

- Disinfectants work best at or above normal room temperature. If disinfection of refrigerated equipment is required, the equipment should be brought to room temperature, or a higher concentration of disinfectant may be used, the disinfectant left in contact for a longer time or an alternative method of disinfection used.

- Since disinfection is not instantaneous and all disinfectants need time to kill microbes. A contact of a few seconds will kill just a few. Although highly dependent on many of the factors listed above, efficient disinfection occurs over minutes and occasionally hours. Disinfection will only take place when the disinfectant is present in solution, so when a disinfectant applied to a surface dries out or evaporates, the killing of microbes ceases.

- Many disinfectants decay once diluted to use strength. Once they have decayed, they are more likely both to fail to kill their target and to become colonized by bacteria. Thus disinfectants should be made up freshly and regularly. Some disinfectants decay on bulk storage; these should be freshly purchased and stored according to the manufacturer's instructions.

- In addition to microbicidal issues, factors such as toxicity, taint and corrosion must be considered. Disinfectants not specifically intended for use in food handling areas must be screened for toxicity and taint-imparting qualities. If there is any suspicion on these grounds, the disinfectant must not be used. Corrosion, especially of mild-steel and carbon-steel, can be initiated and accelerated by certain disinfectants. This can be an expensive error.

Disinfectants

Although there are many disinfectant preparations on the market, they are formulated from a limited range of active ingredients. When confronted with an unfamiliar disinfectant, you should find out the active ingredient so that its advantages and drawbacks can be ascertained and its suitability for a particular task determined. All disinfectants used in food production areas must not impart taint to food: this is important even when they are used on non-food contact surfaces.

Chlorine-based disinfectants are among the most useful disinfectants for food hygiene. They are also called chlorine bleaches and hypochlorites. The most common presentations of this group are liquid bleaches (solutions of sodium hypochlorite) and dry powders and tablets made from sodium dichloroisocyanurate (NaDCC) which release hypochlorite when dissolved. The liquid forms can be unstable on storage; the dry forms are stable on long-term storage but decay once made up to use dilution.

The strength of a hypochlorite solution is best expressed in terms of parts per million available chlorine (ppm av Cl) rather than as a percentage. Commercial products are formulated by manufacturers and supplied as ready-to-use solutions or with dilution instructions and contact times.

- **Advantages:** Wide microbicidal range, low toxicity at use dilutions, cheap.
- **Disadvantages:** Can be corrosive to some metals, low concentrations are inactivated by organic matter, do not mix with strong acids (chlorine gas is released which is highly toxic).

Peroxygen and hydrogen peroxide compounds are oxidizing disinfectants with a wide microbicidal range. They are sometimes formulated with a compatible detergent for use as a combined cleaner-disinfectant. The activity of different formulations may vary.

- **Advantages:** Wide microbicidal range, low toxicity at use dilutions.
- **Disadvantages:** Some undiluted products can be irritant, low concentrations inactivated by organic matter.

Quaternary-ammonium compounds (QACs) are a family of surface active (and therefore detergent) molecules, all based around a similar molecular structure. They are easy to use and combine the functions of both cleaning and chemical disinfection. Their main disadvantage is related to their surfactant property. If confronted with substances that attract surfactants (such as fabrics and many types of organic matter in solution or suspension), the QAC molecules will combine with this matter, leaving little remaining in true solution. This process inactivates QACs as disinfectants. It follows that, despite being cleaning agents, they work best as disinfectants in already clean environments.

- **Advantages:** Easy to use, stable, little corrosion, low toxicity, all have detergent action.
- **Disadvantages:** Easily inactivated, narrower microbicidal range than hypochlorites.

Iodine-based disinfectants are sometimes used in connection with food. As iodine itself is unsuitable for general use, the disinfectants contain iodine as a complex with other molecules or a complex with detergent molecules. Both these formulations allow only a small amount of iodine to be free in solution, thus diminishing undesirable effects of the iodine. Once the small amount of free iodine has been used up, more will be released from the complex to take part in disinfection.

- **Advantages:** Wide microbicidal range, most have detergent properties, some can be corrosive to certain metals, stable on storage.
- **Disadvantages:** Can be expensive, concentrated solutions can be viscous.

Hand disinfection

Bacteria that normally inhabit skin ('resident' microbes) are, for the most part, harmless (see the section on hand hygiene in Chapter 8). Pathogenic microbes that are picked up by touch (such as handling raw chicken) are easily removed by washing (i.e. disinfection by cleaning). Chemical skin disinfectants have no routine role to play in food hygiene.

STERILIZATION

This is the process leading to the *complete* elimination of *all* microbes. The most common method of sterilization is by steam under pressure. Bacterial spores can survive hours of boiling at atmospheric pressure ($100\,°C$) and steam above this temperature requires a pressurized vessel. Sterilization is only relevant in the control of food

poisoning and spoilage in the process of canning. After a can has been sealed, it is heated by steam in a large pressurized vessel to sterilize the contents. This is necessary to kill the heat resistant spores of the bacterium *Clostridium botulinum* which, if left in a high protein, low acid food such as meat or fish, can produce a lethal toxin (see Chapter 4, p. 85, for more details on botulism). Sometimes chemical disinfectants are referred to by those selling them as 'sterilants'. This is misleading. Although in well thought-out laboratory tests such products can achieve sterility, in normal practice they can be relied on, at best, to give disinfection.

CLEANING

In the context of food hygiene, cleaning is the process which removes those microbes, which can cause poisoning and spoilage, from contact with foodstuff, as well as removing dirt that prevents removal of these microbes and provide nutrients for their proliferation. Cleanliness is often regarded as the fundamental process of food hygiene. This is perhaps not the absolute concept that it is often accepted to be since (for reasons given below) knowledge, rational thought and action all have to be co-ordinated to achieve best practice.

Cleaning includes both hygienic and aesthetic considerations. **Hygiene** refers to practices as they relate to the maintenance of health. For food hygiene this centres around the exclusion and elimination of harmful microbes or their products from the diet. **Aesthetics** refers to perceptual factors related to the senses. These include the outward appearance of food or its surroundings and acceptability. These two concepts do not always equate. A kitchen can be scrupulously clean and yet contain food items which will cause food poisoning when consumed; a sparklingly clean oven does not prevent a chicken from being undercooked. However, their is often a behavioural association between maintenance of an aesthetically acceptable environment and good food hygiene.

As an example, consider the importance of the state of cleanliness of a kitchen floor to food hygiene. Should the floor be either scrupulously clean or grossly dirty, in either case, were food dropped on it, it would (in an ideal world) no longer be considered fit for consumption. A second example is the chopping board. Here the same surface may be used for potentially hazardous foods (e.g. uncooked meat) and foods which require no further preparation before being eaten. So chopping is safely done by the use of separate boards for these two products but if necessary, the same board can be cleaned between processes. In the latter situation, the quality of cleaning of the surface is vital to the hygiene. If a decontamination process is important for food hygiene, it must always be carried out efficiently, i.e. **quality control** of the process is important.

Certain processes in the series of steps that lead to a safe food product are more relevant than others. If the processes can be controlled at these points, the safety of the end product can be assured. (See Chapter 10 for principles of **Hazard Analysis and Critical Control Points [HACCP] system**). For example, in the safe production of pasteurized milk, factors that contribute to the hygiene of the milk are:

- health of the cows
- hygiene of the milking process
- conditions of storage and transport of the raw milk
- efficacy of its pasteurization
- prevention of recontamination
- post-pasteurization temperature and time control
- hygiene of packaging.

The most critical event in this sequence is pasteurization which rids the milk of pathogens such as *Mycobacterium tuberculosis*, *Brucella abortus*, *Salmonella* or *Campylobacter*, and after which the introduction of such organisms is highly unlikely. Thus, the process of pasteurization is that stage in milk production where quality control is highest and where the most intensive monitoring occurs. Controls for pasteurization are precise, 'fail safe' precautions are highly developed, and there are post-process checks. This is an example of a **critical control point** when applying the HACCP procedure (see Chapter 10).

Similar considerations should be made to cleaning when it makes a definite contribution to food hygiene and so has to be of the highest assured quality. To return to the example of the chopping boards, if there are separate and segregated chopping boards for uncooked meats and ready-to-eat food, the cleaning of the respective boards is not such a critical process. But where the same board is to be used for both tasks, the quality of cleaning has to be ensured. In practice, the best ways are either to use a good quality dishwashing machine or have competent, well-instructed staff washing by hand.

Specific cleaning areas

Floors

As contact between floors and food should not occur, floor cleaning is not closely related to food hygiene. Surprisingly little transfer of contamination takes place between floors and work-surfaces in a kitchen except by vectors such as insects or vermin, floor cleaning with pressure hoses, or lifting food containers from the floor onto a work surface. Floor cleaning serves two purposes:

- **safety of the workers**: a build-up of grease can result in a slippery surface
- **vermin control**: food residues on the floor provide nutrients for the complete range of kitchen pests.

Floor cleaning must be done with cleaning materials (cloths and mops) different from those used on surfaces or utensils associated with food contact. Should there not be a segregation, cleaning can be the cause of, rather than a solution to, food contamination.

Drains and gullies

The reasoning here is similar to that of floor cleaning. Dirt or smells from drains may be aesthetically offensive but they are not related to food poisoning except where they act as food for pests. Acceptability of drains and gullies is usually a combination of cleanliness and good plumbing. Should their appearance or smell be offensive, first clean them using hot water with a degreasing agent, and if this fails, an inspection for blockages or faulty plumbing should be done. Use of disinfectants in this situation will not be helpful.

Kitchen utensils

Kitchen utensils include knives, forks and spoons, all manner of slicers and mixers, bowls, chopping boards and so on. Wherever possible, if they are to be used for raw foods which may harbour food poisoning or spoilage microbes, they should be separate from those used for ready-to-eat food. If this is not possible or practicable, they must be thoroughly washed, then quickly and efficiently dried before re-use.

Eating and drinking utensils

Here aesthetic appreciation is readily made by consumers and, should cleanliness of eating and drinking utensils be found to be lacking, consumers will draw conclusions about other aspects of hygiene in an establishment. Lack of cleanliness of these utensils is only a minor food poisoning hazard, microbial inocula are likely to be small and the contamination immediately before or during food consumption, but there is a person-to-person risk. Should the previous user have had an acute infection of the mucous membranes of the mouth, for example a rhinovirus (common cold) infection, contact with the next user's oral mucous membranes may well be sufficient to transfer the infection. This is true for only those microbes that can be transmitted through saliva, and is not true of all microbes. Other viruses, such as the human immunodeficiency virus (HIV), will not be transferred in this way.

Cleaning utensils, cloths, etc.

Items used for kitchen cleaning are mobile and can come into contact with many different surfaces and utensils over a comparatively short time period. This process can itself act as a transfer mechanism for the microbes that it is attempting to curb. Thus segregation and decontamination of cleaning items is an essential component of food hygiene.

Aesthetic and hygienic considerations coincide with floor cloths and work surface cloths. It goes without saying that they are not interchangeable. The dangers of using a clean-looking cloth – which happens to have been used to mop up a minor spill from thawing raw poultry in a refrigerator – on the blade of a knife that is then used to cut a cream cake, may not be immediately apparent. Yet this is probably a far more efficient way of causing food poisoning than the transfer of contamination from the floor. Cloths can be colour coded by their category of use: dirty environment (floors); potentially contaminated foodstuff and their utensils; ready-to-eat foods and their utensils. If the cloths are to be re-used they must be hot washed, rinsed and thoroughly dried at regular intervals (at least daily). Cloths for different categories of purpose must not be mixed, even in the washing process. In

many ways it is both easier and safer to use single-use wipes which are disposed after a single task, so ensuring that they do not transfer contamination.

Counter tops and work surfaces

Like floors, these are cleaned *in situ*. Unlike floors, counter tops may legitimately make contact with food prior to consumption. Should this contact be sequentially with raw and then cooked or ready-to-eat food, the counter top can transfer contamination from one to the other. Any cleaning process must be compatible with the surface material and not cause damage leaving cracks and crevices that can harbour bacteria, which are then safe from attempts to remove or kill them. Manual cleaning requires a degree of diligence and application. A quick, haphazard wipe will not contribute to food hygiene. Cleaning should take place between preparation of items and not just at the end of a session.

Food storage containers

As storage containers may have prolonged contact with foods that will support growth of bacteria responsible for both food poisoning and spoilage, their initial cleanliness is important. Where mechanical dishwashing is feasible for containers, it is preferable. When manual washing is used, it must be thorough, followed by efficient drying prior to storage or re-use.

Cooking vessels

Although heat disinfected during the cooking process, cooking vessels should be cleaned after each use, and stored dry.

Hand hygiene

All skin surfaces carry bacteria. Bacteria for which the skin is the permanent habitat are, in general, harmless. They are present both on the surface of the skin and in the various pores and follicles deep inside the skin and so can never be fully eliminated (i.e. skin cannot be sterilized). These bacteria are referred to as **residents** of the skin. The other category of micro-organism found on skin are known as **transients**, their home is not the skin but they have been acquired by touch, for example by handling contaminated foodstuffs, and are present only on the surface layers of the skin. This superficial location means that they stay on the skin for a short time and are easily removed. Transients can be removed either by touch or by washing. To be lost by touch means that the bacteria can be transferred via hands from contaminated raw foods to ready-to-eat foods. Washing in between handling these foods will prevent this transfer.

Hands are a vehicle for transfer of food poisoning organisms and are just as important as chopping boards and other pieces of equipment. By the same logic, it is pointless to attempt food hygiene by whole-body showering before starting work in catering or on a food production line. This may remove (or re-arrange) a small proportion of the resident microbes (i.e. those not relevant to food hygiene) but subsequent hand-transfer of potentially pathogenic transient organisms will not be affected. As a case in point, surgeons pay scrupulous attention to hand hygiene but do not shower before operations as a hospital infection control measure.

The only microbe sometimes be found on skin that can cause food poisoning is *Staphylococcus aureus* (see Chapters 4 and 5). It is unusual to find this organism as a resident inhabitant of the skin on hands unless there are skin lesions, but it can be a permanent resident of nostrils. Thus when preparing food, the nostrils should not be touched and hands should be washed after blowing the nose.

It is increasingly the practice to wear gloves during food preparation. This does not stop hands transferring transient contamination on the surface of the glove rather than on the skin of the ungloved hand. Gloves are only useful if they are changed between tasks (i.e. gloves are changed in situations where the equivalent ungloved hands would be washed).

THE PRACTICE OF CLEANING

Materials

Cleaning is the practice of getting rid of dirt or 'soil' in cleaning jargon. The degree to which soil should be removed varies, as does opinion about what constitutes 'clean'. One person's idea of cleanliness, as we have all experienced, is not necessarily another's. 'Soil' (any matter present that is not be part of an item) can be a wide variety of substances or mixtures of substances. Soil can be broadly classified into three groups:

- water soluble
- fat soluble (and water insoluble)
- fat and water insoluble.

The last group comprises those substances that are innately insoluble (such as charred deposits from burnt food) and those that were initially soluble (such as proteins in blood) but are **denatured** by heat and thus become insoluble and fixed onto surfaces. Soil can be removed in a variety of ways depending on its nature. (see Table 12.1).

The common aim of food-linked cleaning processes is to dissolve and disperse the soil in water and then to dilute and remove it. Dilution in water will remove water-soluble substances. Other forms of soil require more complex forms of removal. There are two ways to remove fat and fat-soluble soils. One is to use liquids that are themselves fatty in nature and in which the fat will dissolve. This is the essence of the process known as 'dry cleaning', as used for fabrics. The solvents used are toxic, volatile and expensive, which make it unsuitable for general use in catering. In catering, microscopic fat particles are suspended in water in the presence of a detergent, so that they can then be removed by dilution.

Detergent molecules have two contrasting characteristics. One end of the molecule is **hydrophilic** (literally 'water-loving') because of charge polarization and is better able to dissolve in water. The other end of the molecular has a long tail and is **hydrophobic** ('water-hating' or sometimes interchangeably lipophilic 'fat-loving'), without significant polarization of charge, and has affinity for other non-polarized molecules such as fats and oils (Figure 12.1). When a solution of detergent molecules in water encounters fat, that portion of each molecule which is hydrophobic will dissolve in the fat, leaving the hydrophilic portion remaining in the water.

Table 12.1 *Hard surface cleaning*

Soil type	Removal options
Water soluble	Water with or without detergent
Fat soluble	Water with detergent Alkali (forms soap *in situ*) Organic solvents (rarely applicable)
Insoluble	Mechanical abrasion with or without detergent Acid (if limescale) Enzymes (if denatured protein)

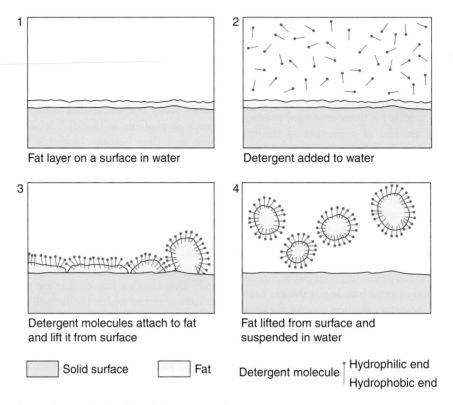

Figure 12.1   *Mechanism of detergent action*

Detergent molecules will eventually surround the fat, lifting it off the surface as a microscopic ball of fat contained within a coating of detergent molecules (see Figure 12.1). These detergent molecules will have their hydrophobic portions buried in the fat and their hydrophilic portions above the fat surface. This will effectively render the exterior surface of the fat hydrophilic and it will dissolve in the water/detergent solution. Detergents also prevent the dissolved fat droplets coalescing with each other and keep them in solution. A water/detergent solution will remove both water and fat soluble soils.

Another way of removing fat-based soils is to use a strongly alkaline preparation. When a fat reacts with a strong alkali such as sodium hydroxide (caustic soda) it forms a soap. This performs a dual function. It renders the reacted fat soluble in water and it makes the fat capable of acting as a detergent to help solubilize and remove unreacted fat. This method of *in situ* detergent formation is most useful for surfaces with fairly solid baked-on grease, within which there may be insoluble carbon particles from

burnt food, as may be found on oven interiors. Care is needed when working with such caustic preparations.

Two further insoluble soils should be considered. Hard water deposits are insoluble in water. They arise through the reaction of dissolved atmospheric carbon dioxide in rainwater as it filters through chalk in the ground. The dissolved carbon dioxide lowers the pH and allows small amounts of insoluble chalk (mostly calcium carbonate) to form calcium bicarbonate, which is carried in solution in water. However when the water is heated, the soluble bicarbonate decomposes back to the insoluble carbonate. This gives rise to hard water deposits in kettles, on glassware and so on. The most practical way to remove these insoluble carbonate deposits is by a chemical reaction that turns them back into a soluble salt, such as by reaction with an acid. Care is needed when working with strong acids.

The other common form of insoluble soil is **denatured protein**. In the natural state, there are both soluble proteins, such as those in blood and milk, and insoluble proteins, such as those found in muscle (i.e. meat). When soluble proteins are heated, their molecules change configuration and become insoluble. As this happens, the proteins firmly adhere to surfaces and in effect become baked on. They can be removed mechanically, i.e. by use of abrasive cleaners on a solid surface, or chemically by use of enzyme-based cleaners if on a delicate surface such as fabrics. Proteolytic (i.e. protein-splitting) enzymes breakdown the large insoluble protein molecules into smaller, soluble units. For example, soluble proteins from uncooked meats on chopping boards or fabrics can be coagulated by washing directly in hot detergent solutions. A preliminary cool or warm wash stage will remove soluble proteins before they are denatured by the hot wash.

Formulation of cleaning agents

Cleaning agents are formulated or 'built' for specific tasks. Decisions about formulation will centre around a number of factors.

Surfactant choice

A detergent is a surfactant that is useful for cleaning purposes. There are four main categories of detergent depend on their molecular charge:

- The largest group of detergents, the anionic detergents, are negatively charged. There are some good cleaning agents within this group but usually they foam.
- Cationic detergents are positively charged, and most have lower cleaning ability; some have microbicidal activity.
- Non-ionic (non-charged) and amphoteric (charge depends on pH of solution) detergents can be good cleaners and tend to have low foaming properties.

Even within these broad categories there are considerable variations. It is best to think in terms of *appropriate* detergents rather than as good or bad. For example when hand dishwashing, a high foaming detergent is acceptable, whereas for a mechanical dishwasher this property is undesirable. The reverse would be true of efficient detergents used in dishwashers that are corrosive to human skin.

Compatibility of components

If detergents with incompatible charges are mixed together, they can react with each other and, in effect, cancel the total activity. The formulation of a built detergent product should be a carefully thought out process so that its components act synergistically. Cleaning products should never be mixed unless the components are compatible.

Water conditioning

Soluble calcium and magnesium salts present in water are responsible for so-called 'hardness'. These metal ions can form insoluble complexes with detergents, which both depletes the amount of active detergent in solution and creates deposits that may adhere to washed articles. Such salts can be 'sequestered', that is removed from effective solution, by a variety of additives to detergents. These chemicals, termed water softeners, include sodium carbonate (washing soda), sodium metasilicate and a variety of sodium phosphate salts. The need for water softeners is reduced if water is naturally soft (a reflection of the geology of the substrata in those areas) or is softened artificially in an ion-exchange resin in which calcium and magnesium ions are exchanged for sodium ions (sodium carbonates and bicarbonates are readily soluble).

pH

Other agents present in formulated detergent preparations can be acidic or alkali according to the function of the preparation and the compatibilities of the surfactant used.

Finishing agents

Another important aspect of cleaning agents for many catering items is the finish. The final stage should leave a smooth water-film on a drying object rather than allowing separate droplets to form, which when dry gives a speckled dirty appearance on what should have been a gleaming surface.

STAGES IN CLEANING

In the ideal situation, cleaning comprises four stages: gross soil removal, fine soil removal, detergent removal, and **drying**. This is only a general outline; in practice cleaning can vary from ultrafine multistage methods used in microelectronics or for surgical instruments to a quick rinse under the tap. Sometimes the stages in the process may not be totally distinct from each other but merge into a graded procedure. There are various types of equipment for cleaning, from a conveyer belt (tunnel) type continuous dishwasher (Figure 12.2) to the manual use of spray heads and sinks (Figure 12.3).

Gross soil removal

In the previous section, detergent molecule action was outlined (see Figure 12.1). Detergent molecules surround hydrophobic particles, lift them off surfaces, break them up into microscopic particles, each in turn surrounded by detergent molecules, and keep them suspended so that a rinse will remove them without re-deposition onto surfaces. This process depends on having an excess of detergent molecules above the equivalent amount of soil present both to remove soil and to keep it in suspension. If this fails due to insufficient detergent, a surface will have remaining and re-deposited soil as it goes from the wash to the rinse stage. So unless objects have little initial associated soil or very high concentrations of detergent are used, washing processes should commence with the removal of gross soil. This will vary, though, according to the

washing process that follows. At its simplest, as in hand dishwashing, it could be pre-rinsing, that is removing the left-over food from plates before they go into the bowl of detergent and water or batch dishwasher. Or it could be the first stage in a conveyer-belt-type continuous dishwasher. The principle is the same: where possible there should be an initial removal of gross soil by water and mechanical action with or without detergent.

Fine soil removal

This is the stage at which all remaining soil is removed. It involves water, detergent and mechanical action and comprises one or more substages. A cool or warm temperature initial wash is desirable to remove protein-based soil which may be denatured and rendered inextricably adherent by heat. The hot wash that follows this will be more effective at removing the other possible soils.

Mechanical action, anything from a washing-up brush to water jets, helps break up remaining lumps of adherent soil so that they can more easily be lifted off a surface by the detergent.

Detergent removal and drying

This is the function of the rinsing stage; it aims to remove any toxicity and taint the detergent may impart. It will also remove remaining soil suspended

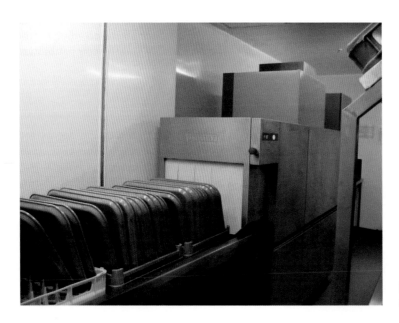

Figure 12.2 *Tunnel washer used in commercial premises*

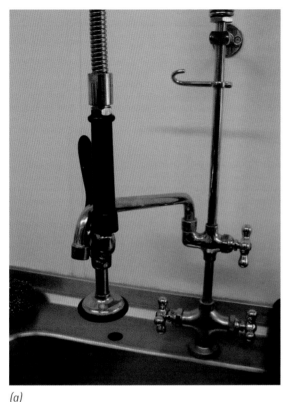
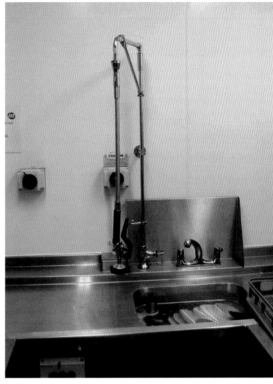

(a)   (b)

Figure 12.3   *a,b Spray heads for removal of gross soil before tunnel washing*

by detergent so that it will not be re-deposited onto a surface when drying. Simultaneous functions may be: adding an anti-smear 'rinsing aid' to prevent the formation of droplets that would leave a speckled or smeary finish in drying and, in the final rinse, including a heating stage. This stage will have the dual function of leaving items warm so that they dry quickly and disinfecting items if the heating is for sufficient time and to a sufficiently high temperature.

Summary

- Disinfection is the reduction or removal of micro-organisms and is achieved by cleaning, chemicals or heat.
- Among the methods of disinfection, heating (as in cooking or dishwashing machines) is the most effective.
- Cleaning and disinfection contribute to food hygiene and must be targeted at critical areas to stop the transmission of hazardous micro-organisms. Aesthetic cleanliness will not achieve food hygiene.
- Physical separation of sensitive items (such as ready-to-eat foods) from sources of contamination (such as raw meats) makes cleaning and disinfection less critical procedures.

SOURCES OF INFORMATION AND FURTHER READING

Bloomfield SF, Scott E (1997) Cross-contamination and infection in the domestic environment and the role of chemical disinfectants. *J Appl Microbiol* **83**: 1–9.

Dillon M, Griffith C (1999) *How to Clean. A Management Guide*. Grimsby: MD Associates.

Gibson H, Taylor JH, Hall KE, *et al.* (1999) Effectiveness of cleaning techniques used in the food industry in terms of removal of bacterial biofilms. *J Appl Microbiol* **87**: 41–8.

Gorman R, Bloomfield S, Adley CC (2002) A study of cross-contamination of food-borne pathogens in the domestic kitchen in the Republic of Ireland. *Int J Food Microbiol* **76**: 143–50.

Hoffman PN, Bradley CR, Ayliffe GAJ (2004) *Disinfection in Healthcare*, 3rd edn. Oxford: Blackwell Publishing.

Sagoo SK, Little CL, Griffith CJ, *et al.* (2003) A study of cleaning standards and practices in food premises in the UK. *Communicable Dis Public Health* **6**: 6–17.

Shapton DA, Shapton NF (1993) Cleaning and disinfection. In: Shapton DA, Shapton NF, eds. *Principles and Practices for the Safe Processing of Foods*. London: Butterworth-Heinemann, pp. 148–90.

13

Food premises and equipment

Rob Griffin

General principles	245	First aid	261
Catering	246	Licensed trade	262
Food storage	259	Food Law Code of Practice/Practice Guidance	262
Cleaning equipment	260	Summary	262
Staff room	261	Sources of information and further reading	262

To protect consumers, particularly in relation to hygiene, controls are required not only for food itself, but also for all food-related activities, food establishments or premises and equipment. Food establishments must comply with legal requirements covering construction, occupational health and safety, and food safety. Establishments must be designed and constructed in ways that prevent contamination and access to pests. Effective design and construction of buildings and equipment help prevent contact between high risk and other foods, and between food and dirt, waste, rubbish, unfit food and toxic materials.

Food business Any undertaking, whether for profit or not, and whether public or private, carrying out any of the activities related to any stage of production, processing and distribution of food (Regulation [EC] No. 178/2002).

Premises Includes any place, any vehicle, stall or moveable structure and, for such purposes as may be specified in an Order made by the Ministers, any ship or aircraft of a description so specified, (Food Safety Act 1990 [as amended]). Following an Order, specified ships and aircraft are now included in the definition of 'premises'.

Establishment Any unit of a food business (Regulation [EC] No. 852/2004).

Food premises Any premises used for the purposes of a food business (Food Safety Act 1990 [as amended]).

Food hygiene The measures and conditions necessary to control hazards and to ensure fitness for human consumption of a foodstuff taking into account its intended use (Regulation [EC] No. 852/2004).

Food law The laws, regulations and administrative provisions governing food in general, and food safety in particular, whether at community or national level; it covers any stage of production, processing and distribution of food, and also of feed produced for, or fed to, food-producing animals (Regulation [EC] No. 178/2002).

GENERAL PRINCIPLES

Food business operators are required by European Union (EU) **food law** to take responsibility for food safety in the part of the food chain in which they are engaged (primary production, transport, manufacturing, processing, importation, distribution, and sale or supply to the final consumer). The General Food Law (Regulation [EC] No. 178/2002) also requires systems to be in place to ensure the traceability of food, or any substance intended to be incorporated into a food, at all stages of production, processing and distribution.

A wide range of structural methods and materials are used in the construction of buildings for food business operations. The basic **hygiene requirements** for all **establishments**, including those exclusively used for primary production, are set out in general terms in Regulation (EC) No. 852/2004 on the hygiene of foodstuffs. Where food business operations require approval by the relevant competent authority under Regulation (EC) No. 853/2004 laying down specific **hygiene rules** for food of animal origin, the requirements for a particular business may be more specific. In general, all food business establishments must comply with satisfactory standards of stability, durability and protection against the weather, which are applicable to all buildings. There are traditional forms of **construction material**, such as brick, concrete, slates and tiles, and also lighter forms of construction supported by steel or concrete frames. Insulation and fire protection must meet the required standards laid down in building and associated regulations. For food business establishments that are movable and/or temporary (e.g. ships, aircraft, trains, market stalls and marquees) there are similar requirements to be met, but regard must be given to the nature of the food operations and design. For example, in aircraft, there are specific constraints in terms of size and shape, and passenger safety.

The layout of any food business depends on the activities undertaken and the need to comply with food law. For example, food business operators need to ensure prevention of cross-contamination and have in place a permanent procedure or procedures based on **Hazard Analysis Critical Control Point (HACCP)** principles. These procedures will depend on the complexity of the activities undertaken by the food business operator – this may range from a relatively small registered food business to a large approved food manufacturer. Account must also be taken to ensure the **health and safety** of employees and any visitors to the food establishment.

Irrespective of the type of food establishment, the **design and layout** of any food production area must consider some basic aspects:

- Location and suitability of the building, i.e. full **planning consent**, with appropriate input from the local environmental health department at the planning stage.
- Adequate space, not only to allow **hygienic practices**, but also to reduce health and safety risks to staff or others who might be in the working environment, such as equipment service engineers.
- Adequate **delivery facilities** including an area for the removal of packaging (while retaining

product information), unprocessed food storage facilities (including refrigerated environments) and staff facilities including office accommodation, and where necessary, toilets and basins for handwashing.

- A work-flow that ensures prevention (or reduction) of **cross-contamination**, preferably through a system which avoids cross-over of staff undertaking different duties, separates raw and ready-to-eat food, and ensures acceptable staff personal hygiene.
- Appropriate **surfaces** to ensure proper care, maintenance and cleaning to prevent them becoming reservoirs of contamination.
- Suitable equipment and machinery for food preparation/processing which is positioned to allow **proper cleaning and maintenance** and reduce any health and safety risks to staff. Where appropriate, equipment and machinery should be moveable.
- The food business operator should ensure that the relevant **requirements of food law** are met, including the supervision, instruction and/or training of staff as well as the proper disposal of waste products of animal origin.
- Before commencing operations in a new food business, the food business operator should seek advice from the local environmental health department and, subject to the proposed activities, apply for **registration or approval of the business** in terms of Article 6 of Regulation (EC) No. 852/2004. Should there be any changes in the nature and operations undertaken by the food business operator, the relevant environmental health department should be notified, in accordance with the aforementioned Article.

CATERING

The catering industry serves millions of meals daily, is large and diverse, and one of the largest employment areas in the UK. This industry has continued to grow – for example in 2005, it was estimated that there were approximately 2.6 million employees in the hospitality and leisure industry compared with about 2 million in 1987. This is probably the most labour intensive sector of the food industry, and a large proportion of staff work part-time.

Interior

A kitchen should, ideally, be on the same storey, adjoining the dining room. The delivery of stores and removal of refuse are easier from the ground floor, but natural lighting, ventilation and outlook are usually better on upper floors.

Kitchen staff should work in congenial surroundings. Fatigue and strain from cramped conditions, inadequate equipment, poor lighting, overwork and noise will predispose to carelessness. Good ventilation and lighting, readily accessible and easily cleaned surfaces facilitate good kitchen hygiene. The design, construction and equipment of commercial kitchens should satisfy certain basic criteria appropriate for the proposed menu, types of food and scale of operation. There should be a logical sequence of safe operations that avoid cross-contamination with suitable and practicable methods of cleaning.

Layout

The minimum size of kitchens serving the public, and certain staff canteens, in common with those of several other kinds of workplace, is subject to requirements laid down by the Workplace (Health, Safety and Welfare) Regulations 1992, and the accompanying Approved Code of Practice (ACoP) and guidance. Rooms must not be overcrowded with the risk of injury to the health of workers. Regulation 10 covers room sizes and requires that every room must be large enough for people to work in it safely. The ACoP sets a minimum of 11 m^3 per employee, accounting for a height of 3 m. These figures refer to basic room capacity rather than to the space available after allowing for equipment. Since kitchen equipment usually occupies a large amount of space compared with the number of persons using it, it seems unlikely that there will be many kitchens 2.4–3 m high where the standards are not met.

Every plan must be subject to the basic legal requirements. The working space requirements will vary according to the menu, the extent that pre-prepared foods are used and the type of equipment installed. For example the requirements of heavy-duty, large-scale installations that provide three full meals each day will be much greater than that for lighter catering establishments. Space standards for food service areas and service facilities (Figure 13.1) are also provided in *Planning and Design Data* (1999). The figures are for use in preliminary sketches and estimates.

The usual trend in kitchens is to install preparation equipment at the side of the room where waste can be conveniently drained away, and to have an island cooking apparatus in the centre where ventilation can be more easily localized. This needs to be divided further into compartments for the preparation of different kinds of food prior to cooking, and for washing up. Work and production should flow without return- or cross-trafficking and progress from delivery of goods to storage, preparation and service.

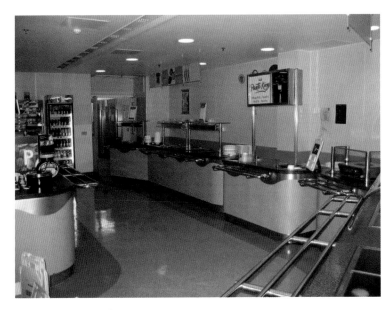

Figure 13.1 *A canteen servery*

Contamination from raw to cooked or ready-to-eat food should be prevented by any means possible. Vegetable storage and preparation should be sited near the point of delivery in an area separate from the other parts of the kitchen to prevent soil from root crops reaching other food. Sections for raw meat and fish should be well separated from those dealing with cooked and prepared products, including pastry. There should be adequate storage for each activity undertaken in the kitchen (e.g. dry, vegetable, raw meat and fish, prepared food and waste).

Most dirt generated in the kitchen comes from food materials, which also attract vermin. Thus the preparation of food should involve processes that will cause least contamination/wastage/scraps/scrapings consistent with the menu. For bulk cooking it may be better to use vegetables pre-prepared and packed by the supplier or pre-packed frozen vegetables, so that production of waste associated with used vegetables is reduced.

In general, the size, design and layout of a kitchen depends on the menu, type of service and method of cleaning (by hand, machine, high-pressure lances). The use of high-pressure lances should be restricted to periodic deep-cleaning to avoid spray and excess water in food handling areas, and where socket outlets and other electrical equipment are suitably waterproofed.

Floors

The main objectives for floors are that they should be impervious, easily cleaned and durable. Floor surfaces should be non-absorbent, anti-slip and without joints and crevices where dirt, bacteria and insects can lodge. They should not be adversely affected by grease, salt, vegetable, fruit acids or other materials used in the preparation of food, and should be capable of being effectively cleaned. Floors should be light in colour. Angles at floor level should be avoided and the junction between the floor and walls coved. The top of the coving sometimes forms a narrow ledge that collects dirt – this should be avoided.

Tessellated quarry tiles are recommended for floors in heavy-duty kitchens because they provide a smooth and hard surface. With light catering and in dining rooms, vinyl sheet tiles at least 3.2 mm thick provide a good floor surface. Sheet vinyls impregnated with graphite particles are available, but may be difficult to clean. Epoxy resin and granolithic (concrete incorporating granite chippings) coverings are more hardy, but epoxy resin is costly and the granolithic coverings may crack. The lifespan of floor finishes and cleaning costs in terms of annual maintenance should be considered. Non-slip floors should be inspected under operating conditions before purchase. Non-slip footwear may be a better investment than supposedly non-slip floors that retain dirt and become slippery from deposits of grease and water. Timber floors, soft or hardwood, are unacceptable because they are absorbent, wear quickly and the joints harbour moisture and dirt. Rubber and cork tiles are unsatisfactory because rubber is slippery when wet and cork is not durable to heavy traffic. A particular floor surface may not be suitable for all rooms and if the floor is graded to a floor gully, care must be taken to avoid the formation of pools.

Walls

Similarly to floors, walls should be smooth, impervious, light in colour and durable. Wall surfaces from floor to ceiling should allow cleaning without deterioration. The basic materials for the wall structure are brick or concrete blocks. Faced stud partition walls of plasterboard should not be used as they tend to harbour vermin which can reach the cavity by gnawing through the plasterboard, skirting or duct work. Some equipment cannot be attached to the stud partitions because of its low strength. A plastered finish will provide a smooth and non-porous surface, especially if the final coat is 'hard' plaster. However, it requires regular maintenance and can be unsuitable in certain areas such as behind sinks or where heat creates problems such as loss of adherence of paint – a source of foreign body contamination to food. Sheet materials with a vitreous face are acceptable, such as standard glazed tiles. Other suitable wall surfaces include stainless steel cladding bonded to the wall (which is long-lasting and easy to clean), resin-bonded fibreglass, ceramic-faced blocks, or rubberized paint on hard plaster or sealed brickwork. Some paints incorporate a fungicidal additive, but absorbent emulsion paint should not be used. The better wall surfaces, such as solid-bedded ceramic tiles, have no hollow places; any spaces should be filled with lightweight concrete. Proprietary wall-cladding materials, if properly fixed, can be a hygienic alternative to the traditional wall surfaces.

In some areas it is necessary to provide localized

protection against damage. Glazed tiles will protect walls behind working surfaces and should extend at least 450 mm above the surface. Depending on their position and the activities undertaken, such tiles can be easily damaged and although providing a smooth hard surface, the grouted joints hold dirt and are difficult to clean. External corners subject to contact with trolleys or other moveable equipment can be protected with suitable polyvinyl chloride (PVC) extrusions, which are fixed to the wall with adhesive. Areas such as trolley parks should be protected by a PVC or timber rail at handle level or at any other height where there are projections liable to damage the wall surface. Stainless steel provides an impervious surface almost as indestructible as tiles or sheets for splash-backs and angles. Galvanized or stainless steel crash rails can be used also. Resin-bonded fibreglass provides a finish that withstands severe impact blows without damage: it remains impervious and withstands heat provided fire-retardant resins are used. Special provision for wall surfaces near sources of heat must be made. When separating walls are provided in food rooms, the tops should be rounded to assist cleaning and to prevent their use as shelves.

Ceilings

A ceiling is necessary in food preparation areas to prevent dust falling from the roof or upper structure. Ceilings should be smooth, fire-resistant, light-coloured, coved at wall joints and easy to clean. They may be solid or suspended. Plasterboard finished with a skim coat of plaster to eliminate joints may be combined with a hot-air blower suspended from a corner of the ceiling to eliminate condensation. Suspended ceilings in absorbent 600 mm square acoustic tiles (fibreboard) may be used. The tiles, laid loose on aluminium bearers, are cheap and easy to replace. Disadvantages include cleaning difficulties, deterioration when saturated, attack by vermin, and corrosion of the alloy suspension grids. There must be access above suspended ceilings for pest-control purposes and service maintenance for extraction ducting, air conditioning, water pipes and water tanks. Services to equipment are usually accommodated in floor zones for easy access. Services to lighting run in the ceiling void; they are usually free from trouble. Insulation to the roof should be placed between the plasterboard or tiles and the structural roof.

Surface finishes for walls and ceilings

Decorative finishes for walls and ceilings protect the wall finish from damage caused by cleaning and provide a visually acceptable and pleasing environment. **Oil-bound eggshell paints** (i.e. semi-gloss paint with a finish mid-sheen between matt and gloss, which is easily cleaned) are the most widely used with a gloss finish on fittings. Other paints may help to reduce condensation, but they may not seal surfaces as well as oil-based paint. White ceilings are generally best since they reflect the light from artificial sources. All-white walls may be hard on the eye, pastel colours with bolder tones on fittings are better. Paints should be used with caution with the danger of flaking and the possible contamination of food in mind. Proprietary ceiling systems are available for food-handling areas and some wall materials may be suitable for ceilings.

Lighting

Good lighting in kitchens improves concentration and safety, and it also deters insects and vermin. Regulation 8 of the Workplace (Health, Safety and Welfare) Regulations 1992 requires suitable and sufficient lighting to be provided. The Health and Safety Executive (HSE) publication *Lighting at Work* (HSG38) deals with lighting and how it affects the safety, health and welfare of people at work. The Industry Guide to Good Hygiene Practice, *Catering Guide*, recommends illumination levels from 150 lux in store rooms to 500 lux in food preparation areas. Information regarding lighting is also available from the Society of Light and Lighting/Chartered Institution of Building Services Engineers (CIBSE). The Society's *Code for Interior Lighting* (2006) recommends levels of 500 lux for food preparation and cooking areas, 300 lux for serveries, vegetable preparation and washing-up areas, and 150 lux for food storage and cellars, with a limiting glare index of 22 lux. Artificial illumination is necessary even though the suggested standard could be met during normal working hours by natural lighting when there is a high window-to-wall ratio. Good natural lighting is desirable, but without glare from direct sunlight causing reflection from polished surfaces. North light is preferable, otherwise overhanging eaves, tinted glass or solar film should be fitted to reduce direct light. Venetian and roller blinds are difficult to clean and should not be used.

The running costs of fluorescent lighting are lower than for tungsten filament and the light is more evenly distributed. The tubes should be fitted with diffusers to prevent glare and also to protect food if there is breakage. Twin tube lamps are recommended for food preparation areas but they lose at least 20 per cent efficiency within a year and should be replaced when flicker and black ends are observed. Light fittings (**luminaires**) should be vapour proof and consideration should be given to the sites of equipment and preparation areas including sinks, stoves and tables. Spotlights can be placed directly over servery counters to complement the overall lighting. Additional lamps may be required to aid cleaning of less accessible dark areas. In kitchens, proofed luminaires are necessary to withstand both the heat and the possibility of explosions if tubes are defective.

Insectocutors are electrified flying insect killers that attract flying insects by emitting ultraviolet (UV) light (see Chapter 14, p. 270). Therefore, because of the natural UV light, such pest control devices should not be placed adjacent to windows or should be placed at least at right angles to them. They should not be placed over food preparation areas, open food displays or in areas with great air movement, but between entry points and production areas. The UV lamps should be changed at least every 12 months as their efficiency diminishes over time. If wall mounted, the height should be approximately 2 m above floor level and if ceiling suspended about 2.6 m (taking account of any particular operations in the area, e.g. fork lift trucks). The dead insect collection tray should be cleaned frequently.

Windows and doors

Window boards and ledges situated behind kitchen equipment are not easily accessible for cleaning. Sills should be higher than equipment and constructed with an angled ledge to prevent their use as shelves. Louvered windows in kitchens are not recommended as they can be difficult to clean and maintain. Fly-screens, where fitted over windows or other openings, should be removable for cleaning purposes. Kitchen windows should not face due south unless precautions are taken to eliminate glare and the effect of solar heat.

Doors should be tight-fitting and self-closing; where necessary they should be proofed against insects and vermin. They should be identified with prominent signage, particularly when entering into 'high-risk' food production environments (Figure 13.2). Doorways must be large enough to allow movement of mobile equipment. Swing doors should have sight panels and also hand and kick plates.

Ventilation

Efficient ventilation and extraction systems are essential. The operations of preparation, cooking,

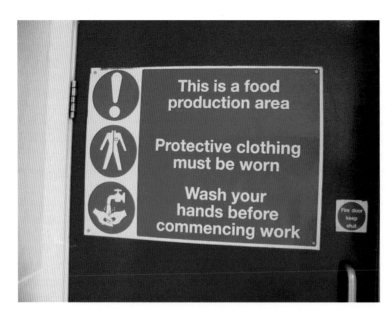

Figure 13.2 *Typical signage on a door for a food production area*

serving and washing-up generate large amounts of water vapour, which, if not extracted will condense, creating moisture that will drip from ceilings or run down walls. In addition to high humidity, the kitchen may also have volatile fats. To control humidity, volatile fats and cooking odours, localized systems of extraction may be used. Extractor fans in ducting should be chosen with care at the design stage and properly maintained otherwise they can give rise to an unacceptable level of noise, which can be a nuisance for kitchen staff or neighbours. Inside the kitchen, if the noise from fans irritates food handlers, they may be switched off. Outlets to extraction systems need to be carefully sited to avoid malodours, which may arise even with proper filters if they are badly maintained.

The commercial fish fryer for fish and chips includes ventilation matched to the equipment, but the system may still contravene the law by releasing objectionable smells. A ventilation system cannot operate without sufficient air for the extraction fans. With gas appliances, adequate ventilation is essential so that the open flames burn steadily. Table 13.1 provides guidelines for ventilation of various food premises.

The grouping of cooking appliances in islands is convenient for the extraction of steam and odours. The arrangement saves space and lends itself to a localized extraction system, but the items cannot be moved for cleaning, and it may be difficult to reach the services. Cantilevered or mobile equipment with approved flexible connections, for example, to gas appliances, will assist cleaning. Fans should be sited outside food rooms and be capable of extracting through grease filters. The filters should be placed so that they can be readily removed for

Table 13.1 *Ventilation for food premises and facilities*

Food premises and facilities	Air changes per hour
Bakeries	20–30
Café and coffee shops	10–12
Canteen and restaurants	8–12
Cellars	3–10
Clubrooms and bars	12+
Dairies	8–12
Kitchens	30+
Shops/supermarkets	8–15
Stores/warehouses	3–6
Showers	15–20
Toilets	6–15

cleaning or replacement, and a spare set should be available. The extraction should be up to 20 m^3/min per m^2 of hood area. The ventilation should flow away from a clean area. Ducts should be as short as possible, and airtight with properly sealed joints. Simple baffle boards are sometimes placed below extraction fans. They are usually made from block-board covered with plastic laminate, are about 1 m^2 and are suspended below the ceiling on adjustable straps. The distance between the board and the ceiling should be fixed so that the desired extraction velocity can be achieved. Such boards can be removed, cleaned and replaced relatively quickly. In small kitchens, extraction fans can be placed in walls or windows. Their position should be carefully chosen to prevent air circulating between window and fan. When the fan is running, windows should be closed. The use of pressure vessels, microwave ovens and increased insulation around ovens will reduce heat production. Air conditioning may be installed.

If the vegetable store is not situated on an outside wall, ducted mechanical ventilation must be introduced. The dry store will also need ventilation although to a lesser degree. Where mechanical extraction units are incorporated in food storage areas to form rapid cooling larders, it is important that air inlets draw in fresh air and not air from the general kitchen area.

Heating

The Workplace (Health, Safety and Welfare) Regulations 1992 ACoP requires that the minimum temperature in workrooms should usually be at least 16 °C, unless much of the work involves severe physical effort in which case the temperature should be at least 13 °C. Usually, heating appliances are necessary only in staff rooms and offices. Where foods are prepared and temperature control is important, the Chilled Food Association recommends that an entire area should be chilled only where it is impractical to have localized product chilling.

Services

Services for kitchens include water, drainage, electricity, gas and ventilation; numerous points are required so that services may be tapped readily. Ducts can provide routes for vermin to enter, leave and infest buildings. Holes for services must be sealed and proofed. Floor ducts liable to be flooded by wash water or to harbour vermin should be filled with lightweight concrete or similar inert material. Services should be chased into walls, where possible, or fitted clear of walls to allow proper cleaning. The use of wooden ducts around services encourages insects. With suspended ceilings, electricity cables may be sited above them. Appliances should not be permanently connected so that proper cleaning and maintenance can be performed.

Legionella is a genus of bacteria responsible for causing legionellosis (Legionnaire's disease). These bacteria are found in both natural water sources and artificial water systems, e.g. humidifiers, spa and whirlpool baths, storage tanks and showers. Dead-legs or pipes with only an inlet connection and hence no water flows through it, should be avoided, as bacteria may survive and multiply. They can survive at low temperatures but proliferate in the temperature range of 20–45 °C particularly when the water is inert or if it re-circulates. High temperatures of >60 °C will destroy the organism. Legionnaires disease is potentially fatal and infection is caused through breathing in contaminated droplets of water, which might be emitted from contaminated water systems such as air conditioning units. The HSE has produced an ACoP (L8) *Legionnaires' disease: the control of legionella bacteria in water systems*. This gives advice regarding the requirements of health and safety legislation and places responsibility on employers to take adequate precautions.

Listeria are widely present in the environment and have been isolated in soil, sewage, silage, dust and water. They can also move through the intestinal tract of humans and animals without causing illness. However, one species, *Listeria monocytogenes*, can cause a serious infection in humans, *viz.* listeriosis (see Chapter 4, p. 75). The organism is remarkably resilient and can survive on cold surfaces and also multiply slowly at low temperatures (4 °C or lower). Adequate cooking temperatures for sufficient time will destroy the organism. Post-processing contamination of food is usually thought to be the cause when the organism is detected on such foods. *L. monocytogenes* may survive well at specific sites within food manufacturing environments (sometimes for many years), particularly those difficult to clean.

Gas

Gas is popular with chefs, but pressure in installations must be carefully balanced using a water gauge. Automatic ignition is essential to reduce waste, and devices that respond to flame failure help prevent accidental build-up of gas. The possibility of explosions can be eliminated by the installation of an alarm system for gas detection.

Flexible supply pipes with bayonet fitting connectors for each appliance have in-built mobility that allows effective cleaning and maintenance. Gas appliances should have governors fitted to prevent variations in gas pressure affecting the operation of the burners. Supply pipes should be mounted clear of the floor, and of other pipes, for cleaning purposes. A gas company or an approved gas installation technician should ensure that the pressure is satisfactory.

Electricity

Electricity may be expensive, but it is the most suitable source of energy for many catering processes. As a fire precaution, one master switchboard, clearly identified, is necessary, indicating the supply to each piece of equipment. This should be situated close to the kitchen. Single-phase electricity may be satisfactory for a few light catering kitchens, but usually a 415 V supply consisting of three phases and a neutral wire is essential for larger operations. Electrical wiring should be either insulated, copper-covered cable or water-resistant heavy gauge conduit with outlets about 1.5 m above the floor. It should be protected by waterproof conduits and switches fitted flush to walls. Main switches should be placed outside the food preparation rooms. Where switch boxes serve individual appliances, they should be splash-proof, readily accessible, and sited away from areas of excessive soiling. There should be no low-level sockets in danger from wet floors (cleaning) and sockets should not be sited above sinks or hand basins.

Water supply

To ensure constant and adequate supply of hot and cold water, pipes should be installed as a ring main, whereby water circulates continuously. Stop taps should isolate every fitting. A direct supply from the mains is required in kitchens except for wash basins, showers, baths and dishwashing machines. A cold water tap for culinary use can be conveniently sited adjacent to the cooking appliances. Softened water will help reduce the amount of detergent used. Boiling of water for tea and coffee rapidly produces scale, hence boilers should be supplied with soft water as well.

An ample supply of hot water, ≥60 °C, is essential, but the actual quantity of hot and cold water needed depends on the types of menu and the scale of equipment. The temperature of the water used for a disinfecting rinse may be raised by means of a thermostatically controlled gas burner or electrical unit, or by steam. This compensates for loss of heat from the rinse water while work is in progress. Alternatively, an independent boiler can provide hot water directly to the disinfection sink as a constant overflow to the washing sink as the water cools. Where a piped supply is not practicable from the main hot-water system, for example, for handwashing, a small gas geyser or electrical appliance is useful.

An external water supply should be available for flushing refuse areas and loading bays. If water is stored on site, such as in tanks in roof spaces, for later use in the food business, its purity should be assured. Where water is sourced from a private supply, it is essential that it is monitored and that it meets the parameters set out in the Private Water Supplies Regulations 1991 (as amended). Dead-legs, which are sometimes created through modifications to the pipework in an establishment, should be avoided. Hot water cylinders should be insulated to avoid unnecessary heat loss and hot water pipes should be lagged for the same reason.

Sanitary and washing facilities

In all premises used for the preparation of food, toilet and washing facilities must be incorporated to satisfy the relevant law. Food authorities are empowered to require that sufficient water closets, urinals and washbasins are provided and maintained in a clean condition at places for public entertainment, or where food and drink is sold to members of the public to take away or for consumption on the premises. The minimum requirement is the provision of one lavatory for up to five employees. For more than five employees, additional toilets must be provided on the basis of the Workplace (Health, Safety and Welfare) Regulations 1992. Low-level water closet cisterns are recommended as they are more readily adapted to a pedal-operated flush.

The siting of toilet accommodation in relation to food preparation areas is subject to statutory control. Lavatories must not open directly into rooms in which food is handled. All toilets should be entered from an intervening and separately ventilated lobby or corridor. Toilet areas should be adequately lighted and ventilated either by natural light or by artificial means. Artificial ventilation should provide at least six air changes per hour, and supply air for fans. Two fans should operate continuously with the availability of a further fan for emergency use. For small places, individual fan units, operated by the light switch and continuing to function 20 minutes after the light is switched off are sufficient. Mechanical ventilation for sanitary facilities must not communicate with other ventilation systems within a building. The Workplace (Health, Safety and Welfare) Regulations 1992 requires washing facilities to be provided in the immediate vicinity of every sanitary convenience which must have a supply of clean hot and cold water. This is in addition to the requirement for an adequate number of flush lavatories and suitably located basins for handwashing under Regulation (EC) No. 852/2004.

Therefore, basins for handwashing must be placed in or adjacent to toilet cubicles as well as in food preparation areas where hands will be soiled from contact with raw food and other materials; foot-operated control is recommended. When food handlers are working on more than one floor of a building, toilets with adjacent handwash basins are desirable on each storey, but if this is not possible, they should be situated so that each serves not more than two floors.

For handwashing, there must be supplies of running hot and cold water, or water blended to a suitable temperature. Where a piped supply of hot water is not available, thermal storage units and small instantaneous water heaters are convenient. Spray taps that discharge water at a temperature of approximately 50 °C are economical in the volume of water delivered and consequently in cost. Lever-arm taps, operated by the elbow or forearm, reduce chances of cross-contamination: alternatively, pedal-operated taps or sprinklers should be used. The automatic tap, whereby water flows at a pre-determined temperature when hands are placed in front of the tap and ceases when the hands are removed, is an alternative to the foot or lever-arm-operated tap. All basins and troughs should be made of stainless steel and connected to drains by trapped waste pipes.

Washing facilities include the provision of soap and some means to dry the hands. Liquid or dry soap dispensed from fitted containers is preferable to tablets of soap in wet dishes. Liquid soap should be provided in disposable containers where it is unlikely that dispensers will be washed and disinfected before re-use. The process of hand washing is also discussed in Chapter 8. Means for drying hands include paper towels, the continuous roller towel providing a clean portion for each person, and electric hot-air blowers. However, a paper towel cassette system, similar to the continuous roller towel, is better than the electric hot-air blower, which may not effectively dry hands without patience.

Male and female sanitary and washing facilities must be separate, unless the number of persons employed does not exceed five at any one time. The facilities provided for customers may be used by employees, but the number must be increased by one extra closet and wash basin when there are more than 10 employees. A notice drawing attention to the necessity to wash hands should be displayed in all sanitary facilities for staff, and also brought to the attention of customers.

Sparge pipes, i.e. a continuous perforated pipe serving a urinal but not a urinal stall, although these are more common nowadays, to ensure thorough flushing of the whole surface, particularly in hard-water areas, should be thoroughly cleaned periodically to remove build-up of scale at the water outlets and subsequent inadequate swilling of urinals leading to malodours.

BS6465–1:2006 Sanitary Installations Code of Practice for the design of sanitary facilities and scales of provision of sanitary and associated appliances covers a range of premises, including restaurants and licensed public houses. The Building Regulations 2000 (SI No 2531), require that in new buildings and ground floor extensions to existing buildings where customer toilets are provided, at least one should be for disabled people.

Sink and washing–up units

Various dishwashing machines and sink units are available for crockery, cutlery, glassware, pots, pans and utensils. A separate sink for vegetables and salad preparation is essential. Guards of 150–300 mm integrated with the back of sink units and preferably made of stainless steel protect adjacent walls. Sinks should be installed under wall-mounted taps with stopcocks fitted at a low level on the water pipes. When the taps and plumbing are not fixed directly on to a sink, the waste trap can be unscrewed and the unit removed to allow cleaning of concealed wall areas.

Articles can be disinfected in a dishwasher or by means of a stainless steel, double-sink unit with the water temperature in the rinse sink maintained at 77–82 °C. An ample supply of deep wire baskets is required. A sink unit with a small section for hot disinfection of knives, choppers and other articles is useful. Usually clean, dry crockery, cutlery and glassware do not need thermal or chemical disinfection. Where disinfection is required, thermal methods are preferable to the use of chemicals: alternatively, single-use items may be used. When dishwashing machines are not used there is a continuing need for sinks with heated water to remove grease and to disinfect eating utensils. Sinks and handwash basins may also be mobile. Automatic lettuce- and vegetable-washing machines with integral dirt filters are available.

Drainage

The design and construction of drainage systems for all classes of buildings have to meet the requirements of the Building Regulations 2000 (SI No 2531). The design drawings must be inspected and approved by the local planning authority before construction. Grease is discharged into kitchen drains mostly from the washing-up area; it is molten as it enters the pipes, but solidifies unless intercepted. **Grease traps** are tanks in the ground that hold sufficient water to cool the inflow of washing-up water to a temperature below the melting point of the grease. The inlets and outlets are submerged so that the solidified grease forms layers that can be skimmed off at regular intervals. Such traps are not entirely satisfactory, but with correct procedures, accumulation of grease can be avoided. It is important for drains to be rodded from the fitting to the entry into a manhole so that any blockage can be cleared easily. Large cast-iron and copper waste pipes should be used, 50–75 mm in diameter.

Plastics, able to withstand high temperatures, are also available. One large pipe can be used to drain several fittings and it should discharge to a back inlet gully. Wherever possible, drainage channels should be avoided and only used where necessary. Where appropriate, floors should be graded and drained to a floor gully (Figure 13.3).

Tilting bratt pans are deep cooking pots with counter-balanced lids that are operated by gas or electricity. They have a tilting feature operated electrically or by hand, so that the contents may be tipped into another container after cooking. Subject to the model, bratt pans are used for braising, boiling, steaming, stewing, deep-fat frying, etc. When bratt pans or similar equipment are in use, a small section of stainless steel floor channel, with widened lip and properly sealed at the edges should be sufficient. The grating should be easily removable and not screwed down. Gullies serving handwash basins and sinks should be sited outside the building and there should be no access to drainage systems in food rooms, or soil pipes passing through them from above. Drainage channels

provided around cooking equipment should be covered with galvanized gratings which can be easily removed. Sinks and basins should discharge via trapped gullies. Items of equipment such as potato peelers, dishwashing machines, or waste disposal units that are connected directly into the drainage system should be trapped to prevent waste pipes acting as vents.

Waste disposal

Unlike the waste from many industrial and commercial processes, kitchen waste is mainly organic and requires particular care pending final disposal. Immediate disposal by disintegration and flushing to the drainage system is the most convenient method. Such disposal units may be fixed under metal sinks or stand in a frame with their own receiving hoppers. An electrically driven macerating unit breaks down the waste food to a fine suspension which is washed away through a trapped waste pipe. One type of machine automatically switches on only when water flows through the grinding chamber. Units for the domestic market have motors of one-third horse power, but heavier duty machines are needed for commercial premises. Where waste disposal units are to be fitted, it may be necessary to obtain local authority approval to ensure that the drainage system is adequate. Commercial waste disposal should also have a fail-safe device so that if, for example, a fork were to fall into the mechanism, it cannot be retrieved until a baffle, held in place by a clamp knob, is removed, which switches off the motor. Machines are available to reduce bulky refuse to a smaller size. Such refuse compaction is economical in large food businesses where skips are provided.

Catering waste includes all waste food including used cooking oils. Its disposal is controlled by the Animal By-Products Regulations 2005. Such waste is subject to this Regulation if it is deemed to be international catering waste, i.e. from means of transport operating from non-EU countries; is destined for animal consumption and/or is intended for use in a biogas plant or for composting (such plants must be approved). Where catering waste is disposed of through landfill or incineration, it must be handled in such a way that livestock and birds can not access it.

Paper or plastic sacks filled with waste are light and clean to handle, they can be sealed easily with a

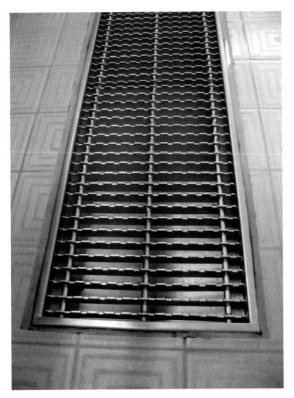

Figure 13.3 *Covered drain in a tiled floor*

bag-twist tool and 254 mm wire twists, both available from agricultural merchants. They should be placed inside bins to prevent attack from vermin, domestic animals and birds. Waste containers should conform to the relevant British Standard Specification. Dustbins should be of a nominal capacity of 90 L. Lids should fit closely with an overhanging lip. Wheeled bins may be used for the collection of waste from business premises, although the heavy lids may be left off and the bins can be difficult to clean. The alternative wheeled 'Eurobins' with four wheels and hinged lids are easier to clean and are bird-proof.

Staff should be aware of the necessity to remove refuse daily and to take care with storage. It is essential to have a properly constructed storage area for refuse, with a concrete floor and suitable hose tap for water to flush the yard and drainage gully fitted with a straining basket. The refuse storage area needs to be graded to the yard-floor gully and if it consists solely of a concreted platform, should include a bund wall to prevent spillage/washings accumulating on the surrounding earth and giving rise to the breeding of flies. The wall surfaces should be smooth, impervious and able to withstand water from high-pressure hoses. Refuse bins need to be washed each time they are emptied and stored inverted to drain dry on metal racks above the yard surface. A daily collection is necessary for large quantities of kitchen waste. If frequent collection is impossible, a secure refrigerated refuse store, away from food, should be provided.

Equipment

Directive 2006/42/EC on machinery updated previous Directives on machinery that were implemented in England by the Supply of Machinery (Safety) Regulations 1992 (as amended). These laws set out Essential Health and Safety Requirements (EHSRs) that must be met before machinery is supplied in the EU or European Economic Area (EEA). There is a section in the Directive on **foodstuffs machinery and machinery used for cosmetics or pharmaceutical products** which contains rules to ensure hygiene. Working groups representative of member states have formulated CEN (European Committee for Standardisation) standards for different types of food equipment/machinery covering hygienic design.

Equipment must be designed and sited so that all surfaces are accessible for cleaning. Every item

should be reached and removed easily. Large equipment should stand free from walls and floor. Mobile equipment with wheels which can be locked facilitates cleaning and also helps to reduce the movement of foods. There should be at least 300 mm space under appliances, otherwise they should be sealed to a solid base such as a concrete plinth approximately 150 mm high, topped with quarry tiles and with a coved tile skirting. Dirt may accumulate in the framework and outer casing, which should be as smooth as practicable, and spaces in the supporting structure totally enclosed and sealed or adequately open for cleaning purposes. For example, legs of standing equipment formed of sealed tubes are better than angle or channel section. The basic material for food equipment must be non-absorbent and resistant to damage by cleaning or disinfection. Temperature controlled trolleys are available and are widely used in institutions. Wooden duckboards and pallets should not be used.

Surfaces

Equipment surfaces should be smooth, continuous, sealed and both easily cleaned and disinfected. Internal angles should be easily cleaned and without voids and dead spaces. Cleaning chemicals or acid foods should not lead to deterioration. For servicing and cleaning, equipment must be accessible or mobile. Tables and worktops should be constructed for ease of cleaning, strength and durability. Stainless steel tables with tubular legs and braked castors are recommended. Working surfaces/tables in 18/10 gauge stainless steel may be cantilevered, centralized or back-to-back. Wood is unsatisfactory because it is porous and cannot be effectively cleaned and disinfected. A stainless steel upstanding back, 150–300 mm, at the rear of worktops, as for sinks, will keep adjacent wall surfaces clean and undamaged. Movable worktops will facilitate cleaning, or if fixed, a space of at least 300 mm should be left behind them.

For storage of small items of equipment and foodstuffs, open shelves made of stainless steel or cantilevered plastic laminate are preferred to cupboards or drawers (Figure 13.4). Fixed shelves sited over cooking equipment should be made of stainless steel and not wood. Hollow plinths under shelves gather dirt and may attract mice for nesting. Free-standing wire shelves allow air circulation and

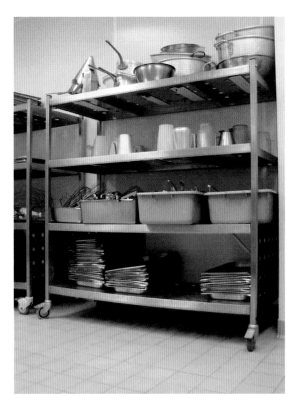

Figure 13.4 *Open storage for kitchen utensils*

dust to fall through, but are unsuitable for open food. Detachable shelves are convenient for cleaning and redecorating.

Cooking equipment

There are many kinds of cooking equipment available: gas, electrical or appliances may be arranged in combination. Some equipment may be wall-mounted or back-to-back with fitted splashbacks. Induction cookers rely on electromagnetic waves to heat cooking vessels directly; thus there is a greater degree of heat control than when using traditional electrical elements. A vitreo-ceramic surface on which the vessels stand, allows simple cleaning and does not become heated in areas where the vessels are not placed.

Polished stainless steel, for example type 302 and thickness 14/16 gauge, is the best material for catering equipment with rounded corners and deburred edges. The design should allow heavily soiled parts to be removed for cleaning. Each piece should fit easily into a sink, or better still, into a

dishwashing machine directly before emptying the tanks (i.e. the wash or rinse tanks of the dishwasher). Several washes may be necessary for heavily soiled trivets, trays and shelves; if the washing process is carried out daily, the finish can be maintained. The traditional method of cooking, using pots and pans on an open ring, is wasteful of energy and can be hazardous because:

- as much as half the heat produced is lost by ventilation
- a large amount of food in one container above several open burners requires much water and constant stirring
- it is hazardous for containers full of hot food to be carried by staff
- excessive heat in the kitchen causes unpleasant and debilitating working conditions and the warmth and humidity encourage microbial growth
- cooking large amounts of food too far ahead of requirements without adequate cooling and refrigeration facilities may lead to **food poisoning**.

Equipment is available to cook food in batches with only small losses of flavour and nutriment, for example, pressure steamers, bratt pans that can be tipped to empty, and forced air-convection ovens. Such equipment should be raised above the floor surface and cleaned underneath. Thus the safety and efficiency of cooking equipment are improved by separating the boiling top from the oven, which should be situated at waist height on movable stainless steel tubular frames. Aluminium or light alloys should not be used for burners and handles because they are difficult to clean and are damaged by caustic agents. Convection ovens, microwave ovens and pressure cookers are described in Chapter 9. Pass-through cabinets, either heated or chilled, allow the easier passage out of the kitchen.

Cooking vessels

Cooking vessels and other utensils are made of a wide range of materials, including various metals and vitreous substances. There have been no reports of illness following the consumption of food prepared in contact with the more common metals such as stainless steel, aluminium and its alloys. Iron and tin cans for food are mostly constructed of tin-plated iron sheet, although aluminium is increasingly used as a can material for a variety of foods as well as soft drinks. Copper can be solubilized by acid foods. Lead is a poisonous metal and the glaze of earthenware vessels, which contains lead oxide, may react with acid products; similarly, zinc may be dissolved from galvanized equipment. Antimony is a component of enamel used for coating food vessels. Cadmium is used for plating utensils and fittings for cookers and refrigerators, and may be a component of earthenware from some countries. Both antimony and cadmium can be poisonous when vessels are used for acid foods; care should be taken with chipped enamel vessels and food should not be laid directly on the shelves of refrigerators. The use of cooking pots and pans that are heavily carbonized wastes energy.

Fryers

Deep-fat fryers hold large quantities of cooking oil. This oil undergoes a physical change at prolonged high temperature so the quality of fried food deteriorates. Fat deposits may build-up in kitchens, in ventilation systems and even outside buildings. The factors that cause breakdown of cooking oils include:

- high-temperature frying and oxidation
- the introduction of excessive moisture, common salt, potato whitener and charring by food particles; charring can be reduced by providing a deep cool zone in frying equipment
- the catalytic action of copper and brass in old chip fryers or filter valves, which rapidly darkens fat or oil.

Portable fat filters may be used for removing suspended particles from the oil or fat. They may also be used to hold the fat while the fryer is being cleaned. Several small-capacity fryers give greater flexibility and better results. All frying equipment should be fitted with thermostatic controls and heat applied slowly. Thermostats should be calibrated and checked against a thermometer at least weekly. Enclosed filter systems are useful for clarifying oil; open systems may oxidize the oil. Manufacturers recommend a minimum level of oil during frying and frequent topping-up with new oil. For fish and doughnuts a complete change of cooking oil is required on a regular basis. All deep-fat equipment needs careful operation and supervision.

Hot cabinets

The hot cabinet is satisfactory for heating plates but not for keeping food warm since food dries quickly, losing flavour and nutritional quality. The appliances are not designed to cook food and the system of holding food in this manner can provide the warm conditions favourable for the growth of food poisoning and spoilage organisms. Nevertheless, provided that heated cabinets or display cases for hot food storage are thermostatically controlled and hygienically designed, they are important for the maintenance of relevant foods at temperatures greater than 63 °C. Generally it is necessary to pre-heat these units prior to use in order to achieve the required temperature. Food should be served directly from cooking appliances, hot **bain maries** and cold cabinets.

Cutting boards

Kitchen equipment traditionally made of wood, such as spoons, and boards, should be manufactured from impervious, easily cleaned materials. Synthetic, non-absorbent polypropylene cutting boards are easily cleaned and disinfected, and can be put in a dishwasher, although they may sustain cuts. Hard synthetic rubber is good although it may be deformed by heat; this can be corrected if it is softened in hot water and allowed to harden on a flat surface. Hardwood, if used, should be constructed without joints.

Separate cutting blocks and boards should be used for different foods to avoid the risk of cross-contamination when raw and cooked foods are prepared in the same area. Cutting boards should be colour-coded as well as the kitchen knives. They should be kept in suitable racks. Hard synthetic rubber chopping blocks or table tops are useful in many food trades, and this surface is suitable for boning meat, cutting pastry and filleting fish without damage to knives. Rubber is impervious, unlike wood, where the cellular structure permits the absorption of food particles and juices. Sandpaper may be used to re-surface rubber pads after prolonged periods of heavy use. Rubber table tops, 25 mm or 50 mm thick, should be supported on stands made of tubular aluminium, stainless steel, or galvanized steel, and should be of adjustable height.

Slicing, mixing and mincing machines

Slicing and mixing machines should never be used for both raw and cooked foods without thorough cleaning in-between. The practice of using one mincing machine for both raw and cooked meat even with washing in between should be discouraged because of the difficulty in the thorough cleaning of the parts of the mincer. All these machines can be responsible for cross-contamination. Food machinery should be designed for easy cleaning and disinfection, and should be readily dismantled and reassembled; safety is also important in the selection of machines. Hygiene and safety considerations should come first in the choice of equipment and outweigh the initial cost.

The risk of cross-contamination will be increased with machines with interchangeable parts and when used for more than one purpose, such as mincing and mixing.

FOOD STORAGE

Refrigeration

The growth and multiplication of bacteria in food will be reduced by **rapid cooling** and **refrigerated storage**. The temperatures at which relevant foods must be kept are laid down in Schedule 4 of the Food Hygiene (England) Regulations 2006. These temperatures are above 63 °C or below 8 °C, subject to the status of the food. Specific temperatures for certain foods are laid down in Regulation (EC) No. 853/2004 and there is a general requirement to keep food at **safe temperatures** in Regulation (EC) No. 852/2004. Hence, if food manufacturers specify a specific storage temperature for the food they have produced, then that temperature should be used.

Refrigerators should provide separate storage space at the temperatures recommended for each particular type of food; thus separate refrigerators may be required. All commercial refrigeration equipment should have in-built thermometers, which need to be checked periodically for accuracy. In some situations it is necessary to have a temperature history of refrigerated foods which may

be in various forms such as electronic recall, as on some vending appliances, to chart recorders. A suitable digital thermometer with appropriate probes should be available together with a supply of disinfectant wipes. This thermometer should be checked for accuracy at regular intervals against a reference thermometer or the sensor checked with a wet ice mixture. Cold-storage facilities should be provided for vegetables and fruit, at a temperature of approximately 10 °C. Cooked and uncooked food should be refrigerated and stored separately, not on the **cold room** floor or beneath other foods that may spill or drip. Cold-store evaporators should be defrosted regularly, otherwise temperature control cannot be maintained and the temperature will rise inside the refrigerator.

Automatic defrosting is recommended. Refrigeration is a heat exchange process and heat removed by the refrigerant must be dissipated elsewhere. Ample ventilation to the condenser is required and no obstruction of the plant should occur. Wherever possible, large refrigerator condensers should be sited outside the building and always outside the kitchen. Refrigeration equipment, if outside the premises, should be sited in such a position that its noise does not become a nuisance for neighbours. This equipment is a source of heat and a good nesting place for mice. A warning device for refrigerator or deep-freeze failure is essential. Two separate monitors are valuable in case one fails. Mobile refrigerated cabinets are recommended for use in large-scale catering with spacious preparation areas. **Blast chillers** and **blast freezers** are required for **cook-chill** and **cook-freeze** catering and are available in several sizes; some allow trolleys holding food to be wheeled in directly. They may also be used with conventional catering, provided the caterer is knowledgeable and has carried out a risk analysis. Such units allow greater flexibility with an even distribution of work, thus avoiding 'peak' periods and menus may be wider and properly planned. The Chilled Food Association (2006) has provided guidance for manufacturers for producing a wide of chilled foods and includes sections on HACCP and shelf-life assessment.

Blast chillers should be able to reduce the temperature of cooked foods to between 0 ° and 3 °C within 1.5 hours and blast-freezers should allow the food to reach −5 °C within 1.5 hours of entering the freezer, and subsequently to reach the storage temperature of −18 °C. Walk-in cold storage facilities do not have a constant temperature or humidity, and verification of appropriate storage conditions should be undertaken at least daily. The relative humidity in a walk-in cold store gives an indication of the balance between the water that has evaporated from the stored food, and its removal by the evaporator. Foods such as vegetables and fruit should not be stored in relatively dry air as moisture evaporates and they would wither, so the humidity of the air can play an important part in respect of the storage of certain foods. Too much humidity can lead to condensation and possible bacterial contamination. However, humidity levels may be affected by the type of food packaging, method of stacking, exposed food products, type of control system, conditions outside the cold store and the working cycle. Periodically, cold stores should be emptied and the ceiling, walls and floor thoroughly cleaned. The floor should be dried before re-use.

Deep freeze

Frozen foods should be maintained at a constant temperature in a cabinet operating at −18 °C; the temperature should be checked frequently. The position of the cabinet should be such that it is not affected by draught, heat from the sun or radiators, and with no obstruction to the compressor, motor and condenser.

Rapid cooling cold room

The provision of facilities for rapid cooling is strongly recommended, particularly for foods refrigerated after cooking. They are especially necessary for meat and poultry dishes intended to be served cold. A room should be allotted on the cold side of the kitchen provided with an extractor fan and means to maintain the temperature at less than 8 °C. Such facilities are also useful for the storage of dairy products. Mobile cabinets provided with fans and air filters are desirable in any situation where food is cooked in bulk for large numbers of people. It cannot be over-emphasized that rapid cooling from cooking temperatures and before refrigeration prevents many outbreaks of food poisoning. However, the provision of this room may no longer be necessary with the availability of blast chillers and consequent stricter temperature control of foods.

Storage of dry goods

Equipment used for the storage of dry goods, such as cereals, should be constructed of inert materials, easily cleaned, mobile and lidded. Shelves should also be mobile, preferably stainless steel and easily cleaned. The lowest shelf should be at least 36 cm above floor level to facilitate cleaning and reduce the risk of infestation by insects and harbourage for vermin. Many foods are labelled 'Store in a cool, dry place' – this should be less than 10 °C; although a temperature is rarely specified.

The **vermin-proof** room or cupboard, depending on the size of the kitchen, for dehydrated and canned goods should have impervious surfaces to the floor, walls and shelves and it should be screened against flies and other insects. Good ventilation can be supplied by 229 mm air bricks in an external wall together with an extractor fan to aid air movement. The inlet and extract vents should be on opposite walls, the inlet at a lower level than the extract to ensure good circulation of air.

CLEANING EQUIPMENT

The various articles used for **cleaning**, although nominally regarded as clean, are often profusely contaminated with bacteria and they should not be stored in food rooms. Cloths, mops and brushes can **recontaminate** otherwise clean surfaces, and it is essential to wash and disinfect them after use in separate facilities. Such equipment should also be **colour-coded** to reduce the risk of **contamination** and the use of the same equipment in toilets and food handling areas.

Provision should be made for racks to drain buckets after washing. There is a risk that spillage of chemicals may contaminate food, therefore separate storage areas are essential for cleaning materials. Sinks and wash basins in kitchens should not be used for the disposal of wash-water used for cleaning. A separate slop sink or gully should be provided together with supplies of hot and cold water, a handwash basin and an extractor fan. If cloths are used to clean equipment, cutlery, surfaces and glasses, they should be disinfected at least daily in boiling water or freshly prepared bleach solution. After disinfection in the bleach solution, cloths must be thoroughly rinsed. Paper towels and single-use cloths are recommended. Single-use towels are preferable because disposable cleaning materials can be misused. Twin bucket trolleys are available for washing floors manually using a mop. One bucket contains detergent water and the dirty water is wrung out into the second bucket. Powered floor-cleaning machines may be used such that hot water is sprayed on the floor with a cleaning agent and a rotating brush loosens the dirt. Some types of machines are able to remove the dirt from grooves in the floor, but it may be necessary to follow the path of a machine with a mop and 'squeegee', particularly if the machine cannot remove dirt from the intersections of the floor and walls or around machinery. Other types of floor-cleaning machines scrub and dry the floor in one operation. A small domestic washing machine is useful in the cleaning equipment storage area/room for washing mops and cloths at a disinfecting temperature.

Cleaning methods may also include the use of foam and high-pressure hoses (Figure 13.5). However, should these be used, consideration needs to be given to the potential for contamination. Although following the use of a hose, surfaces may appear to be visibly clean, dirt might have splashed onto surfaces during use of the hose, and aerosols created, which can contain pathogens, thus compromising food safety. Although disinfectants may be used, they might not be effective if incorrectly used. Hence, the use of hoses for cleaning purposes should be carefully considered,

and they should be used only in appropriate places, such as an external waste collection area.

STAFF ROOM

Facilities away from food rooms must be provided to store and dry outdoor clothing of employees. Where lockers are provided they should be adequately ventilated to keep them dry, eliminate odours and prevent mould growth, and situated close to the staff sanitary and washing area. Secure facilities should be made available such that jewellery can be removed before entering food production areas.

It may be preferable to hang clothes freely on rods and to supply a source of heat for drying purposes. Showers for the staff and a receptacle for discarded protective clothing are desirable. Facilities may also be required for the additional protective clothing provided for employees who work in cold stores or in refrigerated rooms, and for the cleaning of special footwear, such as Wellington boots.

FIRST AID

The provision of first-aid materials is a legal requirement laid down in the Health and Safety (First Aid) Regulations 1981 (as amended). A general duty is placed on employers to ensure adequate equipment, facilities and personnel to deliver initial

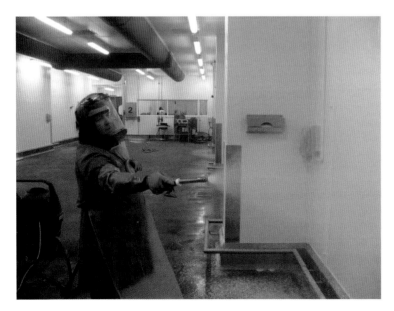

Figure 13.5 *Deep-cleaning of an empty food production area using foam*

first aid to employees. The HSE's (2004) ACoP, *First Aid at Work*, gives guidance on these regulations.

LICENSED TRADE

In public houses or hotel bars there may be a mixture of business and domestic arrangements. However, the preparation of food intended for customers should be separated from domestic occupations. Laundering should be done in a separate room away from food preparation.

Food displayed on bars, or elsewhere, should be kept cold and a rapid turnover assured.

FOOD LAW CODE OF PRACTICE/PRACTICE GUIDANCE

The Food Standards Agency has issued (under Section 40 of the Food Safety Act 1990, Regulation 24 of the Food Hygiene [England] Regulations 2006 and Regulation 6 of the Official Feed and Food Controls [England] Regulations 2006) a Food Law Code of Practice and accompanying Practice Guidance which updates existing enforcement issues and takes account of directly applicable EU legislation. These documents also cover temperature control requirements. Food law enforcers must give regard to the statutory Code of Practice while undertaking their duties. The devolved administrations have their own implementing legislation and have issued similar codes of practice and accompanying practice guidance.

Fire prevention

Food business operators are required to comply with the Management of Health and Safety at Work Regulations 1999 (as amended) in respect of fire prevention and specifically the Fire Precautions (Workplace) Regulations 1997 (as amended). It is essential to have adequate supervision in kitchens, as they are regarded as high-risk areas. The proper use of deep fat fryers, and frying in general, is particularly important, as well as ensuring that ventilation ducting and filters are cleaned periodically to prevent a build-up of waste. As part of the overall health and safety risk assessment for the workplace, the food business operator should undertake a fire risk assessment. Suitable notices indicating emergency routes, exits and the location of fire fighting equipment should be provided. The Home Office, HSE, Northern Ireland Department of the Environment and the Scottish Executive have produced advice for employers entitled *Fire Safety: An Employer's Guide*.

Summary

- The requirements for management and control of the structure of food premises and equipment aim to create the correct hygienic environment in which food can be safely produced, processed, cooked, served, stored or transported.
- There are legal provisions for building design, including social welfare such as the provision of toilet facilities, changing rooms, and rest rooms.
- Different types of premises have a spectrum of requirements because of differing hazards and risks.

All websites cited below were accessed in April 2007.

SOURCES OF INFORMATION AND FURTHER READING

Adler D (ed) (1999) *Planning and Design Data*, 2nd ed. London: Architectural Press, 1999.

British Standards Institute (2006) BS 6465-1. *Sanitary Installations. Code of Practice for the Design of Sanitary Facilities and Scales of Provision of Sanitary and Associated Appliances*. London: British Standards Institute.

European Hygienic Engineering & Design Group (www.ehedg.org).

Campden and Chorleywood Food Research Association Group (www.campden.co.uk).

Chilled Food Association (2006) *CFA Guidelines for Good Hygienic Practice in the Manufacture of Chilled Foods – 4th edition*. London: The Stationery Office.

Health and Safety Executive (1998). HS(G)38 *Lighting at Work*. London, Health and Safety Executive.

Health and Safety (First Aid) Regulations 1981 SI No. 917. London: Office of Public Sector Information.

Home Office, Health and Safety Executive, Northern Ireland DoE, Scottish Executive (1999) *Fire Safety: An Employer's Guide*. London: The Stationery Office (available at: http://www.archive.official-documents.co.uk/document/fire).

Industry Guide to Good Hygiene Practice (1997) *Catering Guide*. London: Chadwick House Group.

Office of the Deputy Prime Minister (2006) *The Building Regulations 2000, Hygiene*. London, NBS. Online version. Available at: www.communities.gov.uk/pub/581/ApprovedDocumentGHygiene1992Edition_id1 165581.pdf.

Regulation (EC) No 178/2002 of the European Parliament and of the Council of 28 January 2002 laying down the general principles and requirements of food law, establishing the European Food Safety Authority and laying down procedures in matters of food safety. Available at: http://europa.eu.int/eur-lex/pri/en/oj/dat/2002/l_031/l_03120020201en00010024.pdf.

Regulation (EC) No 852/2004 of the European Parliament and of the Council on the hygiene of foodstuffs. Available at: www.food.gov.uk/multimedia/pdfs/hiojregulation.pdf.

Regulation (EC) No 853/2004 of the European Parliament and of the Council laying down specific hygiene rules for food of animal origin. Available at: www.europa.eu.int/eur-lex/pri/en/oj/dat/2004/l_226/l_22620040625en00220082.pdf.

Society of Light and Lighting/Chartered Institution of Building Services Engineers (2006) *Code for Interior Lighting*. London: Chartered Institution of Building Services Engineers.

Workplace (Health, Safety and Welfare) Regulations 1992 SI No. 3004. London: Office of Public Sector Information (available at: http://www.opsi.gov.uk/SI/si1992/Uksi_19923004_en_1.htm).

14

Control of infestation

Richard Elson

Legal provision	264	Summary	274
Pests of premises	264	Sources of information and further reading	274
Pests in food	273		

Pests damage food and buildings. They also introduce pathogens to areas where food is produced, stored or processed. Pests can also introduce pathogens to food animals. As well as being a potential source of infection, the presence of pests in food premises is repugnant and is likely to lead to formal action by a food authority. Infestation by pests can be prevented by appropriate design, construction and maintenance of buildings. Most pests require food, water and shelter to survive. Hence, if pests do gain access to a building, they can be managed by denying harbourage and sources of food and water. This will also prevent re-infestation. Pest control is closely linked to the lifecycle of the pest and appropriate treatment and advice should be sought from pest contractors.

Pests Animals, rodents, birds or insects whose presence in food or food premises is unwanted.

Infestation The process of inhabitation by pests or presence of pests.

LEGAL PROVISION

In Europe, Regulation (EC) No. 178/2002 makes it an offence to sell unsafe food. Unsafe foods include those unfit for human consumption due to contamination with extraneous matter. Food may become contaminated with the hairs, faeces or bodies of pests, which can lead to action being taken under this provision. Under the European Regulation (EC) No. 852/2004, food premises must be designed, sited and constructed to permit good food hygiene practices, including protection against contamination and in particular, pest control. Operators of food businesses are also required to have adequate procedures in place to control pests. These procedures range from regular visual inspection of the premises to employing a contractor to provide this service. Further guidance is provided in the 'Industry Guides to Good Hygiene Practice'. There are also specific requirements to prevent pests contaminating food at the primary production level, but this requirement takes into account any subsequent processing, such as sorting, grading and cleaning, that the foods will undergo. Other legislative and occupational health requirements relating to the safe use of pesticides and rodenticides are beyond the remit of this chapter, and expert advice should always be sought when attempting to identify or control an infestation.

PESTS OF PREMISES

Rodents

There are many species of rodents (from the Latin *rodere*, to gnaw or corrode). All of these share the characteristic features of a pair of long and prominent incisors (which are extremely effective for gnawing) and a gap in the place of canine teeth (which gives the incisors room to manoeuvre). The teeth grow continuously and remain sharp through wear.

Rats and mice are common rodent pests. However, in certain situations, squirrels can also present a risk to food safety. It is possible that the estimate of the material damage caused by rats and mice is often overstated, and their contribution in the spread of infection in the developed world is probably not considerable. Nevertheless, the presence of such animals in and around food premises can be a source of material loss and a potential danger to health.

Rats

Two species of rats are commonly encountered as pests of food premises: the brown rat (*Rattus norvegicus* [Figure 14.1]) and the black rat (*Rattus rattus*). The brown rat is the most common, black rats being mainly confined to large seaports. Table 14.1 lists the physical differences that distinguish the two species. Brown rats are omnivorous but have a preference for cereals. Both species of rats are neophobic (fear new things) and this is important when considering methods for their control. Brown rats are also burrowers and construct elaborate tunnel systems in, beneath and around buildings. They also colonize sewer systems and take advantage of defective pipe work and disused drainage systems to develop exits from otherwise secure environments. In contrast, black rats are rarely seen below ground and are expert climbers.

Mice

Compared with rats, mice (*Mus musculus/domesticus* [Figure 14.2]) are much smaller and less habitual.

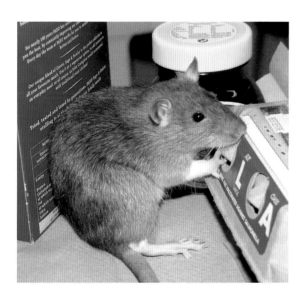

Figure 14.1   *A brown rat* (Rattus norvegicus) *(image courtesy of David Cross, Igrox Ltd)*

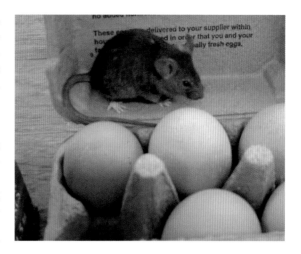

Figure 14.2   *A mouse* (Mus musculus/domesticus) *(image courtesy of David Cross, Igrox Ltd)*

They are less suspicious of unfamiliar objects, and less consistent in travel routes and established feeding points. (See also Table 14.1.)

Signs

Rats and mice are nocturnal animals, and so are rarely seen during the day unless they are disturbed by building or other work. However, infestation can be identified without actually seeing these animals. Rats and mice produce large numbers of droppings that differ in size and shape. The numbers can provide an indication of the size of an infestation (Figure 14.3).

Rats are creatures of habit and follow established routes, thus trails can be found in soft ground or grass, particularly at the boundaries of buildings. Their fur is greasy and will sometimes leave smear marks on walls and other surfaces over a period of time. Gnawed food, food packaging, equipment and surfaces provide evidence of an infestation, and the size and shape of the toothmarks may also assist in species identification.

Prevention

As stated above, rodents require food, water and shelter to survive, so denying any or all of these will discourage infestation. Material which is likely to be suitable for rat food, e.g. cereals, starchy vegetables and fatty compounds (including soap), should be kept in rodent-proof metal/plastic bins or containers. Refuse of the same type must be collected in properly covered metal/plastic dustbins which

Table 14.1 *Distinguishing features of rats and mice*

Characteristic	Brown rat	Black rat	Mouse
Time to attain sexual maturity (months)	2–3	2–3	1.5
Average gestation (days)	23	22	19
Average number of young per litter	6–12	6–8	5–6
Average number of litters per year	4–7	4–6	8
Weight of adult (g)	250–500	225	15–25
Total length – nose to tip of tail (cm)	30–45	35–45	15–19
Head and body	Blunt muzzle, heavy thick body, 18–25 cm	Pointed muzzle, slender body, 16–20 cm	Small, 6–9 cm
Tail	Shorter than head plus body, carried with little movement, 15–20 cm	Longer than head plus body, whip-like movement, 19–25 cm	Equal to or a little longer than head plus body, 8–10 cm
Ears	Small, close set, appear half buried in fur	Prominent, large, stand well up from fur	Prominent, large for size of animal
Fur	Coarse, generally red-brown to grey-brown	Black to slate grey; tawny above, grey-white below; or tawny above, white to lemon belly	Silky, dusky grey
Droppings	Lozenge-shaped and blunt at ends	Banana-shaped and tapered at one end	Thin and spindle-shaped

Sources: DuPont Animal Health Solutions (www.antecint.co.uk) and Bassett WH (ed.) (2004) *Clay's Handbook of Environmental Health*, 19th edn. London: Spon Press.

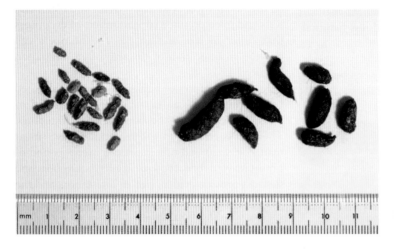

Figure 14.3 *Mouse (left) and brown rat (right) droppings*

are frequently emptied. Food should be stored tidily in sealed containers, preferably off the ground and away from walls so as not to provide a source of food if a rodent enters the premises. Regular cleaning of food storage areas and spillages, particularly in inaccessible areas, will also help prevent build-up of food. Access to water should also be denied by

mending dripping taps and having grids on gully traps. This is particularly relevant to rats, as mice obtain sufficient water from their food.

Good housekeeping is important. When unused for some time, food preparation equipment and items such as storage boxes may provide harbourage and should not be allowed to accumulate or remain undisturbed for more than a few weeks. Anything which affords cover to rats and mice should be removed from buildings and attached yards.

Rodents are able to pass through small gaps by flattening their bodies, hence buildings should be designed and constructed to prevent access to rodents. Stony and metallic materials have advantages over fibrous material such as wood. However, rats have been observed to gnaw through concrete. Structural harbours may occur below hollow floors, in hollow walls and partitions, in pipe ducts and casings, and less commonly in roof spaces above false ceilings. All possible access routes should be considered and closed off (Box 14.1)

Box 14.1 Access routes for rodents
- Apertures where service pipes enter and leave buildings – should be filled
- Drains – should be maintained in good repair
- Inlets, manholes, and rodding eyes – should be properly sealed or covered
- Doors – should be close fitting and protected against gnawing where necessary

---

Figure 14.4 illustrates some of the common defects mentioned above and some of the means by which rodents move from one part of a building to another (for example, from a sub-floor space to the room above). To proof a building against rats, openings must be sealed by cement mortar, sheet metal, or mesh (Figure 14.5). Similar materials are needed to reinforce vulnerable points such as door edges and junction points of walls and floors. Coarse wire wool should be embedded in the cement and used to block holes in walls. Metal plates can be used in the base of ill-fitting doors.

Control

It is important to remember that rodent infestations are rarely isolated to one part of a building, and attempts to control an infestation by treating an individual area will be unsuccessful. Concerted action over the whole infested territory or block is necessary before all the rats and mice can be eliminated. This may be achieved through a contract with the local authority or a **commercial pest control organization**. An infestation may extend below ground to drains and sewers, so vertical control schemes must include treatment for the destruction of rats in underground pipes as well as in the buildings above. Black rats may

be present in the roof and brown rats at ground level.

Individual traps may be useful for controlling mice as they are less suspicious of new objects, and traps can be used for individual rats or small rat infestations. The spring break-back type of trap is frequently used although it has the disadvantage that once sprung it is of no further use until reset. Treadle or plate-based traps are better for holding bait than a prong, as cereals such as oatmeal, dried fruit, nuts or chocolate may be used, and, contrary to popular belief, they are more attractive to mice than the traditional cheese. It is preferable to place traps at right angles against walls so that they will be sprung from either direction, and the treadle should be nearest the wall or vertical surface.

For many years, rodents were controlled using **rodenticides**, usually in the form of anticoagulants, most commonly warfarin. Anticoagulants interfere with the blood clotting process causing the animal to die from internal or external haemorrhage. These may be single dose (lethal after one feed) or multi-dose (lethal only after sufficient rodenticide has been consumed over a period of time). Rodenticides that interfere with other metabolic pathways are also available. However, resistance to common rodenticides, particularly warfarin, has emerged among some rat populations. This resistance has developed from the ingestion of sub-lethal doses of poison.

Rodenticides are usually laid as bait, and may be combined with a foodstuff attractive to the rodent (cereals or grains such as barley) or as manufactured pellets and pastes. Commercial pest control companies employed by most food businesses use pellets or pastes as opposed to more traditional forms of bait due to their convenience and reduced risk of contamination in these environments. The placing of bait is important and a pest control operative will usually survey a site before deciding where to lay bait or traps. As rats are habitual creatures, bait is normally laid in known feeding areas or along established runs. To encourage feeding, bait should be kept dry and covered to prevent access by humans or other animals such as birds.

Birds

Birds are a hazard in food establishments because their droppings can contaminate food and equipment with pathogens such as *Salmonella* spp. In

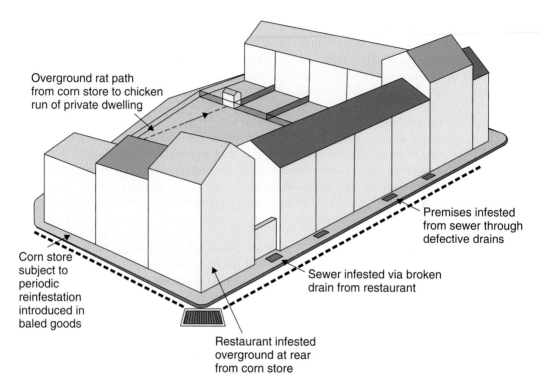

Overground rat path
from corn store to chicken
run of private dwelling

Premises infested
from sewer through
defective drains

Corn store
subject to
periodic
reinfestation
introduced in
baled goods

Sewer infested via broken
drain from restaurant

Restaurant infested
overground at rear
from corn store

Figure 14.4   *Examples of related infestations in separate buildings which require simultaneous treatment*

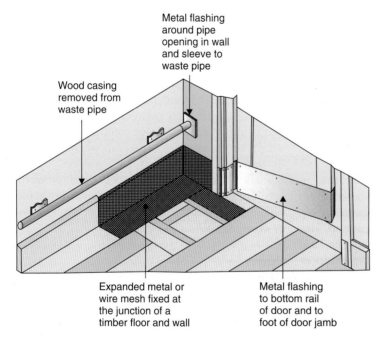

Metal flashing
around pipe
opening in wall
and sleeve to
waste pipe

Wood casing
removed from
waste pipe

Expanded metal or
wire mesh fixed at
the junction of a
timber floor and wall

Metal flashing
to bottom rail
of door and to
foot of door jamb

Figure 14.5   *Rat-proofing: methods of protecting some vulnerable points*

addition, their nests can introduce other pests, such as insects, which spoil stored products.

Prevention

Birds usually congregate where there is a readily accessible food supply and/or suitable roosting sites. If these attractions are controlled or eliminated, birds are unlikely to take up residence and become pests. Audible or visual scaring devices may be of use in remote areas but are not acceptable, and unlikely to be effective, in urban or predominately built-up areas. Screens on windows and doors help to exclude birds, but this may be impractical in larger premises. The treatment of windowsills and other surfaces with gels or tensioned wires or spikes deters some birds from alighting. However, these need to be maintained and may be less effective for smaller birds.

Control

The Wildlife and Countryside Act 1981 (as amended) provides general protection for birds and there is no legal definition of a 'pest' bird. However, the UK Department for the Environment, Food and Rural Affairs (Defra) annually grants general licences for authorized persons to kill or take birds, or to take or destroy their eggs, for many purposes including preventing the spread of disease, preserving public health or safety and preventing damage to foodstuffs for livestock, crops, vegetables and fruit. Birds that may be covered by these licences are the Canada goose, collared dove, crow, gull (great/lesser black backed and herring), jackdaw, jay, magpie, feral pigeon, rook and woodpigeon.

Population control is rarely successful but can be effective where a defined group of birds needs to be dealt with. Options for control are shown in Box 14.2.

> **Box 14.2 Methods of bird population control**
> - Egg control – eggs are removed or treated so they do not hatch
> - Cage trapping
> - Humane destruction of trapped birds
> - Shooting
> - Mist trapping
> - Baits

Mist trapping and shooting are commonly used methods in food premises although birds such as sparrows, robins and blackbirds must only be dealt with by trained and licensed operators.

Insects

Cockroaches

A huge number of species of cockroaches can be found in diverse environments worldwide: they are almost universally reviled. Cockroaches seek warm, moist environments and will readily infest food premises. These insects usually feed at night and may occur in food premises in large numbers. They contaminate food both with their faeces and by regurgitating the contents of their stomach onto the food. They will eat almost anything with an organic content, including food and refuse. Cockroaches also live in and around drains and sewers. They need water to survive, and obtain this from moist foods.

The females produce egg cases; the number of eggs within each egg case varies among the species. Eggs hatch into nymphs which progress through a number of stages before maturation, depending on the species and sex. The two species of cockroach commonly found in Europe are the german cockroach (*Blatta germanica*) and the oriental cockroach (*Blatta orientalis*). The identifying features of these two species are given in Table 14.2.

Table 14.2 *Distinguishing features of common European cockroaches*

Characteristic	Oriental cockroach	German cockroach
Colour	Dark brown/black	Mid-light brown. Two dark bands in front of the wings
Length	20–25 mm	15 mm
Lifespan	Up to 10 months	~4 months
Number of eggs per ootheca	Up to 16	30–40
Number of nymphal stages	Males – 7	Males – 5
	Females – 10	Females – 7
Preferred temperature	20–29 °C	15–35 °C
Other	Poor climber. Females have small wings	Prefer high humidity. Good climbers

Source: Bassett WH (ed.) (2004) *Clay's Handbook of Environmental Health*, 19th edn. London: Spon Press.

Signs

Cockroaches are rarely seen during the day unless disturbed when equipment is moved or they are flushed out by the application of **insecticide** sprays. However, the presence of egg cases and faecal deposits are indicative of infestation. Infestations are usually accompanied by the presence of a distinct sour smell. Infestations can be discovered or monitored with sticky traps.

Prevention

Good design, construction and maintenance of premises is essential to prevent infestation. Good housekeeping is also essential as access to food and water will encourage and support infestations of cockroaches. Routine baiting or insecticide treatments contribute to preventing an infestation and sticky traps can provide a monitoring tool to enable rapid treatment should an infestation become apparent.

Control

Since cockroaches inhabit inaccessible areas, treatment needs to be carefully planned and must have regard for the lifecycle of the species. Treatment usually involves application of a residual insecticide to wall and floor surfaces. In food preparation areas, gel and paste baits may be used to prevent contamination of foodstuffs. The residual effect should be maintained for at least three months to ensure that newly hatched nymphs are killed. Treatments should be reapplied after cleaning.

Flies

Several different species of fly are important in and around food premises (see Table 14.3). Flies such as the housefly (Figure 14.6) and bluebottle (Figure 14.7) readily move between faeces, refuse and fresh

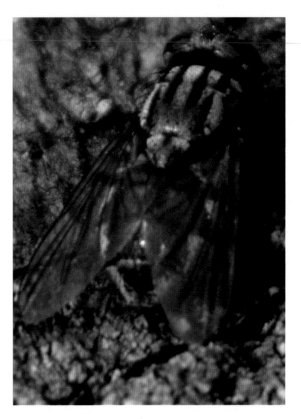

Figure 14.6 *A housefly (image courtesy of Dr G Nichols, HPA)*

food while feeding and are known to carry pathogens on and in their body. During feeding, flies regurgitate their gut contents onto food and defecate randomly. The danger of flyborne contamination of food must not be underestimated and all steps must be taken to deny flies access to food intended for human consumption. However, this must not divert attention from other essential safeguards such as

Table 14.3 *Distinguishing features of flies*

Characteristic	Housefly	Bluebottle	Fruit flies
Length	6–9 mm	10–15 mm	2 mm
Wingspan	13–15 mm	25 mm	3–4 mm
Colour	Grey-black in male. Yellow and black in females	Iridescent dark blue	Yellowish grey
Feeding habit	Decaying animal and vegetable matter, faeces and fresh food	Fresh meat or fish, decaying animal and vegetable matter, faeces and fresh food	Fermenting matter such as decaying fruit, vegetables alcohol and yeasts

Bassett WH (ed.) (2004) *Clay's Handbook of Environmental Health*, 19th edn. London: Spon Press.

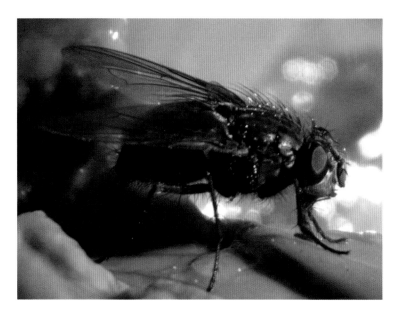

Figure 14.7   *A bluebottle (image courtesy of Dr G Nichols, HPA)*

personal and factory cleanliness, and temperature control.

The life cycle of the fly has four stages (Box 14.3). The time spent in each stage depends on the species and the ambient conditions, especially temperature.

Box 14.3 Stages in the life cycle of the fly

- **Egg** – laid by the female in some material which provides food for the larva
- **Larva** – or maggot – hatches from the egg after 8 hours to 3 days. The larva burrows into its food supply, eating voraciously until fully grown, which takes from 42 hours to 8 weeks, when it seeks a dry and cool spot in which to pupate
- **Pupa** – or chrysalis – remains motionless in its early stages (puparium) for a maturation period of 3 days to 4 weeks
- **Fly** – emerges from the pupa

Signs of infestation are usually self-evident from the presence of adult flies, larvae or pupae in or around food premises.

Prevention

Prevention is achieved by not allowing food and refuse to accumulate, either inside or outside the building, and keeping these items covered until disposed of. Providing fly screens to windows that open, on lower floors of buildings, and self-closing devices and/or vertical plastic strips on doors helps prevent access (Figure 14.8).

Control

The most vulnerable stage in the fly's lifecycle is that of the adult. Although there are many forms of flytrap and many insecticides, the most effective way to destroy adult flies is by sprays containing natural or synthetic **pyrethrins**. However, care should be taken when applying insecticide, ensuring that all food and food preparation surfaces are not contaminated, and sprays should only be used as a last resort in addition to physical controls. There is a danger that flying insects affected by insecticides may drop into food and escape detection.

Fly killers are widely used in food premises and work by attracting flies to an ultraviolet light surrounded by an electrified metal frame (Figure 14.9). These units are provided with a collection tray for bodies and debris. However, some research has shown that bacteria can survive this process and the process of electrocution can distribute parts of the fly beyond the collection tray so great care should be taken when siting this equipment in food rooms.

Ants

Two kinds of ants occur in buildings: garden ants which nest outside but enter in search of food; and Pharaoh's ants, which nest in warm buildings. Garden ants are not known to be of public health importance, but are a nuisance in kitchens and other food premises. Pharaoh's ants have been shown to transmit human pathogens and constitute a health hazard in hospitals by roaming from open

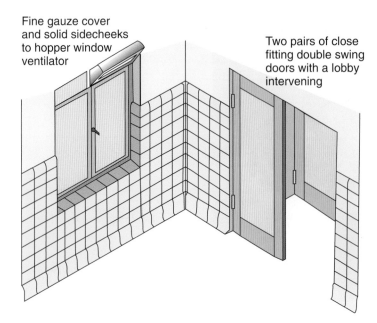

Fine gauze cover
and solid sidecheeks
to hopper window
ventilator

Two pairs of close
fitting double swing
doors with a lobby
intervening

Figure 14.8   *Fly-proofing: protecting common places of entry*

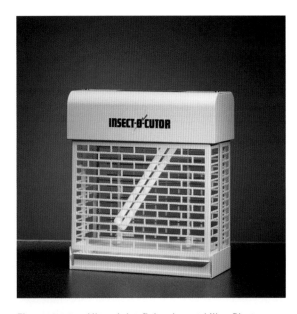

Figure 14.9   *Ultraviolet flying insect killer. Photo courtesy of eeeee.co.uk*

wounds and soiled dressings to sterile equipment and dressings or to food.

Prevention

As with most pests, much can be done to avoid attracting ants by careful observance of cleanliness, removal of waste food (even the smallest crumbs), and the repair of structural cracks and crevices in walls and floors which afford nesting sites.

Control

Established infestations of Pharaoh's ants indoors will involve many nests over a large area, each with several queens. Control must be performed systematically. Treatment should start beyond the infested area and consists of applying bands of insecticide at the wall/floor junction of rooms and corridors, around pipe exits, sinks, air vents, cracks, sills and on the undersides of cupboard shelves in infested buildings.

Wasps

Wasps are easily recognized and can be a nuisance in food premises, although there appears to be no evidence that they are involved in the spread of foodborne infections. From mid-summer onwards, foraging workers are attracted by and feed on fruit juice, sugar, syrup and other sweet substances, but in early summer they will also take insects, fresh and decaying meat and fish to feed the grubs in the nest.

Prevention

Measures taken to prevent flies entering food premises also apply to wasps. However, wasps can enter premises usually regarded as fly-proof, although they cannot penetrate mesh as fine as 3 mm (1/8 inch).

Control

The workers range a mile or more from their nest. When an infestation occurs a search should be made for nests in the vicinity and steps taken to destroy them. This work is best performed in the evening when most of the wasps are in the nest and drowsy, and it is a wise precaution for the operator to wear gauntlets and a beekeeper's hood. When the nest is in a suitable position it can be soaked with a rapid 'knock-down' liquid insecticide and burnt or broken up. Where it is impossible to find or to deal with the nests, attractive baits set outside the premises will often intercept and divert wasps from the building. The bait may be jam, syrup, molasses, fermenting fruit or beer, mixed with enough water in a wide-mouthed jar to drown the insects. The ultraviolet light traps used for flies are also effective against wasps inside buildings.

PESTS IN FOOD

Several species of insect pests live on or in food, particularly during storage. These insects are not known to be vectors of human illness, however their presence can cause food to deteriorate in appearance and taste unpleasant. See Table 14.4 for insect pests of importance and the foods they usually attack.

Prevention

Infestations can be prevented by inspecting incoming food and food ingredients for infestation and rejecting those where an infestation is found. Good stock rotation is essential to prevent recurring problems. Foods stored for long periods of time should be inspected for sign of damage and infestation.

Control

Badly infested goods should be destroyed and affected areas either sprayed with a residual insecticide or fumigated.

Table 14.4 Insect pests of foodstuffs

Insect species	Preferred food	Comments
Larder beetle	Meat, bone, hides	Presence indicates poor hygiene
Flour beetle	Flour and animal feeds	Also infest dried fruit, spices and nuts. Adults produce secretions that taint food with a bitter taste
Saw-toothed grain beetle	Stored grain	Also eats rice and other dried food
Flat grain beetles	Cereals	Prefers warm environments
Biscuit beetle	Cereal products and dried vegetable products	Larvae can chew though packaging to gain access to contents
Spider beetle	Grain, flour, spices, dried animal feeds nuts and dried fruit	Found in birds' nests
Mealworm beetles	Cereals and cereal products	Also feed on dead insects, birds and rodents. Found in birds' nests
Grain weevils	Stored grain	Lays eggs inside grain. Larvae feeds on contents and then exits through a small hole producing large amounts of waste material
Mites	Moulds on stored products	Favours moist environments

Bassett WH (ed.) (2004) *Clay's Handbook of Environmental Health*, 19th edn. London: Spon Press.

Summary

- Pests are unwanted visitors to food premises and may cause physical damage to buildings and food.
- Their presence in food preparation areas is unacceptable and may lead to formal action on discovery.
- Prevention is better than cure and if buildings are designed, constructed and maintained with pests in mind, infestations are unlikely to develop.
- The owners of food businesses are under a legal obligation to prevent infestations and control them when they do occur.

All websites cited in this chapter and below were accessed in November 2006.

SOURCES OF INFORMATION AND FURTHER READING

Bassett WH (ed.) (2004) *Clay's Handbook of Environmental Health*, 19th edn. London: Spon Press.

National Pest Advisory Panel website (www.cieh-npap.org.uk).

Department for Food, the Environment and Rural Affairs. Wildlife management and licensing advice (available at: www.defra.gov.uk/wildlife-countryside/vertebrates/default.htm).

Pesticides Safety Directorate website (www.pesticides.gov.uk).

15

Legislation

Christine Little

Food safety legislation	276	Communicable disease legislation	297
Food hygiene legislation	282	Summary	299
Official controls	293	Sources of information and further reading	300

Food hygiene and food safety legislation cannot be viewed in an exclusively national context – it is a worldwide issue. The European Commission (EC) has been involved in food legislation since 1964. The central goal of the EC is the achievement of the highest possible level of health protection for the consumers of Europe's food. The Commission also ensures that all EC laws are compatible with the international obligations of the European Union (EU) under the World Trade Organization (WTO) Sanitary and Phytosanitary and Technical Barriers to Trade Agreements. The production, processing, distribution, retail, packaging and labelling of food stuffs are governed by a mass of laws, regulations, codes of practice and guidance.

This chapter is intended only as a general outline of the most important legislation relating to food safety and hygiene. It is not intended to provide explicit detail since legislation is constantly changing, and regard must be had of any new legislation introduced since this book was published. Up-to-date information on food law can be sourced from the websites of the EC (http://ec.europa.eu/food/), Food Standards Agency (FSA) (www.food.gov.uk), and Office of Public Sector Information (www.opsi.gov.uk) websites.

Types of EC legislation There three types of legislation in the EC (Regulation; Directive; Decision). These are defined below.

Regulation A legal act which has general applications and is binding in its entirety and directly applicable to the citizens, courts and governments of all Member States of the EU.

Regulations do not, therefore, have to be transferred into national laws and are chiefly designed to ensure uniform law across the Community. However, in some places, the regulations permit or require EU Member States to make national legislation to provide for powers and responsibilities of enforcement and enforcement authorities, the creation of offences and penalties for failure to comply, powers of entry and rights of appeal. Such national legislation in the UK would be in the form of a **statutory instrument** under the **Food Safety Act 1990**.

Directive A binding law directed to one or more Member States. The law states objectives that the Member State(s) are required to conform within a specified time. A directive has to be implemented by Member States by amendment of their national laws to comply with the stated objectives: in the UK this is done in the form of statutory instruments. This process is known as '**approximation of laws**' or '**harmonization**' since it involves the alignment of national policy throughout the Community.

Decision An act which is directed at specific individuals, companies or Member States, and which is binding in its entirety. Decisions addressed to Member States are directly applicable in the same way as Directives.

Types of UK legislation Laws are made by Parliament or with Parliamentary authority (see below).

Acts of Parliament These are statutes passed by Parliament that can only be modified by parliamentary procedure. Acts are normally concerned with principles of legislation and must pass through both Houses (Commons and Lords) before receiving Royal Assent.

Regulations and orders (statutory instruments) These are delegated legislation made by the appropriate minister, who is empowered to do so under a specific Act. Regulations normally deal with specific premises or commodities in much greater detail than acts.

FOOD SAFETY LEGISLATION

General food law – principles and general requirements regarding food safety

General Food Law Regulation [EC] No. 178/2002 (http://europa.eu.int/eur-lex/pri/en/oj/dat/2002/l_031/l_03120020201en00010024.pdf), lays down the general principles (Articles 5 to 10) and requirements of food law, establishes the European Food Safety Authority (EFSA), and lays down procedures in matters of food safety. The Regulation also establishes the principles of risk analysis in relation to food and the structures and mechanisms for the scientific and technical evaluations undertaken by EFSA.

General objectives

Regulation [EC] No. 178/2002 came into force on 21 February 2002, although certain key provisions applied only from 1 January 2005. The aim of this Regulation is to provide a framework to ensure a coherent approach in the development of food legislation. At the same time, it provides the general framework for those areas not covered by specific harmonized rules but where the functioning of the internal market is ensured by mutual recognition. It lays down definitions, principles and obligations covering all stages of food/feed production and distribution. It applies to all stages of production, processing and distribution of food and feed, but there is an exemption for primary production for private domestic use, and the domestic preparation, handling, or storage of food for private domestic consumption.

From 2005 onwards this Regulation placed a clear responsibility on food and feed businesses to:

- ensure that food is safe
- establish systems to ensure that they can trace food throughout the food chain
- withdraw or recall food from the market where it does not comply with food safety requirements
- notify authorities of any action they have taken to secure withdrawal or recall of food or feed.

This Regulation also covers the safety of animal feedstuffs to ensure that this does not indirectly cause illness or harm when humans consume animal products.

The food law aims at ensuring a high level of protection of human health and consumers' interests in relation to food, taking into account the protection of animal health and welfare, plant health and the environment. This integrated farm to fork approach is now considered a general principle for EU food safety policy. Food law, both at national and EU level, establishes the rights of consumers to safe food and to accurate and honest information. The EU food law aims to harmonize existing national requirements to ensure the free movement of food and feed in the EU. The food law recognizes the EU's commitment to its international obligations and will be developed and adapted taking international standards into consideration, except where this might undermine the high level of consumer protection pursued by the EU.

Definition of food
Article 2 defines food as

> any substance or product, whether processed, partially processed or unprocessed, intended to be, or reasonably expected to be ingested by humans.

Food includes drink, chewing gum and any substance, including water, intentionally incorporated into the food during its manufacture, preparation or treatment.

Food does not include:

- feed
- live animals unless they are prepared for placing on the market for human consumption

- plants prior to harvesting
- medicinal products
- cosmetics
- tobacco and tobacco products
- narcotic or psychotrophic substances
- residues or contaminants.

Food Business Operator and Food Business

Food Business Operators (FBOs) are:

> natural or legal persons responsible for ensuring that the requirements of food law are met within the food business under their control. (Article 3.2)

A food business is:

> any undertaking, whether for profit or not, and whether public or private, carrying out any of the activities related to any stage of production, processing and distribution of food. (Article 3.3)

This includes seasonal and sporadic businesses. Stages of production, processing and distribution are defined in Article 3.16 and covers all stages from and including primary production (as defined in Article 3.17) up to and including sale or supply to the final consumer. Therefore, the activities of, for example, farmers, importers, manufacturers, wholesalers, distributors, transporters, retailers and catering outlets, are covered.

Article 3 lists other definitions used in the Regulation, such as placing on the market, risk, hazard, and traceability.

Risk analysis (Article 6)

Food law must be based on risk analysis in order to achieve the general objective of a high level of protection of human health and life. Risk assessment must be based on the available scientific evidence and undertaken in an independent, objective and transparent manner. Risk management must take into account the results of risk assessment, the opinions of EFSA, other legitimate factors and the precautionary principle.

Precautionary principle (Article 7)

In specific circumstances where, following an assessment of available information, the possibility of harmful effects on health is identified but scientific uncertainty persists, provisional risk management measures necessary to ensure a high level of health protection may be adopted, pending further scientific information for a more comprehensive risk assessment.

Measures adopted must be proportionate and no more restrictive of trade than is required to achieve the high level of health protection, regard being given to technical and economic feasibility and other factors regarded as legitimate. The measures must be reviewed within a reasonable period of time, depending on the nature of the risk to life or health identified and the type of scientific information needed to clarify the scientific uncertainty and to conduct a more comprehensive risk assessment.

Principles of transparency (Articles 9 and 10)

The Regulation establishes a framework for the greater involvement of stakeholders at all stages in the development of food law and establishes the mechanisms necessary to increase consumer confidence in food law. There must be open and transparent public consultation, directly or through representative bodies, during the preparation, evaluation and revision of food law, except where the urgency of the matter does not allow it.

Better communication about food safety and the evaluation and explanation of potential risks, including full transparency of scientific opinions, are of key importance. Where there are reasonable grounds to suspect that a food or feed may present a risk for human or animal health, then, depending on the nature, seriousness and extent of that risk, public authorities must take appropriate steps to inform the general public of the nature of the risk to health, identifying to the fullest extent possible the type of food or feed, the risk that it may present, and the measures that are taken or about to be taken to prevent, reduce or eliminate that risk.

Consumer confidence is an essential outcome of a successful food policy and is therefore a primary goal of EU action related to food. Transparency of legislation and effective public consultation are essential elements of building this greater confidence.

General obligations of food trade

Food and feed imported into the Community (Article 11)

Food and feed imported into the EU for placing on the market must comply with the relevant requirements of food law. Alternatively, compliance can be obtained with these requirements either by conditions recognized by the Community to be at least equivalent or by a specific agreement between the Community and the exporting country.

Food and feed exported from the Community (Article 12)

Food and feed exported or re-exported from the Community for placing on the market of a third country must comply with the relevant requirements of food law, unless otherwise requested by the authorities of the importing country or established by the laws, regulations, standards, codes of practice and other legal and administrative procedures as may be in force in the importing country.

General requirements of food law

Food and feed safety requirements (Articles 14 and 15)

Food must not be place on the market if it is unsafe. Food is deemed to be **unsafe** if it is considered to be: **injurious to health; or unfit for human consumption.**

In determining whether a food is unsafe regard shall be had to:

- the normal conditions of use of the food by the consumer and at each stage of production, processing and distribution
- the information provided to the consumer, including information on the label, or other information generally available to the consumer concerning the avoidance of specific adverse health effects from a particular food or category of foods.

In determining whether a food is injurious to health, regard shall be had:

- to the probable immediate and/or short-term and/or long-term effects of that food on the health of not only the person consuming it, but also subsequent generations
- to the probable cumulative toxic effects
- to the particular health sensitivities of a specific category of consumers where the food is intended for that category of consumers.

In determining whether a food is unfit for human consumption, regard shall be had to whether the food is unacceptable for human consumption according to its intended use, for reasons of contamination by extraneous matter or otherwise, or through putrefaction, deterioration or decay.

Feed shall not be placed on the market or fed to food-producing animals if it is unsafe. Feed shall be deemed to be unsafe for its intended use if it is considered to:

- have an adverse effect on human or animal health
- make the food derived from food-producing animals unsafe for human consumption.

Where any food/feed which is unsafe is part of a batch, lot or consignment of the same class or description, it is presumed that all the food/feed in that batch, lot or consignment is also unsafe, unless following a detailed assessment there is no evidence that the rest of the batch, lot or consignment is unsafe.

Responsibilities (Article 17)

The Regulation establishes the basic principle that the primary responsibility for ensuring compliance with food law, and in particular the safety of the food, rests with the food business. This principle is similarly applies to feed businesses. To complement and support this principle, there must be adequate and effective controls organized by the competent authorities of the Member States.

Traceability (Article 18)

Regulation [EC] No. 178/2002 defines traceability as the ability to trace and follow food, feed, and ingredients through all stages of production, processing and distribution. The identification of the origin of feed and food ingredients and food sources is of prime importance for the protection of consumers, particularly when products are found to be faulty. Traceability facilitates the withdrawal of foods and enables consumers to be provided with targeted and accurate information concerning implicated products.

The Regulation contains general provisions for traceability (applicable from 1 January 2005) which cover all food and feed, all food and feed business operators, without prejudice to existing legislation on specific sectors such as beef, fish, genetically modified organisms, etc. Importers are similarly affected as they will be required to identify from whom the product was exported in the country of origin. Unless specific provisions for further traceability exist, the requirement for traceability is limited to ensuring that businesses are at least able to identify the immediate supplier of the product in question and the immediate subsequent recipient, with the exemption of retailers to final consumers (i.e. **one step back – one step forward**). This information must be made available to competent authorities on demand. Food and feed which is placed on the market or likely to be placed on the market in the Community must be adequately labelled or identified to facilitate its traceability, through relevant documentation or information in accordance with the relevant requirements of more specific provisions.

Guidance on implementation of the general food law main requirements

An EC guidance document on the implementation of the general food law main requirements (Box 15.1) has been developed (http://europa.eu.int/comm/food/food/foodlaw/guidance/guidance_rev_7_en.pdf).

Box 15.1 General food law – main requirements

● Traceability of food and feed products
● Responsibility of operators
● Withdrawal of unsafe food or feed from the market
● Import requirements
● New rules on food hygiene and official food controls
● Notification to the competent authorities

The guidance aims to assist all players in the food chain to better understand the Regulation and to apply it correctly and in a uniform way.

European Food Safety Authority (Chapter III)

The EFSA (www.efsa.eu.int), was legally born from the Regulation (EC) No. 178/2002, and is based in Parma, Italy. EFSA is the keystone of EU risk assessment regarding food and feed safety. It provides independent scientific advice on all matters linked to food and feed safety, including animal health and welfare and plant protection, in relation to Community legislation. EFSA's risk assessments provide risk managers (consisting of EU institutions

with political accountability, i.e. EC, European Parliament and Council) with a sound scientific basis for defining policy-driven legislative or regulatory measures required to ensure a high level of consumer protection with regard to food safety. EFSA is also responsible for monitoring **zoonoses** across the EU. The Authority also communicates to the public in an open and transparent way on all matters within its remit.

Rapid Alert System for Food and Feed, crisis management and emergencies (Articles 50–57- Chapter IV)

Rapid Alert System for Food and Feed

The Rapid Alert System for Food and Feed (**RASFF**) is a system which has been in place since 1979. The legal basis of the RASFF is now the general food law **Regulation [EC] No. 178/2002**. Article 50 of this Regulation establishes the RASFF as a network involving the Member States (EU, European Free Trade Association [EFTA] or European Economic Area), the Commission and EFSA. On 1 May 2004 the number of countries of the RASFF network increased to 28 (the 25 Member States and the three EFTA countries: Norway, Iceland and Liechtenstein). The Commission publishes a weekly overview of alert and information notifications (see http://europa.eu.int/comm/food/food/rapidalert/index_en.htm).

RASFF was established to provide the control authorities with an effective tool for exchange of information on measures taken to ensure food safety. Whenever a member of the network has any information relating to the existence of a serious direct or indirect risk to human health, this information is immediately notified to the Commission under the RASFF. The Commission immediately transmits this information to other members of the network. Without prejudice to other Community legislation, the Member States shall immediately notify the Commission under the rapid alert system of:

● any measure they adopt which is aimed at restricting the placing on the market or forcing the withdrawal from the market or the recall of food or feed in order to protect human health and requiring rapid action
● any recommendation or agreement with professional operators aimed at, on a

voluntary or obligatory basis, preventing, limiting or imposing specific conditions on the placing on the market or the eventual use of food or feed on account of a serious risk to human health requiring rapid action

- any rejection, related to a direct or indirect risk to human health, of a batch, container or cargo of food or feed by a competent authority at a border post within the EU.

The Commission must inform a third (non-EU) country to allow it to take corrective measures and thus avoid repetition of the problem in the following circumstances:

- if it is known that a product subject to an alert notification has been exported to that country

or

- when a product originating from that country has been the subject of a notification.

The Member States shall immediately inform the Commission of the action implemented or measures taken following receipt of the notifications and supplementary information transmitted under the rapid alert system. The Commission shall immediately transmit this information to the members of the network.

Participation in RASFF may be opened up to applicant countries, third countries or international organizations on the basis of agreements.

Emergencies

Regulation (EC) No. 178/2002 (Article 53) confers special powers to the European Commission for taking **emergency measures**. Such measures can be taken where it is evident that a feed and food originating in the EU, or imported from a third country, is likely to constitute a serious risk to human health, animal health or the environment, and that such a risk cannot be contained satisfactorily by means of measures taken by the Member States. Such action can be initiated by the Commission itself, or be requested by a Member State. Depending on the gravity of the situation, emergency measures can take one of two forms (Box 15.2).

> **Box 15.2 Emergency measures (Regulation [EC] No. 178/2002 [Article 53])**
>
> - *For products of EU origin.* Suspension of the placing on the market or use of the product in question, imposition of special conditions and adoption of any other appropriate interim measure
> - *For products imported from a third country.* Suspension of imports, imposition of special conditions and adoption of any other appropriate interim measure.

In emergencies, the Commission alone may provisionally adopt the necessary measures, after consulting the Member State(s) concerned and informing the other Member States. In such a case, the provisional measures in question must, within 10 working days at most, be confirmed, amended, revoked or extended in the context of the Standing Committee on the Food Chain and Animal Health.

If, following information from a Member State on the need to take emergency measures, the Commission does not initiate the procedure for the adoption of emergency measures at Community level, the Member State in question may adopt interim protective measures. The Member State may maintain its national interim protective measures until a Community decision has been adopted concerning the extension, amendment or abrogation of the emergency measures.

Crisis management

Regulation [EC] No. 178/2002 provides for the establishment of a general plan for food/feed crisis management and the creation of a **crisis unit**. This crisis unit will be set up by the Commission in cases where the Commission identifies a serious direct or indirect risk to human health deriving from food and feed and the risk cannot be managed adequately by application of existing provisions, in particular the emergency procedures. EFSA will participate in the crisis unit and provide scientific and technical assistance.

In close co-operation with the Authority and the Member States, the Commission has drawn up a **general plan** for crisis management, specifying the situations entailing direct or indirect risks to human health not provided for by the Regulation, and setting out the practical procedures necessary for managing a resultant crisis (Commission Decision concerning the adoption of a general plan for food/feed crisis management 2004/478/EC). The crisis unit will be responsible for collecting and evaluating all relevant information and identifying the options available to prevent, eliminate or reduces the risk. The crisis unit will keep the public informed of the risks involved and the measures taken.

Execution and enforcement of EC Regulation 178/2002 in the UK

Although as a Regulation it is directly applicable in Member States, new enforcement and penalties in relation to the new obligations on food and feed businesses in Articles 14–20 have been introduced into national law. The necessary changes to national food law have been effected by means of statutory instruments under the Food Safety Act 1990 and the European Communities Act 1972. These are the Food Safety Act 1990 (Amendment) Regulations 2004 (www.opsi.gov.uk/si/si2004/20042990.htm) and the General Food Regulations 2004 (as amended) (www.opsi.gov.uk/si/si2004/20043279.htm).

The Food Safety Act (Amendment) Regulations 2004 SI No. 2990

The Regulations entered into force on 7 December 2004 and align the definition of 'food' in the Food Safety Act 1990 with that in Regulation [EC] No. 178/2002. The key difference is that unlicensed medicinal products are excluded from the new definition of 'food' as they are medicinal products within the meaning of the Medicines Directive 2001/83/EC. The new definition of 'food' applies to other areas of legislation that uses the Food Safety Act definition, for example the Food Standards Act 1999 and Environmental Protection Act 1985, as well as to Regulations and Orders made under all these Acts.

These Regulations also narrow the scope of the public consultation requirement in Sections 40 and 48 of the Food Safety Act 1990 so that it does not apply in cases where the public consultation requirements of Article 9 of Regulation [EC] No. 178/2002 apply. The FSA has issued Guidance Notes for these Regulations (www.food.gov.uk/multimedia/pdfs/generalfoodsafetyguide2.pdf).

The General Food Regulations 2004 SI No. 3279

The purpose of these Regulations is to provide new enforcement powers with regard to the new obligations of Articles 14, 16, 18 and 19 of Regulation (EC) No. 178/2002, and applied from 1 January 2005. The FSA has issued Guidance Notes for these Regulations (www.food.gov.uk/multimedia/pdfs/generalfoodsafetyguide2.pdf).

Food Safety Requirements

The new food safety requirements (Article 14 of Regulation [EC] No. 178/2002) are broadly similar as those in Section 8 of the Food Safety Act 1990, which no longer applies because of the new provisions in Article 14 of Regulation (EC) No. 178/2002. However, food may be injurious to health under Article 14 in circumstances not previously covered by section 8(2)(a) of the Food Safety Act which only referred to food that had been rendered injurious to health by means of certain operations.

The food safety requirements in Article 14 apply to sales and supplies, including one-off sales and supplies free of charge. The requirements of this Article are not limited to FBOs. The aim is to protect public health by covering all eventualities, with the exception of private domestic consumption, which is allowed an exemption by virtue of Article 1.3. The extent to which home producers fall within the definition of 'food business' will need to be decided on a case-by-case basis as suggested by the FSA's Guidance Notes.

Responsibilities for food: food business operators

Article 19.1 of Regulation [EC] No. 178/2002 requires that where an FBO considers or has reason to believe that a food it has imported, produced, manufactured or distributed is not in compliance with the food safety requirements, and has left the immediate control of the initial food business, it should be withdrawn from the market and the action notified to the competent authorities.

Businesses are required to notify both the FSA and relevant enforcement authority when food is not in compliance with the food safety requirements, and has left the immediate control of the initial food business. A form has been produced by the FSA for use by both food and feed business operators. Businesses should return the completed forms to the FSA Food Incidents Branch, to the local authority where the food business is based, and in the case of imports, to the relevant port health authority.

Enforcement

Regulation 3 of the General Food Regulations designates food authorities, port health authorities and the FSA as the **competent authorities. Enforcement authorities** are specified in Regulation 6 as food authorities or port health authorities in relation to Articles 14, 16, 18 and 19 of Regulation [EC] No. 178/2002, but the FSA is specified as an additional enforcement authority in relation to Articles 14 and 19 in certain circumstances.

This means that port health authorities or local authorities are responsible for enforcing all provisions. The FSA is an additional enforcement authority in relation to the enforcement of the food safety requirements, and also recall, withdrawal and notification requirements under certain circumstances.

Regulations 4 and 5 of these Regulations also specify offences in relation to the above requirements and impose penalties for these offences.

FOOD HYGIENE LEGISLATION

The primary objective of the EU food hygiene legislation is to optimize public health protection by consolidating and simplifying previous legislation. The new legislation maintains, and sets out more clearly, the duty of FBOs to produce food safely. The legislation introduces a 'farm to fork' approach to food safety, by including, for the first time, all primary production (i.e. farmers and growers) in food hygiene legislation. In practical terms, the requirements on primary producers amount, in the main, to fairly basic hygiene procedures. As EU regulations (Box 15.3), they are directly applicable law. The new legislation requires FBOs (except primary producers) to implement a permanent procedure, or procedures, based on **Hazard Analysis Critical Control Point (HACCP)** principles. It should be stressed, however, that the legislation is structured so that it can be applied flexibly and proportionally according to the size and nature of the business.

> **Box 15.3 EU food hygiene regulations**
> - Regulation (EC) No. 852/2004 of the European Parliament and of the Council on the hygiene of foodstuffs (http://eur-lex.europa.eu/LexUriServ/site/en/oj/2004/l_226/l_22620040625en00030021.pdf)
> - Regulation (EC) No. 853/2004 of the European Parliament and of the Council – laying down specific hygiene rules for food of animal origin (http://eur-lex.europa.eu/LexUriServ/site/en/oj/2004/l_226/l_22620040625en00220082.pdf)
> - Regulation (EC) No. 854/2004 of the European Parliament and of the Council – laying down specific rules for the organization of official controls on products of animal origin intended for human consumption (http://eur-lex.europa.eu/LexUriServ/site/en/oj/2004/l_226/l_22620040625en00830127.pdf)

The general hygiene requirements for all FBOs are laid down in Regulation [EC] No. 852/2004. Regulation [EC] No. 853/2004 supplements Regulation [EC] No. 852/2004 in that it lays down specific requirements for food businesses dealing with food of animal origin. Regulation [EC] No. 854/2004 relates to the organization of official controls on products of animal origin intended for human consumption.

There are two other parts to the **hygiene package**:

- Directive 2002/99/EC laying down the animal health rules governing the production, processing, distribution and introduction of products of animal origin for human consumption.
- Directive 2004/41/EC repealing certain directives concerning food hygiene and health conditions for the production and placing on the market of certain products of animal origin intended for human consumption and amending Council Directives 89/662/EEC and 92/118/EEC and amending Decision 95/408/EC.

Directive 2004/41/EC repeals the previous legislation and Directive 2002/99/EC (which fall under Department for Environment, Food and Rural Affairs [Defra] policy responsibility) lays down the animal health rules on products of animal origin for human consumption.

The revised hygiene rules are based on the following key measures:

- implementation of a 'farm to table' approach
- introduction of a HACCP system in all sectors of the food business except for the primary sector
- registration or approval for certain food establishments
- development of guides to good practice for hygiene and for the application of HACCP principles
- set-up of a special provision to ensure flexibility for food produced in remote areas and for traditional production methods.

The overall aim of the new hygiene package is to create a single, transparent hygiene policy applicable to all food and all food operators, together with effective instruments to manage food safety and potential food crises, throughout the food chain. The new legislation applies from 1 January 2006.

General hygiene: Regulation (EC) No. 852/2004 on the hygiene of foodstuffs

General provisions
This Regulation lays down general rules for FBOs on the hygiene of foodstuffs. The Regulation applies to all stages of production, processing and distribution of food and to exports, without prejudice to more specific requirements relating to food hygiene.

The Regulation is based on risk assessment, and elimination or control of food safety hazards. It precludes HACCP systems from being used as a form of self-regulation, or as a replacement for **official food control**. Official food controls will still be required to check compliance with the legislation, and FBOs will be required to co-operate with such controls.

Basic principles
The obligations the Regulations imposes on FBOs take account of the following principles:

- Primary responsibility for food safety rests with the FBO.
- Food safety must be ensured throughout the food chain.
- The importance of the cold chain.
- Procedures based on HACCP, along with good hygiene practice, should reinforce FBOs' responsibility.
- The relevance and utility of **guides to good**

hygiene practice in assisting FBOs achieve compliance with the legislation and with the application of HACCP principles.
- The necessity to establish microbiological criteria and temperature control requirements based on scientific risk assessment.
- The necessity to ensure that imported foods are of at least the same hygiene standard as food produced within the EU, or are of equivalent standard.

The primary objective of the Regulation, and the hygiene package as a whole, is to ensure a high level of consumer protection with regard to food safety. The Regulation recognizes and builds on the objectives laid down in Regulation [EC] No. 178/2002 (General Principles and Requirements of Food Law), including protection of human life and health, and the free movement of food within the EU.

To meet the objective of the Regulation, FBOs are required to adopt hygiene measures to comply with specified **microbiological criteria for foodstuffs** (Regulation [EC] No. 2073/2005), as well as measures deemed necessary to meet other targets set to achieve the objectives of this Regulation. Hygiene measures are also required of FBOs to meet temperature control requirements, to maintain the cold chain, and to undertake sampling and analysis.

Farm to fork – to a certain extent
The necessity of an integrated approach, from primary production (farmer, fisherman, hunter of wild game) to placing on the market or export, is emphasized. However, the Regulation does *not* apply to:

- primary production for private domestic use
- domestic preparation, handling or storage of food for private domestic consumption
- direct supply, by the producer, of small quantities of primary products to the final consumer or to local retail establishments directly supplying the final consumer
- collection centres and tanneries that fall within the definition of food business only because they handle raw material for the production of gelatine or collagen.

Primary producers will also not be covered by the HACCP requirements of the legislation. However, the Regulation specifies the use of guides to good practice to encourage good hygiene practice on farms. These guides may be supplemented by specific hygiene rules.

Risk assessment in food production

With respect to HACCP requirements themselves, these are intended to be consistent with principles contained in **Codex Alimentarius**. They are also intended to assist FBOs achieve a higher level of food safety through elimination or effective control of hazards. FBOs, therefore, are required to establish and operate food safety programmes and procedures based on the principles of HACCP. The wider application of HACCP requires staff to be trained.

The application of HACCP principles is also expected to be sufficiently flexible to apply to small businesses. However, the Regulation recognizes that critical control points cannot always be identified, and that, in some cases, their monitoring can be replaced by good hygiene practice. The Regulation makes provision for the development of guides to good practice for hygiene and the application of HACCP principles, both at national and Community level. The use of these guides, however, is not mandatory.

Small- to medium-sized enterprises (SMEs) and traditional production

Additional flexibility may also be provided for small businesses – critical limits need not be specified in terms of numerical absolutes, and the requirements for retaining records may be varied. Flexibility, without compromising on food safety, may also be appropriate to support traditional methods of food production especially in regions subject to geographical constraint (i.e. remote areas). The application of the flexibility or adaptation elements of the Regulation are subject to a special procedure set out in the Regulation.

Registration of food businesses (Article 6(2))

Food establishments, following a site visit, will have to be registered. FBOs will also be required to notify their **competent authority (CA)** of any changes to their business and ensure the CA has up to date information about their operations.

Primary food production requirements – details

Annex 1 to the Regulation details the obligations for **primary production**. In this context primary production includes:

- transporting, storing and handling of primary products at the place of production, provided they are not substantially altered or processed
- transporting live animals, to achieve the objective of the Regulation
- transporting primary products (such as crops, fishery products, and wild game) from the place of production to an establishment.

Annex 1, Part A contains requirements on:

- protecting primary products from contamination, including keeping buildings, vehicles, etc. clean
- the hygiene provisions to be observed, including requirements in relation to the health status of the staff
- record keeping, including records of feed, veterinary medicines and biocides.

Annex 1, Part B contains recommendations on guides to good hygiene practice.

Hygiene requirements further down the food chain

Where Annex 1 does not apply, Annex 2 will, and specifies requirements for:

- fixed and permanent food premises, including the requirements for design, layout, surfaces, and facilities
- moveable and temporary premises, market stalls, and vending machines
- domestic houses (where food is regularly prepared for placing on the market)
- transport and equipment
- food waste, water, wrapping and packaging
- heat treatment of food placed on the market in hermetically sealed containers (e.g. cans)
- personal hygiene and staff training.

Annex 2 also specifies provisions applicable to foodstuffs and, among other things, prohibits FBOs from accepting raw materials or ingredients, known or suspected to be, contaminated to such an extent that, the final product would be unfit for consumption.

The European Commission has published guidance documents on the implementation of Regulation (EC) No. 852/2004 on the hygiene of foodstuffs (see http://ec.europa.eu/food/food/biosafety/hygienelegislation/guidance_doc_852-2004_en.pdf), and on implementation of HACCP principles (see http:// ec.europa.eu / food / food / biosafety / hygiene legislation/guidance_doc_haccp_en.pdf).

More specific rules for certain products (e.g. meat, fish, etc.) are contained in Regulation (EC) No. 853/2204.

Specific hygiene: Regulation (EC) No. 853/2004 laying down specific hygiene rules for food of animal origin

This Regulation builds on the rules laid out in the Regulation on the Hygiene of Foodstuffs ([EC] No. 852/2004). It applies to all processed and unprocessed food of animal origin produced, imported into, or exported from the European Union from 1 January 2006. A specific Regulation for food of animal origin (Box 15.4), in addition to the generally applicable Regulation on the Hygiene of Foodstuffs, is considered to be necessary because of the specific hazards to human health that are potentially present in such food. The Regulation is intended to address these specific microbiological and chemical hazards.

Box 15.4 Food of animal origin

- Meat (i.e. the edible parts of specified animals, including blood), meat products, minced meat and mechanically separated meat
- Poultry
- Rabbits, hares and rodents
- Wild and farmed game
- Live bivalve molluscs, live echinoderms, live tunicates, live marine gastropods intended for human consumption
- Fishery products and mechanically separated fishery products
- Milk and dairy products
- Eggs and egg products
- Frogs legs and snails
- Honey

This legislation builds on principles already confirmed in previous legislation (now repealed) as being effective. The Regulation will not apply to primary production for private domestic use, or to the domestic preparation of food for domestic consumption. As with the Regulation on the Hygiene of Foodstuffs, the supply of small quantities of primary products or certain types of meat (poultry, rabbit and game), supplied directly by the producer to the final consumer or to a local retail premises, is a matter dealt with through national, rather than Community law.

This Regulation is intended to cover wholesale activities, although the provision exists for Member States to extend this Regulation to cover retail activities in certain circumstances. Retail activities, though, are generally governed by the Regulation on the Hygiene of Foodstuffs. Member States may also limit the application of this Regulation, where it is considered that the provisions of the Regulation on the Hygiene of Foodstuffs are sufficient, and where the supply of food of animal origin from a retail premises to another premises is a marginal, localized and restricted activity.

As with previous laws, establishments producing food covered by this legislation will require approval or registration, and will be required to apply their health mark to any products they place on the market, in accordance with the requirements set out in the Regulation. To be approved, an establishment must meet the requirements laid out in the Regulation on the Hygiene of Foodstuffs, and this Regulation. However, establishments only engaged in primary production, transport operations, the storage of products not requiring temperature control, or retail operation outside the scope of this Regulation, do not require approval. Competent authorities are required to visit an establishment before granting it approval or conditional approval.

The traceability provisions of the Regulation build on those already in Regulation (EC) No. 178/2002 (general principles and requirements of food law). This Regulation, however, creates additional requirements in the areas of HACCP-based procedures and food chain information. The structural and hygiene requirements of the Regulation will apply to all businesses, regardless of size. The Regulation also includes requirements for fishing vessels. However, flexibility, without compromising on food hygiene objectives, may be appropriate to facilitate the ongoing use of traditional methods of food production especially in regions of 'geographical constraint' (i.e. remote areas). The application of the flexibility or adaptation elements are subject to a procedure set out in the Regulation.

Specific allowance is also made for hunted wild game to ensure its proper inspection without adversely impacting on certain traditions associated with hunting. Additionally, further allowances are provided for raw milk and cream. Member States may, through national law, prohibit or restrict the placing on the market of raw milk and raw cream intended for direct human consumption. With respect to imports, food must come from countries, and establishments within those countries, listed in accordance with the Regulation. The food itself must also meet the requirements of this Regulation.

Some of the general obligations placed on FBOs include:

- a requirement to comply with the legislation
- use only water or an approved substance to remove surface contamination
- co-operating with the relevant CA
- ceasing operation, where approval is withdrawn, or where conditional approval is not made full.

Further requirements may be introduced by way of a committee procedure in areas such as the transport of meat while warm, additional health standards for live bivalve molluscs, and the use of raw milk not meeting the criteria laid down in the Regulation to manufacture specified dairy products.

The extensive Annexes to the Regulation detail the requirements relating to the nature, preparation and handling of each category of food, and the establishments in which these activities take place. They also cover identification marking of food of animal origin, HACCP-based procedures, food chain information and transport of live animals.

The Annexes also include requirements to be applied to the collection and processing of rendered animal fats and greaves; the treatment of stomachs, bladders and intestines; the manufacture of gelatin; and the manufacture of collagen.

The European Commission has published guidance documents on the implementation of Regulation (EC) No. 853/2004 (see http://ec.europa.eu/food/food/biosafety/hygienelegislation/guidance_doc_853-2004_en.pdf).

Official controls: Regulation (EC) No. 854/2004 laying down specific hygiene rules for the organization of official controls on products of animal origin intended for human consumption

This Regulation lays down the specific rules for the organization of **official controls** by CAs on products

of animal origin intended for human consumption. The Regulation is additional to the rules laid out in Regulation on the Hygiene of Foodstuffs ([EC] No. 852/2004) and the Regulation laying down Specific Hygiene Rules for Food of Animal Origin ([EC] No. 853/2004), and will apply where Regulation (EC) No. 853/2004 applies. Official controls are defined as any form of control that the CA performs for verification of compliance with food law. This includes verification of compliance with animal health and animal welfare rules. Specifically, official controls may include audits of good hygiene practices and HACCP-based procedures to ensure that they are being applied correctly by FBOs.

Member States are expected to have sufficient staff to carry out these controls in a manner consistent with the Regulation. The nature and intensity of official controls should be proportionate to the degree of risk presented to public health. Their nature and intensity should also relate to animal health and welfare (where that is appropriate), as well as the type and throughput of the processes carried out by the FBO. Where non-compliance is detected, CAs are required to take action to ensure the situation is rectified. The action taken should reflect the nature of the non-compliance and the FBO's history.

Official controls should also be based on the most recent relevant information available and should be adaptable to reflect changes in the state of the knowledge in this area. However, as with the other Regulations mentioned above, flexibility without compromising on food safety may be appropriate, for example:

- to facilitate the ongoing use of traditional food production methods
- in regions of 'geographical constraint'
- to allow pilot projects to take place to test new hygiene controls on meat
- to meet the needs of low throughput premises.

The application of the flexibility or adaptation provisions are subject to limitations, and must be applied in accordance with a procedure detailed in the Regulation.

On specific types of food of animal origin, the Regulation specifies particular official controls expected to be applied. For example, extensive details on the controls to be applied in the production of meat are detailed in Annex I of the Regulation. These additional official controls for meat are expected to include audits of activities and inspections, including checks on establishments' own controls. Such official controls are required to ensure FBOs are complying with food law and meeting relevant legislative criteria and targets. **Official veterinarians (OVs)** will be expected to carry out audits and inspections of slaughterhouses, game handling establishments, and certain cutting plants. The matter of who will deal with other types of establishments has been left to individual Member States. In the UK, this is carried out by the **Meat Hygiene Service** and/or **food authorities**. The Regulation also contains provisions allowing slaughterhouse staff to provide limited assistance with official controls, under the supervision of the OV and only in the case of poultry, lagomorphs (rabbits, hares), fattening pigs and fattening veal. The general aim is to prevent the introduction or spread of animal diseases or zoonoses from products of animal origin to humans or livestock. Official controls aimed at live bivalve molluscs target relaying and production areas as well as the end product (Annex II).

Annex III details the official control applicable to fishery products. These include hygiene checks at the time of landing and first sale, fishing vessels and approved establishments. Such controls should include organoleptic examination, testing for histamine, residues and contaminants, microbiological examination, checks for parasites and checks to ensure poisonous species are not being marketed. Similar controls on the production of raw milk target milk production holdings and raw milk on collection (Annex IV).

The requirements described above introduce clearer legal principles to prevent, eliminate or control the contamination of food with pathogens with the aim of reducing or preventing the occurrence of foodborne infections. In addition, they will assist in tracing food during an outbreak of foodborne infection and also clarify situations when food should be withdrawn from sale to protect public health.

In approving establishments, CAs will be required to make a site visit, and only approve an establishment once the FBO has demonstrated that they have met all the relative legislative requirements. That is, the FBO and the establishment must meet all the relevant requirements in Regulations (EC) No.

852/2204 and No. 853/2004. The Regulation, however, does allow for **conditional approval** where an establishment has met the necessary equipment and infrastructure requirements, but other requirements of food legislation, for example in relation to HACCP, remain outstanding. Conditional approval may only be granted for a maximum period of 6 months, or 12 months in the case of certain fishing vessels. Another site visit must be carried out before full approval can be granted. Approved establishments will be required to be issued with an approval number. Additional codes may be added to this number to indicate the types of products of animal origin manufactured by the establishment.

In the conduct of official controls in approved establishments, CAs are required to keep the approval under review. Should serious deficiencies be identified or there are persistent problems for which the FBO cannot give adequate guarantees as to their resolution, the CA is expected to withdraw the establishment's approval. There also exists provisions for an establishment's approval to be suspended if deficiencies cannot be resolved within a reasonable time. Procedures concerning imports are also set out in the Regulation. Food from outside the EU may only be imported from **listed establishments** in **listed third countries**. The requirements for listing are specified in the Regulation. The Regulation also lays down procedures for the development of **implementing measures** to deal with specific issues, such as methods for communicating inspection results or rules for laboratory testing.

EU implementing measures and transitional arrangements

In October and December 2005 the remaining implementing and transitional measures that support the application of EU hygiene legislation were published. They are also applicable from 1 January 2006, and are:

- Regulation (EC) No. 2073/2005 of 15 November 2005 on microbiological criteria for foodstuffs
- Regulation (EC) No. 2074/2005 of 5 December 2005 laying down implementing measures for certain products under Regulation (EC) No. 853/2004 and for the organization of official controls under

Regulation (EC) No. 854/2004 and Regulation (EC) No. 882/2004, derogating from Regulation (EC) No. 852/2004 and amending Regulations (EC) No. 853/2004 and (EC) No. 854/2004

- Regulation (EC) No. 2075/2005 of 5 December 2005 laying down specific rules on official controls for *Trichinella* in meat
- Regulation (EC) No. 2076/2005 of 5 December 2005 laying down transitional arrangements for the implementation of Regulations (EC) No. 853/2004, (EC) Nos 854/2004 and 882/2004 and amending Regulations (EC) Nos 853/2004 and 854/2004
- Regulation (EC) No. 1688/2005 of 14 October 2005 implementing Regulation (EC) No. 853/2004 as regards special guarantees concerning salmonella for consignments to Finland and Sweden of certain meat and eggs.

Microbiological criteria for foodstuffs

Regulation on the Hygiene of Foodstuffs, (EC) No. 852/2004 provides the legal basis for the proposed microbiological criteria. Article 4(3)(a) requires food business operators to comply with micro-biological criteria for foodstuffs and Article 4(4) stipulates how the criteria are to be adopted. This is part of the package of linked measures which aim to optimize public health protection by improving and modernizing existing European food hygiene legislation.

Foodstuffs of animal and plant origin may present intrinsic hazards, due to microbiological contam-ination. Microbiological criteria are tools that can be used in assessing the safety and quality of foods. Due to reasons related to sampling, methodology and uneven distribution of micro-organisms, micro-biological testing of finished food products done alone is, however, insufficient to guarantee the safety of a foodstuff tested. The safety of the foodstuffs must principally be ensured by a more preventive approach, such as product and process design and the application of **good hygiene practices** (GHPs) and **good manufacturing practices** (GMPs) and the HACCP principles.

The Community microbiological criteria for foodstuffs have been revised and certain important new criteria have also been set down. The

Commission Regulation on microbiological criteria for foodstuffs ((EC) 2073/2005; http://europa. eu.int/eur-lex/lex/LexUriServ/site/en/oj/2005/l_ 338/l_33820051222en00010026.pdf) applicable from 1 January 2006, lays down **food safety criteria** for certain important foodborne bacteria, their toxins and metabolites, such as *Salmonella*, *Listeria monocytogenes*, *Enterobacter sakazakii*, staphylo-coccal enterotoxins and histamine in specific foodstuffs. These criteria are applicable to products placed on the market during their entire shelf-life. In addition, the Regulation sets down certain **process hygiene criteria** to indicate the correct functioning of the production process (see Chapter 16). These criteria are applicable at the site of food production as well as in the framework of import control and Intra-Community trade.

The Commission Regulation on the Microbio-logical Criteria for Foodstuffs complements the food hygiene legislation and will apply to all food businesses involved in the production and handling of food. It should be stressed that the Regulation is flexible in its approach, in that sampling and testing plans should be determined on the basis of risk, size and type of business. The microbiological criteria can be used by the food business to validate and verify their food safety management procedures and when assessing the acceptability of foodstuffs or their manufacturing, handling and distribution processes. The competent authority is required to ensure that the food business operator is complying with the criteria and to apply the criteria for official control purposes. A guidance document has been produced by the FSA to help food businesses comply with the Regulation (*General Guidance for Food Business Operators*. EC Regulation No. 2073/2005 Microbiological Criteria for Foodstuffs [www.food.gov.uk/multimedia/pdfs/ecregguidmicro biolcriteria.pdf]). Guidelines are also being developed by the Commission for the use of microbiological criteria for official control purposes.

Execution and enforcement of EC hygiene legislation in the UK

The Food Hygiene (England) Regulations 2006 SI No.14 provide for the execution and enforcement of the Regulations (EC) Nos. 852/2004, 853/2004, 854/2004, 1688/2005, 2073/2005, 2074/2005, 2075/2005, and 2076/2005, designate competent authorities and enforcement authorities, and make provision for offences and penalties. The Regulations also address aspects where the EU Regulations either require or allow Member States to adopt certain provisions in their national law. These are:

- bulk transport in sea-going vessels of liquid oils or fats
- bulk transport by sea of raw sugar
- temperature control requirements
- direct supply of poultry and lagomorphs (rabbits, hares) slaughtered on farm
- restrictions on the sale of raw milk.

Restrictions on the sale of raw cow's milk intended for direct human consumption in England have been retained mainly on public health grounds. Raw cow's milk can only be sold at or from a farm, where the milk was produced, to: the ultimate consumer; a visitor to the farm premises or as part of a meal or refreshment; or a distributor (who can only sell direct to the final consumer). The raw milk must meet set microbiological standards (Regulation 32).

Temperature control requirements at Regulation 30 do not apply in relation to any food business operation to which Regulation EC (No) 853/2004 applies or carried out on a ship or aircraft. Chilled food is required to be held at less than 8 °C and hot food at over 63 °C with defences regarding time limitations and manufacturers' guidance. These control requirements relate to potential risks of growth of pathogenic micro-organisms or the formation of toxins within the shelf-life of the food product.

The FSA has produced a number of guidance documents to the new Regulations to help food businesses understand the legal requirements they have to comply with. This includes a main general guidance to the law and summary guides to the law for certain food sectors (www.food.gov.uk/multimedia/pdfs/fsaguidefoodhygleg.pdf). These guides should be read together with the EU and national legislation. The FSA has also produced a guide for the meat industry. Other guidance is also available including some from the EC on various aspects of the legislation (www.europa.eu.int/comm / food / international / trade / interpretation_imports.pdf).

Provisions of the Regulations relating to powers of enforcement and food safety requirements are that:

- The FSA is the competent authority for the purposes of the Community Regulations except where it has delegated competences as provided for in the Community Regulations. The FSA shall enforce and execute the Regulations in so far as the operator is carrying out primary production and associated operations listed in paragraph 1 of Part AI of Annex I to Regulation 852/2004. The food authority in whose area the FBO carries out operations shall enforce and execute the Regulation in those areas not enforced and executed by the FSA
- A range of enforcement measures to be available in respect of a FBO, namely: **hygiene improvement notices, hygiene prohibition notices, hygiene emergency prohibition notices and orders**, and remedial action notices and detention notices
- In the proceedings of an offence, it shall be a defence for the accused to prove that they took all reasonable precautions and exercised all **due diligence** to avoid the commission of the offence
- Procurement and **analysis of samples** by enforcement officers
- The Secretary of State may issue **codes of recommended practice** as regards the execution and enforcement of the Regulations and that any such code shall be laid before Parliament after being issued
- When an authorized officer of an enforcement authority has certified that any food has not been produced, processed or distributed in compliance with these Regulations and the Community Regulations, it shall be treated for the purposes of Section 9 of the Food Safety Act 1990 as failing to comply with food safety requirements.

Requirements of food hygiene legislation

Registration of establishments by FBOs
The objective of Article 6(2) of Regulation [EC] No. 852/2004 is to provide information for food authorities about food businesses in their area so that they can target enforcement resources more effectively. It is intended that food authorities should use the information provided by registration

to help plan their inspection programmes. The obligation to register and to notify changes to the authority falls on the proprietor of the food business (or the owner of premises used by more than one food business). There is no charge for registration and food authorities cannot refuse to register premises. Registration does not need periodic renewal, but changes in the nature of the business or a change of proprietor must be notified. Any new business has to apply to be registered at least 28 days before it opens. Seasonal businesses also must register and provide the period which they intend to be open each year.

Registration does not apply to those establishments for which approval only is required (Article 6(3) of Regulation [EC] No. 852/2004). Food business establishments that handle food of animal origin must, with certain exceptions, be approved by the CA.

Food Safety Act 1990

The Act covers Great Britain and provides the framework for all its food legislation. It has been amended by the Food Safety Act 1990 (Amendment) Regulations 2004 and the General Food Regulations 2004 as regards Regulation (EC) No. 178/2002 (see Section on UK execution and enforcement of EC Regulation 178/2002).

Powers to deal with contaminated food

Sections 7, 8 and 9 of the Food Safety Act, 1990

These provide substantial powers for local authorities to deal with offences caused by foods, which may have been contaminated with food poisoning organisms.

Section 7

This provides that it is an offence for food to be rendered injurious to health. In determining whether any food is injurious to health regard shall be had to the matters specified in Regulation (EC) No. 178/2002 (see Section on General Food Law). This Section allows food authorities to deal with situations such as occurred in 1989 when an unsuitably processed ingredient (hazelnut purée) was used in yoghurts produced by a number of farm dairies.

Section 8 provides that the sale of food not complying with food safety requirements is an offence. Foods fail to comply with food safety requirements if they are unsafe within the meaning of Article 14 of Regulation (EC) No. 178/2002 (see Section on General Food Law).

Regulation 23

This Regulation of the Food Hygiene (England) Regulations 2006 applies Section 9 of the Food Safety Act 1990 in that it empowers an authorized officer of a food and/or enforcement authority to inspect any food intended for human consumption and if it appears to fails to comply with food safety requirements, food can be seized or required not to be moved for up to 21 days pending investigations. If the authorized officer of a food enforcement authority is satisfied that it does not meet food safety requirements, it may be taken before a Justice of the Peace (JP) with a view to its being destroyed or otherwise disposed of. A prohibition can be imposed on removal of the food and its use for human consumption without inspecting it if it appears that the food is likely to cause food poisoning or other communicable disease. This power might be exercised for example as a preventive measure in response to a food alert received from the FSA that a particular batch of food was implicated in a food poisoning outbreak in the UK or another member country.

Compensation may be payable to any owner of the food in such cases where the authorized officer has detained or seized food which subsequently is found to be fit for human consumption. The reference in Section 9 to 'any disease communicable to human beings' allows action to be taken in respect of parasitic infections such as *Cryptosporidium* or *Giardia*, which do not necessarily fall under the definition of 'food poisoning' (see Chapters 4 and 7).

The Food Safety (Ships and Aircraft) (England and Scotland) Order 2003 (SI No. 1895)

This gives the power of entry to ships and aircraft (where it does not exist already) by authorized officers for the enforcement of certain Regulations of the Food Hygiene (England) Regulations 2006 SI No.14.

Section 13 of the FSA 1990 – emergency control orders

The FSA uses its food alert procedure in situations where nationally distributed foods are found to be hazardous. Food-enforcement authorities follow up with the wholesale, retail and catering outlets involved to ensure the removal of the food from distribution points, supermarket shelves and kitchens.

Section 13 empowers the minister to issue emergency control orders to prohibit commercial operations concerning food, food sources or contact materials where these may involve an imminent risk of injury to health. Such action would apply where the normal voluntary procedures for the withdrawal of food are not appropriate. Where necessary, ministers can direct food authority staff such as **environmental health officers** or **trading standards officers** to act to implement the terms of an order.

The Food Hygiene (England) Regulations 2006 – enforcement action related to premises

Regulation 6 – hygiene improvement notices
This Regulation provides the power to authorized officers to serve a **hygiene improvement notice** when they have reasonable grounds for believing that the proprietor of a food business is failing to comply with regulations relating to hygiene or to the processing or treatment of food. The notice must state the grounds for non-compliance, and specify the contraventions and measures necessary to secure compliance within a specified period of not fewer than 14 days. Failure to comply is an offence.

Regulation 7 – hygiene prohibition orders
This deals with 'health-risk conditions' in the operation of a food business. A health-risk condition is one that involves the risk of injury to health. A court is able to apply a prohibition on the use of equipment, a process, part of a premises, or the whole premises where it is satisfied that risk of injury to health applies. In addition, an order can be applied by the court on the proprietor or manager managing any food business to prevent them controlling the premises or any food business for a period of not less than 6 months.

When the health-risk condition is no longer fulfilled, the proprietor must apply for a certificate lifting the prohibition. There is a right of appeal against any decision of the local authority not to lift the hygiene prohibition order.

Regulation 8 – hygiene emergency prohibition notices and orders
Under this Regulation authorized officers of an enforcement authority can take necessary and immediate action themselves where conditions pose an imminent risk to health. The service of a hygiene emergency prohibition notice may impose the appropriate immediate prohibition on equipment, a process or the whole premises, but the notice must be followed up by an application to the court for a hygiene emergency prohibition order within 3 days. Any food authority not complying with the procedural requirements in Regulation 8 will be liable for compensation to the proprietor of the business. This may apply also if the court feels that the health-risk condition was not fulfilled. There will also be a liability to compensate if the court does not declare itself satisfied as to the existence of the health-risk condition at the time of the service of the notice.

Regulation 11 – the defence of due diligence
Most offences against the Food Safety Act 1990 are of strict liability. This means it is not necessary for the prosecution to prove that someone set out to commit an offence. As a consequence, a statutory due diligence defence is included at Section 21 of the Act and also at Regulation 11 of the Food Hygiene (England) Regulations 2006. It is therefore a defence for people to prove that they 'took all reasonable precautions and exercised all due diligence to avoid the commission of the offence by himself/herself or a person under his/her control'.

Less onerous conditions apply to businesses such as retailers, who neither prepare the food nor import it into the European Union. The purpose is to assign greater responsibility to those who have the greatest influence over the final product.

Regulation 24 – codes of recommended practice
This Regulation empowers ministers to issue codes of recommended practice to guide food authorities on the execution and enforcement of the Hygiene Regulations. The objective of issuing codes of recommended practice is to ensure more even and consistent standards of enforcement across the UK. The **Food Law Code of Practice and Guidance** is published on the FSA's website (www.food.gov.uk/ multimedia/pdfs/codeofpracticeeng.pdf). This Code is mandatory and as such, food authorities must comply with its requirements. In addition to the

Code, a good practice guide has been issued to food authorities. The Guide contains useful non-mandatory guidance for food authorities to help them discharge their functions under the Hygiene Regulations. Likewise, a new code of practice on the enforcement of animal feedstuffs legislation in the UK has been published.

Section 23 of the FSA 1990

Food authorities are enabled to provide training courses on food hygiene for food handlers within or outside their area.

The microbiological examination of food – food examiners

Regulations 12–13 of the Food Hygiene (England) Regulations 2006 empower an authorized officer to purchase or take samples of food, food sources, contact materials or any article or substance required as evidence from food premises and submit them for analysis by a public analyst or examination by a food examiner, who shall provide a certificate specifying the result of the analysis or examination. The EC Regulation on the microbiological criteria for foodstuffs ([EC] No. 2073/2005 [as amended]) provides for statutory sampling of food to verify the implementation of food safety systems by FBOs, such as HACCP. Samples of food have been traditionally collected during epidemiological investigations into foodborne disease and food poisoning outbreaks to assist in the identification of food vehicles.

The FSA 1990 created the entity of a food examiner to perform the statutory function of microbiological examination of food. In this task the food examiner will correspond to the role of the public analyst who has a long-standing traditional role in carrying out statutory chemical analysis of food samples related to nature, substance and quality, correct labelling and description of food being sold. Evidence by food examiners (including formal certificates) can be used by authorities to support prosecution cases in legal proceedings following microbiological contamination of food. Such evidence could also be used by the defence.

The Food Safety (Sampling and Qualifications) Regulations 1990 (SI No. 2463) sets out the procedures to be followed by enforcement offices, when taking samples for analysis or microbiological examination. They also stipulate qualification and practical experience requirements for public analysts and food examiners.

Good practice guides

The aim of good practice guides is to support effective application of the EC hygiene regulations. Article 7 of Regulation (EC) No. 852/2004 on the hygiene of foodstuffs provides for the development of national Guides to Good Hygiene Practice and the Application of HACCP principles (known as good practice guides). These guides are developed by individual food sectors, in consultation with interested parties. Food business operators may choose to use recognized good practice guides to help them comply with the requirements of Regulation (EC) No. 852/2004, Regulation (EC) No. 853/2004 (as amended) and related measures, including relevant UK hygiene regulations. However, good practice guides are voluntary and businesses therefore may demonstrate compliance with legislation in other ways. Several good practices guides have been developed for food sectors (Box 15.5).

Box 15.5 Some examples of good practice guides

- Bottled water
- Catering
- Flour milling
- Retail
- Vending and dispensing
- Wholesale distributors
- Markets and fairs
- Demersal fishermen
- Pelagic fishermen
- Nephrops fishermen
- Dairy UK

Demersal fish, such as haddock or cod, live in the lower water column; pelagic fish are migratory species of tuna, herring, mackerel, and smaller species such as sardines and anchovy; nephrops are prawns.

Article 9 of Regulation (EC) No. 852/2004 provides for the development of Community guides. These will have EU-wide status and be approved by the EC. Details of any such Community guides will be included in the FSA's list of good practice guides (www.food.gov.uk/multimedia/pdfs/practiceguidanceeng.pdf).

OFFICIAL CONTROLS

Regulation 882/2004 of the European Parliament and of the Council of 29 April 2004 on official controls performed to ensure the verification of compliance with feed and food law, and animal health and animal welfare rules

The Regulation (http://europa.eu.int/eur-lex/pri/en/oj/dat/2004/l_191/l_19120040528en00010052.pdf) lays down general obligations for official controls by Member States and has been applicable since 1 January 2006. It sets out the approach that competent authorities of Member States must adopt for official controls, i.e. for monitoring and enforcing compliance of businesses with feed and food law and with animal health and welfare rules. Such checks include, for example, inspections, audits, surveillance, sampling and analysis, etc. It also provides the legal basis for the European Commission, through its Food and Veterinary Office, to assess the effectiveness of national enforcement arrangements. The underpinning aim of the Regulation is to improve the consistency and effectiveness of official controls within Member States and across the EU and consequently to raise standards of food safety and consumer protection as well as preventing the spread of animal disease and improving animal welfare. The Regulation also aims to provide a greater degree of transparency for consumers about enforcement arrangements.

The Regulation describes in more detail how the basic principles of food and feed controls (outlined in the General Food Law Regulation (EC) No. 178/2002) are to be implemented in practice. It sets down the general principles and approach that the enforcement authorities should take. It takes a farm to table approach and covers controls at all stages of production, processing and distribution. It relates to foods produced within the EU and those exported to or imported from non-EU countries. New harmonized rules on checks on third country imports of non-animal products and for those considered 'high risk' are introduced, the new requirements are similar to those for animal products.

Article 41 of the Regulation requires Member States to prepare a single, integrated, 'multi-annual', national control plan. The purpose of this is to ensure effective implementation of official controls

in respect of feed and food law, animal health and welfare rules and, as appropriate, plant health law. The plans will also provide a basis of assessments of the performance of national control systems by the Commission's Inspection Services (the Food and Veterinary Office). Each Member State must have a national control plan in place by 1 January 2007 and, thereafter, must keep this under review and report to the Commission on its implementation on an annual basis. Article 42 of the Regulation sets out the general information that the control plan must include and there are also Commission guidelines for Member States to assist them in the preparation of their control plans (Article 43). The national control plan must cover the activities of all competent authorities within Member States that have responsibilities for official controls in respect of feed and food law, animal health and welfare rules and plant health law.

The Regulation sets down the principles that competent authorities should follow in undertaking official controls (Box 15.6).

Box 15.6 Requirements for official controls

- Adopting a risk-based approach
- Complying with certain operational procedures, e.g. having a sufficient number of suitably qualified and experienced staff, having appropriate legal powers, ensuring that staff are free from conflict of interest, and having and using documented control procedures
- Carrying out internal audit or having external audits undertaken
- Having contingency plans in place to deal with emergencies
- Ensuring that recognized methods of analysis are used and that **Official Food and Feed Control laboratories** meet certain standards (are accredited)
- Taking action where businesses are infringing legal requirements
- Being transparent by publishing information on control activities and their effectiveness.

An EU guidance document has been published on certain key questions related to import requirements and the new rules on food hygiene and official controls (www.europa.eu.int/comm/food/international/trade/interpretation_imports.pdf).

Official food control laboratories

The mutual recognition of microbiological results obtained by different control bodies is an essential pre-condition to unrestricted trade in food between the Member States. Under the terms of Regulation 882/2004 only official food control laboratories can examine **official control samples**. These laboratories will be accredited by their national accreditation organization according to the EN ISO/IEC 17025: 2005 and EN ISO/IEC 17011:2004 series of standards, and the Regulation also proposes that such laboratories participate in a proficiency testing scheme. In the UK this will mean accreditation by the United Kingdom Accreditation Service (UKAS), plus participating in a food microbiology quality assessment (proficiency testing) scheme, such as that provide by the Health Protection Agency.

Execution and enforcement of EC Regulation 882/2004 in the UK

The main legal measures to apply Regulation [EC] No. 882/2004 are included in the **Official Feed and Food Controls (England) Regulations 2006** (SI No. 15) and equivalent legislation in Scotland, Wales and Northern Ireland apply, which came into force on 11 January 2006. These legal instruments identify the authorities that are responsible for organizing and undertaking official enforcement checks and provide them with the powers to ensure that they are able to meet their obligations under the EU Regulation. They also provide for the enforcement of the new harmonized rules on non-EU country imports of feed and food of non-animal origin (e.g. vegetables, cereals, nuts, mushrooms, fruit and products made from these) as well as animal feeding stuffs. Non-EU country imports of food of animal origin are covered by the **Products of Animal Origin (Third Country Imports) (England) (No.4) Regulations 2004** (SI No. 3386). However, the Official Feed and Food Controls Regulations do apply to composite products that may contain a small (or limited) amount of product of animal origin. Importers will need to provide prior warning to the authorities of arrival of consignments and import them through specific ports (**border inspection posts**). The Official Feed and Food Controls Regulations also make provision for offences and penalties, checks on products, procurement and analysis of samples by authorized officers and food examiners, respectively.

The FSA has published guidance notes for feed and food businesses on the imports provisions for products of non-animal origin (www.food.gov.uk/multimedia/pdfs/offcindustryguidance.pdf). Similarly there is guidance for enforcement officers on the import provisions included in the **Food Law Code of Practice** (www.food.gov.uk/multimedia/pdfs/codeofpracticedraft.pdf) and **Practice Guidance** and the **Feed Law Code of Practice** (www.food.gov.uk/multimedia/pdfs/feedcop05.pdf).

In the UK, the FSA is the lead department with regard to matters relating to EU Regulation [EC] No. 882/2004 and has overall responsibility for application of the Regulation in respect of official controls for monitoring and enforcing feed and food law. The Department for Environment, Food and Rural Affairs (Defra) has overall responsibility for applications with respect to animal health and animal welfare. Although overall responsibility for official control for feed and food law and for animal health and welfare rules are held centrally, in practice, day-to-day responsibility for enforcement functions is divided between central and local government. The central authorities include the FSA, Defra, and the devolved agriculture departments and their agencies (e.g. the Meat Hygiene Service, Veterinary Medicines Directorate, Pesticides Safety Directorate, Dairy Hygiene Inspectorate, Egg Marketing Inspectorate, and State Veterinary Service). At the local level, much of the enforcement of feed and food law and animal health and welfare rules is carried out by local authorities. Responsibility for implementing and enforcing plant health controls in England rests with Defra. The devolved agriculture departments, and their agencies, have similar responsibilities in relation to Scotland, Wales, and Northern Ireland. Local port health authorities at ports (sea or air) are responsible for checking food imports at borders. In addition, there are 30 authorized border inspection posts with responsibility for controls on products of animal origin entering the UK from third countries.

The FSA has issued Q&A notes for enforcement authorities on the new EU Regulation on official feed and food controls (882/2004; www.food.gov.uk/foodindustry/regulation/europeleg/feedandfood/offcfaq). The Q&A notes are designed to explain the provisions of the Regulation and to provide informal and non-statutory advice. They are aimed primarily at the enforcement authorities in the UK, but may also provide useful information for the feed and food industries, and for consumers.

Overview of the general food, hygiene and official food control Regulations

Table 15.1 provides an overview of the UK execution and implementation of the EC General Food Law, the hygiene package, and implementation and transitional measures and official food controls. The various bodies involved in UK food safety and hygiene legislation for England are shown in Figure 15.1. There are similar bodies in the devolved administrations (Wales, Scotland, Northern Ireland).

Table 15.1 *General food law, food hygiene, and official food controls*

Food law	EC legislation	UK execution and enforcement
General food law	EC General Food Law Regulation [EC] No. 178/2002	Food Safety Act (Amendment) Regulations 2004 SI No. 2990 The General Food Regulations 2004 SI No. 3279 (as amended)
Food hygiene package	Regulation (EC) No. 852/2004 of the European Parliament and of the Council on the hygiene of foodstuffs Regulation (EC) No. 853/2004 of the European Parliament and of the Council laying down specific hygiene rules for food of animal origin (as amended) Regulation (EC) No. 854/2004 of the European Parliament and of the Council laying down specific rules for the organization of official controls on products of animal origin intended for human consumption (as amended) Directive 2002/99/EC laying down the animal health rules governing the production, processing, distribution and introduction of products of animal origin for human consumption	The Food Hygiene (England) Regulations 2006 (SI No.14) (as amended) provide the framework for the EU legislation to be enforced in England. There are equivalent regulations in Wales, Scotland and Northern Ireland
Food hygiene implementing measures and transitional arrangements	Regulation (EC) No. 2073/2005 of 15 November 2005 on microbiological criteria for foodstuffs (as amended) Regulation (EC) No. 2074/2005 of 5 December 2005 laying down implementing measures for certain products under Regulation (EC) No. 853/2004 and for the organization of official controls under Regulation (EC) No. 854/2004 and Regulation (EC) No. 882/2004, derogating from Regulation (EC) No. 852/2004 and amending Regulations (EC) No. 853/2004 and (EC) No. 854/2004 (as amended) Regulation (EC) No. 2075/2005 of 5 December 2005 laying down specific rules on official controls for *Trichinella* in meat (as amended) Regulation (EC) No. 2076/2005 of 5 December 2005 laying down transitional arrangements for the implementation of Regulations (EC) No. 853/2004, (EC) Nos 854/2004 and 882/2004 and amending Regulations (EC) Nos 853/2004 and 854/2004 (as amended) Regulation (EC) No. 1688/2005 of 14 October 2005 implementing Regulation (EC) No. 853/2004 as regards special guarantees concerning *Salmonella* for consignments to Finland and Sweden of certain meat and eggs	The Food Hygiene (England) Regulations 2006 (SI No.14) (as amended) provide the framework for the EU legislation to be enforced in England. There are equivalent regulations in Wales, Scotland and Northern Ireland
Official food controls	Regulation (EC) No. 882/2004 of the European Parliament and of the Council of 29 April 2004 on official controls performed to ensure the verification of compliance with feed and food law, and animal health and animal welfare rules	The Official Feed and Food Controls (England) Regulations 2006 (SI No. 15) provide the legal measures to apply Regulation [EC] No. 882/2004. There are equivalent regulations in Scotland, Wales and Northern Ireland

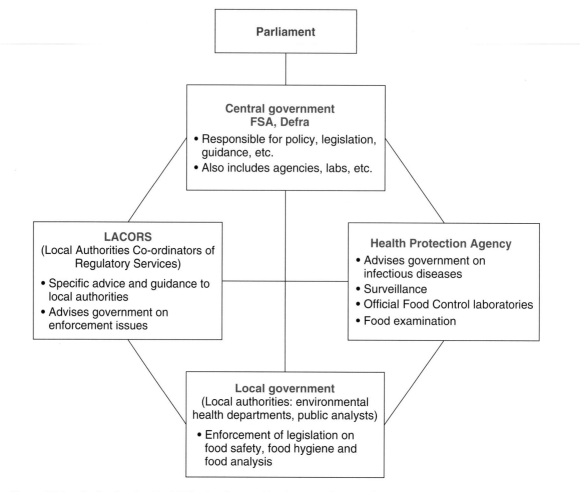

Figure 15.1   *Bodies involved in UK food safety and hygiene law (England)*

Food Standards Act 1999

The main purpose of this Act was to establish the FSA, provide it with functions and powers, and to transfer to it certain functions in relation to food safety and standards under other Acts. The FSA (www.food.gov.uk) is an independent government department set up by this Act in 2000 to protect the public's health and consumer interests in relation to food. The FSA provides advice and information to the public and government on food safety from farm to fork, nutrition and diet. The FSA has overall responsibility in the UK for the enforcement of food law, thereby protecting consumers through effective food enforcement and monitoring.

General Product Safety Regulations 2005

The General Product Safety Regulations 2005 Statutory Instrument (SI) 2005 No. 1803 came into force on 1 October 2005 and revoke the General Product Safety Regulations 1994 SI 2328 and implement into the UK the provisions of Directive 2001/95/EC, on General Product Safety.

These Regulations impose requirements concerning the safety of products intended for consumers or which are likely to be used by consumers. They set in place a **general safety requirement** meaning that only safe products should be on the market. The Regulations also require producers to inform consumers about the risk of products and to monitor the risk that their products pose.

As food is subject to a specific safety requirement under the General Food Law Regulation, the General Product Safety Regulations will not apply directly to food products. However, the safety of, for example, packaging and adverse reactions to food as a result of food allergies/intolerances would be dealt with under these Regulations as it is the food product as a whole, not the safety of the food itself, that is addressed. The Regulations also give enforcement authorities the power to issue safety notices of varying kinds (Box 15.7).

Box 15.7 Safety notices

- **Suspension notices** – to suspend the supply of product
- **Requirements to mark** – which require warnings to be marked on a particular product
- **Requirements to warn** – those who have already been supplied with a particular product
- **Withdrawal notices** – requiring products not to be placed on the market or supplied
- **Recall notices** – requiring the recall from consumers of products that have already been supplied to them

---

COMMUNICABLE DISEASE LEGISLATION

Communicable disease legislation in the UK

The core legislative tools concerning communicable disease in England and Wales are the Public Health (Control of Disease) Act 1984 and the Public Health (Infectious Diseases) Regulations 1988. Similar provisions exist in Scotland and Northern Ireland. They provide UK local authorities wide-ranging powers to control communicable disease. Local authorities exercise these powers in one of two ways: either by direct action or through the proper officer. The proper officer is an officer appointed by the local authority for a particular purpose. For communicable disease control issues, the proper officer is usually the **Consultant in Communicable Disease Control (CCDC)**.

The diseases notifiable under the provisions of the Public Health (Control of Disease) Act 1984 include **food poisoning**. There are also diseases notifiable under the provisions of the Public Health (Infectious Diseases) Regulations 1988, including dysentery (amoebic or bacillary), paratyphoid fever, typhoid fever, and viral hepatitis. The provisions most widely used (Sections 19, 20 of the Act) exclude persons from work if they know they have a notifiable disease yet carry on a trade, business or occupation that is likely to spread the disease. The proper officer may request such persons to discontinue work. Likewise Schedule 4 of the 1988 Regulations empowers the local authority to stop someone working with food. This applies to anyone suffering from food poisoning or found to be a carrier of food poisoning organisms including those able to give rise to typhoid and paratyphoid fevers, salmonella or shigella infections or staphylococcal intoxication; the local authority may take any measures as advised by the proper officer to prevent the spread of infection. The local authority must compensate persons who suffer financial loss.

Other powers within the Act allow application to a JP for the medical examination of a person or persons believed to be suffering from a notifiable disease or infection. The JP may order the removal of such persons to hospital. The **District Health Authority**, the **Chief Medical Officer** of the **Department of Health**, and the FSA must immediately be informed of any serious outbreak of food poisoning or any case of serious foodborne disease. Medical expertise is provided by CCDCs who are employed by the Health Protection Agency in England, but act as local authority officers when they are needed in outbreaks of foodborne disease and to provide medical support. CCDCs are accountable to **directors of public health**, who are responsible for the control of communicable disease (including food poisoning) in health authority districts.

The Health Protection Agency (www.hpa.org.uk) is a national organization, which was created on 1 April 2003 to protect people's health by minimizing risks from infectious diseases, poisons, chemicals, biological and radiation hazards. It consists of a number of centres such as the HPA Centre for Infections, Centre for Emergency Preparedness and Response, Centre for Radiation, Chemical and Environmental Hazards, the Local and Regional Services and the Regional Laboratory Network. The Agency is responsible for:

- advising the government on public health matters
- delivering services to protect public health

- providing impartial advice and information to professionals and the public
- providing a rapid response to health protection emergencies
- improving knowledge of health protection through research, development, education and training.

Communicable disease legislation in the European Union

The EC has gradually strengthened co-operation in public health, especially in communicable disease surveillance and control. Since the end of 1998, a co-operative framework has been enshrined in law by a decision of the European Parliament and of the Council establishing the **Community Network for the Epidemiological Surveillance and Control of Communicable Diseases** (Decision No. 2119/98/EC). This has organized the co-ordination of national surveillance systems and institutes/agencies on the basis of a common list of diseases under surveillance (Decision 2000/96/EC), common case definitions and common laboratory methods (Decision 2002/253/EC). Moreover, it put in place the **Early Warning and Response System** (EWRS) (Decision 2000/57/EC) of the European Community which connects the competent authorities of all the EU Member States responsible for formally notifying outbreaks of disease on the common list and for communicating information on counter-measures, or information on measures already taken if these had to be taken without delay.

Building on how best to improve surveillance and outbreak investigation, and capacity for advice and training, the Council and the European Parliament adopted enabling legislation (Regulation [EC] No. 851/2004) to create a **European Centre for Disease Prevention and Control** (ECDC) in 2004. This new EU agency (www.ecdc.eu.int/), based in Stockholm (Sweden), will provide a structured and systematic approach to the control of communicable diseases and other serious health threats which affect EU citizens. The ECDC will also mobilise and significantly reinforce the synergies between the existing national centres for disease control.

The initial focus of the Centre will be on communicable diseases and outbreaks of disease of unknown origin. The ECDC will enable Europe to pool its disease control expertise more effectively, allowing EU disease outbreak investigation teams to be put together quickly and efficiently. It will ensure the results of their investigations are available to the public health authorities around the EU; and it will produce authoritative advice and recommendations to guide EU and national decision makers.

Control of zoonoses

Animal health is an important factor in food safety because some diseases (zoonoses; diseases that can be transmitted from animals to humans) such as brucellosis, salmonellosis and listeriosis, can be transmitted to humans in particular through contaminated food. The European Commission has adopted a **zoonoses package** of legislation aimed at reducing the incidence of foodborne disease in the EU. The legislation is made up of two laws, and came into force in November 2003.

The first law **Directive 2003/99/EC** replaces earlier EC legislation on monitoring zoonoses and zoonotic agents, and EFSA will be instrumental in assessing information on the sources and trends of pathogens. **Decision 2004/564/EC** provides EFSA with the responsibility for collating, assessing and reporting data on zoonoses, zoonotic agents (any bacteria, virus, parasite or other biological agent likely to cause a zoonoses), and antimicrobial resistance to these agents. EFSA's *First Community Summary Report on Trends and Sources of Zoonoses, Zoonotic Agents and Antimicrobial resistance in the European Union in 2004* was published in December 2005 (www.efsa.eu.int/science/monitoring_zoonoses/reports/1277_en.html).

The aim of the second law **Regulation (EC) No. 2160/2003** is to ensure that effective measures are taken to detect and control *Salmonella* and other zoonotic agents at all relevant stages of production, processing and distribution, and once prevalence of these pathogens in Member States has been investigated, targets will be set to reduce them. *Salmonella*, particularly in poultry products and eggs, has been identified as the priority target. EU Member States will have to adopt national control programmes and encourage collaboration from the private sector in order to achieve the reduction targets, the first of which was set in late 2004. Certification of *Salmonella* status will be compulsory for trade between Member States and third countries.

Earlier legislation ensured compulsory monitoring of salmonellosis, brucellosis, trichinosis, and tuberculosis due to *Mycobacterium bovis*, and laid down rules for voluntary monitoring of other zoonotic agents. Foodborne outbreaks and antimicrobial resistance monitoring were not covered. The new directive will enable harmonization of such schemes. It will introduce control measures in more types of animal populations, and for more types of *Salmonella* and other zoonotic agents.

International Health Regulations

On 23 May 2005, a new set of **International Health Regulations 2005** (IHR) was approved by the World Health Assembly (a supreme decision-making body of the World Health Organization [WHO]), and will formally come into force in 2007. These Regulations are a legally binding code of practices and procedures designed to prevent the international spread of infectious diseases, while minimizing interference with world travel and trade. The current regulations were first agreed by the Member States of the WHO in 1969 and include procedures for notification of certain diseases, health-related rules for international travel and trade, procedures and practices at ports and borders and documentation requirements. For some time, however, the regulations have been recognized to be inadequate for the challenges posed by the twenty-first century global village, and, for example, have contributed little in the face of newly emerging infections such as severe adult respiratory syndrome (SARS) and avian influenza. They set out roles and responsibilities for the WHO and its Member States, but only in relation to three diseases: infectious cholera, plague, and yellow fever.

The new Regulations reflect internationally accepted good practice. They set out rules and operational mechanisms for a more co-ordinated international response to the spread of disease. Countries will have much broader obligations to build national capacity for surveillance and response as well as routine preventive measures (such as public health actions at ports and for means of transport). A particular emphasis is on developing the ability to detect and respond to public health emergencies of international concern and share information about them, with a code of conduct for notification and response. Specific attention is placed on detecting the emergence of new diseases or novel variants of diseases. There is also provision for detecting deliberately released agents. The regulations include a list of diseases such as smallpox, polio and SARS, whose occurrence must be notified to the WHO, but also include a matrix to help national authorities decide whether other incidents constitute public health events of international concern. Consideration is given to whether an outbreak is serious, unusual or unexpected, if there is a significant risk of international spread and if there is a significant risk of international travel or trade restrictions.

Summary

Food safety is a high profile matter attracting a great deal of attention. All too often it has been elevated to public attention by a catastrophic incident. The law which seeks to promote food safety is necessarily complex, and FBOs must know the rules and regulations, and must work daily to ensure the safety of the food products entering the market. Members of the public also depend on competent authorities to ensure verification and compliance of FBOs with the Regulations. Since 1 January 2006, food hygiene legislation has applied to farmers, growers and other producers, in many cases for the first time, as part of the 'farm to fork' approach to food safety. The overall impact of the developments in EC legislation outlined in this chapter should optimize public health protection. Legislation is constantly changing: the law and guidance detailed here is current as of 25 February 2006.

All websites cited in this chapter and below were accessed in November 2006.

SOURCES OF INFORMATION AND FURTHER READING

Atwood B (ed.) (2000) *Butterworth's Food Law*. London: Butterworths, 2000.

Bassett WH (ed.) (2004) *Clay's Handbook of Environmental Health*, 19th edn. London: Spon Press, 2004.

Campden & Chorleywood Food Research Association Group (eds) (2002) *UK Food Law Notes*. Chipping Campden, UK: Campden & Chorleywood Food Research Association Group.

European Commission Food and Feed Safety. Food Safety – From the Farm to the Fork (available at: http://europa.eu.int/comm/food/food/index_en.htm).

European Food Safety Authority (www.efsa.eu.int/).

Food Standards Agency (www.food.gov.uk).

16

Microbiological criteria

Christine Little

Introduction	301	Sampling plans, limits and analytical methods	306
Development of criteria	301	Appropriate level of protection and food safety	
Application of microbiological criteria	304	objectives	309
Responsibility of food businesses	304	Summary	311
Role of competent authorities	305	Sources of information and further reading	311

The purpose of establishing microbiological criteria is to protect the health of the consumer by providing safe, sound and wholesome products, and to meet the requirements of fair practices in trade. Microbiological criteria provide guidance on the acceptability of foodstuffs and their manufacturing processes. Microbiological testing alone cannot guarantee the safety of the foodstuff, but criteria for interpreting test results provide objectives and reference points to assist food business operators (FBOs) and competent authorities in their activities to manage and monitor the safety of foodstuffs. Of equal, or greater, importance is the use of Good Hygiene Practice, in conjunction with the application of Hazard Analysis and Critical Control Point (HACCP) principles, to ensure that undesirable organisms are eliminated as far as is practical. Microbiological criteria can be used in validation and verification of HACCP procedures and other hygiene control measures.

Microbiological criteria These provide objectives and reference points to assist **FBOs** and **competent authorities** to interpret results of tests to manage and monitor the safety of foodstuffs, respectively. These criteria can be categorized as **standards, guidelines** and **specifications** according to the intended application.

Microbiological standard This criterion is contained in law or regulation where compliance is mandatory. As well as being an offence, products not complying with the standards are rejected as unfit for their intended use.

Microbiological guideline This criterion is applied at any stage of food processing that indicates the microbiological status of the sample. These are usually intended to guide the manufacturer and help to ensure good hygienic practice. Significant deviations from a target guideline usually indicate the need for investigation and attention before control is lost. Investigative action is required to identify and rectify problems.

Microbiological specification This criterion is applied to a purchase agreement between a manufacturer and a purchaser to check that foods are of the required quality. These criteria may include pathogens, toxins, spoilage or indicator organisms. Non-conforming products will need to be investigated to determine the cause.

INTRODUCTION

This chapter will cover international principles of developing **microbiological criteria** but confines consideration of **microbiological standards** to European Union (EU) legislation.

DEVELOPMENT OF CRITERIA

Several international organizations are concerned with the establishment and application of microbiological criteria (Box 16.1) for foods. These include the European Commission (EC), the World

Health Organization (WHO), the International Commission on Microbiological Specifications for Foods (ICMSF) and the Codex Alimentarius Commission. According to the Codex Alimentarius:

> a **microbiological criterion** for food defines the acceptability of a product or food lot, based on the absence or presence, or number of microorganisms including parasites, and/or quantity of their toxins/metabolites, per unit(s) of mass, volume, area or lot.

Box 16.1 Main principles for developing microbiological criteria

- Microbiological criteria should be established and applied only where there is a definite need and where their application is practicable
- A mandatory microbiological criterion shall only apply to those products and/or points of the food chain where no other effective tools are available, and where it is expected to improve the degree of protection offered to the consumer
- The micro-organisms included in the criterion should be widely accepted as relevant pathogens or as indicator organisms to the particular food and technology

---

The need to set microbiological criteria for the causative agents of foodborne illnesses of most concern, such as *Salmonella*, *Campylobacter*, and *Listeria monocytogenes*, means that FBOs must comply with these requirements. They also have to take into consideration sampling and testing of the pathogen in their HACCP systems.

Existing criteria are revised on the basis of the latest scientific advice and international principles, taking into account new microbiological hazards and developments in food technologies and methods of analyses. Setting of criteria is a risk management measure which not only increases consumer protection, but also increases competitiveness between FBOs including third (non-EU) country importers by a fair and transparent set of EU rules. According to Codex, to establish microbiological criteria, consideration should be given to the following:

- evidence of actual or potential hazards to health (e.g. epidemiological evidence or the outcome of a microbiological risk assessment)

- the microbiology of raw materials
- the effect of processing
- the likelihood and consequence of contamination and growth during handling, storage and use
- the category of consumers at risk
- the cost–benefit ratio of the application
- the intended use of the food.

These considerations are of a very general nature and apply to all foods. When dealing with specific foods, however, decisions must be made about where criteria are to be applied in the food chain and what would be achieved by applying them.

Traditionally, control of micro-organisms in a food has been demonstrated by microbiological testing of food samples at various stages of production and of the final product. Criteria have been developed to provide some degree of assurance that food is safe and of suitable quality. It must be recognized that microbiological testing can never give an absolute assurance of product safety, particularly because of the problems involved in product sampling and the distribution of micro-organisms in food. Used sensibly however, microbiological testing is a valuable tool to validate and verify that critical control points remain under control in HACCP-based systems in the food industry. Microbiological criteria relate:

- directly to the hazard
- to other organisms that, if present, are considered to correlate with the presence of the hazard (i.e. **indicator organisms**)
- to loss of quality as suggested by total aerobic counts, and/or the presence of spoilage bacteria.

Microbiological criteria can be used to design products and processes and to indicate the required microbiological status of raw food materials, ingredients or end-products at any stage of the 'farm to fork'. Criteria are developed by regulators charged with protecting consumer health and ensuring the quality of foods or by food manufacturers to formulate design requirements or examine end-products for verification of a HACCP system. Therefore, criteria are used either by those concerned with the role of the regulatory authorities in protecting consumers and stated as legal requirements or by those in the industry for meeting legal requirements and to establish and maintain internal targets.

In international trade, microbiological criteria are also used as a means of assessing product safety at the '**port of entry**' because usually little is known of the methods of production or the efficacy of food safety systems operating in the country of origin. But previously, many problems arose through the application of these criteria. The lack of harmonized Community criteria led to different interpretations concerning the acceptability/rejection of batches of food produced in the Community or imported and also caused problems for border-control as well as intra-Community trade. In addition, before 2006, criteria in Community legislation were applicable at the site of food production and were used for import control and intra-community trade, but not at retail level, with the exception of the criteria set for natural mineral waters. Furthermore, there were no criteria for food of non-animal origin in previous Community legislation. The great need to harmonize criteria for the trade of foodstuffs led to the development of the Commission Regulation on microbiological criteria for foodstuffs, and these came into force in January 2006.

Commission Regulation on Microbiological Criteria for Foodstuffs

Microbiological criteria in the EU have been harmonized in Community legislation by the European Commission Regulation on Microbiological Criteria for Foodstuffs ([EC] No. 2073/2005) which has been applied since 1 January 2006. It relates to the Regulation on the Hygiene of Foodstuffs ([EC] No. 852/2004) that also applies since 1 January 2006, and to the General Food Law Regulation ([EC] No. 178/2002) that came into force on 1 January 2005. In addition, the Regulation laying down specific rules for food of animal origin ([EC] No. 853/2004 contains criteria for marine biotoxins for live bivalve molluscs, raw milk, and *Trichinella* in meat [see Chapter 15]).

The Regulation on Microbiological Criteria for Foodstuffs (Box 16.2) seeks to modernize and revise existing criteria and ensure that they are consistent and relevant to consumer health protection. The Regulation applies to all food businesses involved in the production and handling of food, including primary producers. To ensure compliance with the microbiological requirements, food businesses need to have a sampling and testing plan as part of their risk-based food safety management plan that is proportionate to the nature and size of their business. In addition, the competent authority (CA) verifies that the FBO complies with the Regulation. The CA may also use microbiological criteria for official control purposes in line with the requirements in the Official Control of Feed and Food Law Regulation ([EC] No. 882/2004), when undertaking sampling and analysis for a variety of purposes. These are then monitored for micro-organisms including those specified in the Regulation, as well as for verification of the food safety management plan, where food is suspected of being unsafe, or in the context of a risk analysis.

Box 16.2 Main objectives of Regulation on Microbiological Criteria for Foodstuffs

- Ensure a high level of consumer protection with regard to food safety
- Establish microbiological criteria only where there is a need and where application is practical
- Lay down microbiological criteria to be complied with by FBOs

---

There are two types of microbiological criteria set out in the Regulation:

- **Food safety criteria** – these define the acceptability of a product or a batch. Food safety criteria apply to the products at the end of the manufacturing process or to products which are already on the market. Non-compliance with these criteria requires notification by the FBO to the CA (in the UK the local authority and Food Standards Agency), in accordance with Article 19 of the General Food Law Regulation [EC] No. 178/2002. The prime focus of food safety criteria for foodstuffs is on *Salmonella* and *L. monocytogenes*.
- **Process hygiene criteria** – these define the acceptability of the process, and include criteria for pathogens and indicator organisms, and apply only during the manufacturing process for the following foods, food components and foodstuffs:
  - meat and meat products
  - milk and dairy products

- egg and egg products
- fish, shellfish and fishery products
- vegetables and fruit and their products.

The Regulation also includes rules for sampling and preparation of test samples. In the absence of more specific rules on sampling and preparation of test samples, the relevant standards of the International Organisation for Standardisation (ISO) and the guidelines of the Codex Alimentarius should be used as reference methods. Analytical methods other than reference methods can be used if they provide at least equivalent results. The Regulation stipulates a certain level of sampling for official control purposes and by the FBO for carcasses, minced meat, meat preparations and mechanically separated meat. Otherwise, sampling frequencies are the responsibility of FBOs and are based on the risks concerned and HACCP procedures.

APPLICATION OF MICROBIOLOGICAL CRITERIA

The Commission has adapted the definition of Codex Alimentarius in Regulation (EC) No. 2073/2005 with an extension to also cover the acceptability of processes. Thus a microbiological criterion for foodstuffs means a criterion defining the acceptability of a product, a batch of foodstuffs or a process, based on the absence or presence or number of micro-organisms (including parasites), and/or quantity of their toxins/metabolites, per unit(s) of mass, volume, area or batch.

A microbiological criterion should consist of the following components:

- a statement of the micro-organisms or their toxins/metabolites of concern and the reason for that concern
- the analytical methods including, when available, the analytical tolerance
- a plan defining the number of field samples to be taken and the size of the analytical sample
- microbiological limits considered appropriate to the food at the specified point(s) of the food chain
- the number of analytical units that should conform to these limits
- the foodstuff to which the criterion applies

- the point of the food chain where the criterion applies
- the actions to be taken when the criterion is not met.

The process hygiene criteria are applicable only to the food business manufacturing, preparing or producing the foodstuff in question. These criteria are set for a product at a specified stage of the process and they do not apply to products already placed on the market. These kinds of criteria are usually used in the monitoring of manufacturing and preparation processes. They are, for example, able to indicate whether good hygiene practices are being followed and may assist in checking if the HACCP procedures are functioning properly.

Criteria set for end-products (food safety criteria) may apply to the products ready to be placed on the market or which are already at the retail stage. These criteria are applicable to both the sale and delivery to final consumers as well as to the retail trade operators. Food safety criteria are also applicable at the point of entry to the EU when imported from countries outside it.

Food safety criteria are mandatory in nature whereas process hygiene criteria take the form of a guideline. Non-compliance with mandatory type of criteria would lead to rejection, sorting, reprocessing or withdrawal from the market of the product or batch in question. Non-compliance with the guideline type of criteria would usually lead to corrective actions in processing or handling of the foodstuffs and the FBO would normally decide on the actions to be taken. The measures required would depend on the risk involved, the point in the food chain and the product in question. The site of application and the actions to be taken in case of non-compliance will always be described in the criterion itself when laid down in the legislation.

RESPONSIBILITY OF FOOD BUSINESSES

The microbiological criteria to be complied with by FBOs in the new hygiene legislation are laid down on the basis of Regulation [EC] No. 852/2004 on the hygiene of foodstuffs. One of the basic obligations is that food businesses shall implement permanent procedures based on HACCP principles to ensure the safety of their products. Food business operators also have to comply with the microbiological criteria and take measures to meet the target set to achieve the objectives of the Regulation.

In addition to checking compliance with regulatory provisions (see Chapter 15), microbiological criteria may be applied by FBOs to formulate design requirements and to examine end-products as one of the measures to verify and/or validate the efficacy of the HACCP plan (see Chapter 10). Such criteria will be specific for the product and the stage in the food chain at which they apply. In addition to comparing the results against the criteria, food businesses can also follow and assess the trends in the results over a longer period of time. This allows them to react before the processes are already out of control and the limits exceeded.

Microbiological criteria are not usually suitable for monitoring critical limits as defined in the HACCP plan. Monitoring procedures must be able to detect loss of control at a critical control point. Monitoring should provide this information in time for corrective action to be taken to regain control before there is a need to reject a product. Consequently, online measurements of physical and chemical parameters are often preferred to microbiological testing because results are often available more rapidly and at the production site (see Chapter 10).

The Regulation on Microbiological Criteria for Foodstuffs is flexible with regard to the actions that may be taken to demonstrate compliance with the criteria. These should be determined by a risk-based approach, which depends on the specific circumstances. The flexibility provided permits food businesses to set sampling and testing plans according to the risk and within the framework of their food safety management procedures, apart from where specified sampling frequencies are provided for in Annex I of the Regulation. Equally it allows the FBO to apply the criteria within their own controls, and allows for alternative indicators to be monitored to ensure the process hygiene criteria are being met. For example, instead of testing as laid down in the Regulation, the FBO might equally monitor time/temperature profiles for a heat treatment process as a means of showing that the process criteria are being met.

The General Food Law Regulation (EC) No. 178/2002, which lays down general food safety requirements, states that where the foodstuffs tested exceed a food safety criterion, FBOs have an obligation not to place on, or to withdraw/recall

unsafe food from, the market. In addition, corrective actions must be undertaken to ensure the criterion is likely to be met with future production. However, where a process hygiene criterion is exceeded, the corrective actions taken should form part of their risk-based management system as well as those corrective actions specified in Annex I Chapter 2 of the Regulation, and that such batches of product may still be placed or remain on the market.

ROLE OF COMPETENT AUTHORITIES

Although the microbiological criteria for foodstuffs are mainly intended to be used by FBOs in the context of their HACCP procedures, CAs are required to verify the compliance of foods with the microbiological criteria laid down in Community legislation. The Regulation devolves competence to the Member States and allows them to decide how they will implement the checks in accordance with the Official Control of Feed and Food Law Regulations (EC) No. 882/2004 when undertaking sampling and analysis for a variety of purposes. In practice, this does not necessarily mean that the CA will take duplicate samples to verify results obtained by the FBO. It is envisaged that samples may be taken when monitoring for micro-organisms including those specified in the food safety management plan, where food is suspected of being unsafe, or in the context of a risk analysis: producer's samples from the market as well as samples from the border inspection point of imported products may be included here.

Within the framework of intra-Community trade or border inspection posts levels *only food safety criteria* are applicable, and the process hygiene criteria would only apply at production establishments where they would be verified by audit by the relevant national CA. Verification of compliance with the Regulation also includes assessment of the HACCP and other control systems operated by the food businesses and examination of documentation kept by the FBOs. In this context, CAs may check the results from microbiological testing and the actions taken in case of unsatisfactory results. In situations of non-compliance with microbiological criteria, depending on the assessment of the risk to the consumer, the point in the food chain and the product-type specified, the regulatory control actions may be sorting, reprocessing, rejection or destruction of product, and/or further investigation to determine appropriate actions to taken.

The Health Protection Agency has published guidelines (www.hpa.org.uk/infections/topics_az/food_sampling/Guidelines.pdf) on ready-to-eat foods at the point of sale to aid food examiners and CAs (e.g. enforcement officers). The purpose of these guidelines is to help determine the bacteriological quality of various ready-to-eat foods at the point of sale and to indicate the level of contamination that is considered to represent a significant potential risk to health. The guidelines are not intended to be prescriptive and have no legal standing in their own right.

SAMPLING PLANS, LIMITS AND ANALYTICAL METHODS

Sampling plans and microbiological limits should reflect the severity of the health hazard, the likelihood of its occurrence, and the expected conditions in which the foodstuff are handled and consumed. The described sampling plans should always be used, as a minimum, when the acceptability of a food batch or process is assessed. More guidance on sampling plans is provided in the ICMSF (2002) *Book 7: Microbiological Testing in Food Safety Management*. The first part of this book deals with the scientific rationale for the development of sampling plans.

Sampling plans

A sampling plan includes the sampling procedure and the decision criteria to be applied to a batch, based on examination of a prescribed number of sample units and subsequent analytical units of a stated size by defined methods. A well-designed sampling plan defines the probability of detecting micro-organisms in a batch, but it should be borne in mind that no sampling plan can ensure the absence of a particular organism. Sampling plans should be administratively and economically feasible. The choice of sampling plans should take into account:

- risks to public health associated with the hazard (severity and likelihood of occurrence of hazard)
- the susceptibility of the target group of consumers (very young or old, immunocompromised, etc.)
- the heterogeneity of distribution of micro-organisms where variables sampling plans are employed
- the acceptable quality level (i.e. percentage of non-conforming or defective sample units tolerated)
- the desired statistical probability of accepting or rejecting a non-conforming batch.

For many applications, **2-class** or **3-class attribute plans** may prove useful, as described below. The sampling method should be defined in the sampling plan.

Attribute plans

The number of samples selected for examination from a batch should be sufficient to indicate the extent of undesirable contamination likely to threaten health or lead to spoilage. In practice, only a small number of units from the batch can be examined, because of limited laboratory capacity and the expenses incurred. When the preliminary sampling of foods has yielded results which are thought to be dubious, careful attention should be paid to them with regard to numbers of samples, frequency of sampling and the interpretation of results. The ICMSF has devised a scheme for sampling which incorporates 2-class and 3-class plans.

The **2-class plan** provides presence or absence criteria for foodborne pathogens, such as salmonellae, from 'n' sample units. It has also been proposed that if the number of samples containing a pathogen ('c') was zero (for example n = 10, c = 0), samples might be bulked to reduce the length of time and amount of media required for tests. However, for epidemiological purposes, examination of individual samples may be necessary to find particular serotypes involved in outbreaks of food poisoning and the intensity of sampling may also be influenced by the degree of hazard arising from particular agents of foodborne disease. Factors to be considered are frequency of incidents, clinical severity, duration of illness, the extent of distribution of the pathogen in the implicated or suspected food, and the previous history of a food as a vehicle of infection or intoxication.

The **3-class plan** is based on enumeration of the general bacterial flora and takes into account minimum and maximum levels. In the ICMSF notation on sampling plans:

- n = the number of sample units
- m = the acceptable level
- M = the rejection level.

Values between m and M are undesirable, but subject to a number ('c' – reached by applying results and experience of previous tests), which can raise the acceptable level to meet the capabilities of the food industry concerned.

The ICMSF distinguishes foodborne pathogens and indicator organisms into five categories according to the degree of hazard (Box 16.3).

Box 16.3 Degrees of hazard

- **Severe hazards** – for (a) the general population or (b) restricted populations, causing life-threatening or substantial chronic sequelae or illness of long duration
- **Serious hazards** – incapacitating but not life-threatening
- **Moderate hazards** – severe discomfort of short duration
- **Indicator** – low indirect hazard
- **Utility** – e.g. general contamination, reduced shelf-life, spoilage

---

The first three categories of hazards and examples as presented in Table 16.1 are based on available epidemiological information, but may need to be reviewed when new data become available.

The other factor that needs to be considered is the likelihood of occurrence of an adverse effect, taking account of the anticipated conditions of use. The ICMSF distinguishes three conditions that:

- reduce the risk
- increase the risk
- do not cause a change in risk.

Combining the levels of severity with the categories of likelihood of occurrence produces different levels of concern called **cases**: case 7 being of lowest concern to food safety and case 15 the highest. Based on these 9 cases, the ICMSF has developed 2- and 3-class sampling plans, numbered according to degree of hazard. Cases 9, 12, and 15 represent the

Table 16.1 *Categories of hazards with examples**

Category of hazard	Pathogenic micro-organisms
Severe – for restricted populations	*Campylobacter jejuni* Enteropathogenic *Escherichia coli* *L. monocytogenes*
Severe – life-threatening for general population	*Clostridium botulinum* *Vibrio cholera* O1 *Salmonella typhi* Enterohaemorrhagic *E. coli*
Serious – incapacitating, not life-threatening	*C. jejuni* *Salmonella* (non-typhi) *Yersinia enterocolitica* *Shigella* (non-dysenteriae I) *L. monocytogenes*
Moderate – severe discomfort, short duration	*Staphylococcus aureus* *Vibrio parahaemolyticus* *Bacillus cereus* *C. perfringens*

* Based on International Commission on Microbiological Specifications for Foods (2002).

highest levels of concern as they refer to situations where pathogens can multiply in the food under expected conditions of handling, storage, preparation, and use (Table 16.2). Cases 7, 10, and 13 represent the lowest levels of concern, because they refer to intermediate situations of concern where the level of the hazard is likely to be reduced before consumption, for example during preparation. Cases 8, 11, and 14 refer to situations where the level of hazard remains the same between the time of sampling and the time of consumption.

Utility tests (tests providing information regarding general contamination, incipient spoilage, or reduced shelf-life) are included in cases 1–3 and include relatively lenient 3-class sampling plans (see Table 16.2). They may involve direct microscopic counts, yeast and mould counts, aerobic plate counts, or specialised tests, such as for cold-tolerant organisms or for species causing a particular type of spoilage, e.g. lactobacilli in mayonnaise. Indicator tests are included in cases 4–6 that are also 3-class sampling plans (see Table 16.2). It is important to recognize that relations between pathogen and indicators are not universal and are influenced by the product and process. Because of the uncertain relation between indicators and specific pathogens, the level of concern is moderate and it is appropriate to apply sampling plans with high stringency for indicator organisms.

Table 16.2 *Sampling plan stringency (case) in relation to degree of health concern and conditions of use**

Degree of concern relative to expected health effect	Conditions in which food is to be handled and consumed after sampling in the usual course of events		
	Conditions reduce degree of concern	Conditions cause no change in concern	Conditions may increase concern
Severe for – (a) restricted populations, or (b) life-threatening for general population	Case 13 2-class n = 15, c = 0	Case 14 2-class n = 30, c = 0	Case 15 2-class n = 60, c = 0
Serious – incapacitating, not life-threatening	Case 10 2-class n = 5, c = 0	Case 11 2-class n = 10, c = 0	Case 12 2-class n = 20, c = 0
Moderate – severe discomfort, short duration	Case 7 3-class n = 5, c = 2	Case 8 3-class n = 5, c = 1	Case 9 3-class n = 10, c = 1
Indicator – low indirect hazard	Case 4 3-class n = 5, c = 3	Case 5 3-class n = 5, c = 2	Case 6 3-class n = 5, c = 1
Utility – general contamination, reduced shelf-life, spoilage	Case 1 3-class n = 5, c = 3	Case 2 3-class n = 5, c = 2	Case 3 3-class n = 5, c = 1

n, number of sample units tested; c, number of defective sample units which can be accepted.
*Based on International Commission on Microbiological Specifications for Foods (2002).

An example of 2- and 3-class tests is provided in the Regulation on Microbiological Criteria for Foodstuffs for cooked crustaceans and molluscan shellfish; it is based on the examination of five samples per product batch. *Salmonella* is a food safety criterion, whereas the criteria for *Escherichia coli* and coagulase-positive staphylococci are process hygiene criteria.

Salmonella: n = 5, c = 0, m = not detected in 25 g

E. coli: n = 5, c = 2, m = 1 CFU/g, M = 10 CFU/g

Coagulase-positive staphylococci: n = 5, c = 2, m = 100 CFU/g, M = 1000 CFU/g

The Commission's intention is generally not to establish sampling frequencies in the Regulation, but based on the risks concerned and HACCP procedures, this would be the responsibility of the FBOs. In many cases the distribution of micro-organisms is not homogeneous and random sampling is not possible most of the time. This clearly illustrates that examination of batches or consignments of products for the presence of pathogens has only limited value as a control measure.

Microbiological limits

Microbiological limits should take into consideration the risk associated with the micro-organism, and the conditions under which the food is expected to be handled and consumed. Micro-biological limits should also take into account the likelihood of uneven distribution of micro-organisms in the food and the inherent variability of the analytical procedure. If a criterion requires the absence of a particular micro-organism, the size and number of the analytical unit (as well as the number of analytical units) should be included.

The microbiological limit defined in a criterion represents the level above which action is required. Levels must be realistic and should be determined from a knowledge of microbiology of raw materials and the effects of processing, product handling, storage and end-use on the microbiology of the end-product. Limits may be derived by determining microbial levels in products where conditions of processing, storage and product characteristics are known. They should take into account the levels that indicate inadequate control and may represent a hazard to health.

Microbiological methods

Preference should be given to methods that have been validated for the commodity concerned, preferably in relation to reference methods elaborated by international organizations. Only the reference methods are laid down in legislation, and preference must be given to **horizontal methods** (applicable to products intended for human consumption and for the feeding of animals, and to environmental samples in the area of food production and food handling) developed by international standardization organizations. Such methods should be used when compliance with regulatory requirements is monitored. Analytical methods other than reference methods can be used if they provide at least equivalent results. Although methods should be the most sensitive and reproducible for the purpose, those used for in-plant testing often sacrifice, to some degree, specificity and reproducibility in the interest of speed and simplicity. They should, however, have been proved to have a sufficiently reliable estimate of the information needed.

Plate counts should be interpreted with understanding and with caution because of the difficulty of obtaining reproducible results. Media and equipment also need to be standardized. Automated systems will relieve the drudgery of repetitive counts and they are likely to improve the reproducibility. The clumping of organisms in food will increase the variability of most probable number (MPN) counts of *E. coli* and of plate counts. The adherence of food particles and organisms to the lumen of pipettes and to other glassware cannot be eradicated entirely by homogenization and dilution. Water is the best medium for the even distribution of organisms. In spite of these drawbacks in the interpretation of results from counting methods, it is observed that the higher the general count as well as that of organisms with potential for food poisoning, the greater the risk. *Clostridium perfringens*, *Bacillus cereus* and *Staphylococcus aureus* are food poisoning agents but which are commonly found in food samples in small numbers. When isolated in large numbers – millions per gram of sample – they are indicative of both the potential for food poisoning and spoilage. Factors leading to growth in food are similar for most organisms.

Where legislation is required for criteria, it might be more appropriately applied to process control rather than to microbiological standardization of the end-product. Laboratory methods would then be concerned with tests for the destruction of enzymes or the change in colour of dyes, indicating reduced oxygen potential from growth of organisms, where such tests are applicable. When a heat process is involved, the destruction of the enzymes phosphatase in milk and α-amylase in liquid egg, for example, can be used to monitor the process. Dye tests are more arbitrary, but economical of time, effort and expense. The methylene blue reductase test is applicable to milk, cream and ice-cream although it is no longer included in the statutory tests for milk. A resazurin test may be used for the oxidation-reduction (redox) potential as a measure of the growth of organisms in foods. The quantitative evaluation of micro-organisms' metabolites, such as microbial adenosine triphosphate (ATP), may be used to monitor hygiene in food production sites. Instruments are available where a swab taken from food equipment or the environment can be assayed directly for ATP giving a virtual immediate measure of surface contamination. This speed and simplicity of ATP determination makes it suitable for routine monitoring of critical control points as part of quality assurance within HACCP.

APPROPRIATE LEVEL OF PROTECTION AND FOOD SAFETY OBJECTIVES

The **appropriate level of protection (ALOP)** is defined in the WHO's sanitary and phytosanitary (SPS) agreement as:

> the level of protection deemed appropriate by the member (country) establishing a sanitary or phytosanitary measure to protect human, animal or plant life within its territory.

The principles of microbiological risk management are currently being discussed in international forums. The new concepts of **food safety objective (FSO)**, **performance objective (PO)** and **performance criterion (PC)** have been introduced by Codex Alimentarius Commission as tools to be used in risk management of microbiological hazards in foodstuffs. However, their application is still under development. The following definitions have been accepted for these new concepts:

- **Food safety objective**: Maximum frequency and/or concentration of a microbiological hazard in a food at the time of consumption that provides or contributes to the ALOP.
- **Performance objective**: Maximum frequency and/or concentration of a hazard in a food at a specified step in the food chain before the time of consumption that provides or contributes to an FSO or ALOP, as applicable
- **Performance criterion**: Effect in frequency and/or concentration of a hazard in a food that must be achieved by the application of one or more control measures to provide or contribute to a PO or an FSO.

Box 16.4 shows an example of how these relate to each other.

In the context of microbiological risk management the ALOP is a reflection of a particular country's expressed public health goals for a microbiological hazard associated with a food. A description of ALOP may be in terms of a probability of an adverse public health consequence or an incidence in disease associated with a particular hazard-food combination and its consumption in a country.

The concept of FSO has been introduced because of the difficulties of relating control measures directly to an ALOP. While ALOP is an expression of a public health risk, an FSO expresses the level of hazard in relation to that risk. As the FSO applies to the time of consumption, it will need to be used in conjunction with performance or other criteria to establish the level of control needed to other parts of the food chain. In most cases the acceptable levels of hazard at the earlier stages of the food chain differ from the FSO. The PC and PO are by definition the required outcomes of control measures at a step or combination of steps to contribute to assuring the safety of food.

Some hypothetical examples of FSOs are:

- Staphylococcal enterotoxin in cheese not exceeding 1 µg/100 µg.
- *Salmonella enteritidis* in eggs not exceeding 1 egg per 100 000.
- Salmonellae in powdered milk below 1 CFU/100 g.

Box 16.4 FSO, PO and PC
- Hazard is *C. botulinum*
- PC is the change in numbers, i.e. 12D reductions (the process criterion is the critical limit of 2.45 min/121 °C)
- PO is <1 spore/10^{12} g after processing (assuming an initial concentration of <1 CFU/g)
- FSO is <1 spore/10^{12} g (when the product is ready for consumption)

Table 16.3 *Characteristics of food safety objectives and microbiological criteria**

Food safety objective	Microbiological criterion
A goal on which food chains can be designed so that the resulting food will be expected to be safe	A statement that defines the acceptability of a food product or batch of food
Aimed at consumer protection	Confirmation that effective good hygienic practices and HACCP† plans are applied
Applies to food at the moment of consumption	Applies to individual batches or consignments of food
Components: 　Maximum frequency and/or concentration of a 　　microbiological hazard 　Product to which it applies	Components: 　Micro-organisms of concern and/or their toxins/metabolites 　Sampling plan 　Analytical unit 　Analytical method 　Microbiological limits 　Number of analytical units that must conform to the limits
Used only for food safety	Used for food safety or quality characteristics

*Based on van Schothorst (2002).
† HACCP, Hazard Analysis and Critical Control Point.

- *L. monocytogenes* in ready-to-eat food below 100 CFU/g.

It is important that the PC be validated. Examples of well-established PCs are:

- 12D reduction of proteolytic *C. botulinum* in low-acid canned foods
- 6D reduction of *L. monocytogenes* in ready-to-eat chilled foods
- 6D reduction of psychrotrophic *C. botulinum* in pre-packed chill-stored foods with extended shelf-life.

As the application of the above concepts is still under development they could not be included in the recent recast of Community hygiene legislation in which targets and criteria have been set to facilitate the implementation of Regulation [EC]

No. 852/2004 on the hygiene of foodstuffs. However, in the future FSOs will be taken into consideration as a basis for Community legislation.

Although microbiological criteria differ in both function and content from FSOs (Table 16.3), there are some similarities in the way they are established. Occasionally the limit in a criterion is the same as a FSO as, for example, in the case of the FSO for *L. monocytogenes* in a ready-to-eat product (<100 CFU/g). Sampling plans are associated with microbiological criteria but not with FSOs. The FSO is (indirectly) an expression of the stringency required in food safety management in view of the level of public health concern. As such, it provides a link to control measures applied by food manufacturers. There will be a relation between a microbiological criterion and a FSO, but it may not be a direct one.

Summary

Microbiological criteria may be used to formulate design requirements and to indicate the required microbiological status of raw materials, ingredients and end-products at any stage of the food chain as appropriate. They may be relevant to the examination of foods, including raw materials and ingredients of unknown or uncertain origin, or when other means of verifying the efficacy of HACCP-based systems and good hygienic practices are not available. Generally, microbiological criteria may be applied to define the distinction between acceptable and unacceptable raw materials, ingredients, products and batches, by regulatory authorities and/or FBOs.

All websites cited in this chapter were accessed in November 2006.

SOURCES OF INFORMATION AND FURTHER READING

Brown M, Stringer M (eds) (2002) *Microbiological Risk Assessment in Food Processing*. Cambridge: Woodhead Publishing.

Codex Alimentarius (2004) *Food Hygiene Basic Texts, 3rd ed 2003*. Rome: Food and Agriculture Organization of the United Nations/World Health Organization.

European Food Safety Authority (2007) Opinion of the Scientific Panel on Biological Hazards on Microbiological Criteria and Targets based on risk analysis. *The EFSA Journal* **462**: 1–29.

International Commission on Microbiological Specifications for Foods (1994) Choice of sampling plan and criteria for *Listeria monocytogenes*. *Int J Food Microbiol* **22**: 89–96.

International Commission on Microbiological Specifications for Foods (2002) Microorganisms in Foods. *Book 7: Microbiological Testing in Food Safety Management*. London: Blackie Academic & Professional.

Institute of Food Science and Technology (1999) *Production of Microbiological Criteria*. London: Institute of Food Science and Technology.

International Life Sciences Institute (2004) *Food Safety Objectives – Role in Microbiological Food Safety Management*. Brussels: International Life Sciences Institute Europe.

van Schothorst M (2002) Implementing the results of an MRA: pathogen risk management. In: Brown M, Stringer M (eds) *Microbiological Risk Assessment in Food Processing*. Cambridge: Woodhead Publishing.

17

Education

Christine Dodd

Introduction	313	Keeping up to date	322
Education	314	Summary	324
Getting the message across	321	Sources of information	324

The production of a safe food depends on, and is the responsibility of, all those involved with foodstuffs, whatever their capacity. Therefore, all those involved with food need to be trained in the principles of food hygiene and how to prevent foodborne disease. The training methods will differ between groups but the basic principles are the same for all disciplines.

> **Food hygiene education** The process of acquiring knowledge and training for the prevention and control of foodborne disease.
>
> **Due diligence** 'a defence for the person charged to prove that he took all reasonable precautions ... to avoid the commission of the offence by himself or by a person under his control.' (Food Safety Act 1990 section 21 subsection 1).

INTRODUCTION

Foodborne disease occurs because organisms or toxins causing disease enter and survive in the food supply chain. The disease-causing agents can enter the food chain at almost any stage, from primary production or processing, through handling and cross-contamination, to inadequate cooking and storage. Thus all individuals involved with food – those with a professional responsibility for food and the consumers – need to be trained in the principles of food hygiene and how to prevent foodborne disease. Even the architects who design plant and equipment and plan kitchens, and the engineers involved in construction of establishments, abattoirs, markets and farms should be aware of their part in controlling the spread of foodborne disease.

Besides training in the basic principles, there is also a need for continued education to maintain food safety – processes and eating habits change, foods can be sourced from different places, and new information on new agents and hazards becomes available. Since the 1980s, *Listeria monocytogenes*, *Escherichia coli* O157:H7 *Salmonella* and *Campylobacter* have all become recognized as significant bacterial foodborne pathogens. Reported numbers of incidents of foodborne disease have shown a steady increase over the same period and the reasons for this are probably multifactorial. Changes in eating habits with an increased incidence of eating out have been suggested as a factor, but changes in food preferences such as increased consumption of ready-prepared meals and salad vegetables have also generated new sources of foodborne disease. Similarly, cooking practices have undergone a change over this period. The move to microwave cooking of prepared meals has changed cooking skills, and the popularity of the barbecue means that cooking is increasingly performed outdoors with less controlled cooking conditions. All these changes indicate there is a need for people to be educated about foodborne organisms and food hygiene, and for this knowledge to be periodically updated as a response to change.

In the UK, the current legislative requirement with regard to food safety, hygiene and general food law has changed in response to European Community harmonization. New food safety legislation was implemented on 1 January 2006, when the

European Union (EU) Food Hygiene Regulations replaced the existing body of food hygiene legislation with more modern, risk-based requirements. The new legislation includes the EC Regulation on the Hygiene of Foodstuffs 852/2004 and The Food Hygiene (England) Regulations 2006. The legislation affects all food businesses, including primary producers (such as farmers), manufacturers, distributors, caterers and retailers, but exactly how will depend on the size of the business. However, the new legislation will require all **food business operators** (FBOs) to provide appropriate documents and records showing how they are applying food safety management procedures based on **Hazard Analysis and Critical Control Point** (HACCP) principles. Employees will therefore require appropriate training to understand their role in the implementation and maintenance of suitable HACCP-based systems. More generally, FBOs must ensure that food handlers are supervised and instructed and/or trained in food hygiene matters commensurate with their work activity.

EDUCATION

The level of training needed varies with the involvement of the individual in food production. Everyone needs to understand the requirement for hygiene in food preparation to ensure personal safety, however, those involved at a professional level in food preparation and production have the additional responsibility of **due diligence** for their actions.

Professional training

Various levels and types of training regarding food safety and hygiene are available depending on the specific needs of particular groups. These range from foundation certificate courses in hygiene to degree and postgraduate level education. In some instances a number of bodies provide equivalent qualifications or new qualifications have been brought in. The National Database of Accredited Qualifications (www.openquals.org.uk/openquals/) provides guidance on courses and their equivalences.

Food hygiene legislation and due diligence require all food handlers to be appropriately trained. In the UK, three organizations provide nationally recognized food hygiene and safety courses: the Chartered Institute of Environmental Health (CIEH) the Royal Institute of Public Health (RIPH) and the Royal Society for the Promotion of Health (RSPH) with the Royal Environmental Health Institute for Scotland (REHIS) providing some aspects of training in Scotland. These organizations provide courses targeted at a wide range of people involved in food preparation, production and catering, as well those managing such professionals. Full details of the nature and availability of these training courses are available via the websites of each organization (see end of chapter for website addresses). Here a brief outline is provided.

The CIEH is concerned with the education and training of environmental health officers (EHOs) and the promotion and regulation of education and training of other environmental health practitioners. A fully qualified EHO will have passed an accredited degree course in environmental health, undertaken practical training and successfully completed a practical training logbook assessment and professional examinations. Accredited courses are currently offered by 11 universities and include undergraduate and postgraduate courses on a full-time or part-time basis. Information on requirements to undertake the degree and details of the content of courses is available on the CIEH website (www.ehcareers.org/).

The CIEH has a series of food safety courses leading to a Certificate in Food Safety at Foundation, Intermediate and Advanced levels (Table 17.1). In addition courses have been developed addressing the specific food safety needs of the catering and hospitality sector (Table 17.1):

- Level 2 Award in **Food Safety in Catering** – which provides fundamental food hygiene knowledge for all food handlers
- Level 3 Award in **Supervising Food Safety in Catering** – designed for those working at a supervisory level. Again, this is a sector-specific food safety qualification tailored for the catering environment
- Level 4 Award in **Implementing Food Safety Management Procedures** – for owners and managers of small- and medium-sized catering and hospitality businesses

All of these courses address the requirements of EU legislation which, since 1 January 2006, requires all

Table **17.1** *Food safety/hygiene courses for food handlers including those in the 'food service' (catering) sector*

Food hygiene/safety qualifications		New 'food service' sector qualifications	
Level 1	Foundation Certificate in Food Safety/Hygiene	Level 2	Food Safety in Catering
Level 2	Intermediate Certificate in Food Safety/Hygiene	Level 3	Supervising Food Safety in Catering
Level 3	Advanced Certificate in Food Safety/Hygiene	Level 4	Implementing Food Safety Management Procedures

businesses producing food to have a documented food safety management system in place based on HACCP principles. Separate courses are also run on HACCP:

- Level 2 Intermediate Certificate in Hazard Analysis Principles and Practice – for training of managers and supervisors in hazard analysis principles and their applications and legal requirements
- Level 3 HACCP in Practice Certificate – for managers, supervisors and owners of food businesses to prepare and implement a HACCP plan.

The CIEH also owns the publishing company Chadwick House Group Ltd, which publishes the Industry Guides to Good Hygienic Practice. Guides for various food producing sectors can be accessed on the internet or as books; for examples the guides for catering (http://archive.food.gov.uk/dept_health/pdf/catsec.pdf), retail (http://archive.food.gov.uk/dept_health/pdf/retsec.pdf) and ships catering (www.british-shipping.org/publications/Catering%20Guide.htm).

All inspectors of higher risk food premises working in a food hygiene enforcement authority in England, Wales and Scotland are required to hold the **Higher Certificate in Food Premises Inspection.** The CIEH accredits courses leading to this certificate in England and Wales. In Scotland, the Scottish Food Safety Officers' Registration Board, a committee of REHIS, administers and maintains the scheme of practical training for food safety officers. These officers are employed and authorized by Scottish local authorities to enforce a range of food safety legislation in a variety of food production premises. They can take the **Ordinary Certificate in Food Premises Inspection** (OC in FPI) or the **Higher Certificates in Food Premises Inspection** (HC in FPI) and **Food Standards Inspection** (HC in FSI), depending on their initial qualification levels.

The RIPH also offers foundation, intermediate and advanced food hygiene/safety courses, and, in addition, offers its qualifications to candidates throughout the world via a range of approved distance learning courses. The **Foundation Certificate in Food Hygiene** (Level 1; formerly the Basic Food Hygiene Certificate) incorporates fundamental food hygiene knowledge for all food handlers. Current industry guidance indicates that handlers of high-risk foods need to be trained to the standard described as Level 1. This qualification is suitable for food handlers in the food service sector, hospitals and food processing.

The intermediate course (Level 2 **Intermediate Certificate in Food Safety**) is designed for those working in all food businesses at a supervisory level including anyone who needs a broad understanding of food hygiene as part of their work, such as potential managers. These could be those involved in quality assurance or in training and those managing small- to medium-sized organizations. Qualification at Level 2 provides evidence of in-depth knowledge and understanding of food hygiene and safety that enables holders to identify and prevent food safety hazards at all stages in food production, preparation and service.

The **Advanced Food Hygiene Certificate** (Level 3) provides a high-level practical training programme with external accreditation and is designed for those with responsibilities for management of food production and with responsibilities for determining training, and supervision of food handlers, i.e. senior staff and managers. This qualification requires holders to apply their knowledge and judgement to problems affecting all aspects of food safety management.

The Level 2 Award in **Food Safety in Catering** is a new award aimed at providing a basic understanding about safety in relation to food preparation and handling within the catering and hospitality sector. It has been developed to meet the new occupational standards in food safety in this sector and recent changes in legislation. This award may also be appropriate for people whose work requires them to enter food premises, e.g. equipment maintenance engineers. Foundation, Intermediate and Advanced Certificates in HACCP Principles are also available.

The RSPH provides a range of training programmes in food hygiene and safety. As well as offering a Foundation Certificate in Food Hygiene and Intermediate and Advanced Certificates in Food Safety, it also offers a new series of accredited awards (accredited by the Qualifications and Curriculum Authority) specifically designed for the catering and hospitality industries. These courses have all been in place since January 2006 (see Table 17.1 for a summary). The Level 2 Award in Food Safety in Catering is aimed at food handlers in the catering and hospitality industries whose training would previously have been addressed through Level 1 Foundation Certificate in Food Hygiene: Option A; it is particularly directed at those working with 'high-risk' foods such as unwrapped or open foodstuffs. The Level 3 Award in Supervising Food Safety in Catering is targeted to food handlers working in the hospitality and catering industries who have a supervisory role; the content is similar to the Level 2 Intermediate Certificate in Food Safety but with a change of emphasis towards those aspects that enable supervisors to identify and rectify problems in the area. The Level 4 Award in Managing Food Safety in Catering is equivalent to the Level 3 Advanced Certificate in Food Safety and is specifically designed for those food handlers in the hospitality and catering industry who have, or are training for, a management role. In particular it emphasizes food safety management systems consistent with HACCP principles and addresses the role of the manager in the development of a food safety culture within the business and communicating risk assessment. Specialist training in the form of courses such as Level 2 Certificate in Wild Game Meat Hygiene is also offered.

The Meat Training Council (MTC) administers a range of courses and training programmes for the red meat and poultry sectors. These include a range of National Vocational Qualifications (NVQs) or Scottish Vocational Qualifications (SVQs) appropriate for all sectors of the red meat and poultry industry, from the abattoir to processing, wholesale,

manufacturing, catering, butchery and independent or multiple retail. Four levels are available:

- Level 1 – for new staff or those with little individual responsibility
- Level 2 – for operative or craft level staff
- Level 3 – for supervisory management/ technical operations
- Level 4 – for technical and production managers.

These courses cover all skills, not just hygiene, needed in the meat industry. Full details of these can be found on the MTC website (www.meattraining.org.uk).

The MTC also administers Vocational Related Qualifications (VRQs) for meat handlers. These include the Foundation Certificate in Meat and Poultry Hygiene (including HACCP awareness), the Advanced Certificate in Meat and Poultry Hygiene (Level 3) and the Meat Safety Certificate and the Basic Meat Safety Certificate which is jointly awarded in England, Wales and Northern Ireland by CIEH and the MTC, with appropriate awarding arrangements for Scotland (www.meattraining.org. uk/pages/msc.htm). A number of HACCP VRQs are also awarded including Intermediate Certificate in HACCP Practice (Meat Plant) and a Meat Managers' Hygiene and HACCP Course designed to assist butchers in HACCP awareness and meeting licensing requirements (www.meattraining.org. uk/pages/haccp.htm).

The Meat Hygiene Service provides verification, audit, and meat inspection services in approved fresh meat premises. Meat hygiene inspectors (MHIs) and poultry meat inspectors (PMIs) work alongside plant staff on the production line at various critical points, and ensure that animal welfare and hygiene standards are observed throughout the production process, under the direction of the Official Veterinary Surgeon. Meat inspectors need to hold the RSPH Level 3 Certificate in Meat Inspection (or, where appropriate, the Certificate in Poultry Meat Inspection). This is a statutory qualification, involving at least 400 hours of training. The RSPH also offers the Level 2 Certificate in Wild Game Meat Hygiene to comply with the latest food hygiene regulations.

University and postgraduate training

At degree level, food hygiene and safety are included as core elements in undergraduate degrees or postgraduate diplomas in dietetics or nutrition and dietetics that have been approved by the Health Professions Council. This is important both for understanding the general risks associated with food preparation and because nutritionists and dieticians will often give food safety advice to specific groups, e.g. pregnant women and the immunocompromised. Undergraduate degrees in microbiology, food microbiology and food science include detailed information on foodborne pathogens, their food associations and transmission of micro-organisms in foods. Food hygiene training is also provided in veterinary and medical degrees as well as in courses for various other professions, some of which are listed in Table 17.2 (e.g. Trading Standards Officer). Some food hygiene and safety training is also included in a broad range of other degrees which may be management based but have a food hygiene element, such as hospitality or tourism management. Foundation degrees and Higher National Diploma (HND) levels are available in many areas encompassing the food industry as well as bachelor of science degrees.

Postgraduate training at MSc and PhD levels is provided at various higher education institutions as well as by non-governmental organizations such as the Health Protection Agency (www.hpa.org.uk), the Veterinary Laboratory Agency and the Institute for Food Research. Specialist MSc training courses covering aspects of food production, policy, law, safety and hygiene management are offered by a range of university departments – engineering, biological or biosciences departments as well as food sciences or microbiology.

The University and College Admissions Service (UCAS) is the central co-ordinating organization that processes applications for full-time undergraduate courses at all UK universities and colleges. Its website allows online course searches as well as online submission of applications. However, MSc and other higher degrees are not centrally co-ordinated in this way and individual higher education institutions supply details of the courses they provide through their websites and application offices.

Food examiners and public analysts

The Food Safety Act 1990 established the role of the **food examiner** to perform the statutory function of microbiological examination of food. In performing this task the role of the food examiner corresponds to the role of the **public analyst**, who has a long-standing tradition of carrying out statutory chemical examination of food samples. Food examiners and public analysts can be described as people designated by an official control laboratory as such on the basis of appropriate qualifications and experience as detailed in the Food Safety (Sampling and Qualifications) Regulations 1990 (SI No. 2463). See Table 17.2 for examples of qualifications for food examiners. To meet the official requirements, a food examiner's experience must include examination of food over a period or periods amounting to at least 3 years in an appropriate laboratory as detailed in the Regulations. The qualifications and experiences are stated so that the competence of the food examiner or public analyst, when asked to provide a statement to a court, is not open to question. Further details can be found in *Requirements of Food Examiners, Expert Witnesses and Witnesses of Fact acting for/on behalf of the Health Protection Agency* (www.hpa-standardmethods.org.uk/documents/qsop/pdf/qsop 50.pdf).

Training in forms other than formal taught courses is also available. The Society of Food Hygiene Technology (SOFHT), for example has developed SOFHT Options in Training. As well as providing a Foundation Level **Certificate in Food Hygiene** in partnership with the RSPH, it has also developed an e-training course, **Hygiene Awareness – Principles and Practice**, which is an interactive CD-based training course covering modules on personal hygiene, food safety, principles of cleaning and waste disposal and pest control.

Educating the public

As already discussed, changes in food preparation, cooking and eating practices mean that traditional approaches for safety are being lost and new sources of foodborne disease are arising. The public's awareness of potential sources of foodborne disease is often based on media reports. Major outbreaks make headline news and a particular food source becomes recognized as a potential problem for a while: however such events are usually transient and thereafter there is a general assumption that the problem has been resolved. Advice to a specific target group who may be at greater risk can have a positive

Table 17.2 *Sources of education and training for individuals involved with food*

	Basic	Continuing
Professions involved with food manufacture and consumption		
Food producers and handlers	Appropriate CIEH, RIPH, RSPH or REHIS certificates at Foundation, Intermediate and Advanced levels. Meat Training Council NJSVQ and VRQs for those involved in all aspects of meat handling	FSA WHO CCFRA Leatherhead Food International Association of Meat Inspectors Food and Drink Federation SOFHT
Caterers	CIEH, RIPH or RSPH certificates at Foundation, Intermediate and Advanced levels	FSA Food and Drink Federation SOFHT
Dieticians and nutritionists	Undergraduate degree or postgraduate diploma in Dietetics or Nutrition and Dietetics approved by the Health Professions Council	FSA Health Protection Agency
Professionals specifically involved with food safety		
Veterinarians	Appropriate veterinary sciences degree	VLA, professional societies, primary research literature
Medical practitioners (GPs, CCDCs, CMM)	Appropriate medical sciences degree	Health Protection Agency, professional societies, primary research literature
Food examiners	May include Fellowship of the Institute of Biomedical Sciences (if gained by passing examinations in medical microbiology); Member of the Royal College of Pathology (in medical microbiology); BSc Hons in Microbiology; MSc (if awarded by examination instead of thesis with at least one paper in microbiology); Fellowship or Membership of the Institute of Food Science and Technology	FSA Health Protection Agency IFST
EHOs	Appropriate CIEH-accredited degree course	FSA CIEH SOFHT
Trading Standards Officer	TSI-accredited qualification programme	Training Standards Institute
Food inspectors	Appropriate CIEH-accredited course in Food Premises inspection	FSA SOFHT
Meat and poultry Inspectors	Appropriate RSPH Meat Inspection Certificate	FSA Association of Meat Inspectors
Food scientists	BSc in appropriate Food science degree	FSA CCFRA Leatherhead Food International SOFHT IFST

Table 17.2 *Sources of education and training for individuals involved with food* (continued)

	Basic	Continuing
Professional specifically involved with teaching		
Teachers	Appropriate undergraduate degree	Microbiology On-line The FSA
University and higher educational lectures	Appropriate undergraduate degree and usually PhD	SfAM, SGM, IFST, FSA, HPA other professional societies, primary research sources
General public and consumers		
Purchaser and preparers	Varied	FSA WHO
School-age children	National Curriculum Key Stages 1 and 2	FSA Foodlink WHO
Vulnerable groups	Varied	FSA HPA The British Dietetic Association

For abbreviations see text and 'Abbreviations used in this book' (pp. **xviii–xx**).

effect in this regard. For example, in the 1980s there was a series of outbreaks associated with *L. monocytogenes* and particular food groups, which was highlighted in the media at the time. The decision was made to target advice, particularly to pregnant women and also to the immunocompromised to:

- not eat soft ripened cheeses of the brie, camembert or blue veined types
- not eat pâté
- reheat until piping hot any bought cooked-chilled meals or ready-to-eat poultry.

This led to a dramatic downturn in incidence among pregnant women (Figure 17.1). This advice is still in place today and rates of listeriosis associated with pregnancy have stayed low. In contrast, in the rest of the population numbers of cases of listeriosis have shown a rising trend (see Figure 17.1). The British Dietetics Association website also provides specific food safety advice for pregnant women (www.bda.uk.com/Downloads/FINALPregnancyFFfeb.pdf).

This does not mean information is not widely available, only that people have to be interested enough to find out. For example, the Food Standards Agency (FSA; www.food.gov.uk) has developed an 'eat well be well' website (www.eatwell.gov.uk) which offers general advice on safe preparation, cooking and storage of foods as well as nutritional advice. More in-depth information can be gained from the 'safe food and health eating for all' section of the FSA's website (www.food.gov.uk/safereating/microbiology). A similar website, food**link** (www.foodlink.org.uk), has been organized by the Food and Drink Federation (www.fdf.org.uk) in association with FSA, REHIS, CIEH, the Local Authorities Coordinators of Regulatory Services, the Departments of Health, Food and Education, the National Farmers Union, the British Retail Consortium and the British Hospitality Association. National Food Safety Week (www.foodlink.org.uk/nfsw.asp) is the point in the calendar for highlighting the importance of food safety and the basic principles of food hygiene. This is sponsored by a number of agencies each year and a calendar of events is published each year on the food**link** website.

The popularity of cookery programmes on the

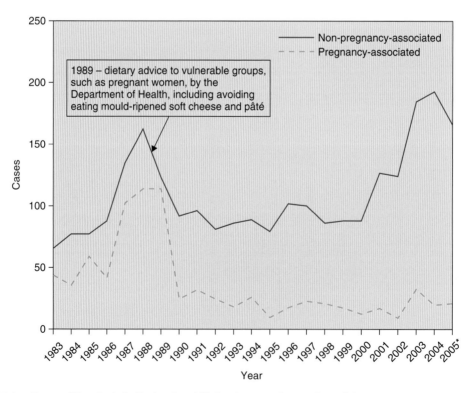

Figure 17.1 *Cases of listeriosis in England and Wales: impact of targeting advice to pregnant women as an 'at-risk' group (source: www.hpa.org.uk/infections/topics_az/listeria/data_ew_gr.htm [accessed 2 November 2005]).*

television has provided an opportunity for good hygiene practices to be demonstrated and some programmes make a point of commenting on the need to wash hands after touching raw meat or using separate chopping boards for different types of food stuffs. The FSA also runs advertising campaigns to highlight the ease with which cross-contamination occurs in the kitchen environment. Advice for safe eating and cooking practices is also given by retailers and manufacturers and sometimes included on the packaging label. This not only includes safe cooking or storage instructions but also dietary advice to specific groups such as warning about avoiding eating soft cheese during pregnancy to prevent listeriosis and not to feed honey to babies younger than 12 months old because of the risk of infant botulism.

Educating children

Schools cover basic food safety and hygiene as part of design and technology and science teaching which are compulsory parts of the National Curriculum for primary school children at Key Stages 1 (aged 5–7) and 2 (aged 7–11). A range of materials is available to support teaching of food hygiene and safety at this level. For example, the FSA has developed Food Hygiene Mission Control as an interactive resource for children aged 7–14 and their teachers. This uses quizzes, games and fact files to support teaching of food hygiene (http://archive.food.gov.uk/hea/index2.html). The eat well, be well website also contains games (such as The barbecue game and Stack the fridge) and quizzes which are appropriate across a range of ages (www.eatwell.gov.uk/info/games). In addition the Agency's Cooking Bus (www.food.gov.uk/healthiereating/nutritionschools/bus/) has been developed together with the Focus on Food campaign to get across healthy eating and food safety messages to school children. For 42 weeks a year the bus, which is a state-of-the-art mobile kitchen, goes to different destinations around the country where its two teachers work with school staff to give hands-on workshop experience to children and highlight the importance of food education, in line with the national curriculum and government health messages.

Similarly the food**link** website has interactive games to teach children about food issues (www.foodlink.org.uk/testyourself.asp); it also pro-

duces a range of resources which can be used to support National Food Safety Week and classroom activities (www.foodlink.org.uk/resources.asp). The Society for General Microbiology together with the Microbiology in Schools Advisory Committee have developed Microbiology On-line (www.microbiologyonline.org.uk), a website dedicated to providing support for microbiology education and teaching resources for microbiology in schools for Key Stages 1–4 and post-16. These include information on foodborne pathogens in foods.

GETTING THE MESSAGE ACROSS

At its essence, food hygiene and safety relies on a few simple principles which, if imparted, allow safe and hygienic food production. To this end, a number of campaigns have been run to instil these basic principles. The FSA's 4 Cs (Box 17.1) food hygiene campaign is designed to reduce foodborne illness by improving awareness and application of the 4 Cs food hygiene principles in the home. This campaign is concentrating on working with schools but it does cover other important groups as well, such as those working with vulnerable groups. It was the focus for the National Food Safety Week in 2006.

Box 17.1 The 4 Cs

- Cleaning
- Cooking
- Cooling
- Cross-contamination

The 4 Cs provide four simple messages:

- Wash hands properly and keep them clean
- Cook food properly
- Chill food properly
- Avoid cross-contamination

Of specific interest with regard to food hygiene, the World Health Organization (WHO) in 2001, after consultations with food safety experts and risk communicators, introduced the 'Five Keys to Safer Food' (Box 17.2), a series of simple rules elaborated to promote safer food handling and preparation practices for all food handlers, including professionals and ordinary consumers (www.who.int/foodsafety/consumer/5keys/en/index.html).

Box 17.2 WHO's five keys to safer food
● Keep clean
● Separate raw and cooked
● Cook thoroughly
● Keep food at safe temperatures
● Use safe water and raw materials

A poster illustrating these is available on the website, with different versions for different geographical areas and in a number of languages. WHO has also developed a Five Keys training manual with tips on how to adapt the training programme for different target groups (food handlers, consumers, school children and women). The training manual will be finalized in 2006 after being field-tested.

KEEPING UP TO DATE

As already discussed, the causes and sources of foodborne disease change over time. New pathogens have been emerging and undoubtedly in the future there will be new micro-organisms that will become a problem. Similarly the foodstuffs associated with disease also keep changing, both as our preferences change and as new technologies emerge. For people working in microbiology or in areas associated with microbiology and food it is important to know about these newly emerging problems.

In addition, in the food industries there is a need for reinforcement of training and staff motivation to ensure hygiene knowledge/standards are maintained.

For professionals

The FSA supplies a wide range of information via its website with specific sections for industry (www.food.gov.uk/foodindustry). This covers a broad range of issues such as guidance notes and regulation changes, food alerts and a range of other information for industry professionals in catering, local authorities, primary producers and retailers, as well as for some specialist groups (e.g. meat producers). A new initiative is **Safer Food, Better Business** (SFBB) (www.food.gov.uk/foodindustry/regulation/hygleg/hyglegresources/sfbb/), packs

which provide a practical approach to food safety management and cover aspects of cross-contamination, cleaning, chilling, cooking and preparation and management. There are two different SFBB packs – one for small catering businesses and one for small retail businesses. The SFBB pack for retailers has been developed to help retail businesses across the UK comply with new regulations introduced in January 2006. The SFBB pack for caterers has been developed to help businesses comply with the new regulations, show how to make food safely, and train staff. FSA Scotland has developed **CookSafe** which is designed to help catering businesses understand and implement a HACCP-based system. **Safe Catering** is FSA Northern Ireland's food safety management pack. It has been prepared to help produce a HACCP plan and to keep appropriate records. All of these can be accessed via links from the SFBB website. In addition the FSA has published a booklet *Food hygiene – A Guide for Businesses* (www.food.gov.uk/news/newsarchive/2006/feb/foodhygguide) which explains good practice in relation to food hygiene and is aimed at restaurants, cafés and other catering businesses, as well as shops selling food. It complements other food safety management packs produced by the Agency and replaces their previous publications *Food Safety Regulations* and *Guide to Food Hygiene*.

In addition, the FSA has also developed a continuing programme of update training for local authority food law enforcement officers. These are only for food law enforcement officers currently employed by local authorities and a full list of the courses and contacts for details are on the website (www.food.gov.uk/enforcement/laresource/lowcost/).

There is also a range of specialist professional bodies that disseminate information to their members, run conferences to update knowledge and may offer training courses on specific aspects. The Health Protection Agency website provides links to training and education delivered by the Centre for Infections (www.hpa.org.uk/cfi/about/training_events.htm), which are of relevance to health sector workers including EHOs. The Campden and Chorleywood Food Research Association (CCFRA) website (www.campden.co.uk) includes details of various conference and training courses available to industry members and others. The Leatherhead Food Research Association

(Leatherhead Food International) also provides a variety of information directed at its members and includes details of forum series. The Food and Drink Federation also runs a series of seminars, events and workshops to keep members informed of current trends and issues.

The Society for Applied Microbiology (SfAM) and the Society for General Microbiology (SGM) are the two main professional microbiological societies in the UK. These societies run regular conferences on specialist themes and publish peer-reviewed scientific journals which contain high-quality research papers and topical review articles. Attendance at conferences not only helps update knowledge in particular areas but also allows scientists from around the country and from abroad to meet and discuss research. The Institute of Food Science and Technology, which is a professional qualifying body for food scientists and technologists, provides information and advisory statements on a range of food issues including food safety on-line. It also publishes a range of books including guidelines for different areas of the industry.

The Association of Meat Inspectors brings together all the authorized officers engaged in meat and poultry inspection. The body publishes a journal, *The Meat Hygienist*, and holds regular residential seminars covering current issues in meat hygiene. The Society of Food Hygiene Technology (www.sofht.co.uk) brings together everyone with an interest in food hygiene issues including food manufacturers, retailers, caterers, EHOs, suppliers to the food industry, consultants, research organizations, training bodies and students. As well as the training packages outlined earlier, the Society provides a series of events, newsletters, publications and other benefits to its members. Scottish Food and Drink provides an information source via their website on various aspects of hygiene, safety and compliance.

Open access information

The internet has become a major vehicle for dissemination of information and has given the subject of food hygiene an international perspective. Websites offering information on food safety and hygiene range from those associated with the professional bodies already mentioned and designed for specialists and those working in the industry, to ones designed for public access and teaching. As has already been indicated in this chapter, some websites, such as the FSA's, have pages which inform a range of groups – so include guidelines and documentation to inform industry on changing regulations and practices as well as pages designed for public information access, including interactive games for children. Similarly the Food and Drink Federation site is directed at providing information to the consumer as well as to industry members.

Some websites are primarily of interest to health and microbiology professionals with a specialist interest in food safety. The WHO site takes a global perspective on food safety, foodborne illness surveillance and emerging foodborne disease (www.who.int/topics/food_safety/en/). This site has a range of downloadable specialist publications and workshop reports on specific health aspects. As an example there is a section on Ensuring Food Safety in the Aftermath of Natural Disasters. The International Life Sciences Institute (ILSI) site also includes information on the food chain including processing and risk and benefit assessments (http://europe.ilsi.org/). The Health Protection Agency site supplies detailed information on infectious disease epidemiology including foodborne organisms and sources. A link from this site is to the weekly publication *Health Protection Report* that reports statistics on foodborne disease outbreaks and highlights organisms and food sources of concern.

Summary

Food continues to be an important vehicle for transmitting disease. New food safety legislation is addressing the problem across the whole of the production chain and the requirement for 'due diligence' means that food producers have a responsibility to provide a safe food supply. However, ultimately, food safety relies not only on those who produce the food but also on those who prepare and cook it. Everyone therefore shares the responsibility in knowing and understanding how to produce safe food. A wide range of materials is available that can provide and help gain the necessary knowledge. On the whole, food hygiene relies on a few simple messages which should be understood by all.

All websites cited in this chapter and below were accessed in November 2006.

SOURCES OF INFORMATION

Sources of information include websites cited in the chapter.

Food Safety Act 1990. London: The Stationery Office (available at: www.opsi.gov.uk/ACTS/acts1990/Ukpga_19900016_en_1.htm).

WEBSITES OF KEY ORGANISATIONS AND AGENCIES

Campden and Chorleywood Food Research Association http://www.campden.co.uk/

Chartered Institute of Environmental Health http://www.cieh.org/

Food and Drink Federation http://www.fdf.org.uk/home.aspx

Food Safety Act 1990 The Stationery Office Limited http://www.opsi.gov.uk/ACTS/acts1990/Ukpga_19900016_en_1.htm

Food Standards Agency http://www.food.gov.uk/

Health Protection Agency http://www.hpa.org.uk/

Institute for Food Research http://www.ifr.ac.uk/

International Life Sciences Institute http://europe.ilsi.org/

Leatherhead Food International http://www.lfra.co.uk/

Meat Hygiene Service http://www.food.gov.uk/enforcement/meathyg/mhservice/

Royal Institute of Public Health http://www.riph.org.uk

Royal Society for the Promotion of Health http://www.rsph.org

Scottish Food and Drink http://www.scottishfood and drink.com

Trading Standards Institute http://www.tscareers.org.uk/

The Association of Meat Inspectors http://www.meatinspectors.co.uk/

The British Dietetic Association http://www.bda.uk.com/

The Institute of Food Science and Technology http://www.ifst.org/

The Meat Training Council http://meattraining.org.uk

The Royal Environmental Health Institute for Scotland http://www.rehis.org

The Society of Food hygiene Technology http://www.sofht.co.uk/

The Society for Applied Microbiology http://www.sfam.org.uk/

The Society for General Microbiology http://www.sgm.ac.uk/

The Veterinary Laboratory Agency http://www.defra.gov.uk/corporate/vla/

UCAS http://www.ucas.ac.uk/

World Health Organisation http://www.who.int/en/

18

Food hygiene in developing countries

Martin Adams

Introduction	326	Street-vended foods	329
Climatic factors	326	Mycotoxins	330
Socio-economic factors	327	Parasites	331
Significance of foodborne illness in developing		Bushmeat	333
countries	327	Summary	333
Childhood diarrhoea and traditional technologies	328	Sources of information and further reading	333

The general principles of food poisoning and food hygiene are the same in developing and developed countries. However, in most developing countries food hygiene is made more difficult by the tropical climate as well as socio-economic problems such as poverty. Diarrhoeal diseases (especially in childhood) are much more common in the developing world and are a significant cause of morbidity and mortality.

Developing countries Countries with low income per capita, poorly developed human resources and a high level of economic vulnerability.

Street-vended or street foods Foods and beverages prepared and/or sold in public places for immediate consumption or later consumption without further processing.

Bushmeat Meat of wild animals hunted by local people for income or subsistence in West and Central Africa. Unsustainable levels of hunting are believed to be threatening the survival of many target species.

Foodborne illness Any illness of an infectious or toxic nature caused by the consumption of food or water.

INTRODUCTION

In previous editions of this book, the chapter 'Food hygiene in the tropics' highlighted that although the basic factors leading to **foodborne illness** in the tropics are the same as elsewhere, there are conditions which enhance the dangers. It went on to list a number of these factors, such as high ambient temperature and humidity, general lack of refrigeration, local habits, impure water, poor sanitary facilities and profusion of intestinal pathogens and parasites. These factors can, however, be assigned into two broader groups; those relating directly to climate (temperature, humidity and sunlight), and socio-economic factors which derive largely from poverty and the associated lack of training and infrastructure. Factors such as lack of refrigeration facilities or universal availability of clean, safe water fall clearly into the second category, and it is these that often have the greatest impact on food safety in tropical **developing countries**.

CLIMATIC FACTORS

Climatic factors generally exacerbate food hygiene problems since **high ambient temperatures** are conducive to increased growth of mesophilic bacterial pathogens. Under these conditions, delays between preparation and consumption will have a greater adverse effect than in cooler climes. High temperatures, coupled with high levels of humidity, can also be particularly favourable for the growth of mycotoxin-producing fungi on agricultural products.

Sunlight can, however, have a positive effect and

there have been numerous reports of its use to disinfect water (Acra *et al.* 1989). Some rely on solar heating to inactivate bacteria, but others have identified ultraviolet (UV) solar radiation as the inactivation principle. The effect has not been fully defined but has been shown to be influenced by factors such as container type and material, water turbidity, and the presence of oxygen or residual chlorine. Experiments where these factors differ or are undefined have yielded conflicting results and generated some debate about the overall efficacy of the process. Despite a lack of understanding of the general principles of this effect, one study in which Masai children (aged 5–16 years) were encouraged to store their contaminated water in plastic bottles in full sunlight, reported significantly reduced episodes of diarrhoea compared with controls (Conroy *et al.* 1996).

SOCIO–ECONOMIC FACTORS

The designation 'developing country' used in this chapter is one of several, not wholly appropriate, terms used to describe poor countries. 'Developing' carries optimistic overtones that imply ongoing improvement and development. This is true for some countries, but can be misleading for many others whose situation has worsened over recent years with increasing rather than decreasing levels of poverty.

Developing countries have the over-riding characteristic of widespread poverty, usually with other common features such as an economy based on the production of primary products for export, rapidly increasing population and large-scale migration to overcrowded cities. Some of the public health problems these countries face are similar to those encountered previously in the developed world during industrialization, and whose solution depended not on new discoveries in medical science, but on investment in improved nutrition, housing, water supplies and sanitation. Currently about 2.6 billion people in the developing world lack even a simple improved pit latrine and 1.1 billion have no access to any source of improved drinking water.

At the individual level, poverty can also exacerbate food safety problems due to the lack of facilities for the hygienic preparation and storage of food, unavailability of fuel and the cost of basic foods.

SIGNIFICANCE OF FOODBORNE ILLNESS IN DEVELOPING COUNTRIES

Attempts have been made to estimate the extent of foodborne illness in particular communities and the degree to which this is reflected in official statistics. Such studies are only feasible in countries where a strong reporting system exists and these have shown that, depending on the pathogen concerned, there is a large but variable degree of under-reporting of diarrhoeal disease. For example, an extensive study in England of the incidence of infectious intestinal disease determined that the true number of *Salmonella* infections was 3.2 times higher than official statistics, but 7.6 times greater for *Campylobacter* and 1562 times higher for norovirus (Wheeler *et al.* 1999).

In developed countries such as the UK, diarrhoeal disease is usually an unpleasant but generally transient experience for otherwise healthy adults. Long-term health problems occur in a small percentage of cases and the consequences are far more serious in the more vulnerable members of the community: the old and the young; the sick; and those who are immunocompromised. The impact of diarrhoeal disease in the developing world is far more severe, but its extent is more difficult to define.

It has been estimated that on a worldwide basis in 2000, 2.1 million people died from diarrhoeal disease, a great proportion of which can be attributed to contamination of food and drinking water (World Health Organization [WHO] 2002a). According to the WHO/UNICEF Global Water Supply and Sanitation Assessment 2000, cited in the *World Health Report* (WHO 2002b), the vast majority of diarrhoeal disease in the world (88 per cent) was attributable to unsafe water, sanitation and hygiene, accounting for approximately 3.1 per cent of deaths (1.7 million) and 3.7 per cent of all **disability-adjusted life years** (DALYS; the sum of years of potential life lost due to premature mortality and the years of productive life lost due to disability) which totalled 54.2 million years. Overall, 99.8 per cent of deaths associated with these risk factors are in developing countries.

In poorer countries, the impact of food and waterborne diarrhoea falls particularly heavily on the very young. In addition to the direct adverse effects of diarrhoea on children, such as dehydration and loss of electrolytes, this condition results in loss of appetite and malabsorption of nutrients. The resulting malnourishment predisposes children to further episodes of diarrhoea and other infections which establishes a vicious cycle of illness and malnutrition, which at least will impede normal development and at worst result in death – a phenomenon known as the **malnutrition infection cycle** (Keusch 2003). Ninety per cent of deaths associated with contaminated water, sanitation and hygiene are in children. The annual number of deaths in children under 5 years of age from diarrhoeal disease over the period 2000–2003 was estimated as 1.76 million: 701 000 of those deaths occurring in Africa, 552 000 in southeast Asia and 178 000 in the Western Pacific (WHO 2005).

CHILDHOOD DIARRHOEA AND TRADITIONAL TECHNOLOGIES

Treatment centres have conducted studies into the causative agents of childhood diarrhoea on many occasions. These usually succeed in isolating and identifying a pathogen from about 70–80 per cent of the stool samples examined and have allowed a general picture of the organisms responsible for childhood diarrhoea to emerge. This was summarized in a WHO publication in 1992 (Table 18.1); more recent studies suggest that the situation has changed little since.

Weaning, the period in which maternal breast

Table 18.1 *Pathogens frequently identified in children with acute diarrhoea in developing countries*

	Pathogen	Percentage of cases
Viruses	Rotavirus	15–25
Bacteria	Enterotoxigenic	
	Escherichia coli	10–20
	Shigella	5–15
	Campylobacter jejuni	10–15
	Vibrio cholerae O1	5–10*
	Salmonella (non-typhoid)	1–5
	Enteropathogenic *E. coli*	1–5
Protozoa	*Cryptosporidium*	5–15
No pathogen found		20–30

*May be higher during epidemics.
Adapted from WHO (1992).

milk with its protective properties is replaced or supplemented with other foods, is a particularly hazardous time for the child. Weaning or complementary food itself appear to be an important source of pathogens, and basic principles for the preparation of safe food for infants and young children have been produced (Box 18.1).

Box 18.1 Basics of safer food for infants and younger children (Motarjemi *et al.* 1994)

- Cook food thoroughly
- Avoid storing cooked food
- Avoid contact between raw foodstuffs and cooked food
- Wash fruit and vegetables
- Use safe water
- Wash hands repeatedly
- Avoid feeding infants with a bottle
- Protect food from insects, rodents and other animals
- Store non-perishable foodstuffs in a safe place
- Keep all food preparation premises meticulously clean

Although these points are applicable anywhere and are general good hygienic practice for safe food preparation, there are often specific socio-economic or climatic factors in tropical developing countries that prevent them from being adhered to and increase risks such as lack of fuel for adequate cooking or reheating. Facilities for cool or chill storage are unlikely to be available in the poorest areas, and in the absence of cool storage, high ambient temperatures allow pathogens to multiply more quickly than in temperate regions. Safe water may not be readily available for washing foods, hands or utensils. The fauna of tropical countries tends to be more numerous and more diverse than in cooler regions, affording greater opportunity for contamination to occur.

In view of the special difficulties faced in developing countries, attention has been given to **traditional food preservation technologies** such as **fermentation** in ensuring food safety. Bacterial lactic acid fermentation of starchy substrates such as maize, millet or cassava is particularly widespread in Africa although the use of fermented foods for child feeding is declining. In Tanzania this has been ascribed to factors such as the time necessary for their preparation and the availability of cheaper, more easily prepared substitutes (Lorri and Svanberg 1995).

The ability of fermentation processes, more specifically those involving the growth of lactic acid bacteria, to inhibit a variety of pathogens is well known and has been thoroughly reviewed (Adams and Nout 2001). Its role as a household technology to improve food safety was also the topic of a Food and Agriculture Organization (FAO)/WHO workshop held in South Africa in 1996 (WHO 1996a). There is considerable evidence that lactic acid fermentation inhibits both the growth and survival of bacterial pathogens, and that traditional fermented products such as cereal gruels have lower counts of pathogens and indicator bacteria than unfermented products. There is, however, little evidence relating to its effect on levels of diarrhoeal disease itself. A prospective study conducted in Tanzania compared the incidence of diarrhoea in children younger than 5 years in two villages: one where a fermented maize product, *magai*, was consumed, and another similar village where it was not. This study found a significantly lower incidence of diarrhoea over 9 months in the village where *magai* was consumed compared with the neighbouring village (Lorri and Svanberg 1994). In another Tanzanian study, the presence of enteropathogens in faecal swabs from children younger than 5 years was significantly reduced by consumption of the fermented cereal *togwa* from 27.6 per cent at baseline to 7–8 per cent 1–2 weeks after feeding commenced. A similar but smaller drop was seen in the control group fed the unfermented cereal *uji* (Kingamkono *et al.* 1999). There is a clear need for further studies of this type to prove the beneficial effect of fermentation in practice.

In addition to their effect on pathogens in foods, there is some evidence that the consumption of high numbers of lactic acid bacteria can have a probiotic role in alleviating diarrhoea. A meta-analysis of reports published between 1996 and 2000 has indicated that consumption of high numbers of *Lactobacillus* reduced the duration and frequency of diarrhoea in children (Van Niel *et al.* 2002).

STREET-VENDED FOODS

Street-vended or **street foods** are foods and beverages prepared and/or sold in public places for immediate consumption or later consumption without further processing (WHO 1996b). This informal food supply system is important throughout the world but has increased markedly in developing countries over recent decades in response to urbanization and population growth. It has been recognized as offering a number of benefits which enhance the security of those involved in the food sector (raw produce suppliers, processors and vendors).

In Bangkok (Thailand) 20 000 street food vendors provide city residents with 40 per cent of their overall energy intake, each vendor purchasing up to US$41 of raw materials per day, whereas in Latin America and the Caribbean, the purchase of street foods accounts for 20–30 per cent of urban household expenditure. In Calcutta (India), the 130 000 street food vendors make an estimated profit of US$ 100 million each year (FAO 1997; 2001a,b). The sector also helps give women some degree of financial independence as the owners or employees are frequently women: in several African countries they represent 70–90 per cent of vendors (Tomlins 2002).

However, street-vended foods are associated with significant health risks (Box 18.2). These arise from the climatic and socio-economic factors outlined previously.

> **Box 18.2 Problems associated with street foods**
> - Foods are frequently prepared early in the morning and stored without refrigeration throughout the day allowing considerable microbial growth to occur
> - Clean water may not be available for washing produce, hands or utensils, and appropriate toilet facilities may also be lacking
> - While on display, foods may not be protected from the flies and rodents that increase the risk of contamination with pathogens
> - Vendors may have poor knowledge of basic food hygiene measures, with no qualified inspectors to regulate their activities
> - A lack of public awareness of the possible dangers associated with such foods

Associations between street-vended foods and diarrhoeal disease have been noted in epidemiological studies. Lim-Quizon and co-workers (1994) cite an unpublished study conducted in the Philippines in 1988 that showed cholera patients were eight times more likely to report having bought street foods than healthy controls. The same authors went on to identify an association between cholera and particular street foods: *pansit* (rice noodles with shrimp, meat and vegetables) and mussel soup. The potential of street vended foods to act as vehicles for foodborne illness has also been supported by a number of microbiological studies. In Mexico City, enterotoxigenic *Escherichia coli* was found in 5 per cent of samples of street-vended chilli sauce whereas *E. coli* and *Salmonella* were present in 43 per cent and 5 per cent of taco dressings, respectively (Estrada-Garcia *et al.* 2004). In India, Kakar and Udipi (2002) found that street-vended meat products in Mumbai were more hazardous than small shop or railway stall samples, all having high viable counts and some containing *Salmonella*. *Salmonella* were also found in 10.1 per cent of 1200 samples of street food in Cameroon and samples of street foods in Zambia (Jermini *et al.* 1997; Akenji *et al.* 2002).

Limited sampling programmes are not guaranteed to detect the presence of pathogens such as *Salmonella* which pose a serious risk even at low levels. Numerous studies have not detected *Salmonella* but have frequently reported high viable counts and the isolation and enumeration of other pathogens such as *Staphylococcus aureus*, *Clostridium perfringens* and *Bacillus cereus*. These are generally present in numbers that are not considered to pose a direct threat to health, although they are indicative of poor hygienic quality with sporadic samples showing dangerously high counts. In a study in Brazil, 35 per cent of the 40 samples were found unsuitable for consumption with *B. cereus* identified as the pathogen posing the greatest risk (Hanashiro *et al.* 2005). Other studies have also described concerns about observed deficiencies in hygienic practices. So even where microbiological data indicate poor quality rather than any immediate health threat, the potential for infection is evident.

Surveys have also assessed food hygiene knowledge of street food vendors. Deficiencies have sometimes been found, but the level of food hygiene understanding is often judged to be good, suggesting that the lack of an appropriate physical infrastructure is the principal cause of the problem. Mahon and co-workers (1999) in Guatemala found that vendors 'demonstrated good knowledge of food safety ... but unsafe practices', and work in the Philippines identified a significant gap between knowledge and practice that was primarily attributed to the tendency of vendors to compromise food safety for financial reasons (Azanza *et al.* 2000). To improve the overall knowledge and hygiene awareness among street food vendors, specifically targeted training materials have been developed in some regions, as, for example, in a collaboration between the FAO and the Government of South Africa (FAO 2001b).

The FAO/WHO Codex Alimentarius Commission has created guidance documents to serve as the basis for national and local regulations on street foods. These have been produced for Latin America, the Caribbean and Africa, setting policies for licensing vendors, establishing street food advisory services and educating consumers about hygienic practices (FAO 2001c). The Hazard Analysis of Critical Control Points (HACCP) concept is now central to the control of foodborne hazards in the food industry in the developed world, and its use in street foods sector has been advocated. Although full application of HACCP to small-scale operations such as street-vended foods may be excessive and unrealistic, some HACCP-based studies have been conducted and this approach has been recommended as a means of focusing strategies on essential safety requirements (WHO 1996b).

MYCOTOXINS

Mycotoxins are toxic metabolites produced by a few species of fungi when they colonize crops in the field or during storage. Depending on their end use, contaminated crops can pose a hazard to animals or humans, and are a problem in both tropical and temperate regions in indigenous and imported crops. Particular problems in the tropical developing countries are associated with **aflatoxins** (mycotoxins produced by a small number of species of the genus *Aspergillus)* in products such as cereals, nuts and oilseeds. For further details see Chapter 4, p. 89.

At high levels, aflatoxins are acutely hepatotoxic and aflatoxin B_1 has been shown to be a potent liver carcinogen in many animal species. A number of epidemiological studies have linked aflatoxins with human liver cancer and there is also potent synergy between hepatitis B virus infection and aflatoxin in the induction of liver cancer (International Commission on Microbiological Specifications for Foods [ICMSF] 1996). Aflatoxins are most notably produced by *A. flavus* and *A. parasiticus*. Although these fungi are ubiquitous, they are most active in warmer climates with optimum temperatures for growth and aflatoxin production of 35–37 °C and 30 °C, respectively (Moss 2002). They grow best at high water activity (~0.99) but can grow down to values around 0.82 (ICMSF 1996). The highest levels of aflatoxins are produced as a result of inadequate post harvest storage when high moisture content, relative humidity and temperature promote growth and toxin production. This can be controlled by appropriate post harvest treatments to reduce moisture content and sound storage under dry, cool conditions. When fungal growth does occur, aflatoxin contamination is not usually homogeneous and overall levels can be reduced in some affected products by physical sorting.

Countries in the developed world import large quantities of crops from the tropics. These crops are susceptible to contamination with aflatoxins. To control this problem, importing countries impose stringent controls on the permissible levels of aflatoxins, particularly on those commodities destined for human consumption. Under such conditions, aflatoxin contamination becomes more of an economic than a health problem. The situation is rather different in producing countries where aflatoxins pose a very real health threat in addition to the economic damage they cause through loss of exports (Williams *et al.* 2004). People living in producing countries are likely to be exposed to higher levels since local inspection and control may be less rigorous, products deemed unsuitable for export may be available more cheaply on the local market and in times of scarcity, poor quality food may be all that is accessible to the very poor. Hence acute aflatoxicosis, which occurs after consumption of highly contaminated products, is only reported from producing countries and even then only occasionally. The largest recorded outbreak occurred in northwest India in 1974 when 400 people were affected and 100 people died as a result of consumption of heavily contaminated maize containing up to 15 000 parts per billion (ppb) aflatoxin (ICMSF 1996). Other smaller outbreaks have been reported from Thailand and Malaysia (Lye *et al.* 2005) but a similar, large outbreak occurred in April 2004 in rural Kenya. This also involved locally produced maize and resulted in 317 cases and 125 deaths. Following the outbreak a survey of 65 markets in Kenya found that 55 per cent of maize samples exceeded the Kenyan regulatory limit of 20 ppb (compared with the European Union limit of 2 ppb), 35 per cent exceeded 100 ppb and 7 per cent exceeded 1000 ppb (Lewis *et al.* 2005).

PARASITES

Most foodborne parasitic infections occur in tropical developing countries. Invariably these are the result of consumption of contaminated foods that are eaten raw, inadequately cooked, or partially processed (such as cured or fermented foods). The principal organisms involved are listed in Table 18.2, however, two examples will be considered here to illustrate how they are controlled. Readers seeking a more comprehensive account are referred to the reviews by Taylor (2001) and Dawson (2003).

Taenia solium, the zoonotic **pork tapeworm**, is endemic in many of the world's poorest countries. It causes cysticercosis in humans infected with the larval stage and taeniasis when infection is with the adult tapeworm. Cysticercosis can lead to a variety of severe neurological symptoms when the larvae develop in the central nervous system. The disease has been either controlled or eradicated in all countries in Europe and North America but is a serious economic problem and public health concern in Latin America, Asia and Africa. As with many other foodborne hazards, control is a function of development requiring improvement in both the general sanitary conditions associated with rearing of animals and the functional slaughterhouse control systems (Gonzalez *et al.* 2003). Reliance on the latter alone is ineffective since rejection or confiscation of pigs detected as having *Taenia* simply drives farmers to unregulated markets. In Peru, pigs are confiscated without payment if cysticercosis is detected, and it is estimated that 55 per cent of pigs are slaughtered illegally (Gonzalez *et al.* 2003).

Foodborne **trematode** infections affect more than 40 million people throughout the world and are particularly prevalent in the southeast Asia and the Western Pacific. They also pose an economic threat to the development of aquaculture in these regions. Human infection occurs when the infective metacercariae, found encysted in fish, crustacea or plants are ingested in a raw, pickled or undercooked state. Clinical manifestations vary with the infective

Table 18.2 *Foodborne parasites*

Parasite class	Parasite	Source of human infections
Protozoa		
Coccidia	*Cryptosporidium parvum*	Animal products, apple juice, water, faecal contamination
	Cyclospora cayetanensis	Fruit, water, salad
	Toxoplasma gondii	Meat, water, faecal contamination
Flagellates	*Giardia duodenalis*	Contaminated water, salads, fruits etc.
Amoeba	*Entamoeba histolytica*	Contaminated food and water
	Blastocystis hominis	Contaminated food and water
Ciliates	*Balantidium coli*	Contaminated food and water
Helminths		
Nematoda (roundworms)	*Angiostrongylus*	Molluscs, contaminated vegetables and salads
	Anisakis	Fish
	Capillaria philippinensis	Fish
	Dioctophyma renale	Fish
	Gnathostoma	Fish, frogs, chickens, ducks, snakes
	Trichinella spiralis	Meat
Cestoda (tapeworms)	*Diphyllobothrium latum*	Fish
	Taenia saginata	Beef
	Taenia solium	Pork
Trematoda (flukes)	*Clonorchis (Opisthorchis) sinensis*	Fish
	Echinostoma	Molluscs, fish
	Fasciola hepatica	Salads, vegetables
	Fasciola gigantica	
	Fasciolopsis buski	Aquatic plants
	Heterophyes heterophyes	Fish
	Opisthorchis viverrini	Fish
	O. felineus	
	Paragonimus	Crustaceans
	Haplorchis	Fish
	Metagonimus	Fish

Adapted from Taylor (2001).

organism and the intensity of the infection but can be life-threatening. About 70 species of trematodes are known to cause infection in humans. An important example is **opisthorchiasis**, caused by the liver fluke *Opisthorchis viverrini* and thought to be responsible for two-thirds of cases of cholangio-carcinoma, a common form of primary liver cancer, in Thailand (WHO 2004). When faeces from an infected person or animal contaminate water, eggs pass through freshwater snails (which act as the first intermediate host) to cyprinid fish (the second intermediate host) in which the organism exists as metacercaria under the scales. It is then transmitted to humans through consumption of improperly cooked or raw fish. Opisthorchiasis is endemic in north and northeastern Thailand and is particularly associated with the product *koi pla* (a traditional dish containing raw fish). Control strategies are based on three inter-related approaches (Jongsuk-suntigul and Imsomboon 2003):

- stool examination to diagnose human cases and initiate treatment
- health education to promote cooked fish consumption
- improved methods for human waste disposal.

BUSHMEAT

Bushmeat is the African term for the meat of wild animals, although the hunting of wild animals for meat is not confined to Africa. It is a worldwide phenomenon that has been practised for at least 100 000 years. For many people in Central and West Africa, particularly those living in rural areas, bushmeat is a major source of animal protein. In some parts of Cameroon it provides up to 98 per cent of the animal protein consumed. In addition to its nutritional importance, the bushmeat trade is significant in providing economic benefits to different groups of people in the commodity chain. The size of the bushmeat trade has been estimated in a number of African countries and ranges per year from US$24 million in Liberia, where it exceeds the timber trade in economic importance, to US$117 million in Côte d'Iviore. However, there is international concern that bushmeat hunting in some areas is threatening some wildlife populations with extinction. Unsustainable levels of bushmeat hunting could harm both the wildlife and the people who depend on bushmeat for food or income.

Studies in Ghana have linked falls in the populations of mammals to the bushmeat trade and changes in the availability of fish. Years of poor fish supply coincided with increased hunting in nature reserves and declines in wildlife species (Brashares *et al.* 2004). Recent increases in bushmeat hunting have been linked to overfishing by EU countries in West African waters. The handling of freshly butchered bushmeat, in particular primates, brings about a risk of transmission of new **zoonoses** (human diseases originating from animals). Pathogens that do not cause disease in their natural hosts can do so in their new hosts, or evolve to do so, as was the case with simian immunodeficiency virus (SIV) and human immunodeficiency virus (HIV).

Of particular relevance to developed countries are the implications of the trade for human and animal health through possible disease transmission from illegal bushmeat imports. Rapid advances in infrastructure and transportation, coupled with increased human migration around the globe, mean that infected people, animals or meat can move further from the source of infection, faster. Illegally imported bushmeat poses a low threat of transmitting a zoonosis to a person in a developed country, such as the UK. However, the main risks to public health from bushmeat are those associated with well-known food pathogens that will be destroyed by cooking.

Summary

Problems of food hygiene in tropical developing countries are not unique but are exacerbated by climatic conditions and, more significantly, the effects of poverty and economic under-development. It is, however, possible to identify particular areas of concern such as childhood diarrhoea, the safety of street vended foods and hazards such as mycotoxins and parasite infections. Measures to control all these problems are well known but implementation often depends on improvements in the economic status of affected countries.

All websites cited below were accessed in November 2006.

SOURCES OF INFORMATION AND FURTHER READING

Acra A, Jurdi M, Allem HM, *et al.* (1989) Sunlight as disinfectant. *Lancet* i: 280.

Adams, MR, Nout MJR (eds) (2001) *Fermentation and Food Safety*. Gaithersburg: Aspen, p. 290.

Akenji TKN, Aduh J, Ndip RN (2002) A study on the prevalence of *Salmonella* in food from road-side cafes in the Buea district of Cameroon. *J Food Sci Technol – Mysore* **39**: 664–6.

Azanza MPV, Gatchalian CF, Ortega MP (2001) Food safety knowledge and practices of street vendors in a Philippines university campus. *Int J Food Sci* **51**: 235–46.

Brashares JS, Arcese P, Sam MK, *et al.* (2004) Bushmeat hunting, wildlife declines, and fish supply in West Africa. *Science* **306**: 1180–3.

Conroy RM, Elmore-Meegan M, Joyce T, *et al.* (1996) Solar disinfection of drinking water and diarrhoea in Maasai children: a controlled field trial. *Lancet* **348**: 1695–7.

Dawson D (2003) *Foodborne Protozoan Parasites*. Brussels: ILSI Press, p. 40.

Estrada-Garcia T, Lopez-Saucedo C, Zamarripa-Ayala B, *et al.* (2004) Prevalence of *Escherichia coli* and *Salmonella* spp. in street-vended food of open markets (tiangus) and general hygienic and trading practices in Mexico City. *Epidemiol Infect* 2004; **132**: 1181–4.

Food and Agriculture Organization (1997) Street food: small entrepreneurs, big business (available at: FAO News and Highlights. www.fao.org/NEWS/1997/970408-e.htm).

Food and Agriculture Organization (2001a) Street food vendors around the world (available at: FAO News and Highlights. www.fao.org/News/2001/010804-e.htm).

Food and Agriculture Organization (2001b) Street foods made safer (available at: FAO News and Highlights. www.fao.org/News/2001/010803-e.htm).

Food and Agriculture Organization (2001c) Setting street food standards (available at: FAO News and Highlights. www.fao.org/News/2001/010805-e.htm).

Gonzalez AE, Garcia HH, Gilman RH, *et al.* and Cysticercosis Working Group in Peru (2003) Control of *Taenia solium*. *Acta Tropica* **87**: 103–9.

Hanashiro A, Morita M, Matte GR, *et al.* (2005) Microbiological quality of selected street foods from a restricted area of Sao Paulo city, Brazil. *Food Control* **16**: 439–44.

International Commission on Microbiological Specifications for Foods (1996) Toxigenic fungi: *Aspergillus*. In: *Micro-organisms in Foods*. Vol 5. London: Blackie Academic & Professional, pp. 347–81.

Jermini M, Bryan FL, Schmitt R, *et al.* (1997) Hazards and critical control points of food vending operations in a city in Zambia. *J Food Protection* **60**: 288–99.

Jongsuksuntigul P, Imsomboon T (2003) Opisthorchiasis control in Thailand. *Acta Tropica* **88**: 229–32.

Kakar DA, Udipi SA (2002) Microbiological quality of ready to eat meat and meat products sold in Mumbai city. *J Food Sci Technol – Mysore* **39**: 299–303.

Keusch GT (2003) The history of nutrition: malnutrition, infection and immunity. *J Nutr* **133**: 336S–340S.

Kingamkono RR, Sjogren E, Svanberg U (1999) Enteropathogenic bacteria in faecal swabs of young children fed on lactic acid-fermented cereal gruels. *Epidemiol Infect* **122**: 23–32.

Lewis L, Onsongo M, Njapau H, *et al.* and Kenyan Aflatoxicosis Group (2005) Aflatoxin contamination of commercial maize products during an outbreak of acute aflatoxicosis in Eastern and Central Kenya. *Environ Health Perspect* (available at: http://ehp.niehs.nih.gov/docs/2005/7998/abstracts.html).

Lim-Quizon MC, Benabaye RM, White FM, *et al.* (1994) Cholera in metropolitan Manila: foodborne transmission via street vendors. *Bull. World Health Organ* **72**: 745–9.

Lorri W, Svanberg U (1994) Lower prevalence of diarrhoea in young children fed lactic acid-fermented cereal gruels. *Food Nutr Bull* **15**: 57–63

Lorri W, Svanberg U (1995) An overview of the use of fermented foods for children feeding in Tanzania. *Ecol Food Nutr* **34**: 65–81.

Lye MS, Ghazali AA, Mohan J, *et al.* (2005) An outbreak of acute hepatic encephalopathy due to severe aflatoxicosis in Malaysia. *Am J Trop Med Hyg* **3**: 68–72.

Mahon BE, Sobel J, Townes JM, (1999) Surveying vendors of street-vended food: new methodological aspects applied to two Guatemalan cities. *Epidemiol Infect* **122**: 409–16.

Mensah P, Yeboah-Manu, Owusu-Darko K *et al.* (2002) Street foods in Accra, Ghana: how safe are they? *Bull World Health Organ* **80**: 546–54.

Moss MO (2002) Toxigenic fungi. In: Blackburn C de W, McClure PJ (eds) *Foodborne Pathogens*. Cambridge: Woodhead Publishing, pp. 479–88.

Motarjemi Y, Kaferstain F, Moy G *et al.* (1994) Contaminated food, a hazard for the very young. *World Health Forum* **15**: 69–71.

Murindamombe GY, Collison EK, Mpuchane SP *et al.* (2005) Presence of *Bacillus cereus* in street foods in Gabarone, Botswana. *J Food Protect* **68**: 342–6.

Taylor M (2001) Microbiological hazards and their control: parasites. In: Adams MR, Nout MJR (eds) *Fermentation and Food Safety*. Gaithersburg, USA: Aspen, pp. 175–217.

Tomlins K (2002) Street foods in Ghana: a source of income but not without its hazards. Ph Action News, No. 5, March 2002, International Institute of Tropical Agriculture.

Van Niel CW, Feudtner C, Garrison MM *et al.* (2002) Lactobacillus therapy for acute infectious diarrhoea in children: a meta-analysis. *Pediatrics* **109**: 678–84.

Wheeler JG, Sethi D, Cowden JM *et al.* (1999) Study of infectious intestinal disease in England: rates in the community, presenting to general practice, and reported to national surveillance. *BMJ* **318**: 1046–50.

World Health Organization (1992) *Readings in Diarrhoea: Student Manual*. Geneva: World Health Organization, p. 8.

World Health Organization (1996a) Fermentation: assessment and research. Report of a FAO/WHO workshop on fermentation as a technology to improve food safety. FAO/FNU/FOS/96.1. Geneva: World Health Organization.

World Health Organization (1996b) *Essential Safety Requirements for Street-Vended Foods*. Food Safety Unit, WHO. WHO/FNU/FOS/96.7. Geneva: World Health Organization.

World Health Organization (2002a) *Food Safety and Foodborne Illness*. WHO Fact sheet No. 237. Geneva: World Health Organization.

World Health Organization (2002b) World Health Report 2002 (available at: www.who.int/whr/2002/chapter4/en/index7.html).

World Health Organization (2004) Joint WHO/FAO workshop on foodborne trematode infections in Asia. Manila: World Health Organization, RS/2002/GE/40(VTN).

World Health Organization (WHO) (2005) World Health Report 2005 (available at: www.who.int/whr/2005/en/Statistical Annexe, p.195).

Williams JH, Phillips TD, Jolly PE *et al.* (2004) Human aflatoxicosis in developing countries: a review of toxicology, exposure, potential health consequences, and interventions. *Am J Clin Nutr* **80**: 1106–22.

19

Food hygiene in the wilderness

Paul R Hunter

Introduction	336	Safe disposal of faeces	344
Diarrhoeal illness associated with wilderness travel	336	Summary	345
Water	337	Sources of information and further reading	345
Food	343		

The wilderness exerts a strong attraction to ever increasing numbers of people for recreation and restoration. By its very nature, the wilderness is remote from the infrastructure of modern society, including treatment of water, prepared food and its storage (including refrigeration) and the safe disposal of faeces. The principles of food poisoning and food hygiene are the same in the wilderness as in other environments, but additional considerations for the drinking of sufficient water are essential for survival. Diarrhoeal illness is probably the most common infection associated with wilderness travel.

Wilderness Wild, uninhabited and uncultivated regions.

Surface waters Waters collected from lakes, rivers and streams.

Bushcraft Ability to survive and obtain sufficient food and water from a wilderness environment.

INTRODUCTION

The term '**wilderness**' covers many different environments including mountain, desert, forest, jungle, polar ice sheets, grasslands, lakelands, etc. Each environment provides its own risks, challenges and dangers, but probably the most challenging are the very dry and the very cold. Deserts pose a major problem for those without their own source of water (or food). As deserts receive less than 25 cm of rain each year, there is very low humidity and it is often very hot during the day and cold at night.

Some environments provide plenty of both food and water for those with the knowledge to find it. Food may stay fit for a long time in some environments but in others it will spoil rapidly. However, food is of secondary concern because the most important factor for survival is access to drinking water, without which death can occur within 2–3 days. In some environments water may be plentiful and in others it may be scarce.

People's experiences of the wilderness differ depending on their reasons for being there. For those who are deliberately travelling through the wilderness prior training, planning and preparation should considerably reduce the risks of food and waterborne disease. Others may find themselves in the wilderness as a result of accident or disaster. Even in these latter circumstances, prior knowledge and preparation may make the difference between survival and death.

This chapter will discuss some of the food and waterborne risks associated with wilderness travel. First, the evidence for diarrhoeal disease associated with wilderness travel will be examined. Second, good water disinfection and food hygiene practices (two of the three essential steps to prevent foodborne illness in the wilderness) are discussed. Finally, behaviours for the safe disposal of faeces are described which, though equally essential, are sadly often neglected probably because it is a taboo subject.

DIARRHOEAL ILLNESS ASSOCIATED WITH WILDERNESS TRAVEL

Most of what we know about the incidence of food and waterborne disease associated with wilderness travel comes from outbreaks and a few prospective epidemiological studies. Diarrhoeal illness appears to be common in people who spend time in the wilderness. Drinking untreated surface water is one of the prime risk factors in the aetiology of infectious diarrhoea in wilderness travellers. Food may also be a risk, especially when prepared with contaminated and untreated water, although this is less clear than the role of water. In part this is because foods carried while travelling in the wilderness tend to be light enough to carry as they are dehydrated or, for the more adventurous, may be caught or harvested during the journey. If perishable foods are carried into the wilderness, these are subject to the same risks as such foods back in civilization and may be subject to further deterioration if inadequately stored. Finally poor hygiene after defecation and during food preparation is also a significant risk. Of note is the importance of choosing wisely where to defecate when in the wilderness (see p. 344).

There is limited information about the relative importance of specific pathogens. The two most frequently reported pathogens from outbreaks and case–control studies in temperate regions are *Giardia* and *Campylobacter*, with additional cases due to *Escherichia coli* O157, *Salmonella* and norovirus. In tropical wildernesses the range of potential food and waterborne infections is greater, and pathogens also include parasites such as *Entamoeba* (the causes of amoebic dysentery) and *Dracunculiasis* (the guinea worm).

Boulware (2004) reported a survey in which 56 per cent of 334 backpackers who walked the Appalachian Trail for at least 7 days developed diarrhoea. The risk of diarrhoea was more than twice as common in people who drank surface water. But in this group, those who consistently treated water prior to drinking, handwashed after defecation and routinely washing cooking utensils had less illness than those who did not. Barbour *et al.* (1976) reported an outbreak of giardiasis that affected 34 of 54 campers on a 2-week trip into the mountains of Utah. The source of infection was not identified, though consumption of untreated water was suspected. A further outbreak among university students and staff on a geology field course in Colorado (Hopkins and Juranek 1991) strongly implicated drinking untreated water as the risk factor. A further prospective case–control study of

giardiasis in Colorado found that about a third of all cases occurring in the state were associated with drinking mountain stream water or camping overnight in the mountains (Wright *et al.* 1977).

Two prospective studies have implicated *Campylobacter* with diarrhoea in wilderness. In the first, *Campylobacter* gastroenteritis in the Grand Teton National Park area of Wyoming was more common among people drinking untreated surface water in the month before illness compared with matched controls (Taylor *et al.* 1983). Another study from Colorado also found that people with *Campylobacter* diarrhoea were more likely to have drunk untreated surface water (Hopkins *et al.* 1984).

Other pathogens that have been associated with camping or wilderness travel include *E. coli* O157, *Salmonella*, *Shigella* and norovirus. Lee *et al.* (2002) reported five people developed *E. coli* O157 infection while camping in California. They drank untreated creek water and used this water to reconstitute foods: members of this expedition reported defecating close to the campsite as well as directly into the creek. In 1999, an outbreak of norovirus infections was reported in long-distance hikers on the Appalachian Trail (Peipins *et al.* 2002). The source of the outbreak was traced to food items prepared in a general store on the trail, and *E. coli* was detected in the water supply suggesting faecal contamination. There was a suggestion that since the supply of water was limited this may have contributed to unsanitary food preparation practices.

WATER

Water is second only to oxygen for survival. At rest and at sea level in a temperate climate a man will need about 1800 mL of fluid a day and a woman a little bit less. This need increases with temperature, low humidity, altitude and exercise. Even in cold climates, water loss can be surprisingly high and many people may not realize that they are getting dehydrated. For example, water loss during Nordic ski racing can be up to 2 L per hour. In a hot desert, water loss can be even higher, especially when trying to walk: survival at 40 °C with 4 L a day is about 3 days.

The ideal source for water during wilderness travel is a potable supply that can be accessed at the start of each day. The only problem is how and what to carry it in, how heavy it weighs, and if it has to be

Table 19.1 *Types of disinfection**

Method	Recommendation (1 L [or 1 Qt] of water)	What it DOES	What it DOES NOT do
Boiling	Bring water to a rolling boil and allow to cool	Kills all pathogens	Does not remove turbidity/cloudiness
Chlorine compounds Household bleach (sodium hypochlorite)	For typical room temperature and water temperature of 25 °C, minimum contact time should be 30 minutes; increase contact time for colder water, e.g. 1 hour at less than 10 °C	Very effective for killing most bacteria and viruses Longer contact time required to kill *Giardia* cysts especially when water is cold	Not effective against *Cryptosporidium* or some other parasites; not as effective as iodine when using turbid water
Sodium dichloroisocyanurate tablet Calcium hypochlorite	Prepare according to package instructions Should be added to clear water or after settling or clarification to be most effective Type and typical dosage: Household bleach (5%) – 4 drops Sodium dichloroisocyanurate – 1 tablet (per package directions) –15 mg/L of clear water Calcium hypochlorite (1% stock solution†) – 4 drops		
Chlorinating-flocculating tablets or sachets	Chlorinating-flocculating tablet (per package directions)	Very effective for killing or removing all waterborne pathogens	Flocculated water must be decanted into a clean container, preferably through a simple fabric filter
Iodine Tincture of iodine (2% solution) Iodine (10% solution) Iodine tablet Iodinated resin Caution: For pregnant women who may be more sensitive, a carbon filter should be used to remove excess iodine after iodine treatment	25 °C – minimum contact for 30 minutes; increase contact time for colder water Not recommended for pregnant women, people with thyroid problems, or for more than a few months continuous use Prepare according to package instructions Type and typical dosage: Iodine 10% solution – 8 drops Iodine tablets – 1 or 2 tablets Triiodide or pentaiodide resin – room temperature according to directions and stay within rated capacity	Kills most pathogens Longer contact time is required to kill *Giardia* cysts especially when water is cold Carbon filtration after an iodine resin will remove excess iodine from the water, replace the carbon filter regularly	Not effective against *Cryptosporidium*

Table 19.1 *Types of disinfection** (continued)

Method	Recommendation (1 L [or 1 Qt] of water)	What it DOES	What it DOES NOT do
Portable filtering devices Ceramic filters Carbon filters. Some carbon block filters will remove cryptosporidia – only if tested and certified for cyst removal Reverse osmosis and ultrafilter type devices Membrane filter devices	Filter media pore size must be rated at 1 μm (absolute) or less for filtration of clear unsafe water	1 μm or less filter pore size will remove *Giardia duodenalis*, *Cryptosporidium* and other protozoa Reverse osmosis and ultrafilter devices can remove almost all pathogens	Most bacteria and viruses will not be removed Many carbon-block filters do not remove pathogens, other than possibly protozoa, even if carbon is impregnated with silver. They must have a specified pore size and be certified for microbe removal

*From World Health Organization (2005). *Preventing Travellers' Diarrhoea: How to Make Drinking Water Safe* with permission of the World Health Organization.
†To make a 1% stock solution of calcium hypochlorite, add to 1 L of water, 28 g if chlorine content is 35%, or 15.4 g if 65%, or 14.3 g if 70%.250

carried through the day. The safety and quality of piped water cannot always be guaranteed for small rural supplies even in developed countries. When piped supplies are not available, bottled water may be available. This offers a safer alternative in many countries, however, it is important to recognize that bottled water itself may not be safe unless purchased from a reputable supplier. It is only too easy to refill bottles. Bottled water can only be relied on if it is from a reputable supplier and sold in a sealed bottle. If in doubt carbonated waters are generally safer than still waters. It is difficult to add the carbon dioxide if refilling at the local stream. When piped and bottled waters are not available, the traveller may have to rely on **surface waters** or water from shallow wells that may be of high turbidity and contaminated with faecal pathogens.

Water treatment has two functions:

- to improve the organoleptic quality of the water, making it more palatable
- to improve safety by removing or killing pathogenic micro-organisms.

Although the former may reduce the bacterial load this cannot be relied on to make water safe from all microbial pathogens. For a comprehensive review of **field water treatment** see Backer (1995, 2001). The World Health Organization (WHO) guidelines for travellers are given in Table 19.1.

Improving aesthetic quality and filtration

If the water is cloudy or contains sediment then it should be filtered or otherwise clarified. Many surface waters are particularly turbid due to inorganic particulates such as clay and silt and/or organic material such as algae. The treatment method is **sedimentation**. Simply fill a container with water and let it stand for an hour or so after which carefully pour off the water into another container for subsequent disinfection. Sedimentation works well for larger but not for small particles, the latter of which are more likely to contain waterborne pathogens. Even so, the bacterial load will be reduced by sedimentation but not sufficiently for the water to be presumed to be safe to drink.

Coagulation/flocculation
This has the advantage of removing smaller particles that will not settle under gravity within an

acceptable time. Coagulation can be achieved by adding a small amount of alum (aluminium sulphate) to the water (about 20 mg/L water). The water is stirred briskly for about a minute, then gently for about 5 minutes before being left to stand for about 30 minutes. Flocs will then settle and the supernatant (water) can be then gently poured into a new container. Coagulation/flocculation will effectively remove small particles and will improve both taste and colour. The process will also remove a substantial proportion of bacteria, protozoa and some heavy metals. However, it cannot be relied on to make water safe from infectious agents and a subsequent disinfection step should always be performed.

Filtration
A wide variety of filtration systems are available to the traveller. All filters require a container, a filter and some means of generating pressure across the filter. The filter medium can also vary and some add disinfectant to the water as it passes through. Some filters are effective at making water safe to drink and these are discussed below. Of particular value is the **Millbank filter** which is a large sock made from a felt-like material (Figure 19.1). This is effective at removing particulate materials and turbidity. If nothing else is available, a sock can be used to filter water (Figure 19.2), though in this author's experience many people have a psychological barrier to drinking water that has been through material worn on the foot.

Filtration alone through a Millbank filter, sock or other material cannot be relied on to make drinking water free from pathogens. It can, however, remove the vectors responsible for transmitting *Dracunculiasis* (Guinea worm) and is a valuable and effecting means of control. Other pathogens are less easily removed. Table 19.1 lists some of the main filter types. The effectiveness of a filter at removing pathogens depends on the effective pore size of the filter and whether there is any associated disinfection step. Low turbidity water that has been through a filtration step is more effectively disinfected by halogen disinfectants than turbid water. With all filters, if the membrane breaks the filter becomes ineffective.

Several filters are effective at removing both bacteria (those with an effective pore size <0.2 µm) and parasites (those with an effective pore size

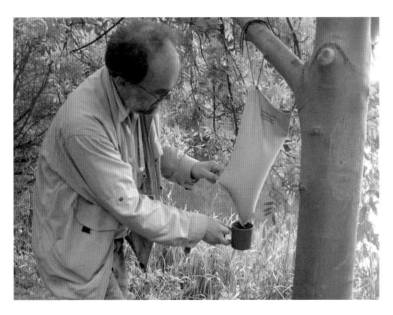

Figure 19.1 *A Millbank filter in use by the author*

1–2 μm) but few can be relied on for viruses. In remote environments where other humans are rare, filtration may be sufficient as waterborne viruses are generally strict human pathogens and faecal contamination is unlikely. **Reverse osmosis** filters can remove viruses and desalinate water but are costly and require high filter pressures. **Granular activated charcoal (GAC)** filters can remove both organic and inorganic chemicals from water but should not be relied on to remove micro-organisms.

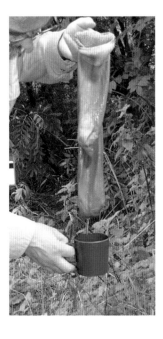

Figure 19.2 *A foot sock being used to filter drinking water*

Improving safety by heat or chemical disinfection

Boiling

Boiling is the most effective means of making water safe from microbial pathogens. All known waterborne pathogens are inactivated rapidly in boiling water, indeed inactivation occurs well below 100 °C. Pasteurization (72 °C for 15 seconds) is a well-recognized method for inactivating most non-sporing pathogens, including relatively heat resistant ones such as *Mycobacterium bovis* (Backer 1995; Mossel *et al.* 1995). In some guidance there remains doubt about whether boiling is adequate and concerns about *Cryptosporidium* contamination of water supplies has led the Centers for Disease Control and Prevention (Atlanta, USA) to advise people with acquired immune deficiency syndrome (AIDS) to boil drinking water for 1 minute rather than 5 minutes (which was the initial recommendation). The reality is that *Cryptosporidium* is inactivated long before the water comes to a boil (Table 19.2) and the advice to do any more than bring to a rolling boil seems unnecessary. The other area of uncertainty about the effectiveness of pasteurization is with regard to the viruses, especially hepatitis A virus (HAV). Table 19.2 shows available data for both. Poliovirus also appears effectively inactivated at 72 °C. There are limited data on HAV above 60 °C, however, inactivation in blood products does occur

Table 19.2 *Evidence for effectiveness of pasteurization for the inactivation of a range of potential waterborne pathogens*

Pathogen	Reference	Conditions	Log inactivation or other end point
Poliovirus	Strazynski *et al.* (2002)	72 °C for 15 s in water	1.11 ± 0.003
		72 °C for 30 s in water	≥5
Hepatitis A virus	Murphy *et al.* (1993)	60 °C for 30 min in tissue culture medium	>3.6
Cryptosporidium	Harp *et al.* (1996)	71.7 °C for 5 s in water	Complete inactivation in mouse model
	Deng and Cliver (2001)	71.7 °C for 5 s in cider	4.8
	Fayer (1994)	72.4 °C for 1 min	>4

at this temperature. All waterborne viruses, including HAV, are likely to be fully inactivated well before water comes to a boil. In any event people trekking in remote countries at high altitude should be protected against HAV through immunization before travelling.

Bringing water to the boil applies even at high altitude where the boiling point is reduced, but this should still be sufficient to ensure safety. In Denver Colorado (1609 m [5280 feet]) water will boil at 95 °C and in Lhasa (Tibet, just over 3360 m [12 000 feet]) water will boil at 87 °C. In Wenzhuan, Tibet, the world's highest town at 5099 m (16 730 feet), water will boil at 82 °C. At Everest base camp (altitude 5340 m [17 520 feet] and boiling point 81 °C) people should be reassured that boiled water is still perfectly safe. However, on the top of Mount Everest (8840 m [29 000 feet]), water boils at 71 °C, so there may be a 'theoretical' risk from HAV, though faecal contamination of snow to be melted for drinking would be unlikely.

Chemical disinfection

If boiling is not practical, a range of other options are available for disinfecting water. The most widely used chemicals are based on the halogens chlorine or iodine, neither of which is effective against *Cryptosporidium* oocysts (see Table 19.1, p. 338). Crucial to the effectiveness of chemical disinfection is using water that is free from turbidity and achieving sufficient contact time. Details for some disinfectants are given in Table 19.1. If water is turbid it should be filtered or clarified before disinfection. It is important to use the appropriate dose of disinfectant and allow the full contact time. Care should be taken to increase the dose or contact time in cold weather. Chlorine has the benefit over iodine of being readily available as household bleach.

However, iodine is more effective in turbid waters, is more stable and effective over a broader pH range than chlorine. Chlorine is generally safe, provided care is taken with the concentrated solution. Iodine should not be used to treat water for pregnant women for extended periods (>1 month), for those allergic to iodine or for those with thyroid dysfunction. Some people dislike the taste of halogens, but waters can be dehalogenated either by passing through a granular activated carbon filter, or by the addition of vitamin C or sodium thiosulphate. The taste of chorine can also be reduced by decanting the water a few times or just leaving it a few hours (covered so as not to allow further contamination).

Silver disinfection is still widely available for water treatment. However, its microbial effectiveness is relatively poor and the WHO does not recommend it as a treatment for potentially contaminated drinking water. It does have a role in preventing bacterial growth in stored water, such as when an expedition returns to stored water in the desert. Potassium permanganate also has disinfectant activities, but despite previous widespread use, owing to the lack of data on its effectiveness against certain pathogens, it is no longer recommended. Potassium permanganate can be carried for other purposes such as treating certain skin conditions and for lighting fires (if mixed with a glycerol-based antifreeze it spontaneously bursts into flame).

Combination filtration and disinfection

Some devices (known as **purifiers**) combine filtration with disinfection and provide a highly effective means of treating water. One model has a two-barrel system, one barrel containing iodine resin and the other GAC (Figure 19.3a). The other type looks like an ordinary drinking bottle but with a filter and disinfectant sleeve in the neck of the

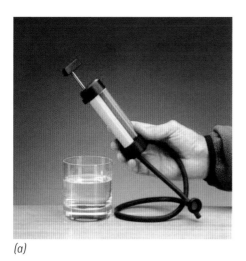 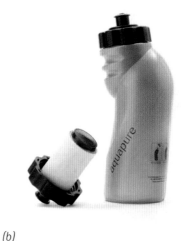

(a)   (b)

Figure 19.3   *Two commercially available combined filtration/disinfection (water purifiers) (a) Travel Well Trekker (published with permission of Pre-Mac International Ltd) (b) Aquapure traveller (published with permission of BW Technologies Limited)*

bottle (Figure 19.3b). These purifiers also remove certain chemical contaminants.

Finding water

Sources of drinking water that are easiest to find in the wilderness are streams, rivers and lakes. However, in deserts and in frozen or mountainous environments, surface water may not be readily available. A range of **bushcraft** skills have developed to enable people to obtain water in these environments (Mears 2003), and some options, ranging from the obvious to the bizarre, are listed in Box 19.1.

Box 19.1 Bushcraft skills to obtain water

- In areas where there is a morning dew, this can be mopped on the ground using a towel which is then wrung out into a container
- A 'gypsy well' may be dug in marshy ground. This will then fill with water which can be filtered and treated. The initial fill may be discarded as subsequent fills are usually less turbid
- Collect rain using a flysheet or polythene sheet
- Melt snow or ice
- Some plants may be useful sources of water, for example bamboo which can be sliced and bent over for sap to drip out, or the barrel cactus which can be sliced open and the contents sucked out with an improvised straw: be sure the plant is not poisonous as many are

---

- Provided the traveller knows how to find them, the water-bearer frog can be squeezed to obtain drinking water
- In extremis, Mears (2003) reports that the stomach contents of large herbivorous mammals can be placed in a cloth to allow the liquid to be squeezed out and drunk: the stomach contents of carnivores should not be drunk due to the increased likelihood of pathogenic bacteria

---

It is never safe to drink sea water or your own urine as both have a higher osmotic pressure than serum and will lead to a worsening of dehydration. If this is all that is available then some form of **distillation** or **reverse osmosis** filter will make this drinkable.

FOOD

Food is less crucial to immediate survival than water, although a lack of food makes it difficult to operate effectively or keep warm in cold climates. In the wilderness, food can be carried, bought en route, or hunted and collected from the land. If wilderness activity is based around a single base camp then there is the opportunity to have a more varied diet with fresh fruit, vegetables and meat.

A wide range of expedition food is available, much of which is expensive. Two factors determine the value of expedition food: its nutrient value and its portability. Most commercially prepared expedition food is dehydrated to reduce weight, stored in water-tight packages and requires mixing with water prior to reheating and serving. Food hygiene issues with such food are unlikely to be significant, provided the food has been safely prepared by the manufacturer, the packaging remains intact, and the contents dry. When fresh fruit, vegetables and meat are used in cooking or where food is hunted or gathered from the surrounding area, then 'normal' food safety issues are equally applicable in as outside the wilderness. Advice on hunting and food collection in the wilderness is beyond the scope of this book but there are many sources of information. However, when intending to live off the land, it is vital that the traveller knows what they are eating and which local foods are safe or dangerous. Good hygienic practices will not help if poisonous mushrooms or other plants are eaten.

Storing and preparing food in the wilderness brings additional problems (Bennett-Jones 2002; see Box 19.2 for preventing foodborne illness in the wilderness). Food storage at camp may be difficult, and refrigerators are rarely available or, if present, unreliable. Perishable foods may spoil in hot humid environments, however in arctic conditions, refrigerators are probably not necessary, but thawing the food can be a problem. When living under canvas, it may be difficult to keep rodents away from foods, and in some places, larger mammals such as bears are attracted to foods. Local cooks may also be the source of infection. Food preparation can also be problematic and decreased care in personal hygiene while in the wilderness increases the potential for contamination of food during preparation. It may be difficult to adequately wash some foods such as salads that are not cooked before consumption, and the lack of utensils makes cross-contamination between raw and cooked food more likely.

Box 19.2 Preventing foodborne illness in the wilderness (based on Bennett-Jones 2002)

- Know what you are eating and whether it is poisonous
- Follow safe food handling practices common to all kitchens
- Do not let people who are ill prepare food for others – especially important if they have diarrhoea or skin infections

---

- Store perishable foods in a cold box/refrigerator or do not take them
- Separate raw and cooked food
- Ensure food is adequately cooked
- Practise good personal hygiene including handwashing after visiting the latrine and before touching food
- Store food in rodent-proof containers or out of their reach
- Keep insects off food by use of nets
- If sharing the wilderness with large mammals such as bears or lions, store food well away from the areas where people sleep
- Do not take foods that are intended to be eaten raw and are difficult to wash such as salad
- Do not take food such as shellfish that are more likely to be the source of infection

---

SAFE DISPOSAL OF FAECES

Good hygiene and safe disposal of faeces is often overlooked and forgotten, possibly because these do not protect the person at toilet, just the rest of humanity using the wilderness. Since diarrhoeal disease in humans is often due to pathogens that were fairly recently excreted in the faeces of another human, keeping people and excreta separate is good wilderness practice. We should not need to refer to the paper by Lee *et al.* (2002) to know it is bad practice to defecate into the river from which people are likely to drink water.

A well-designed camp layout is vital. In static camps with sufficient transport, chemical toilets may become an option. A chemical-free alternative for static camps is the pit latrine which should be cited away from the main camping and food preparation areas and in an area away from surface water. The pit should be dug to a depth of about 1.25 m and covered with a large rock or leaf to prevent flies getting in. After defecation into the latrine, some of the soil from the hole should be replaced. When finished, the remainder of the soil should be replaced into the hole and, in grassland, the sod replaced. Disinfectants should never be added to a pit latrine.

Latrines should be sited away from the sleeping and cooking areas and should, wherever possible, be placed downhill of the main campsite. During heavy rain it is preferable for the contents to flow away from sleeping areas. It is also preferable to build camp up hill and away from sites where previous campers have dug their own latrines. It is also essential that the latrine is in a place where it will not contaminate streams or rivers that could be used for recreation or a source of drinking water. Enteric organisms can survive for long periods before percolating through soils. In one study in an alpine environment (Backer 1995), exploration trenches dug through the sites of pit latrines 1–2 years after they had been closed showed little decomposition with most of the mass being recognizable as faecal material with high levels of faecal coliforms.

When on the move, a pit latrine is impractical. However, there is a general responsibility to choose carefully where to defecate. Defecation should be away from the trail and in a place at least 30 m away from watercourses from which others may drink. If possible, faeces should be buried 25 cm below ground, but since in rocky environments this is not always practical, some authorities advocate that it is better to smear faeces across rocks to allow desiccation and ultraviolet disinfection (Backer 1995). Some people would find this somewhat disconcerting to have to do. A more detailed discussion of the most environmentally sound approaches to daefecating in the wilderness is given by Meyer (1994) in her classic and aptly named book *How to Shit in the Woods*.

To end this chapter – a final reminder about the importance of handwashing with soap and water in the wilderness after visiting the toilet and before touching food.

Summary

The reader should be in no doubt of the importance of good food hygiene practices while in the wilderness. The additional concerns about water safety and availability need meticulous attention and can be essential for survival. Diarrhoeal illnesses are the most frequent infection acquired in the wilderness and the three essential steps to prevent foodborne illness in the wilderness are:
- good water disinfection
- good food hygiene practices
- safe disposal of faeces.

All websites cited in below were accessed in November 2006.

SOURCES OF INFORMATION AND FURTHER READING

Backer H (2002) Water disinfection for international and wilderness travellers. *Clin Infect Dis* **34**: 355–64.

Backer HD (1995) Field water disinfection. In: Auerach PS (ed.) *Wilderness Medicine; Management of Wilderness and Environmental Emergencies*, 3rd edn. St. Louis: Mosby, pp. 1060–91.

Barbour AG, Nichols CR, Fukushima T (1976) An outbreak of giardiasis in a group of campers. *Am J Trop Med Hyg* **25**: 384–9.

Bennett-Jones H (2002) Base camp hygiene and health. In: Warrell D, Anderson S (eds) Royal Geographical Society Expedition Medicine, 2nd edn. London: Profile Books, pp. 93–103.

Boulware DR (2004) Influence of hygiene on gastrointestinal illness among wilderness backpackers. *J Travel Med* **11**: 27–33.

Deng MQ, Cliver DO (2001) Inactivation of *Cryptosporidium parvum* oocysts in cider by flash pasteurization. *J Food Protect* **64**: 523–7.

Fayer R (1994) Effect of high temperature on infectivity of *Cryptosporidium parvum* oocysts in water. *Appl Environ Microbiol* **60**: 2732–5.

Harp JA, Fayer R, Pesch BA *et al.* (1996) Effect of pasteurization on infectivity of *Cryptosporidium parvum* oocysts in water and milk. *Appl Environm Microbiol* **62**: 2866–8.

Hopkins RS, Juranek DD (1991) Acute giardiasis: an improved clinical case definition for epidemiological studies. *Am J Epidemiol* **133**: 402–7.

Hopkins RS, Olmsted R, Istre GR (1984) Endemic *Campylobacter jejuni* infection in Colorado: identified risk factors. *Am J Public Health* **74**: 249–50.

Lee SH, Levy DA, Craun GF, *et al.* (2002) Surveillance for waterborne-disease outbreaks – United States, 1999–2000. *MMWR CDC Surveill Summ* **51**: 1–47.

Mears R (2003) *Essential Bushcraft.* London: Hodder & Stoughton, pp. 55–75.

Meyer K (1994) *How to Shit in the Woods*, 2nd edn. Berkeley, California: Ten Speed Press.

Mossel DAA, Corry JEL, Struijk CB *et al.* (1995) *Essentials of the Microbiology of Foods.* Chichester: John Wiley and Sons, p. 231.

Murphy P, Nowak T, Lemon SM *et al.* (1993) Inactivation of Hepatitis A virus by heat treatment in aqueous solution. *J Med Virol* **41**: 61–4.

Peipins LA, Highfill KA, Barrett E, *et al.* (2002) A Norwalk-like virus outbreak on the Appalachian Trail. *J Environ Health* **64**: 18–23.

Prats G, Mirelis B, Miro E *et al.* (2003) Cephalosporin-resistant *Escherichia coli* among summer camp attendees with salmonellosis. *Emerg Infect Dis* **9**: 1273–80.

Strazynski M, Kramer J, Becker B (2002) Thermal inactivation of poliovirus type 1 in water, milk and yoghurt. *Int J Food Microbiol* **74**: 73–8.

Taylor DN, McDermott KT, Little JR *et al.* (1983) Campylobacter enteritis from untreated water in the Rocky Mountains. *Ann Intern Med* **99**: 38–40.

World Health Organization (2005) *Preventing Travellers' Diarrhoea: How to Make Drinking Water Safe.* Geneva: WHO (available at: www.who.int/water_sanitation_health/hygiene/envsan/sdwtravel.pdf).

Wright RA, Spencer HC, Brodsky RE *et al.* (1977) Giardiasis in Colorado: an epidemiological study. *Am J Epidemiol* **105**: 330–6.

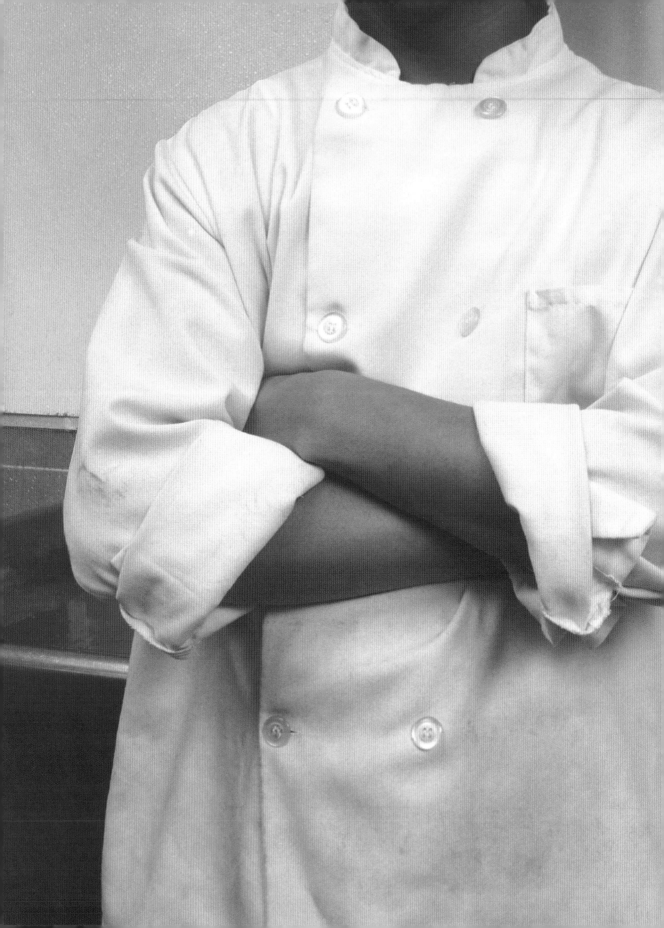

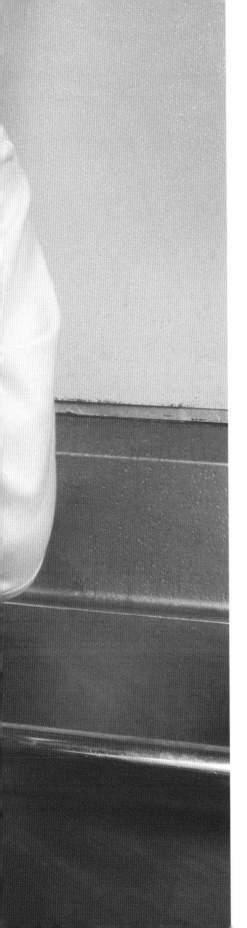

CONTRIBUTION TO FOOD POISONING AND FOOD HYGIENE IN SPECIFIC SETTINGS AND BY SPECIFIC PROFESSIONAL GROUPS

The final part of this book outlines the contribution to prevention of food poisoning and how food hygiene is achieved in specific settings and by various professional groups not dealt with in detail earlier in the text. This part is concluded by a description of how food-poisoning outbreaks are detected, investigated, controlled and managed.

20

Food service sector including healthcare and educational institutions, small retailers and domestic caterers

Richard Elson

The food service sector	351		Domestic catering	353
Hospitals, schools and residential care homes	351		Sources of information and further reading	354
Small retail and catering businesses	352			

This chapter covers the contribution of the food service sector to reducing food poisoning and ensuring food hygiene in addition to those retailers not already covered in Chapter 11.

THE FOOD SERVICE SECTOR

The food service sector can broadly be described as the provision of meals outside the home. It is also known as the catering sector and is estimated to be the fourth largest service market in the UK. The food service sector can be split into cost and profit sectors. The cost sector is also known as public sector procurement and includes schools, hospitals, prisons and care homes. The profit sector is made up of, for example, restaurants, fast food outlets, pubs and hotels. Business contract catering lies between the cost and the profit sectors as many businesses subsidize these activities in the cost sector but the catering company providing them can still make a profit.

The supply chain to each sector is largely the same and is met either by wholesalers or through commercial suppliers. Large companies or chains usually source ingredients and products from suppliers who provide food to the specification of the company concerned. Smaller companies, particularly those that are independent enterprises,

may source from a supplier or through wholesalers. One of the benefits of obtaining food from a supplier is that they can usually provide full traceability from the source.

The food service sector can be further divided into production, sourcing, processing, manufacture, distribution, point of sale and consumption. Different hygiene rules may be applicable to each stage, emphasizing the importance of a 'farm to fork' approach. The size and complexity of the food service sector can therefore present numerous challenges to food safety. This section will cover the catering trade and sectors of the food service that pose particular challenges to food safety owing to the nature of the population which they serve.

HOSPITALS, SCHOOLS AND RESIDENTIAL CARE HOMES

Hospitals, schools and residential care homes are worthy of particular mention with regard to food safety due to the vulnerable populations which they often serve. Following committees of inquiry into a major outbreak of salmonellosis at Stanley Royd Hospital in Wakefield in the 1980s, guidance was issued to the NHS on the arrangements for communicable disease control. These reports recommended the development and adoption of plans for the management of major incidents of infection, including such incidents occurring in NHS premises, and prompted the lifting of Crown immunity from inspection for such premises.

Public sector catering is usually provided by a primary care trust or local education authority through the following means:

- **Cook-serve** – food prepared either from fresh ingredients or pre-prepared in traditional on-site kitchens and served directly, pre-plated or through a trolley service, as in the case of healthcare facilities.
- **Cook-chill** – food prepared in a centrally located kitchen and transported to various schools or hospitals within the area for reheating in on-site kitchens.
- **Cook-freeze** – as for cook-chill but food is frozen before delivery and reheated in on-site kitchens.

The method employed often depends on the layout of a particular site, the type of buildings, kitchen space, staff skill mix, the patient population, the number of meals required and the budget allocated to catering by individual trusts or local authorities.

Food hygiene requirements apply to all three food supply methods, however, each presents different hazards. The Department of Health has provided guidance, albeit now dated, for cook-chill and cook-freeze practices. Local authorities are responsible for food hygiene enforcement in NHS hospitals and schools.

SMALL RETAIL AND CATERING BUSINESSES

Small retailers or catering businesses include those which are not part of a large chain, whether or not they are part of a franchise. Small retailers include small convenience stores, 'corner shops', confectioners, tobacconists and newsagents. Small caterers include takeaways, fast-food shops, cafés and restaurants. The role of small businesses in preventing food poisoning may be underestimated as they are usually the penultimate stage in a long and sometimes complicated food chain. The diverse nature of these operations also presents difficulties in applying consistent advice and enforcement.

Many small retailers sell long shelf-life, low-risk products such as tinned foods. However, most also stock high-risk foods such as cooked meats, milk, cheese, sandwiches and eggs. An increasing number of specialized small retailers are selling high-risk foods and there are also retailers that sell freshly cooked items such as rotisserie-cooked meat and poultry, and 'baked off' goods such as pastries, which require careful attention and special storage, particularly at chilled temperatures. Foods that rely on refrigeration to assure their safety may be produced and distributed under strictly controlled conditions with the assumption that these conditions will be observed until the point of sale. However, if the small retailers do not observe or fully understand the significance of these controls, food safety and quality can be compromised, with resultant effects for both consumers and the business.

Commercial catering organizations are hugely varied in size and operation but are subject to the same food hygiene requirements throughout the European Union. The management of food safety and hygiene is simpler through national or multi-national chains or franchise operations. However, many catering outlets are individual enterprises with varying levels of management experience, a high turnover of staff and low profit margins resulting in overall lower levels of food hygiene. Enforcement of food hygiene requirements in these premises is the responsibility of local authorities.

Managers of food business of this size are unlikely to have access to the same food safety knowledge as larger retailers. Although some are members of trade groups (the Federation of Small Businesses [FSB] represents over 200 000 companies nationally), these may only represent commercial interests rather than directing the food safety policy of their members. Smaller retail and catering businesses therefore require support and training from local authority professionals and private training enterprises. The Food Standards Agency (FSA) initiative 'Safer Food Better Business', launched in 2006, is primarily aimed at smaller businesses and recognizes that this sector requires support in order to comply with the requirements of food safety and standards legislation. Additional guidance for setting up a catering business has also been produced by the FSA and covers areas such as food safety management procedures, food hygiene, and food law.

'Safer Food Better Business' concentrates on ensuring that managers of small businesses have access to a standardized framework relating to food safety (the fours Cs: **cooking**, prevention of **cross-contamination**, **cleaning** and **chilling**; see Chapter 17). The guide also encourages managers to perform regular checks and to maintain a diary for recording unusual events as well as actions taken to rectify them. This provides a record for enforcement officers to audit and evidence of due diligence (see Chapter 17). The FSA is providing grants to local authorities to boost existing training of small retailers and caterers in food safety.

It has been routine practice in a number of countries for many years, notably in Singapore and the USA, to post the last inspection report of catering and retail businesses in a conspicuous place for public scrutiny. This approach has been debated and advocated for a number of years in the UK, and is now being introduced as a pilot scheme known as 'Score on the Doors'. Its introduction has been precipitated by a combination of increased consumer awareness of food safety issues and the introduction of legislation such as the Freedom of Information Act 2000, intended to increase public access to information traditionally regarded as confidential.

The aim of the scheme is to drive food hygiene standards up by informing customers of the standards of food safety and hygiene found at the last inspection of the premises. The information is displayed on the door or window in each food outlet, supported by information on a website maintained by the local authority. Consumers can then assess the outlet before deciding to use it.

DOMESTIC CATERING

Domestic catering is not a large industry, yet there is potential for outbreaks and food poisoning incidents. Domestic catering premises are subject to the same requirements in law as other catering organizations, however, legislative control for domestic catering is not as rigid as for commercial premises. For example, in certain circumstances, domestic caterers are not required to register with the local authority. However this is based on frequency of use and the risk presented by the foods that are prepared on the premises. A person who occasionally bakes wedding cakes to order from home presents a different magnitude of risk to somebody who caters for large wedding parties on a regular basis.

The term 'home caterer' is used to describe those who prepare food in a domestic kitchen on a commercial basis. Food prepared in the home is eaten elsewhere, for example, at business premises or village halls and community clubs. Domestic premises are not usually designed to cater for large numbers of people, and are not a large industry, but there is potential for outbreaks and food poisoning incidents. When compared with outbreaks associated with non-domestic premises, outbreaks attributed to catering for large numbers of people from domestic premises indicate that most outbreaks are caused by poultry, eggs or sauces containing salmonellas. Outbreaks associated with such premises occurred more frequently during the summer. Inappropriate storage, inadequate heat treatment and cross-contamination have all been cited as contributory factors.

The domestic environment can easily be adapted for commercial use. However, the presence of family members and pets or the continuation of domestic activities may present challenges to food safety and hygiene not usually experienced in commercial premises. It is preferable, therefore, that the food room is used solely for food preparation and not for domestic activities such as washing soiled linen or eating. Pets should not be allowed into the room during food preparation. All surfaces must be disinfected before any possible contact with food. Domestic and commercial operations can be either separated physically, by locating domestic cooking facilities elsewhere, or separated by time, i.e. commercial food preparation only takes place in the afternoon.

All websites given below were accessed in December 2006.

SOURCES OF INFORMATION AND FURTHER READING

Food Standards Agency (2006) Safer food better business (available at: www.food.gov.uk/foodindustry/regulation/hygleg/hyglegresources/sfbb).

Department of Health (1989) *Chilled and Frozen. Guidelines on Cook-Chill and Cook-Freeze Catering Systems*. London: The Stationery Office.

Food Standards Agency (2006) *Starting Up. Your First Steps to Running a Catering Business*. London: Food Standards Agency (available at: www.food.gov.uk/multimedia/pdfs/startingup.pdf).

21

Food safety on ships and aircraft

Rob Griffin

Introduction	355	Aircraft	357
Home authority principle	355	UK military ships and aircraft	359
Background and relationship to inspections	355	Sources of information and further reading	359
Ships	356		

The general considerations and actions required for achieving food safety on ships and aircraft are the same as for almost all the other settings described elsewhere in this book. However, ships and aircraft have some unique features and constraints imposed by their physical structure, security considerations and more limited opportunity for sourcing of food and water.

INTRODUCTION

Port health officers at seaports and environmental health officers working at airports have long been able to board ships and aircraft under public health legislation. However, access to ships and aircraft was not permitted for food law enforcement purposes under the Food Safety Act 1990 as these were not defined as premises under food law. Consequently, food hygiene issues relating to ships and aircraft were undertaken on a voluntary and unofficial basis. To rectify this anomaly, the Food Safety (Ships and Aircraft) (England and Scotland) Order 2003 (SI 2003 No. 1895) extended the meaning of 'premises' to ships and aircraft so as to give authorized officers the power of entry. Similar legislation has been enacted in Northern Ireland and Wales.

After the advent of consolidated and updated European Union (EU) food law, particularly Regulation (EC) No. 852/2004 on the hygiene of foodstuffs and the national implementing legislation enforceable from 1 January 2006, the Food Law Code of Practice and Practice Guidance produced by the Food Standards Agency were reviewed. Authorized officers must have regard to this Code. The Code and the Guidance both have a chapter on food safety issues that need to be considered when inspecting ships and aircraft, including cruise liners, passenger ferries, merchant ships, Royal Navy vessels, training yachts and all types of aircraft on which food is served.

HOME AUTHORITY PRINCIPLE

For enforcement of food safety, where possible, the Local Authorities Co-ordinators of Regulatory Services (LACORS) Home Authority (HA) principle should be used to assist with the dissemination of relevant information about airline or shipping company procedures. If such arrangements are agreed, the HA should ensure that all appropriate documentation is made available to it by the company for liaison and information purposes with other relevant authorities. Strategies for the frequency of inspections should be formulated by the HA, and these are usually based on considerations of the type of craft, and its origin and history. Previous inspection reports should be obtained by HAs to ensure that, where appropriate, follow-up inspections are undertaken and unnecessary inspections avoided.

BACKGROUND AND RELATIONSHIP TO INSPECTIONS

Under the Aviation and Maritime Security Act 1990, security clearance is necessary for authorized officers when they enter secure areas at ports and airports to undertake their duties. Authorized officers must take account of any health and safety issues which might affect them and also have regard to requirements of the port authority and the shipping or airline company during any inspection of a ship or an aircraft.

The types of food hazard on shipboard/aircraft environments are likely to be different from those found in land-based food premises. Apart from the 24-hour nature of operations on board ships and aircraft, there are potential hazards associated with methods of storage of both food (dry, chilled and frozen) and water on board, and these are usually only available from when the vessel/aircraft is in port. There are often restrictions to possible improvements because of the fixed layout of food handling areas which cannot be expanded or changed due to the structure and safety of the vessel, as well as its age, condition, and the need for proper maintenance.

Food safety standards on ships and aircraft are covered by the relevant articles and the chapters in Annex II of Regulation (EC) No. 852/2004 on the hygiene of foodstuffs. When a serious condition(s) is found, the service of a hygiene improvement notice or hygiene emergency prohibition notice under the national implementing legislation (The Food Hygiene [England] Regulations 2006 [SI 2006 No. 14]) – similar implementing legislation applies in the devolved administrations – is undertaken if the aircraft or ship is registered in the UK. Other non-food aspects considered by port health officers, subject to the type of vessel, includes public health risks such as infectious disease control, accommodation, swimming pools/spa pools, waste disposal and general hygiene.

If the craft is registered in another EU Member State or non-European country, then liaison with the relevant competent authority in the other country on serious food safety deficiencies may be undertaken via the Food Standards Agency.

SHIPS

Preparation for inspection

Food production and handling on board vessels varies greatly depending on the type of vessel and number of passengers and crew, e.g. some cruise liners may have as many as 900 passengers and 800 crew, whereas smaller vessels may be crewed by only 10–15 personnel.

Since the shipboard environment is a closed community, problems associated with food production on large vessels, such as cruise liners, can have a major impact on both passengers and crew. Food contaminated by food poisoning bacteria or toxins can be extremely disruptive, and even on smaller vessels, an outbreak of food poisoning can have a significant impact on the safety of the vessel because of severe incapacitation of critical crew members.

Inspection frequency

An authorized officer usually considers the frequency of inspection of premises based on a risk rating system outlined in the statutory Code of Practice. Frequency of inspection of vessels for food safety purposes also depends on the information available. That is, consideration should first be given to any documentation that might be available from the ship's master and identification of all food and water-related activities undertaken on the vessel (Box 21.1).

Box 21.1 Factors to consider when determining the frequency of inspection of a vessel

- Name, type of vessel and flag state
- Age/condition/history of vessel
- Number of crew and passengers
- Vessel's trading pattern and previous port(s) of call
- Date and port of last food safety inspection
- Available documentation, e.g. food specifications and suppliers, Hazards Analysis and Critical Control Points (HACCP) records, water sample results, food handlers' training records
- Confidence in the available documentation
- Recent reports of food-related problems on the vessel
- Reports from previous inspections and level of compliance
- Valid ship sanitation control certificate, where appropriate

---

To avoid unnecessary inspections, the authorized officer should ascertain when, and the extent, of the vessel's last inspection, and decide if and when re-inspection should occur. This may be undertaken by requesting a copy of the last inspection report from the ship's master or from the relevant port health authority. Then the officer should decide if there is a need for a primary inspection for food safety purposes, although he or she may consider that only other public health aspects need checking. If no report is available, and after taking into account other factors, such as the date and time of sailing, the officer might decide that a full inspection is appropriate. Issues for possible inclusion in respect of food safety include:

- specifications and sourcing of food and water
- transport of food and water to the vessel and loading
- facilities for food storage and preparation, including storage of water used in food areas or for drinking purposes
- water treatment
- adequacy of any HACCP system
- temperature control of food, as required by Regulation (EC) No. 852/2004, and the methods of monitoring
- food handlers' knowledge of food hygiene appropriate to their activities and their health status
- results of food and water sampling
- records of cases/outbreaks of gastrointestinal illness etc.
- cleaning and pest control activities
- waste disposal.

Action on conclusion of the inspection

The findings of an inspection should be discussed with the ship's master or a delegated representative, giving the expected timescale of any required corrective actions and the vessel's proposed movements. If possible, the authorized officer should also prepare an inspection report for the ship's master before leaving the vessel. Where appropriate, a copy of the report should also be sent to the relevant shipping company and the HA, if appointed, kept informed.

Maritime and Coastguard Agency

Authorized officers at seaports maintain contact with the Maritime and Coastguard Agency (MCA). This Agency is responsible throughout the UK for co-ordinating search and rescue at sea, preventing coastal pollution and ensuring ships are safe (including the welfare of crew and their accommodation), and taking action for breaches of Merchant Shipping legislation. The Food Standards Agency has facilitated a Memorandum of Understanding (MoU) between the MCA, LACORS and the Association of Port Health Authorities (APHA) to assist in joint working. This MoU does not cover military vessels, and was reviewed as the Food Hygiene (England) Regulations 2006 and the directly applicable EU food law and came into force on 1 January 2006.

The MCA has the power under merchant shipping legislation to prevent ships from leaving port should there be a major issue relating to maritime safety. Consequently, this power is covered in the MoU, so that if a port health officer or environmental health officer finds food safety issues that are of major concern and considers that there is an imminent risk, arrangements can be made with the relevant marine surveyor, an officer employed by the MCA, for appropriate action.

AIRCRAFT

Preparation for inspection

For aircraft food safety, it might be inappropriate for inspections to take place on a regular basis, if suitable information has been obtained from the relevant airline company and/or the HA for the airline, and such information has been verified. When there is a HA arrangement, airline companies should be aware of their responsibilities in relation to providing information. When requested, HAs should provide information to other appropriate authorities on an airline's general food safety policy and procedures. Verification of the information is essential and might also require liaison with other food authorities depending on the location of the food supplier(s). If verification shows that such information is satisfactory and that food safety practices meet requirements, there may be no need to board the aircraft on a frequent basis. Nonetheless, it is essential to confirm that the information provided is valid through occasional on-board checks. If there is no HA arrangement, direct liaison with airline companies should be undertaken to obtain the necessary information on how food safety systems are operated both before and after food is loaded. Confirmation of the systems used typically includes no changes to both the in-flight caterers or the water supplier, etc.

Information to be obtained to assist inspection procedures

There are now many airline companies, some of which have large fleets. Therefore, to assist in assessing food safety, the information shown in Box 21.2 should be obtained where appropriate.

Box 21.2 Pre-inspection checklist for aircraft
- Contact details of airline staff who deal with enquiries – this could be a food safety advisor employed by the airline company
- Number and type of aircraft, and home base
- Routes flown, including long/short haul and destinations
- Airline food safety policy/procedure documents or manual
- Type of menu (in-flight menus can assist in the assessment of whether high-risk foods are handled and/or prepared on board)
- Food safety knowledge of food handler/cabin staff – this includes up-to-date guidance notes/explanatory sheets and/or proof of appropriate training commensurate with the food handling activity. Information for the staff should cover personal hygiene, own health status and exclusion from work policy, hygienic food handling, cross-contamination issues arising from other duties, pest awareness, food temperature monitoring and control
- Flight caterers, and/or nominated companies assembling and/or transporting meals to the aircraft, used by the airline
- Specifications for the supply of food to aircraft including the accepted temperature for delivery
- Details of food/water safety arrangements when supplied to an aircraft in another EU Member State or third country
- Flights or routes with return flight catering, times involved and storage arrangements
- Potable water supply, source, use of bowsers, cleaning/disinfection of storage tanks and the frequency/effectiveness

---

- Reports of analysis/examination of food and potable water on aircraft arranged by the airline
- Pest control contract and monitoring procedures
- Cleaning contractor, with details of contracts and monitoring of the effectiveness of the cleaning regimen

---

This information will enable an officer to assess the frequency and need for actually boarding a particular type of aircraft for inspection purposes. In practice, having obtained appropriate information from the airline company and/or the relevant HA, the need for an inspection for food safety purposes, of particular types of aircraft is typically once every 18 months to 2 years, unless there are convincing reasons to undertake such inspections in the intervening period.

Inspection of aircraft

Occasionally cabin crew prepare food and hence should have had appropriate training. There are, for example, possible cross-contamination issues related to their other on-board duties, such as handling flight sick bags, and their personal hygiene practices. If inspections are undertaken at departure/arrival points, then they should be before passengers board the aircraft and ideally after cleaning of the aircraft, when food is on board and when airline staff are able to provide assistance and information. However, inspections can, after perusal of the relevant documentation provided by the airline company, be undertaken at other times such as when the aircraft is at the maintenance base.

Items for consideration in relation to food safety on aircraft

Following a check of the airline documents, the following on-site factors should be considered/confirmed, where appropriate:

- information on operations and facilities of the flight caterers
- transport and temperature control of food and loading into the aircraft
- storage of food on the aircraft – this typically includes the use of insulated containers and ice-packs, the maximum stated period until serving and/or re-heating, taking account of

the trips undertaken by the aircraft, e.g. long or short haul, and the type of food served

- the preparation of food on the aircraft and the facilities available for such operations, e.g. reheating/cooking
- personal hygiene facilities for crew, e.g. provision of disposable gloves for certain duties and disinfectant wipes
- return flight meals taking account of the shelf-life of the food and storage facilities
- temperature control and monitoring during flights
- pest control
- water supply source, potability and cleaning of tanks
- procedures for cleaning food handling areas, trolleys/carts
- sampling of food and water
- waste food disposal.

The actual time spent on an aircraft should be short, as most of the food safety issues are standard operating procedures covered in airline company documentation. However, if there are any issues of concern relating to food safety, the authorized officer should notify the relevant company and HA, if designated, that improvements should be made and enhanced inspections undertaken, e.g. assessment of galley cleanliness, increased water sampling for analysis/examination, etc.

Action on conclusion of the inspection

Following an inspection, a report should be sent to the relevant airline company, with a copy sent to the HA, where this arrangement exists. If it is found that food hygiene law is being contravened, for example cabin crew display insufficient knowledge of food hygiene issues, full details of the type of aircraft and flight number should be recorded to allow a follow-up investigation.

Unnecessary delays to aircraft are costly and authorized officers should not cause disruptions to operations, unless, in the unlikely event, there is an imminent risk to the health of the passengers or crew. Inspections of aircraft in transit should only be undertaken if absolutely necessary. This might be based on information received from another authority about the flight caterer, type of food, temperature control, etc. Authorized officers should consider the practicalities of their inspection schedule and endeavour to work with the relevant crew/ground staff to avoid unnecessary difficulties, and should bear in mind the primary objective of an airline company is the safety of the aircraft, passengers and crew.

For the information of vulnerable passengers, e.g. those who might have allergies or food intolerances, authorized officers may request flight caterers to advise their customers of details of meal ingredients. Such information can then be made available to relevant passengers via the cabin crew.

UK MILITARY SHIPS AND AIRCRAFT

Since security must be considered when an authorized officer visits UK military ships and aircraft, prior notification must be given, as unannounced entry is not possible. The three Services have individual HAs that deal with any general issues with implications for food safety. Authorized officers should liaise with the relevant HA, as well as the environmental health leads within the relevant Service. Military policy, procedures and practices must be considered, and authorized officers should remember the ultimate purpose of military ships and aircraft. Hence galley design might have constraints for operational reasons.

The Defence Catering Group representing the three Services has produced a Defence Catering Manual, which is available on each HA's website and is a good reference document.

All websites cited below were accessed in November 2006.

SOURCES OF INFORMATION AND FURTHER READING

Food Standards Agency (2005) *Food Law Code of Practice*. London: Food Standards Agency.

Food Standards Agency (2005) *Food Law Practice Guidance*. London: Food Standards Agency. Both documents are available online at www.food.gov.uk/enforcement/foodlaw/foodlawcop.

LACORS (2002) *LACORS Home Authority Principle – Standards*. London: LACORS. Online. Available at: www.lacors.gov.uk

Ministry of Defence. Joint Service Publication (JSP) 456 – *Defence Catering Manual: Volume 3 Defence Food Safety Management*, 3rd ed. Defence Catering Group (available at: www.mod.uk/NR/rdonlyres/867F871F-4447-473C-B0D5-35BB76F097F6/0/20061020JSP456Vol3U.pdf).

The Food Hygiene (England) Regulations 2006. (SI 2006 No. 14) (available at: www.opsi.gov.uk/si/si2006/20060014.htm). (There is similar legislation for Scotland, Wales and Northern Ireland.)

22

Food trade associations

Kaarin Goodburn

Introduction	361	Umbrella organizations	362
Role of food trade associations	361	Who does what	362
Membership criteria	361	Incident management	362
Operating standards and guidelines	361	Information flows	362
Horizontal and vertical organizations	362	Conclusion	363

Food trade associations (FTAs) are organizations which represent member companies involved with specific parts of the food supply chain, e.g. growing, manufacturing, distribution, wholesaling, catering, or retailing. FTAs act as representatives for specific food industry sectors or professions, support and promote best practice and standards, and provide an interface for the provision and exchange of information with others such as the government, researchers and the media.

INTRODUCTION

Food trade associations (FTAs) are privately funded organizations. Knowledge of FTA activities and roles assists in identifying industry guidelines, standards and certification systems that may be applied to their memberships. FTAs also assist the government and its agencies in reaching businesses directly involved in or impacted by specific issues.

ROLE OF FOOD TRADE ASSOCIATIONS

FTAs play an important role in representing an industry or profession and working among their members/sector, the government, the media, other interest groups and researchers. Information and advice is provided to members; FTAs also develop industry-wide best practice or standards, fund research, publish members-only and publicly available documents, lobby and co-ordinate responses to consultations and provide comments on behalf of their members to external audiences.

MEMBERSHIP CRITERIA

Some FTAs require third party or self-certification with industry guidance, codes or guides as a membership requirement. However, this is usually confined to national sectoral FTAs as the memberships of umbrella bodies are generally mixed and a single certification approach is not appropriate. Indeed, in some countries such as the USA, the application of such membership criteria is considered anti-competitive and therefore illegal. UK-based FTAs often have a significant role in driving standards in their sector.

OPERATING STANDARDS AND GUIDELINES

FTAs play a major role in promoting food safety assurance through the establishment of best practice guidance, guides for the interpretation and compliance with European Union (EU) hygiene legislation, codes of practice and accreditation schemes. Participation in these activities may be a requirement for membership. Much effort goes into ensuring that issues do not arise which would adversely impact on the sector. FTAs may therefore also fund scientific and other research to ensure that broad issues affecting their members are fully explored and that solutions to potential problems are proactively identified. Such research can also be reactive to pre-existing problems within areas covered by an association. FTAs are therefore a good source of technical information for the government and its agencies.

HORIZONTAL AND VERTICAL ORGANIZATIONS

FTAs can represent either a 'vertical' or 'horizontal' sector. Horizontal sectors include those where a technology (e.g. chilling) or a common activity (e.g. growing) is the key factor even where a large variety of foods are produced or handled by members. However, particularly for ambient foods or food ingredients, which represent some of the longest-standing sectors, these are represented by numerous 'vertical' FTAs, e.g. cereals, spices or seasonings.

UMBRELLA ORGANIZATIONS

Many, but not all, FTAs belong to 'umbrella bodies' which aim to represent an entire link of the food supply chain, e.g. Food and Drink Federation for manufacturers, British Retail Consortium for retailers. Umbrella bodies can be national or international. National umbrella bodies are often also members of international organizations, e.g. the Confederation of Food and Drink Industries in the EU (CIAA) and Eurocommerce (retailing) in Europe. However, umbrella bodies do not usually establish best practice standards for their sectors and only play a significant role in incidents where more than one member is involved.

Particularly well-developed sectors (i.e. those that are present in a number of EU Member States) have established their own European FTAs. These in turn may be members of, for example, the CIAA.

National sectoral membership of these EU-level organizations is often through their membership of national umbrella bodies, e.g. the Food and Drink Federation (FDF). However, membership can be structured such that individual companies rather than FTAs are the lead members, for example comprising the Board.

WHO DOES WHAT

The focus of activities of FTAs depends on the nature of their members' business, and can include food hygiene and safety, regulatory matters, marketing, or all of these (Table 22.1). In the manufacturing sector

there is often overlap between the memberships of various FTAs as companies may be involved in one particular product area and manufacturing type (e.g. frozen red meat could be covered by the British Frozen Food Federation or the Meat and Livestock Commission). However, an FTA's activities are generally in discrete areas, being demarcated either by the scope of the FTA or the types of company included in membership. Despite the potential for competition between FTAs there is often close co-operation between them, particularly during an incident or on specific technical or legal issues.

INCIDENT MANAGEMENT

Some FTAs play an active role in incident management, for example by:

- providing information to members to assist in managing an incident and facilitating a co-ordinated response to a specific issue
- acting as a communications hub for its industry sector, seeking information from authorities or agencies and ensuring that relevant members are kept informed of important issues throughout the incident
- representing the sector to the government and its agencies, providing information on technical matters, industry standards and systems including supply chain information
- generating media statements including questions and answers
- providing spokespeople.

However, the extent of these activities differs for each FTA, dependent on resourcing, the nature and number of members involved with an incident, and policy.

INFORMATION FLOWS

The Food Standards Agency has published, with the input from industry and the FTAs, guidelines for preventing and responding to food incidents, the aim of which is to outline the roles and responsibilities of all key players in preventing and responding to food incidents in the UK.

In the UK, retailers' own-label products form a significant proportion of the food market. This can add complexity to the identification of the most appropriate party to be contacted for a specific

Table 22.1 *Some food trade associations*

Name	Area/sector of the food supply chain	Web site address
British Retail Consortium	Retailing, including food	www.brc.org.uk
Food and Drink Federation	Food and drink manufacture, food ingredients	www.fdf.org.uk
British Frozen Food Federation	Frozen food production, distribution and sale	www.bfff.co.uk
British Sandwich Association	Sandwich manufacture, catering and retailing	www.sandwich.org.uk
British Soft Drinks Association	Production of soft drinks, fruit juices and bottled waters	www.britishsoftdrinks.com
Chilled Food Association	Retailed chilled prepared food	www.chilledfood.org
Dairy UK	Dairy products	www.dairyuk.org
Confederation of Food and Drink Industries in the EU (CIAA)	Food and drink manufacture (European trade body)	www.ciaa.be
Eurocommerce	Retailing, wholesaling and international trade (European trade body)	www.eurocommerce.be

All websites were accessed in November 2006.

issue. However, food manufacturers are legally responsible for the safety of the products they make and technical decisions regarding the placing on the market of their products should rest with them. Commercial realities mean that retail customers inevitably provide a key role in such decisions and it is the brand owner (e.g. retailer whose name appears on the own label product pack) who should report an issue to the competent authorities.

CONCLUSION

Much of the work of FTAs aims to drive, support and promote best practice standards in their sectors and to thereby minimize the likelihood of adverse incidents or issues arising.

FTAs represent discrete or distinct sectors of the industry but there may be overlap depending on the breadth of an issue. However, FTAs work together on common issues and play important roles as the interface between a sector, other organizations, researchers and the media, usually acting as the primary point of contact for provision and exchange of information.

23

The environmental health practitioner

Richard Elson

History	364	Sampling	365
Environmental health and food safety in the twenty-first century	365	Training and advice	366
		Response	366
Inspection	365	Sources of information and further reading	366

Environmental health practitioners (EHPs) have an important role in society and are responsible for the protection of public health and the maintenance of a healthy environment. They are highly qualified professionals who ensure that food is safe and of good quality, and also safeguard standards of workplace health and safety.

HISTORY

The evolution of the traditional inspector of nuisances to the present day profession of the EHP regarding food safety began as a response to the huge social changes that occurred in the UK following the agricultural and industrial revolutions of the eighteenth and nineteenth centuries. Towns rapidly expanded and quickly became insanitary. Epidemics of cholera and typhoid were common and, as towns grew, they became more remote from their food supply allowing ample opportunity for food to be adulterated or substituted fraudulently. In the absence of controlled slaughterhouses and modern cold chain facilities, the supply of milk and meat to urban populations was prone to abuse and also provided ideal conditions for transmission of infectious diseases. Cattle were kept in crowded conditions and often slaughtered in back street slaughterhouses under little or no supervision and without post-mortem inspection. The term 'never buy a pig in a poke' is thought to arise from the unscrupulous practice of substituting a valuable piglet, commonly sold in markets in sacks or pokes, with a worthless cat. To 'let the cat out of the bag' is thought to originate from the purchaser discovering or revealing this fraudulent activity. Government, administrative and legislative reform was therefore needed to prevent fraud and control infectious disease related to food and water. This process began with the Public Health Act of 1848 which introduced powers to form local boards of health which could appoint an officer of health and inspectors of nuisances, and require the registration of both slaughterhouses and common lodging houses.

The Adulteration of Food Act 1860 was the first piece of legislation passed in response to public concern over food adulteration. However, it did not provide powers to sample, merely allowing the appointment of public analysts to respond to complaints from members of the public, who had to pay for their services. Public agitation led to further legislation in the form of the Adulteration of Food, Drink and Drugs Act 1872, which introduced the concept that food sold must be of the 'nature, substance or quality' demanded by the purchaser and introduced sampling powers both for inspectors of nuisances and private individuals. The Public Health Act 1875 authorized medical officers of health and inspectors of nuisances to inspect food intended for sale, powers to seize food as well as to enter slaughterhouses and premises where meat was sold. Compulsory notification of 'food poisoning' was introduced in 1938 along with the concept of a food hygiene code.

Following the Second World War, large-scale food processing became more widespread and food adulteration less of an issue. However, food poisoning increased and this was largely attributed to changes in dietary and social habits as well as poor food hygiene. Following the UK's entry to the then European Economic Community in 1973, most UK food safety legislation was consolidated and amended to bring it in line with Europe. Two notable food safety incidents, the Stanley Royd Hospital outbreak of salmonellosis and the *Salmonella* in eggs crisis, both in the 1980s, prompted further change which culminated in the Food Safety Act 1990, much of which remains in force today. Along with general local government reform in the 1970s, many environmental health departments and practitioners moved away from a generic approach to environmental health and became increasingly specialized, especially in food safety.

ENVIRONMENTAL HEALTH AND FOOD SAFETY IN THE TWENTY-FIRST CENTURY

The present day role of EHPs (Box 23.1) is, therefore, a far cry from that of their predecessors, the underpowered inspectors of nuisances of the nineteenth century. EHPs in food safety in the twenty-first century have specialized training and an array of legal powers. Most EHPs are employed by local government.

Box 23.1 The main tasks of EHPs

- Inspect and register all food businesses to ensure that food is prepared hygienically and sold correctly described. This role includes providing advice on the requirements of food safety legislation as well as using powers of enforcement when necessary
- Provide advice and training on food safety for people setting up new food businesses and people managing existing food businesses, as well as members of the public
- Sample food from food businesses and institutions
- Respond to complaints about food safety or hygiene, outbreaks of foodborne illness, and notifications of food poisoning

---

INSPECTION

The purpose of inspection is to ensure that food sold to the public has been produced safely and hygienically, and that food law is being followed. The Food Law Code of Practice (2006; www.food.gov.uk/multimedia/pdfs/codeofpracticeeng.pdf) includes a risk-rating scheme that requires premises of higher risk to be inspected more frequently than those presenting lower risks. Inspections include a physical examination of the premises and an audit of food safety systems including Hazard Analysis and Critical Control Points (HACCP) (see Chapters 10 and 11), pest control and staff training. Where contraventions are noted, the owner is informed of these in writing along with a recommendation on work needed to rectify the contravention, with a time limit. These may be informal letters or formal notices. Contravention of the requirements of a formal notice may result in prosecution and/or imprisonment and prohibition from running a food business. EHPs also have the power to close businesses where they are satisfied that there is an imminent risk to health presented by the premises or food. EHPs are instrumental in delivering the Food Standards Agency (FSA) policies such as 'Safer Food Better Business' (www.food.gov.uk/foodindustry/regulation/hygleg/hyglegresources/sfbb/) directly to caterers, retailers and smaller businesses who may not be represented by trade organizations.

SAMPLING

Sampling is usually carried out for the following three reasons:

- **Routine inspections or as part of specific sampling visits**. Routine sampling of foods is carried out to monitor compliance with specific food hygiene requirements by food business operators and to verify the food safety systems in place. In addition, samples of particular foods, i.e. of animal origin, are taken at ports of entry in the UK to monitor imported foods.
- **Structured co-ordinated studies**. Such studies are identified locally or in local authority food liaison groups and are usually intended to assess the microbiological or compositional quality of particular foodstuffs. The programme of national Health Protection Agency (HPA)/Local Authority Co-ordinators of Regulatory Services (LACORS) studies primarily provides a co-ordinated approach to sampling (see Chapter 30,

p. 384). The studies also provide invaluable data on the microbiological quality of food and are particularly used to fill knowledge gaps identified through epidemiological surveillance.

- **In response to outbreaks of foodborne illness.** Samples provide evidence of the implicated food vehicle(s) responsible for causing the outbreak. Samples are also taken in response to food complaints received from consumers.

TRAINING AND ADVICE

Training of food handlers and managers is a mandatory requirement of the Food Hygiene (England) Regulations 2006. EHPs are well placed to provide this training, usually through formal vocational training packages on food hygiene, co-ordinated by the Chartered Institute of Environmental Health (CIEH). Courses on risk assessment and HACCP are also provided on a regular basis and informal advice and training is also given to food businesses during inspections. Health promotion, aimed particularly at members of the public on topics such as domestic hygiene, also fall within the remit of the EHP.

RESPONSE

EHPs, along with local health protection units of the HPA, are closely involved in responding to notifications of food poisoning and outbreaks of infection related to food and water. Their main role is to prevent further infections and this may range from interviewing sporadic cases of food poisoning to investigating large outbreaks of foodborne illness. EHPs are well placed to assist in these situations as they have powers to enter premises associated with the outbreak, inspect records, take formal statements, sample and seize food, make recommendations for further improvements and, in exceptional circumstances, secure closure of premises where a threat to health is imminent or ongoing. During outbreaks, EHPs take stool samples to confirm diagnosis in infected individuals as well as to exclude people from work who may be infected or carriers of infections. EHPs have detailed local knowledge and regional networks to promulgate information during outbreaks. EHPs also routinely collect information on sporadic cases of infection in their districts and, together with the HPA and other professional groups and organizations, contribute to surveillance. The investigation of food complaints is also a key responsibility and this may range from food that is incorrectly labelled to the investigation of malicious contamination of food during production.

EHPs are also employed by national governmental and non-governmental agencies such as the FSA, LACORS, the Local Government Association, the CIEH and the HPA. EHPs employed by these agencies are involved in setting food safety policy, auditing the activity of local authority food safety services and developing food poisoning surveillance systems. Safe food is the product of a variety of professional inputs, including the contribution made by EHPs, who continue to be at the forefront of food safety.

All websites cited in this chapter and below were accessed in November 2006.

SOURCES OF INFORMATION AND FURTHER READING

Bassett WH (2004) *Clay's Handbook of Environmental Health*, 19th edn. London: Spon Press.

Chartered Institute of Environmental Health (www.cieh.org).

Frazer WM (1950) *History of English Public Health 1834–1939*. London: Bailliere, Tindall and Cox.

24

Seaport and airport health

Sandra Westacott

Introduction	367	Infectious disease control	368
Port health authorities	368	Imported food safety control	369
Airports and non-port health authority local authorities	368	Other functions of port health authorities	370

Foodborne and infectious diseases are an enormous global health problem that does not respect borders. Nations wishing to remain disease free and reduce the increasing burden of foodborne illness must establish effective strategies for minimizing the risks of introduction of disease-causing agents transported in food from other countries.

INTRODUCTION

The UK is the fourth largest food-importing nation in the world. Thousands of tonnes of food arrive daily and many millions of passengers pass through our ports and airports every year. Both passengers and food volumes are expected to increase in parallel with globalization and consequent international trade. In addition, food and people now travel over far greater distances than ever before, creating the conditions necessary for widespread and rapidly occurring outbreaks of disease. Infectious diseases such as cholera persist and return, and recent decades have shown an unprecedented rate of emergence of new **zoonoses**. Examples of imported diseases in the UK associated with international travel and the risks associated with imported foods are shown in Tables 24.1 and 24.2.

Table 24.1 *Some foodborne and waterborne disease-causing agents associated with international travel*

Risk/control	Example of infectious agent/contaminant
Inadequate disinfection of bunkered water	Pathogenic *E. coli*
Bunkering of contaminated potable water supplies	*Cryptosporidium, Legionella*
Poor controls on sourcing and purchasing of food	Norovirus, *Cyclospora*, marine biotoxins
Poor food preparation techniques	*Salmonella*, pathogenic *E.coli*, staphylococcal enterotoxins
Presence of pests (e.g. rodents, insects)	*Salmonella, Campylobacter*, pathogenic *E. coli*

Table 24.2 *Risks associated with imported food*

Risk	Examples of contamination
Contamination with pathogenic micro-organism	*Salmonella* , pathogenic *E. coli, L. monocytogenes*
Biotoxins	Staphylococcal enterotoxin, marine biotoxin, mycotoxins
Poor production methods and controls	*C. botulinum*
Environmental contaminants	Heavy metals, dioxins, polychlorinated biphenyls (PCBs)
Presence of excessive pesticides and veterinary drug residues	Organochlorine and organophosphate poisoning
Excessive preservatives	Sulphur dioxide involved in asthma attacks
Irradiation of food contaminated with pathogenic micro-organisms	Pre-formed irradiation-resistant staphylococcal enterotoxin

PORT HEALTH AUTHORITIES

Port health authorities (PHAs) were constituted with the primary objective of preventing the international dissemination of dangerous epidemic diseases through shipping activity without creating unnecessary interference with world trade. They trace their origin back to the Public Health Act 1872 when it was deemed necessary to control the importation of disease through ports.

As ports generally extended over the area of more than one local authority, the Act empowered the constitution of port sanitary authorities with permanent jurisdiction over the port. These statutory powers are now embodied in the Public Health (Control of Disease) Act 1984.

The Act defines a port as one established for 'Customs' purposes in the Customs and Excise Management Act 1979, and empowers government ministers to make Orders to constitute port health districts which may be part or all of one or more ports. The Orders establish PHAs for those districts which may be served by one or more local authorities.

AIRPORTS AND NON-PORT HEALTH AUTHORITY LOCAL AUTHORITIES

Many UK airports lie within port health districts, whereas because of the 'Customs' definition of a 'port', others, including the largest international ones, do not. At airports which are not defined as ports and at coastal or inland waters where there is no PHA, the local authority is responsible for infectious disease control and food safety/enforcement.

INFECTIOUS DISEASE CONTROL

The Public Health (Control of Disease) Act 1984 assigns powers for applying controls for health, disease and waste disposal to PHAs and local authorities.

Powers for applying health controls on ships are contained in the Public Health (Ships) Regulations 1979. These Regulations provide for notification by the ship's master of health conditions on board; inspection of incoming ships by PHAs; examination of people; and authorizes measures to be taken for preventing danger to public health.

The application of additional measures appropriate to specified diseases particularly dangerous to public health are subject to the International Health Regulations 2005. The International Health Regulations (IHRs) 2005 address the multiple and varied health risks that face the world today. The IHRs broaden the scope of the previous 1969 Regulations to cover existing, new and re-emerging diseases, including emergencies caused by non-infectious agents and will be transposed into domestic legislation in 2007. New reporting procedures are aimed at expediting the flow of timely and accurate information to the World Health Organization about potential public health emergencies of international concern. People on outgoing ships may also be examined and special measures taken to prevent disease spreading.

Port health authorities work alongside the Maritime and Coastguard Agency (MCA), which has detention powers in respect of vessels with considerable hygiene problems. The MCA also has an important role with regard to the development of port waste management plans including food waste, which is extremely important as a possible vector of animal disease. The MCA is also responsible for the control of disposal of ship's ballast water, which has been implicated in the dispersal of alien phytoplankton into UK waters – leading to toxic algal blooms and infectious diseases such as cholera.

Powers for applying health controls on aircraft are contained in the Public Health (Aircraft) Regulations 1979, and define the responsible authorities charged with enforcing and executing the Regulations. The development of commercial flying and the speed with which people can move around the world to and from infected areas are reflected in the scope of the Regulations. Authorized officers prepare and update lists of aerodromes, and other infected or believed to be infected areas, with diseases subject to the International Health Regulations. Provisions are made for measures to be taken for both incoming and outgoing aircraft and their passengers with a view to preventing danger to public health and the spread of infection, including detention of the aircraft, passengers, stores, equipment and cargo.

When outbreaks of infectious disease are associated with international travel, PHAs and local authorities liaise with the Consultant Physician in

Health Protection, formerly the Consultant in Communicable Disease, employed by the Health Protection Agency in England and Wales. Similar arrangements exist for the devolved administrations in Scotland and Northern Ireland, excepting that in Scotland this service is provided by the local health boards.

IMPORTED FOOD SAFETY CONTROL

Local authorities and PHAs are responsible for food standards and food safety checks on imported foods at points of entry. Import controls on food arriving into the UK are usually applied to countries outside the European Union (EU). The types of check depend on the country of origin and the type of product. These are either **products of animal origin** (POAO), such as honey, eggs, meat, fish, hides, or **food not of animal origin** (FNAO), such as nuts, spices, confectionery, fruit and vegetables.

Imported food legislation is primarily driven by UK implementation of European Community law, e.g. Directive 97/78/EC that draws up the veterinary checks regimen and is implemented in England by the Product of Animal Origin (Third Country Imports (England) Regulations), which are often revoked and re-enacted. The Regulations implement a range of controls for all POAO imported from outside the EU to protect both public and animal health. POAO can only be imported through approved points of entry, i.e. **border inspection posts** (BIPs), and must come from an approved establishment in an approved third country outside the EU and comply with animal and public health conditions. A point of entry can only be designated as a BIP if it meets the approval requirements laid down in Commission Decision 2001/812/EC relating to the provision of facilities for the checking of products and application of procedures for controlling their import. If a health risk is identified with a particular food from an approved third country, the EU may subject it to safeguard measures that specify import restrictions or a ban, e.g. presence of antibiotic residues in foods, foot and mouth disease. Following the outbreak of foot and mouth disease in 2001, the UK government empowered Her Majesty's Revenue and Customs (HMRC) with powers to control the import of smuggled POAO in Customs-approved areas at seaports, airports and international rail terminals.

Since 1 January 2006, import controls on FNAO have been harmonized at European Community level by Regulation [EC] No. 882/2004 on official controls that are performed to ensure the verification of compliance with feed and food law, animal health and animal welfare rules. The provisions of the Regulation are implemented in the UK by the Official Feed and Food (England) Regulations 2006 (SI 2006/15) (and parallel legislation in Scotland, Wales and Northern Ireland).The Regulations include a mechanism for ensuring that where there is a serious or imminent risk to public health, control measures may be invoked to ensure that emergency decisions made at EU level are implemented without delay. Only a small percentage of the total tonnage of imported FNAO is checked on arrival on entry. Most checks are carried out on products that are subject to emergency controls, such as pistachio nuts from Iran for aflatoxins. Consignments are detained and sampled to check that they meet food safety requirements. Emergency Control Regulations (ECRs) may suspend or specify conditions of import. Consignments subject to ECRs may only be imported through designated points of entry.

Regulation [EC] No. 882/2004 provides that the Commission may issue a list of 'high-risk' FNAO. These products will be identified on the basis of known or emerging risk, and will be subject to enhanced import controls at point of entry, including pre-notification, import through designated ports only and specified documentary and physical checks. A list has not yet been prepared, and in the meantime PHAs and local authorities carry out checks other than those for ECRs. These checks are based on intelligence gathered as a result of national or EU surveys, and information from inland authorities and other member states via the EU Rapid Alert System for Food and Feed (RASSF), which gives them reason to suspect that there may be a problem.

The Imported Food Division of the Food Standards Agency provides a focal point for advice, information, training and funding for additional sampling and surveillance of imported food by PHAs and local authorities. PHAs and local authorities work closely with food examiners from the Health Protection Agency and public analysts who analyse samples of imported food and provide expert advice on the safety of the food for human consumption.

OTHER FUNCTIONS OF PORT HEALTH AUTHORITIES

Various pieces of legislation in the field of public and animal health designate PHAs as the competent authority for enforcement. The Prevention of Damage by Pest Act 1949, the Environmental Protection Act 1990 and Clean Air Act 1993 require PHAs to inspect their districts to ascertain there are no statutory nuisances, illegal smoke or dust emissions or any infestations of rats or mice. In addition, the Animal Health Act 1982 provides for the functions relating to imported animals to be enforced by PHAs.

The Food Safety Act 1990 designates PHAs as food authorities, which are responsible for controlling shellfish layings within their district, taking water and shellfish samples to establish classifications of shellfish layings, monitoring seawater and shellfish for the presence of marine biotoxins and controlling the harvesting and marketing of shellfish for human consumption.

PHAs and local authorities work with a number of different professions, government agencies and departments to carry out effective preventive and enforcement controls (summarized in Table 24.3).

Table 24.3 *Summary of roles of professions, government departments and agencies in England associated with sea and airport food safety*

Control area	Policy	Enforcement associates
Products of animal origin	Defra International Animal Health	Legal Imports – AH Illegal Imports – HMRC
Food not of animal origin	FSA	PHAs/LAs HPA, PA
Infectious disease control	Department of Health, Department of Trade and Industry	HPA, MCA
Shellfish	FSA	HPA, CEFAS, EA
International catering waste	Defra International Animal Health	AH, MCA

AH, Animal Health; Defra, Department of the Environment, Farms and Rural Affairs; HMRC, Her Majesty's Revenue and Customs; FSA, Food Standards Agency; PHA, port health authority; LA, local authority; HPA, Health Protection Agency; PA, port authority; CEFAS, Centre for Environment, Fisheries and Aquaculture Science; EA, Environment Agency; MCA, Maritime and Coastguard Agency. There is slight variation in enforcement associates in other devolved nations within the UK.

25

The medical practitioner

David Tompkins

Introduction	371	Consultants in communicable disease control	373
General practitioners	371	Conclusions	373
Clinicians in hospitals	372	Sources of information and further reading	373
Consultant medical microbiologists	372		

This chapter describes the roles of English health professionals in regard to food safety and foodborne diseases.

INTRODUCTION

All medical practitioners undergo basic training in medical microbiology and food hygiene as a small part of their undergraduate medical education. In the UK, after graduation junior doctors go through a period of general medical and surgical training and then specialize as hospital consultants or public health doctors or general practitioners (GPs), also known as primary care physicians. This may vary in other countries, depending on the healthcare system.

GENERAL PRACTITIONERS

Symptoms of food poisoning or foodborne infection closely resemble those of other intestinal infections spread by water or close personal contact, and non-infectious diseases. Individuals who have symptoms of **infectious intestinal disease** (IID) such as acute diarrhoea, vomiting and abdominal pain, will seek advice from their General Practitioner (GP) if the illness is severe or prolonged, or if they have alarming symptoms such as blood in the stool. A large study of gastroenteritis was carried out in 70 GP practices in England from 1993 to 1996. This is generally referred to as the IID Study (Wheeler *et al.* 1999). It found that about 1 in 5 people experienced symptoms of

IID every year, and of these about 1 in 6 presented to their GP for advice. The subsequent introduction of a national telephone advisory service staffed by nurses (NHS Direct) may have reduced GP consultations (Box 25.1).

> **Box 25.1 Roles of GPs**
> - Diagnosis, differentiation from other infections
> - Treatment
> - Early identification and reporting of incidents and outbreaks
> - Surveillance through notification to public health physicians
> - Identification of cause and surveillance by submitting faeces specimens for microbiological tests

A GP in a 10-minute consultation will, on the basis of symptoms described and possibly a physical examination, decide on a possible diagnosis. In the IID study 1 in every 4 patients who consulted a GP had a specimen of faeces submitted to the laboratory for microbiological examination. The GP will usually ask for a microbiology test if the patient is more severely ill, if food poisoning is suspected or if the patient has recently returned from travel abroad where unusual pathogens might have been acquired. These details will be given on the request form submitted to the laboratory with the specimen. As the results of laboratory tests will not be available for at least 2 working days, they have no impact on the immediate management of the patient.

Treatment is usually the same for all cases of IID. Maintenance of a good fluid intake to avoid dehydration is the main priority, with a mixture of glucose and salts to replace losses from the gastrointestinal tract. Oral rehydration salts are available from pharmacies. In general, young children and elderly people are the most susceptible to the complications of IID. The minimal potential benefits of antimicrobials in reducing the duration of symptoms are usually outweighed by the risk of side effects and contribution to resistance. Advice for management of gastroenteritis is available on the internet for GPs at the Clinical Knowledge Summaries website (www.cks.library.nhs.uk).

It is the statutory responsibility of the medical practitioner who clinically diagnoses food poisoning to formally notify the case to the **Proper Officer** for the local authority, usually the **consultant in communicable disease control** (CCDC; see Box 25.3). However, IID caused by food poisoning is clinically indistinguishable from IID caused by organisms that are waterborne or spread directly from person to person. Outbreaks of food poisoning are more easily identified than individual cases.

If GPs are aware of incidents involving more than one individual, or cases of public health importance in food handlers, healthcare staff or children attending nurseries, the CCDC should be 'notified' informally but urgently by telephone.

CLINICIANS IN HOSPITALS

Occasionally, patients with IID may present to accident and emergency departments when GP services are not easily accessible or if the onset of symptoms is severe. Patients with severe illness and those having recently travelled abroad may be referred to a specialist in infectious diseases. These specialists are usually based in teaching hospitals or large centres. Very few are based in district general hospitals. The roles and public health responsibilities for hospital doctors are the same as those for GPs (see Box 25.1).

CONSULTANT MEDICAL MICROBIOLOGISTS

Consultant medical microbiologists (CMMs; Box 25.2) undergo several years of specialist training in the diagnosis, treatment and control of infections and usually will have taken the examination giving membership of the Royal College of Pathologists. Most CMMs are based in public hospital laboratories (National Health Service), which also serve general practices and community health services in the surrounding areas. CMMs are involved in devising standard operating procedures (SOPs) and quality standards for their laboratories, working closely with healthcare scientists employed as laboratory managers. In most hospitals they are the local experts on all aspects of infection.

Box 25.2 Roles of CMMs

- Accurate identification of causative micro-organisms by setting laboratory standards and selecting appropriate tests
- Advice on treatment and control of infection in hospital and community
- Surveillance by sending micro-organisms to reference laboratories for typing, and reporting laboratory findings to the Health Protection Agency (HPA)
- Rapid reporting to HPA of cases of public health significance

---

For economy it is not possible to test every faecal specimen submitted for every possible microbial cause of IID. Specimens from patients in the community will usually be examined for the presence of *Salmonella, Shigella, Campylobacter, E. coli* O157, *Cryptosporidium* and (in children) rotavirus. Other tests will be included according to the clinical details on the request form. The CMM is responsible for ensuring that written reports have sufficient interpretive comments and that urgent findings e.g. '*E. coli* O157 detected', are telephoned to the sending clinician.

Managers of microbiology laboratories also have public health responsibilities which have been defined by the **Inspector of Microbiology** at the **Department of Health**. Relevant bacterial isolates should be sent to reference laboratories for typing and the CCDC should be informed by telephone of all laboratory findings of public health importance. This is accepted good practice and not a statutory notification. The CMM is usually the laboratory representative who liaises with clinicians, CCDCs, the **regional epidemiologist**, the **regional micro-**

biologist, environmental health officers and **reference laboratory** staff when investigating more complex and unusual cases or outbreaks of IID.

Many CMMs are also **infection control doctors**, heading infection control teams in hospitals. Viral gastroenteritis and *Clostridium difficile* are the major causes of IID in hospitals but foodborne infection has to be excluded when outbreaks of IID occur. Organisms such as *Salmonella* and *E. coli* O157 spread easily from person to person and may cause severe illness in frail hospital inpatients. The CMM reports outbreaks of IID in hospital to the CCDC who is a member of the **outbreak control team**.

A few CMMs with a special interest in public health microbiology are employed by the HPA at regional laboratories and advise CCDCs and other CMMs.

CONSULTANTS IN COMMUNICABLE DISEASE CONTROL

CCDCs (Box 25.3) are medical practitioners who have trained in public health medicine and have a particular interest in health protection. They will have taken the examination of membership of the Faculty of Public Health of the Royal College of Physicians. The need for these specialists was recognized in a review of the public health function in the late 1980s by the then Chief Medical Officer, Sir Donald Acheson. In 2003 CCDCs and their teams of nurses and support staff were split from other public health colleagues and moved into the HPA.

Box 25.3 Roles of CCDCs

- Strategic leadership and co-ordination of local programmes for communicable disease control
- Leading investigations and management of incidents and outbreaks
- Proper Officer to local authorities
- Local surveillance of communicable disease

The Public Health (Control of Diseases) Act 1984 places responsibilities and powers for infection control on local government. Each local authority is required to appoint a Proper Officer, usually the CCDC employed in the HPA. Some diseases, including food poisoning, must be notified to the Proper Officer who has various powers of investigation and control. CCDCs work closely with environment health officers in the prevention and investigation of food, water and environmental incidents.

CCDCs now work in teams in **health protection units** (HPUs) serving populations of 1–2 million. They receive laboratory reports and notifications for surveillance and also act on regional and national information gathered by the HPA. Reports on local surveillance are published by HPUs. CCDCs lead investigations into incidents and outbreaks of IID, when necessary forming and chairing outbreak control teams. The CCDCs are the leaders of the 'front-line' teams of the HPA, and local advisers on communicable diseases to healthcare professionals and organizations, and the public.

CONCLUSIONS

Medical practitioners have significant roles in the diagnosis, treatment, control and surveillance of foodborne infection and food poisoning. However, they only treat a minority of cases, as many do not present for healthcare.

All websites cited below were accessed in November 2006.

SOURCES OF INFORMATION AND FURTHER READING

Food Standards Agency (2000) *Report of the Study of Infectious Intestinal Disease in England*. London: The Stationery Office.

Health Protection Agency (www.hpa.org.uk).

Health Protection Agency Local and Regional Services (www.hpa.org.uk/lars_homepage.htm).

Wheeler JG, Sethi D, Cowden JM *et al.* (1999) Study of infectious intestinal disease in England: rates in the community, presenting to general practice, and reported to national surveillance. *BMJ* **318**: 1046–50.

26

The veterinarian's contribution to food safety

John D Collins

The veterinary approach to food safety throughout the food chain	374	Reducing the extent of exposure of consumers to foodborne hazards	376
Longitudinal integrated safety assurance schemes	375	Conclusion	376
The veterinary contribution to the formulation of food law	375	Source of information and further reading	376

Veterinarians have an essential role in the prevention and control of food poisoning incidents, in providing support to reduce exposure of consumers to foodborne hazards and in contributing to the formulation and implementation of food law.

THE VETERINARY APPROACH TO FOOD SAFETY THROUGHOUT THE FOOD CHAIN

A sustained supply of safe food demands vigilance. The respective roles of the medical profession, particularly those specializing in occupational medicine, public health and epidemiology, along with veterinary specialists in these fields, are pre-eminent. In this context, the pivotal role of risk analysis and the application of Hazard Analysis and Critical Control Point (HACCP)-based systems of prevention throughout the food chain have been emphasized in all recent international trade agreements. The risks involved are very real when one considers the persistence of **zoonoses** (diseases or infections transmitted naturally between humans and other vertebrates) such as human parasitic (e.g. trichinosis, taeniasis) and bacterial (campylobacteriosis and salmonellosis) conditions, which are invariably associated with exposure to infected or infested food. The concern is not limited to human

diseases alone. Rather, a major driving force in recent world trade negotiations has been the aim of preventing the risk of introduction of 'exotic diseases' into countries through trade in contaminated meat and meat-based products. In developed countries, the recent epidemic of bovine spongiform encephalopathy (BSE) in the UK and other countries has brought the realization that the incorporation of contaminated meat-based products (ruminant meat and bone meal) in the diet of cattle may have serious consequences for the health of national cattle populations over a number of years, with disastrous consequences for trade. The human health implications of this tragedy are considerable and remain a continuing cause for concern requiring a concerted and sustained approach at all levels (including on the farm, in the meat plant and at retail), so as to prevent exposure of the consumer to the causal agent.

The effective prevention and control of outbreaks of foodborne diseases and intoxications associated with foods of animal origin require an holistic approach to the identification of the origin and causes of such outbreaks. This requires an in-depth knowledge of the pre- and post-harvest factors involved, as well as of the causal agents of disease. Specialists working in **veterinary public health** engage actively in the control and prevention of such diseases and intoxications. Risk analysis is the basis for on-farm and in-plant programmes for the prevention and, where required, management of such problems. The specialist skills of the veterinary public health professional include an understanding of the dynamics of spread of diseases within populations throughout the food production, processing and distribution stages. This expertise is of particular value in the context of the multidisciplinary approach now being adopted by public health agencies when investigating and controlling incidents of foodborne diseases.

The contribution made by the veterinarian as a member of a multidisciplinary team engaged in the investigation and control of foodborne diseases is considerable, because of the part played by on-farm conditions as risk factors in the development of outbreaks. The profession has long held a respected position in such situations, and there is now an increasing awareness of the need for an integrated longitudinal approach to the prevention, investigation and management of food-borne diseases and intoxications.

LONGITUDINAL INTEGRATED SAFETY ASSURANCE SCHEMES

The application of **longitudinal integrated safety assurance schemes** (LISA) in food animal production within a commercially viable framework has come to be regarded as a worthwhile and in some cases an indispensable component of the modern retail trade. These schemes are incorporated with the delivery of a focused programme of veterinary food hygiene and food inspection service, and form the basis for a sustainable veterinary contribution to public health. The schemes provide a platform for consumer confidence in the safety and quality of the food supply and help to sustain the future viability of food animal and agricultural production in general. Many members of the veterinary profession have long been engaged, and continue to be engaged, in the practice of veterinary public health and food safety as it relates to the provision of a healthy food supply, as:

- providers of advice to producers
- food hygienists in meat and dairy plants
- food scientists
- members of the regulatory agencies throughout Europe.

The current expectation of the consumer and the demands of the market are such that there is an established and increasingly more relevant role for veterinarians in population medicine and food safety in this field of public health.

An emphasis on the prevention of contamination of the food product with microbiological, chemical and pharmaceutical hazards, rather than a total reliance on traditional 'detection inspection', is intrinsic to the implementation of food safety control programmes at factory or 'post-harvest' level, and remains a primary objective. In achieving product protection at the 'pre-harvest' level in integrated systems of beef, pig and poultry production, these principles will already have been applied by the field veterinarian in the course of assessing, for example:

- water and feed quality
- animal health and performance records
- animal welfare conditions
- the level of safety applied in the choice and use of therapeutic agents
- the clinical condition of the food animals
- the safety of the environment as affected by the standard of animal effluent management and utilization on the farm.

On this basis a reasoned conclusion can be reached concerning the degree of risk, if any, posed by the food animal and its suitability for slaughter for human consumption. Such information is a basic requirement of a truly integrated food safety assurance scheme and can readily be provided by the attending veterinarian as part of LISA-based programmes.

THE VETERINARY CONTRIBUTION TO THE FORMULATION OF FOOD LAW

There is a defined and recognized need for specialist veterinary advice throughout the various Member States of the European Union (EU) on the implications of impending legislation affecting:

- food safety
- zoonoses control
- herd and flock health in terms of the epidemiological aspects of disease identification, management, control and prevention.

This need extends to non-EU legislative measures imposed for the purposes of world trade. The provision of such advice, where practicable, is also required at the formative stages of legislation so as to take account of local circumstances. In the case of the **epizootic diseases** (epidemics affecting animals) such as avian influenza, the success of disease control measures adopted by the EU relies on a clear understanding, at national and international levels, of the detailed nature of the control measures involved and of the best means of their implementation. Legislation introduced to deal with such issues as the relation between BSE and food safety, and consequences of the use of antimicrobials in veterinary medicine and food animal production, offers further examples of the distinctive nature of the veterinary contribution to public health and food safety at EU as well as national levels.

REDUCING THE EXTENT OF EXPOSURE OF CONSUMERS TO FOODBORNE HAZARDS

The European Commission's White Paper on Food Safety (Commission of the European Communities 2000), acknowledged the need to ensure that all the elements of risk analysis are applied to each phase of the food chain, including the pre-harvest phase. The requirements of pre-harvest risk analysis mean that on-farm food safety risk management programmes have to be developed and implemented. While these programmes are more advanced in the dairy industry, there still remains a concern regarding the level of risk of exposure to such agents as *Listeria monocytogenes*, *Campylobacter* spp. *Salmonella enterica* serovars and, in some countries, *Brucella* spp., *Mycobacterium bovis* and *Mycobacterium paratuberculosis*, associated with the consumption of raw (non-heated) milk and milk products and to vulnerable groups in particular. The safety of food of animal origin with respect to the potential risks posed by BSE has again defined the importance of sound data on the quality and safety of animal feedstuffs, traceability of food animals and their products and an appreciation of the dynamics of internal trade of animals in each country and

region. Active surveillance of transmissible spongiform encephalopathies in animals now provides further data on the regional and national incidence of these diseases for use in the strategic design of control and preventive measures based on quantitative risk analysis for animal health, and where relevant, for consumer protection.

This proactive approach has an immediate application in the assessment of the risk posed by foodborne agents such as *Campylobacter* spp., *Toxoplasma gondii* and *L. monocytogenes* associated with meat products and norovirus, *Anisakis* spp. and *Vibrio parahaemolyticus* associated with fish and other marine products. Also, although not usually regarded as a cause of disease in animals per se, the enterocytotoxin producing strains of *Escherichia coli*, including verocytotoxin producing *E. coli* (VTEC), and their distribution and potential for spread to consumers, have been the subject of recent studies, the final outcome of which is as yet unclear. VTEC represents a real challenge for the primary producer, as well as the processor. On-farm conditions and the carriage and pre-slaughter conditions of food animals, as well as the contamination of carcasses at meat plants, are likely to be the critical factors in determining the risk of exposure for the ultimate consumer. Accordingly, there is every reason for the direct involvement of veterinary graduates engaged in food animal practice and those in veterinary public health, food hygiene and epidemiology and as well as other scientists in the elucidation, management and control of the risk factors that contribute to the exposure of the consumer to these pathogens at each level of food production, processing and distribution.

CONCLUSION

The veterinary contribution to the sustainability of a safe food supply is widely acknowledged as an integral component of food safety assurance throughout the food chain and complements the contributions of other recognized disciplines in this field of public health.

SOURCE OF INFORMATION AND FURTHER READING

Commission of the European Communities (CEC) (2000) *White Paper on Food Safety*. Brussels: Commission of the European Communities.

27

Commercial laboratories

Melody Greenwood

Introduction	377	Sources of information and further reading	379
Functions of commercial laboratories	377		

Commercial laboratories work with food manufacturers to ensure the production of safe food that fulfils its expected shelf-life. Most commercial laboratories examine large numbers of both food and water samples for a relatively restricted number of microbiological parameters. These tests are mainly used to demonstrate compliance with food safety management programmes, such as Hazard Analysis and Critical Control Points (HACCP), and client specifications.

INTRODUCTION

Commercial food testing may be undertaken by in-house laboratories funded and operated by the **food business operator (FBO)** or by contract laboratories independent of the food business operations. Because it is inadvisable to have potential pathogens on food production sites, it is common practice for on-site laboratories to restrict their testing activities to enumeration of indicator organisms. Pathogen testing is usually undertaken by sending samples to contract laboratories located away from food production sites.

FUNCTIONS OF COMMERCIAL LABORATORIES

Microbiological testing by commercial laboratories is done to:

- demonstrate the safety of the product
- demonstrate conformity with legislative specifications
- demonstrate conformity with client specifications, e.g. supermarket specifications

- verify that ingredients are of the microbiological standard required
- monitor trends in order to respond rapidly to a potential problem
- monitor environmental contamination
- demonstrate good hygiene or efficacy of a cleaning regimen and monitor trends for rapid response
- verify that critical controls are in place and under control as part of the HACCP plan or other risk assessment
- demonstrate due diligence (see Chapter 15).

Usually ingredients, end-products and environmental samples are tested. However, samples may also be taken from any point in the production line to monitor trends and identify accumulation of contamination so that remedial action can be taken before more serious interventions may be required. Testing of ingredients is particularly important if the production process is not expected to reduce the microbial load and kill pathogenic organisms. Ideally this should be done before the ingredients are used in food production – not only to prevent the use of poor-quality ingredients or ingredients contaminated with pathogens but also because detection of unwanted organisms in the ingredient is easier at this stage than when the ingredient has been incorporated into a food.

End-product testing is performed mainly to demonstrate conformity with client specifications and compliance with legislation. Microbiological specifications set by clients are usually more stringent than those found in legislation. They are set at levels that are usually achieved by **good**

manufacturing practice (GMP) and designed to ensure that the product is both safe and of organoleptically acceptable microbiological quality throughout its shelf-life and beyond. It is in the interests of the manufacturer to be able to achieve as long a shelf-life as possible, and this is possible only by ensuring good microbiological quality. Further end-product sampling may also be done to establish an appropriate shelf-life, for example as part of new product development, or to verify that the assigned shelf-life is achieved on a continuing basis.

Environmental monitoring is an important element of a HACCP plan and constitutes a significant proportion of commercial testing, particularly for the presence of *Listeria*. Current European Union (EU) legislation requires FBOs who produce ready-to-eat food that may pose a risk for public health to monitor the processing area, equipment and surfaces for *L. monocytogenes* as part of their sampling programme. Similarly there is a requirement for producers of dried infant formula milks and dried foods for special medical purposes intended for infants younger than 6 months of age, which pose an *Enterobacter sakazakii* risk, to monitor the production environment for the presence of Enterobacteriaceae as part of their sampling programme. Regular environmental monitoring for the presence and levels of hygiene indicator organisms together with regular trend analysis of results can help identify potential hygiene problems before the end-product is significantly affected.

For food commodities that are shelf-stable or have a relatively long shelf-life, a positive release system is feasible to ensure the absence of pathogens such as *Salmonella* before distribution. However, positive release systems should not be used in the absence of a risk assessment scheme (such as HACCP) to ensure food safety. The costs of storage before release and the curtailing of the remaining shelf-life imposed by the time taken for conventional microbiological methods to obtain a negative result may dictate the use of rapid detection methods such as enzyme-linked immunosorbent assay (ELISA)-based screening tests and polymerase chain reaction (PCR) techniques. This is feasible if only a relatively narrow spectrum of sample types is to be examined as the testing regimen needs to be validated for each sample matrix. Rapid methods are, however, particularly suitable for testing of environmental samples, for example to detect *L.*

monocytogenes. The additional costs of equipment purchase and the testing kits and reagents are compensated for by the reduction in storage costs of product and the maximization of the available shelf-life at the point of sale. A positive release scheme is not realistic for fresh products that have only a short shelf-life and so the producer needs to ensure the safety and quality of the ingredients used, particularly from new sources.

Contract laboratories typically receive large numbers of samples for examination of a relatively narrow range of microbiological parameters, so automated and rapid detection methods are used frequently by these laboratories. The commercial nature of activities, large numbers of samples processed and the significant use of more automated methods means the number of well-qualified staff capable of undertaking diagnostic work in commercial laboratories is relatively low compared with the number of staff employed in the general processing of samples.

There is an increasing requirement for commercial testing laboratories to be accredited against a recognized standard. To compete commercially, contract laboratories need to hold accreditation against the International Organization for Standardization (ISO/IEC) 17025, thus also operating in compliance with ISO 9001. In the UK, this accreditation is performed by the United Kingdom Accreditation Service (UKAS). In-house laboratories may opt for less stringent accreditation such as the CLAS or LabCred schemes. Table 27.1 lists some examples of accreditation schemes used in the UK. Accreditation requires participation in an **external proficiency testing scheme** to verify and demonstrate competence in an independent manner. In general, as mentioned above, commercial laboratories have a comparatively restricted scope of accredited test methods and frequently restrict enumeration testing methods to the identification of presumptive target organisms only.

The prime function of the commercial testing laboratories is to provide presence/absence or enumeration results, usually in as short a time as possible. Some laboratories will also provide trend analysis derived from their results. These laboratories will promptly notify results that are out of specification, but interpretation of those results or advice about remedial action is usually not included. If FBOs require additional information or expertise they may

Table 27.1 *Examples of accreditation schemes in the UK*

ISO/IEC 17025: 2005	General requirements for the competence of testing and calibration laboratories	An international standard that describes the requirements that laboratories need to meet to demonstrate competence and achieve accreditation
ISO 9001: 2000	Quality management systems – requirements	Applicable to all types of organization
CLAS	Campden Laboratory Accreditation Scheme	An accreditation scheme for food and drink microbiology laboratories. It addresses the requirements and principles of ISO/IEC 17025 and promotes the use of valid methods supported by appropriate quality control checks and good laboratory practices
LabCred	Bodycote laboratory accreditation scheme	An accreditation scheme to assess the operation of chemistry and microbiology industry in-house laboratories
UKAS	United Kingdom Accreditation Scheme	An independent body recognized by the government to assess, against internationally agreed standards, organizations that provide certification, testing, inspection and calibration services

commission the services of a food research association such as Campden and Chorleywood Food Research Association (www.campden.co.uk) or Leatherhead Food International (www.leather headfood.com). These organizations also carry out research and development projects to help ensure the safety and quality of novel foods and food production processes.

All websites cited in the chapter and below were accessed in November 2006.

SOURCES OF INFORMATION AND FURTHER READING

Bodycote Health Sciences Europe (www.healthsciences.bodycote.com).

Campden and Chorleywood Food Research Association (www.campden.co.uk).

European co-operation for Accreditation. EA–4/10. Accreditation for microbiology laboratories (available at: www.european-accreditation.org/n1/doc/EA-4-10.pdf).

International Organization for Standardization (www.iso.org).

Leatherhead Food International (www.leatherheadfood.com).

Roberts D, Greenwood M (2003) *Practical Food Microbiology*, 3rd edn. Oxford: Blackwell Publishing.

United Kingdom Accreditation Service (www.ukas.com).

28

Public sector laboratories

Melody Greenwood

Introduction	380	Sources of information and further reading	382
Functions of public sector laboratories	380		

Public sector food and water laboratories work closely with the local authorities to monitor microbiological safety of food available to the general public. They also have an important role in surveillance and investigation of foodborne diseases.

INTRODUCTION

In the UK, government-funded laboratories such as Health Protection Agency (HPA) laboratories, HPA collaborating laboratories, National Public Health Service laboratories in Wales and public analyst laboratories undertake food and water testing on behalf of local authorities, port health/border inspection post authorities and occasionally on behalf of the Food Standards Agency. They may also undertake limited commercial testing and frequently undertake testing on behalf of hospitals, but this is in addition to their core function. Many of these laboratories are designated as **Official Food Control laboratories** and act to support the Official Food Control function of the local authorities. Each Official Food Control laboratory needs to have at least one qualified **food examiner**. Official Food Control laboratories must be accredited against ISO 17025 and have their Official Food Control activities audited. Because of the breadth of the activities undertaken, government-funded laboratories tend to perform a wider range of more demanding tests than commercial contract laboratories, and consequently participation in more varied external quality assessment (proficiency testing) schemes is required. It is common for public sector laboratories to take part in up to six such schemes, some of which may

be tailored for specific foods, e.g. dairy products or shellfish, or for the detection of specific groups of pathogens, e.g. *Vibrio* spp.

FUNCTIONS OF PUBLIC SECTOR LABORATORIES

Government-funded laboratories usually work in close collaboration with local authorities to help them in their role of ensuring food safety. Samples are taken by local authority personnel from manufacturing premises to verify that the production process is under control and likely to produce safe food. The local authorities may also take samples from retail premises and catering premises such as restaurants, public houses and mobile vendors as part of their inspection programmes and structured surveys organized on a European, national or local basis. Most samples are of ready-to-eat food and results from testing help to ensure that food is produced, handled and stored in a hygienic and appropriate way to maximize safety. Samples of uncooked food such as raw shell eggs, raw meat and poultry are tested as part of specific structured surveys to help identify the source and prevalence of specific food poisoning organisms.

Currently there is also an increased emphasis by local authorities on environmental sampling in catering premises. Environmental samples usually consist of swabs from food contact surfaces and cloths used in commercial kitchens, the results of which are used to demonstrate the need for improved hygiene during food preparation. Most government-funded laboratories also examine water samples from a range of sources; food production premises need to have a supply of potable water, and water in containers is defined as food under European Union (EU) legislation, so these samples also come under the remit of Official Food Control. In addition, water from private water supplies (which may be untreated) that is used for drinking must be of potable quality (for further details see Chapter 7).

One of the key functions of food examiners is to interpret results of microbiological testing and give an opinion on the safety and quality of the food sample submitted. This helps the local authority personnel to identify the source of a problem and thus assist the **food business operator** (FBO) to identify and implement corrective action. The food examiner may also be called to review food production procedures with respect to safe production of food, particularly if the food has been imported and a site visit is not feasible. The food examiner must be prepared to give testimony in a court of law in support of a prosecution taken by the local authority for infringement of food safety laws; it is therefore most important for the food examiner to develop and maintain expertise through a programme of **continuous professional development** (CPD). Government-funded laboratories tend to employ a higher proportion of science graduates than commercial testing laboratories because of the emphasis on food examiner expertise, the role in protection of public health, and the part played by food examiners in research and development.

Another important function of government-funded laboratories is to perform testing in response to a food poisoning incident or as a result of a food complaint. Microbiological evidence is crucial in these investigations in tracing the source of the contamination, and the laboratories have an essential role in establishing clear scientific evidence of the causes of local and national food, water and airborne outbreaks of infection. In addition to testing samples, food examiners may accompany local authority personnel on site visits to try to identify the source of a pathogen or other contamination, or to help verify the proper operation of the food production process, for example that of a milk pasteurizer. Results obtained from routine sampling or specific investigations may then be used to formulate advice on good practice, to help prevent recurrence of the same problem and to form the basis of scientific publications that can help disseminate such informa-

tion. Further support to the local authority teams may be in the form of training in sampling techniques, appropriate sample transport procedures, interpretation of results or education on microbiological topics.

The Official Food Control or frontline laboratories are supported by government-funded **reference laboratories** that provide facilities for confirming the identity of suspected pathogens and typing these organisms for epidemiological purposes (see Chapters 2 and 9). Typing schemes include:

- serotyping
- phage typing
- plasmid profile analysis
- gene detection
- genetic profiling
- patterns of antibiotic resistance.

The accumulation of specific typing information can lead in itself to identification of foodborne outbreaks and the source of the causative pathogen. Preventive measures can then be put in place so that further cases of illness can be avoided. This may happen on a local, national or international basis and is increasingly important with global food transport. Reference laboratories may also provide specialist testing facilities for rare tests that are not usually performed in frontline testing laboratories, for example tests for detection of microbial toxins such as staphylococcal enterotoxin, histamine in scombroid fish such as tuna, and detection of foodborne pathogens such as *Clostridium botulinum*.

Government-funded laboratories may also take part in validation studies to support method development for microbiological tests. This is an important role in advancing method development in food and water testing for the purposes of public health, both nationally and internationally. The laboratories may also initiate or participate in surveys of various food commodities for a variety of reasons as described previously, that include seeking to identify the cause or source of an unusual increase in reports of illness due to a specific pathogen.

Because of the breadth of sample types examined by publicly funded laboratories, the use of routine automated methods in these laboratories is not yet common. This is likely to change in the near future with the advent of simple, commercially available systems based on molecular microbiology techniques that will allow real-time detection of common foodborne pathogens. The official nature of the work undertaken dictates the use of methods that closely follow the International Organization for Standardization (ISO) and other international reference standards. Thus the cost of testing food samples in these laboratories may be significantly greater than that in commercial testing laboratories, which use a simple test that may only identify a presumptive presence. The Official Food Control laboratories, in collaboration with the reference laboratories and others, undertake research and development on topics such as emerging pathogens, microbiological risk assessment, food quality, disease surveillance, environmental contamination including sewage, waste disposal, private water supplies and enhanced surveillance. Results from these investigations have led to changes in public health practices, improved food safety and development of new methods for microbiological testing.

All websites cited below were accessed in November 2006.

SOURCES OF INFORMATION AND FURTHER READING

Health Protection Agency (www.hpa.org.uk).

HPA External Quality Assessment / Proficiency Testing Schemes (available at: www.hpa.org.uk/cfi/quality/eqa/default.htm).

International Organization for Standardization (www.iso.org).

29

Reference laboratories

Jim McLauchlin

Specialist and reference microbiology services	383	Advice, training, research and responding to health alerts	385
Surveillance, microbial epidemiology and investigation of outbreaks	384		

Reference laboratories perform a broad spectrum of work including specialist and reference microbiology services, surveillance, microbial epidemiology, investigation of outbreaks, advice, training, research and responding to health alerts.

SPECIALIST AND REFERENCE MICROBIOLOGY SERVICES

Specialist and reference microbiology laboratories provide essential national and international services by performing both specialist tests on primary samples as well as secondary tests on referred specimens, often using sophisticated methods. **Specialist tests** are needed where there is limited demand or equipment for primary testing in frontline laboratories. An example of this is the provision of tests for detection of *Clostridium botulinum* neurotoxin in foods and patient specimens during the investigation of cases of botulism. Because of the rarity of botulism and the specialist skills and equipment needed for primary toxin detection tests, national (and indeed international) reference laboratories have been established for provision of these tests.

As well as specialist testing, **secondary tests** are also done in reference laboratories on samples referred from primary laboratories. Secondary tests are carried out for confirmation of the results from the primary laboratory as well as for comparative (fingerprinting or typing) analyses for strain characterization, differentiation and interpretation of such differences. Isolate typing is used to establish likely relationships between samples collected from different places or at different times as well as for the identification of rare or 'difficult' variants. An example of a series of secondary tests is the typing of *Salmonella* isolates. This typing allows:

- confirmation of species
- fingerprinting
- identification of a strain from both multiple patients affected in an outbreak, and food and animals associated with the original sources of contamination.

Sometimes typing (Box 29.1) provides clues about the possible country, environmental site or host animal for a specific strain. In addition, as more becomes known about the mechanisms for pathogenicity of pathogens, strain typing (especially the analysis of virulence genes) will be increasingly used to provide information on the ability of a organism to cause disease. For example, *Clostridium perfringens* is part of the normal faecal flora, but it is also found in the faeces of patients with diarrhoeal disease in whom this bacterium produces an enterotoxin in the enteric tract. Only a small proportion of *C. perfringens* contain the enterotoxin gene, therefore molecular typing by detection of fragments of this gene by polymerase chain reaction (PCR) is invaluable in distinguishing isolates that have the potential to cause food poisoning from those that do not.

Other reference laboratory functions include the provision of characterized strains and other control material, often from culture collections, and facilities for the identification of rare or difficult pathogens which require higher levels of containment for safe laboratory analysis. An example of this latter category is the identification of *Bacillus anthracis*, which can cause a gastrointestinal illness and requires high containment. In the UK licensed status is required to manipulate this pathogen.

An additional quality function of reference laboratories is in the operation of both internal quality control schemes, provision of national and international quality assurance schemes, and production of standard operating procedures. These activities are integral with accreditation of laboratory activities by external assessors. Accreditation helps improve quality and to put 'confidence limits' on diagnosis and on interpretation of surveillance data.

Advances in technology have allowed establishment of networks between reference laboratories in different countries (Box 29.2) and rapid exchange of surveillance and typing data. This has allowed rapid investigation of foodborne disease outbreaks where cases are geographically very widely distributed. Further advances in technology, particularly the ability to rapidly generate DNA sequence data are likely to result in greater local (or regional) analysis, for example to achieve rapid strain characterization. Reference microbiology laboratories are increasingly involved in 'dry laboratory' work with the capture of such information and computer-assisted analysis (bio-informatics).

SURVEILLANCE, MICROBIAL EPIDEMIOLOGY AND INVESTIGATION OF OUTBREAKS

Reference microbiology for food and waterborne disease is predominantly related to investigation and prevention of adverse events usually on a population basis. These events can span regional, national and international boundaries, and include investigation of outbreaks of food poisoning due to any agent, analysis of unusual antimicrobial resistances in isolates of *Salmonella typhi*, and detection and investigation of rare infectious diseases such as listeriosis. A key feature of reference laboratory activities is their close integration with surveillance activities. Constant monitoring of reports from both front-line laboratories as well as from reference laboratories are used not only to identify unusual incidents (which could reflect undetected outbreaks) but also to highlight more long-term trends and patterns in the spread of foodborne infections. Analysis of collected reports is used to supply surveillance data which is made available for specific reports, or on the internet and in peer-reviewed articles.

This single co-ordinated team approach to public health investigations facilitates generation of timely and quality information with evidence-based advice allowing targeting of the most appropriate interventions. An example of this process is: confirmation that the strain of *Salmonella* in faecal samples from affected patients and in contaminated food products is the same, followed by advice to withdraw the affected product. Surveillance activities are covered further in Chapter 30.

ADVICE, TRAINING, RESEARCH AND RESPONDING TO HEALTH ALERTS

National reference laboratories have wide-ranging expertise on clinical, microbiological, technical and epidemiological aspects of food poisoning and microbiological food safety. Reference laboratories work in partnership with national and international public and privately funded bodies as well as academia involved with food poisoning and food safety. The work undertaken by reference centres contributes to national and international guidelines and policy development.

Reference laboratories also deliver high-quality training. This can be in-house training for staff both within and between reference units, as well as for trainees seconded from front-line laboratories and external organizations. Training is essential in maintaining competency and improving scientific and technical skills both nationally and internationally. This is particularly true for areas where the skill base is narrow and where a reference unit can serve as a focal point to support training.

Another function of reference laboratories is research and development to improve the understanding of infectious disease and public health interventions. With regard to foodborne microbial pathogens, the focus is on improvements in strain characterization, improved diagnosis and detection (including kit development and expert evaluation), seroepidemiology, understanding pathogenicity mechanisms, improved surveillance tools, evaluating effectiveness of interventions and risk analysis.

International transport and sourcing of foods together with increased air travel has led to global health threats to safe food supply. Reference laboratories have a vital role in national and international protection against foodborne diseases and provide, as well as respond to, early warnings, alerts and assistance calls from other national centres as well as the World Health Organization.

30

Surveillance of food and communicable disease

Christine Little

| Communicable disease surveillance | 386 | Communication | 389 |
| Microbiological food surveillance | 388 | | |

Surveillance is the ongoing systematic collection, analysis and interpretation of outcome-specific data, closely integrated with the timely dissemination of these data to those responsible for control and prevention. The effectiveness and efficiency of public health action is directly related to the quality and, for many purposes, the quantity of relevant surveillance data.

COMMUNICABLE DISEASE SURVEILLANCE

Surveillance has been described as information for action. **Communicable disease surveillance** is the continuous monitoring of the frequency and the distribution of disease and death due to infections that can be transmitted either from humans to humans or from animals, food, water or the environment to humans, and the monitoring of risk factors for those infections. The first step in the control of any communicable disease, regardless of whether it is a prevalent disease or a newly emerging one (including those associated with bioterrorism) is prompt recognition and identification. To achieve this goal, organized systems of surveillance for all prevalent diseases are essential. Communicable disease reporting is the first line of alert for the prevention and control of communicable diseases: all public health and healthcare workers should be aware of diseases that need to be reported as well as how and why reporting is achieved.

Control of infectious intestinal disease requires an understanding of the epidemiology of that disease as well as reliable surveillance data on its prevalence and distribution. Communicable disease reporting is just one part, but an essential component, of any comprehensive public health surveillance system. To allow effective control, surveillance systems should be ongoing, practicable, consistent, timely and have sufficient accuracy and completeness (for further details see Chapter 6). The collection of national (and indeed international) data on infectious intestinal disease allows centres to:

- monitor the long-term trends in disease patterns – to detect significant trends
- detect outbreaks – to identify which parts of the population are most affected (e.g. children or elderly people, males or females, people living in particular areas of the country)
- estimate the burden of disease
- evaluate the application of prevention and control measures
- alert appropriate professionals and organizations to infectious disease threats.

'Internet-based' surveillance is a new and developing approach to the collection of data. Web-based reporting is used in national and international networks, and the internet is also used as a source of data and information.

National surveillance centres (Box 30.1) such as the Health Protection Agency Centre for Infections

(HPA CfI) undertake national surveillance of bacterial, viral and other enteric diseases. Results from laboratories are transmitted daily to HPA CfI so that multidistrict outbreaks can be detected at an early stage and preventive action instituted. Data on enteric diseases acquired abroad by residents of the UK are also collected. The HPA CfI also investigates national and international outbreaks and provides expert advice and support on the investigation and control of outbreaks of foodborne disease to regional epidemiologists, environmental health officers, and infection control teams in hospitals. Priority is given to the field investigation of newly recognized infections and diseases of increasing or sustained high incidence. Advice is available on appropriate outbreak investigation plans, including questionnaire design and statistical analysis. Important findings that require immediate action, such as outbreaks or significant increases in the number of cases in one or more parts of the country, are also communicated directly to consultants and microbiologists working in laboratories, public health departments, and hospitals, and to the Food Standards Agency (FSA) (www.food.gov.uk) if necessary. The FSA will co-ordinate the national response to any food hazard and this may include issuing appropriate food alert notices (see Chapter 32).

Box 30.1 Examples of national surveillance centres

- England and Wales: Health Protection Agency Centre for Infections, London (www.hpa.org.uk)
- France: Institut de Veille Sanitaire (www.invs.sante.fr)
- USA: Centers for Disease Control, Atlanta, Georgia (www.cdc.gov)

A key feature of surveillance is its close integration with specialist and reference microbiology activities. National reference microbiology services for communicable disease provide an essential support function in surveillance and a primary function in microbial epidemiology, as well as infection prevention and control advice. This integrated approach to public health reduces risk, facilitates generation of quality information and evidence-based advice, and provides an immediate and co-ordinated response to infectious intestinal disease outbreaks and foodborne incidents.

Infectious diseases do not respect national boundaries and outbreaks have the potential to involve more than one country. This is being increasingly recognized with the rise in both international travel and trade, as well as in free trade areas where goods and people circulate freely. The World Health Organization (www.who.int/en/) has been responsible for collecting international data on infectious diseases, and administering the International Health Regulations, which have been the mainstay of the international response to communicable disease. However, new patterns of collaboration are required if countries are to be able to respond appropriately to international threats to health through sharing data and skills such that appropriate action can be taken at international level.

Within the European Union (EU), collaborations have developed between national surveillance centres (Box 30.2). These have shown some remarkable successes in identifying outbreaks which would probably not have been identified otherwise, in assisting in the response to international outbreaks and in developing the framework for international collaborative action. These collaborations are based around experts in particular infections and infrastructure developments. The collaborators described are largely funded by the European Commission.

Box 30.2 Examples of international collaborative networks

Enter-net
- International network for the surveillance of human gastrointestinal infections, which involves all countries of the EU, plus Australia, Canada, Japan, South Africa, Switzerland and Norway
- Conducts international surveillance of salmonellosis and verocytotoxin producing *Escherichia coli* (VTEC) O157, including antimicrobial resistance
- Website: www.hpa.org.uk/hpa/inter/enter-net_menu.htm

Eurosurveillance
- EU project dedicated to the surveillance, prevention and control of infectious and communicable disease. Eurosurveillance produces a weekly and a monthly bulletin
- Website: www.eurosurveillance.org

Med-Vet-Net
- European network of excellence working for the prevention and control of zoonoses and foodborne diseases
- Website: www.medvetnet.org

Building on this, a European Centre for Disease Prevention and Control (ECDC) (www.ecdc.eu.int) was created in 2004 to provide a structured and systematic approach to the control of communicable diseases and other serious health threats which affect EU citizens. The ECDC will also mobilize and significantly reinforce the synergies between the existing national centres for disease control. The European Food Safety Authority (EFSA) (www.efsa.eu.int), created in 2002, is the keystone of EU risk assessment regarding food and feed safety. It provides independent scientific advice on all matters linked to food and feed safety. EFSA is also responsible for monitoring zoonoses across the EU by reporting data collected from national centres in Member States.

MICROBIOLOGICAL FOOD SURVEILLANCE

Microbiological food surveillance compiles data from laboratory analyses and other sources and helps establish sound evidence on which to base advice. The results from such surveillance can be used to monitor trends, assess risks in food safety and judge the effectiveness of regulation. Information from food surveillance can also form part of the science base for the development of food policy. Examination of foods for the presence of potentially pathogenic bacteria is also an important part of government-funded surveillance activity. Intervention measures also require that their efficacy is tested by examination of samples for the presence of pathogens. Furthermore, the effectiveness and efficiency of public health action is directly related to the quality and, for many purposes, the quantity of relevant surveillance data. Information regarding the influence of season, geographical area, processing methods and other parameters can also be obtained.

There is a comprehensive food surveillance programme in the UK, with over 120 000 analyses carried out each year for a wide range of microorganisms (pathogens and indicator organisms). The Local Authorities Co-ordinators of Regulatory Services (LACORS) and the HPA implement a national programme of co-ordinated food studies in partnership with Local Authority Food Liaison Groups. The programme focuses on foods of concern associated with: food production; the food service sector; and retail foods that are identified by environmental health officers and HPA public health

microbiologists. These studies produce national data on the microbiological quality of ready-to-eat food and also on raw food samples examined within the UK. They also create national information on specific important areas, such as organic foods, butcher shop hygiene, and spices. Another purpose of food surveillance studies is to develop ways of targeting specific food hygiene problems and investigating ways of monitoring and improvement.

The annual European Commission (EC) Coordinated Programme for the Official Control of Foodstuffs, requires Member States to carry out inspection and sampling of specified categories of food items related to food safety, for example dried herbs and spices for *Salmonella*. This programme is designed to:

- test compliance with public health regulations
- to guarantee fair trade
- protect consumer interests.

At the behest of the EC and FSA, the HPA analyses the majority of samples examined under this programme within the UK.

Food surveillance is initiated in response to the recognition of public health issue. This may be a local or national issue, depending on the problem concerned. An example of such surveillance is the public health investigation of raw shell eggs related to catering premises implicated in a large number of *Salmonella* Enteritidis outbreaks in the UK during 2002–04.

The FSA's microbiological surveillance programme aims to identify the need for action which ensures microbiological safety of food. Surveys are performed on a regular basis and focus on particular foods or food processes. The FSA commissions surveys for information gathering purposes and monitoring, but not for law enforcement. However, the Agency liaises with the enforcement authorities if an urgent food safety problem is found, and, consequently, survey results are made available to enforcement authorities prior to publication so that follow-up action can be taken where appropriate. Surveys are important because they perform checks on retail foods and can therefore alert the FSA to potential food safety issues.

These surveillance exercises collectively contribute to a greater understanding of the microbiological problems associated with food, and of how food safety may be improved. In addition, food studies provide data on the relationships between indicator organisms and pathogens, and on the significance of indicator organisms in determining risk. The results of many of these studies have provided a resource to support the provision of authoritative advice, for example the HPA Microbiological Guidelines for various ready-to-eat foods sampled at the point of sale, and microbiological risk assessments. In addition, these food studies also provide a resource for linking data on food and data on human disease. For example, a study of retail bagged ready-to-eat salad vegetables performed during 2001 detected a national outbreak of *Salmonella* Newport infections.

Food studies provide considerable useful data on the sources of food poisoning organisms. The free movement of foods within Europe, the larger and more intensive farming and manufacturing processes, and the continuing rise in reported food poisoning cases, continue to offer a challenge to public health professionals. Although Hazards Analysis and Critical Control Points (HACCP) is important in limiting the risks of food poisoning, well-organized food surveillance provides essential information on the safety of food.

COMMUNICATION

The internet is an increasing source of surveillance and outbreak-related information. National surveillance centres disseminate data on the occurrence and spread of communicable diseases via websites and through reports, e.g. the HPA publishes a weekly electronic *Health Protection Report* (HPR). The HPA is also involved with the publication of authoritative reports, information to trade associations, outbreak control team reports as well as peer-reviewed articles in scientific journals. Much of the HPA's resource is devoted to the continued delivery of high-quality surveillance and the information outputs that stem from this surveillance activity (Table 30.1).

The communication of information about European communicable disease prevention and control has been facilitated by the development of a monthly journal, *Eurosurveillance Monthly* and a weekly e-mail newsletter. *Eurosurveillance Monthly* publishes summaries of information and completed reports of field investigations and studies, whereas the weekly newsletter presents information of breaking and current events. In North America this has also been facilitated by weekly electronic reports: the *Mortality and Morbidity Weekly Report* (MMWR, www.cdc.gov/mmwr) in the USA and the *Canada Communicable Disease Report* (CCDR, www.phac-aspc.gc.ca/publicat/ccdr-rmtc) in Canada.

The international dimension of communicable disease surveillance makes it essential that national surveillance centres in different countries liaise with each other and exchange information, and also communicate with the World Health Organization, EFSA and ECDC. Sources of surveillance information are described in Chapter 6.

All websites cited in this chapter were accessed in November 2006.

Table 30.1 *Examples of Health Protection Agency key surveillance outputs*

Output	Public health purpose
Communicable Disease Report (CDR) *Eurosurveillance Weekly* Human disease chapters of UK Zoonoses report	Dissemination of public health outputs and bulletins on significant infectious disease incidents in England and Wales, and Europe Integration of human, food and veterinary surveillance information, where possible, to better inform prevention strategies. In support of the Food Standards Agency's disease reduction target
Reports from Local Authorities Co-ordinators of Regulatory Services/Health Protection Agency studies Reports from private water supplies surveillance	Provide information for risk-based public health assessments and interventions
Review of infectious intestinal disease outbreak investigations Royal College of General Practitioners and National Health Service (NHS) Direct information on gastrointestinal disease	Inform control and prevention of gastrointestinal infection

31

The Food Standards Agency

Judith Hilton

| Regulation and advice | 390 | Sources of information and further reading | 392 |
| Food emergencies | 391 | | |

The Food Standards Agency (FSA) is the government department in the UK that has responsibility for protecting the health of the public and the interests of consumers in relation to food.

REGULATION AND ADVICE

The FSA was set up on 1 April 2000, under the Food Standards Act 1999, as an independent body, to:

> put an end to the climate of confusion and suspicion about the way that food safety and standards issues have been handled.

The Agency, which operates on a UK basis, assumed central government responsibilities for food safety and standards previously shared by the agriculture and health departments. Its remit also covers nutrition (jointly with the UK health departments) and consumer protection. The Agency is a non-ministerial department which means that, although it is a government department, decisions on its policies are taken by a board appointed to act in the public interest and not to represent particular sectors. It is also free to publish any advice it issues. These two characteristics mean that it operates 'at arm's length' from the rest of Government. At the same time, the Agency is accountable for its activities to Parliament through health ministers, and to the devolved administrations in Scotland, Wales and Northern Ireland.

Regulatory work is an important aspect of the Agency's remit as it is responsible for preparing legislation as well as developing policies on food safety and standards. Since most food law stems from the European Union, the Agency has a significant role in negotiating legislation in Brussels. The Agency is also responsible for implementation of food legislation. However, with the exception of the work of the **Meat Hygiene Service**, which is an executive Agency of the FSA, enforcement responsibilities lie outside the Agency, with Local Authority Environmental Health and Trading Standards departments, and Port Health Authorities. In line with the principles set out in the government's guide to better regulation (*The Better Regulation Guide*), regulatory activity is reserved for those situations in which no other approach is likely to be effective. Alternatives, such as codes of practice and best practice guidance, are considered preferable, and are part of the proportionate approach to risk that the Agency seeks to adopt in all situations.

Much of the FSA's activities relate to food hygiene (Box 31.1) and the prevention of food-borne disease is based on partnerships with industry to secure the adoption of best practice at all stages of the food chain. Most of this work has been developed within the framework of the Agency's Foodborne Disease Strategy, designed initially to deliver the target of a 20 per cent reduction in foodborne disease by April 2006. The strategy encompasses a wide range of measures, from farm to fork, aimed at reducing pathogens in raw foods and ingredients, improving food safety management throughout the food chain, and promoting better hygienic practice in both commercial and domestic kitchens.

Some of the measures designed to reduce pathogen levels in raw foods, namely the introduction of Hazard Analysis and Critical Control Points (HACCP) in slaughterhouses, are legal requirements. Others, such as improved biosecurity in poultry meat and egg production, and vaccination of poultry breeding flocks and laying flocks against *Salmonella*, are requirements of industry assurance schemes. The consolidated Food Hygiene Regulations, that came into force on 1 January 2006, require all food businesses to adopt food hygiene management approaches based on HACCP principles. To help small- and medium-sized businesses in the catering and hospitality sector to comply with this requirement, the Agency developed tool kits and provided grants for local authorities to help train businesses in their use.

To promote good kitchen hygiene, the Agency has developed a multifaceted Food Hygiene Campaign with activities that include TV and radio advertising, production of food safety videos for caterers and schools, working with schools through the medium of a mobile classroom (the

so-called 'cooking bus') and the funding of local food safety initiatives through a local authority grant scheme.

FOOD EMERGENCIES

The FSA also has a role in protecting the public from immediate risks to health in the shape of food hazards or outbreaks of foodborne disease. Under the EC General Food Law Regulation ([EC] No. 178/2002), there is a requirement for businesses to inform the competent authority, in this case the FSA, of any problems they detect that might compromise food safety. Local authorities are also obliged by the Food Standards Act 1999 to inform the Agency of any serious local or non-local food hazard. Responsibility for the management of food hazards lies with local authority environmental health departments. It is the responsibility of the FSA to satisfy itself that the appropriate action has been taken to prevent further exposure of consumers to the hazard that food source represents. Where the hazard involves a nationally distributed food, the home authority for the food producer or the Agency itself will take the lead in discussing appropriate action with the producer. If the food is considered to be **unfit** or **injurious to health, withdrawal** from the distribution system may be required, accompanied in many cases by warnings to consumers who may already have purchased the product (**product recall**). Where foods are withdrawn or recalled, the Agency also issues food alerts to local authorities and, where foods have been traded with other countries, the Agency is responsible for notifying other Member States through the European Commission Rapid Alert System for Food and Feed (RASFF).

Outbreaks of foodborne disease are normally identified locally through the statutory notification system or local laboratory reports. Local authorities have a responsibility, enshrined in the Food Law **Code of Practice**, to inform the FSA of serious local outbreaks of foodborne illness. Where cases are more geographically dispersed, it is often the Health Protection Agency (HPA) that identifies the outbreak as a result of isolates referred for subtyping to the reference laboratory. In such cases, the HPA informs the FSA under provisions in the Concordat between the two organizations.

Statutory responsibility for the investigation and management of outbreaks lies with the **outbreak** control team (OCT) convened by a proper officer of the local authority. This is derived from the Public Health (Control of Disease) Act 1984 and the Food Safety Act 1990, and their associated Regulations. Where cases occur in more than one local authority area, a national OCT to co-ordinate investigations may also be convened by the HPA.

Where investigations by the local OCT reveal a suspected food source, that source is then dealt with in the same way as a food hazard whereby it is the responsibility of the FSA to satisfy itself that the appropriate action has been taken to protect public health. In cases other than minor, localized incidents, the Agency has a role in advising local OCTs and the food producer on the appropriate course of action and, where foods are withdrawn and/or recalled, in issuing food alerts and RASFFs. Producers are themselves encouraged to withdraw and/or recall food. Failing this, local authority environmental health departments can take action under the Food Safety Act 1990 to ensure compulsory withdrawal and/or recall.

All websites cited in this chapter and below were accessed in November 2006.

SOURCES OF INFORMATION AND FURTHER READING

Cabinet Office, Better Regulation Unit (1998) *The Better Regulation Guide*. London: The Cabinet Office.

European Commission. Rapid Alert System for Food and Feed (RASFF) (available at: http://ec.europa.eu/food/food/rapidalert/index_en.htm).

Government White Paper on the Food Standards Agency (1998) *A Force for Change*. Cm3830. London: The Stationery Office.

Food Standards Agency. Foodborne Disease Strategy 2001–2005 (available at: www.food.gov.uk/multimedia/pdfs/fdscg-strategy-revised.pdf).

Food Standards Agency (2006) Food Law Code of Practice and Practice Guidance for England (available at: www.food.gov.uk/enforcement/foodlaw/copengland).

Regulation (EC) No. 178/2002 of the European Parliament and of the Council of 28 January 2002 laying down the general principles and requirements of food law, establishing the European Food Safety Authority and laying down procedures of food safety (available at: http://europa.eu.int/eur-lex/pri/en/oj/dat/2002/l_031/l_03120020201en00010024.pdf).

32

Investigation, control and management of foodborne outbreaks

Richard Elson, Judith Hilton, Christine Little, Jim McLauchlin

Recognition and preliminary investigation	393		Conclusion of outbreaks	397
Investigation	395		References and further reading	397
Control and management	396			

Foodborne outbreaks can differ markedly in the pathogens, toxins, vehicles of infection, ways of spread and reservoirs involved, as well as in their settings and numbers affected. However there are common features relating to the management, investigation and control of outbreaks. The following account is based on systems used in England and Wales (Department of Health, 1994). However, since the underlying principles of control do not differ, details of this process in other countries will be very similar, if not identical.

The stages, from discovery, investigation and ultimate control, include the following:

- ***recognition and preliminary investigation**, including the prompt recognition of the outbreak and its extent and formation of an outbreak control team*
- ***investigation,** the identification of the source and means of spread*
- ***control and management**, the prevention of further illness by eliminating any continuing hazards which will reduce the likelihood of further primary or secondary cases.*

In England, local authorities, the Health Protection Agency (HPA), the Food Standards Agency (FSA) and, less directly, the Department of Health (DH), are primarily involved in the detection, investigation and management of foodborne outbreaks. The major roles, duties and actions taken by these organisations are summarised in Table 32.1, although these have been discussed in greater detail in earlier chapters.

RECOGNITION AND PRELIMINARY INVESTIGATION

Ideally the recognition of outbreaks and potential food poisoning problems should be as rapid as possible and this can occur via a series of diverse routes including:

- local recognition by GPs, clinicians and hospital staff (microbiologists, accident and emergency staff, infection control doctors or nurses), local authority staff, laboratory staff or other public health professionals
- local recognition by members of the public
- recognition by public health professionals from regions outside the outbreak
- analysis of local or national infectious disease surveillance data
- microbiological examination of food samples and food surveillance data
- analysis of reference microbiology (typing) data
- results and follow up from food industry quality control, complaints or recalls
- international hazard alerts and recognition of outbreaks in other countries.

When an outbreak of disease occurs, effective communication is important and a group of relevant experts should be pulled together forming an **Outbreak Control Team (OCT)** when necessary, but particularly when the disease poses

Table 32.1 *Principal roles, duties and activities of organizations primarily involved in the management of foodborne outbreaks in England and Wales*

Organizations	Roles and statutory responsibilities	Activities
Local authorities	Provide prevention and control of food- and waterborne diseases and enforcement of food safety legislation	• Inform "the proper officer" (Consultants of Communicable Disease Control, CCDCs) of anyone in the district who is "suffering from food poisoning which may be caused by an infection" or "is suffering from, or is a carrier of, any infection mentioned" • Inform the Food Standards Agency of all serious outbreaks of foodborne disease and food contamination incidents • Directly investigate outbreaks including interviewing individuals and collecting clinical and food samples • Exercise legal enforcement powers including entering and inspecting premises, sampling food, product or the environment, excluding food handlers, seizing and detaining food, close premises and prosecute offenders • Instigate remedial actions which will prevent a recurrence of the incident.
Health Protection Agency	Provide an integrated approach to public health through the provision of support and advice to the NHS, local authorities, emergency services, the Department of Health, the Food Standards agencies and other public health bodies	Inform the Food Standards Agency and the Chief Medical Officer (CMO) at the Department of Health of all serious outbreaks of foodborne disease. Regional Health Protection Units (including CCDCs): • manage communicable disease incidents at regional level • provide surveillance of communicable diseases and infections • support local authorities. Clinical and food, water and environmental public health microbiology laboratories: • microbiological examination of clinical and food samples. Centre for Infections: • manage communicable disease incidents at national level • provide national surveillance data • centralised statistical and epidemiological support • confirmation and epidemiological typing of isolates • specialist laboratory diagnostic services.
Food Standards Agency	Protect the public's health and consumer interests in relation to food including the management and control of foodborne disease	• Central competent authority for food safety and hygiene legislation • Provides national and international rapid alerts • Leads on discussions with the food industry and advises on dealing with implicated foods • Ensuring that the public are aware of significant food hazards and outbreaks of foodborne disease.
Department of Health	Protect the health of the public	Setting strategy and policy for the prevention, treatment and control of infectious diseases.

an immediate health hazard, there are a large number of cases, or there is advance warning of a serious incident affecting food. The suggested membership of OCTs is outlined in Box 32.1.

The purposes of the OCT are to:

• review evidence and decide whether an outbreak has occurred

• develop a strategy to deal with the outbreak
• initiate investigations to determine the nature, vehicle, and source
• prevent further cases by ensuring that the cause is removed and the source controlled
• provide a source of information for other professionals, the media and the public.

Box 32.1. Membership of an Outbreak Control Team

Usual membership:
- Consultant in Health Protection and/or other Local Health Protection Unit representation
- Chief Environmental Health Practitioner
- Food Examiner/Microbiologist
- Consultant Microbiologist
- Administrative and secretarial support
- Press and Communications Officer

Optional additional representation depdending on the size and nature of the outbreak:
- Member of State Veterinary Service
- Virologist, bacteriologist, parasitologist, toxicologist
- Representative(s) from national surveillance and/or reference centres such as the Health Protection Agency
- Infection control doctor or nurse
- Technical expert of a suspect food or commodity
- Food Standards Agency, Department of the Environment, Food & Rural Affairs

Any public messages issued from the OCT via the media should be accurate and consistent and designed to prevent further cases of infection. It is important not to cause unnecessary alarm through public messages, so these should be targeted, as much as possible, to provide appropriate and reassuring messages about the control of an individual incident as well as to give general food safety information. Proactive publicity may reveal the hypothesis under investigation which may bias epidemiological studies, however this should be balanced against the more important purpose of disease prevention.

INVESTIGATION

Outbreaks may already be over by the time they are discovered and, if there is good evidence that there is no continuing public health risk, a decision may be made as to whether or not a full investigation is justified. However, without further enquiry it may be difficult to reach firm conclusions about the source of the contamination, or the vehicle or mode of transmission. The next stages of an outbreak investigation are likely to involve:

- review of the case definition and ensuring that the affected patients are all suffering from the same illness
- reviewing what evidence there is for an association between the cases
- interviewing the patients
- arranging for appropriate specimens to be collected from the patients for laboratory investigation
- reviewing descriptive epidemiological evidence, and, if possible, formulating a **preliminary hypothesis** as to the cause and mode of spread
- agreeing further plans and responsibilities for investigation.

Depending on the level of evidence available, it may be possible at this stage to apply interventions such as the removal of suspect food from retail sale or from the premises of any food business associated with the outbreak. If there is evidence that the food vehicle of infection is linked to a specific location, the premises involved should be visited as soon as possible and this may identify additional cases among food handlers, customers and clients. Early site visits are important since the amount of physical evidence will diminish with time. The types of investigations may include examination of:

- menus, the food used, production schedules, food sources and supplies
- the food preparation practices including cooking, storage, possible cross-contamination, temperature records and other records including work schedules
- details and records of any Hazard Analysis and Critical Control Point (HACCP) or Risk Assessment systems
- staff details including sickness absence
- policies on pest control, cleaning, hygiene and medical screening of food handlers.

Those at risk during outbreaks should be identified and data from as many cases as possible obtained by standardized interviews. There is also an urgent need to identify affected persons, such as food handlers, who pose a risk of further spread. At this stage of the investigation all existing data should be consolidated, validated and reviewed, ensuring that undue emphasis is not placed on any particular part of the dataset.

All outbreaks of foodborne disease warrant a descriptive study, because this evidence is usually needed if lessons are to be learnt to prevent similar outbreaks occurring in the future. These studies provide detailed descriptions of outbreaks together with any associations of time, place and person, setting, onset, size and progress as well as categorization of cases by age and gender. Descriptive studies also allow the development of more detailed hypotheses as to the source and mode of spread, and may suggest the need to collect further clinical, food or environmental samples for laboratory investigation, or the need to perform further laboratory or epidemiological studies.

If it is decided to conduct an analytical study, expert advice should be sought for the design, analysis and subsequent interpretation of results from cohort or case-control studies. A particular food may be implicated either by laboratory or epidemiological studies, but neither type of evidence should be considered conclusive in isolation. In order for a causal relationship to be inferred from epidemiological evidence, the following criteria are recommended:

- the investigation should have obtained evidence from most of the people in the study (a response rate of at least 60 per cent and preferably more than 80 per cent, achieved if necessary by 'chasing up' non-responders)
- the time-relationship between the consumption of the food item and the onset of illness is consistent with the incubation period of the disease under investigation
- the probability of the association being due to chance is less than 1% (p = 0.01) if there are several food items being tested, or less than 5% (p = 0.05) if the study began with a hypothesis of an association with a single food item. In a small outbreak interpretation may be difficult as these levels of significance may not be achieved and a high relative risk (odds ratio of more than 5) should not be discounted if it is consistent with the results of environmental and laboratory investigations
- there are no important causes of bias in the conduct of the investigation. Bias can occur in the type of investigation pursued, in the way questions were asked, the choice of controls, in the analysis of data and in the presentation of results.

CONTROL AND MANAGEMENT

A systematic approach to the outbreak investigation and the rigorous application of scientific method allows control measures to be implemented with greater confidence of success. The control measures will differ with each outbreak and will depend on the mode of spread and may be directed at the source (animal, human or environment), the vehicle, or both. Continued monitoring, both of the control measures themselves and to identify any further cases of illness associated with the outbreak, is essential to ensure that the measures are working. Possible control measures include:

- exclusion of infected people from work
- seizure, detention and destruction of food
- closure of premises
- withdrawal or recall of food so that it is no longer available for consumption
- vaccination (although this is not available for the majority of food poisoning agents)
- Recommendations regarding personal hygiene to prevent secondary spread.

A further part of the management of outbreaks involves wider communication to public health professionals, informing food authorities of the withdrawal of large quantities of food, or to require enforcement officers to ensure that the product has been withdrawn. In the UK the **Food Alert System** is operated by the FSA and is the FSA's way of letting local authorities know about problems associated with food and, in some cases, providing details of specific action to be taken.

Food businesses have a duty to notify the FSA, via local authorities, of any problems which render food unsafe. If the food is widely distributed, the FSA has procedures to enable urgent action to be taken at any time. The FSA has two categories of alert:

- **Food Alert For Action** (FAFA), which requires action by enforcement officers
- **Food Alert For Information** (FAFI), which is for information only, usually informing enforcers that a withdrawal or recall has taken place.

Food Alerts are issued by fax and electronically to each local authority or by other means including to dedicated mailboxes and pagers. They are also published on the FSA's website, thus alerting the public as well to the problem, and are also archived at http://www.food.gov.uk/enforcement/alerts/.

In the EU the **Rapid Alert System for Food and Feed (RASFF)** provides the control authorities with an effective tool for exchange of information on measures taken to ensure food safety. Whenever a member of the network has any information relating to the existence of a serious direct or indirect risk to human health affecting more than one Member State, this information is immediately notified to the European Commission under the RASFF. The Commission immediately transmits this information to the members of the network. In the UK, the FSA is the Competent Authority (CA) concerned for the RASFF. Further information on the RASFF is provided in Chapter 15.

CONCLUSION OF OUTBREAKS

The outbreak control team should decide when an outbreak is over and hold a final 'debriefing' meeting to consider any lessons which can be learnt and discuss dissemination of information to prevent similar occurrences in the future. A report of the outbreak and its investigation should be written upon its conclusion and circulated to appropriate local and national authorities and individuals. Reports can be invaluable to policy-making decisions at all levels locally as well as nationally. The report should examine the effectiveness of the investigation and control measures, and draw out any lessons that have been learnt. However, care should be taken while legal proceedings are in progress since publication of a report may contravene the rule of sub-judice or otherwise prejudice legal proceedings.

REFERENCES AND FURTHER READING

Department of Health (1994). Management of outbreaks of foodborne illness. London: Department of Health.

US Department of Health and Human Services. Principles of Epidemiology in Public Health Practice: An introduction to applied epidemiology and biostatistics. Third edition. Self Study Course SS1000. Available from: http://www.cdc.gov/mmwr/preview/mmwrhtml/mm5542a5.htm.

Index

Note: page numbers in italic refer to boxes, tables or figures.

acidity of foods 51–2
    delicatessen products 225
    food preservation *42*, 52, 102,
        328–9
adenosine triphosphate (ATP) 18,
    181, 309
adenoviruses 151
aerobes, growth 26, 52, 53
aflatoxins *83*, 89–90, 107, 153,
    330–1
agar 29, *30*, *32–4*
age distribution, food poisoning
    122
agricultural land 157, *158*, 161
air, food poisoning agents in 111
air conditioning 252
aircraft 290, 355–6, 357–9, 368
airport health 367–70
algae 26, 27–8
    toxins 9–10, 26, 81, 84, 108,
        153
    see also ciguatera poisoning;
        diarrhoetic shellfish
        poisoning; paralytic
        shellfish poisoning
alimentary toxic aleukia 153
alkalinity of foods 51–2
allergens *211*, 224, 227, 229
almond kernels 9
amino acids 17
amnesic shellfish poisoning (ASP)
    82, 84, 108
amoebic dysentry 12, *176*, 297
anaerobes, growth 26, 52, 53–4
analytical studies *115*, 125–9,
    396
animals
    bushmeat 333
    cycling of organisms 160, 162
    dairy products 105
    feedstuffs 98, *158*, 277–81, 293,
        294, 376
    food contamination routes 12,
        98, *99*, 110, 162
    food hygiene legislation 282,
        283, 285–7
    longitudinal integrated safety
        assurance schemes 375
    official controls 293, 294
    as parasite hosts 27
    prion disease 13, 90, 91

as reservoirs of infection 95,
    98–100
veterinary public health 376
waste management 160, 161
water 149, 158, 160
zoonoses control 298–9, 333,
    374, 376
see also pests; wild animals
Anisakis 108, *109*, 151–2
antibiotics
    for enteric fever 78
    use in food processing 55
antigenicity 22, 35
ants 271–2
Appert, N 7
appertized foods *42*, 43
appropriate level of protection
    (ALOP) 309, 310
apricot kernels 9
Aspergillus 30, 83, 89–90, 153,
    330, 331
attack rates (ARs) 122, 123,
    126–7
attribute plans 306–7
attribution 129–31

Bacillus
    bakery products 227–8
    food handlers *176*
    spores 26, 43, *44*, 87, 182
    *see also Bacillus cereus; Bacillus
        subtilis*
Bacillus cereus
    control measures 47, 49, *51, 88*
    cooking 191, 194
    food types *103*, 105, 111
    intoxications 11, *83*, 87–8, 142,
        194
    laboratory cultures *32*
    level of outbreak involvement
        133
    in milk 190
    routes of infection *96*
    shape *21*
    spoilage of food 43
    street foods 330
Bacillus subtilis 83, 87, 88, *133*
bacteria 21–6
    antigenicity 22, 35
    burden of disease *14*, 132, 148
    cell organization 19, *20*

detection 29–36, 37, *38, 39*,
    309
extra-gastrointestinal infections
    9, 12, 75–9
factors in outbreak involvement
    133
flora of the hand 169–70
food contamination routes *99*,
    162
food preservation 43, 44, 45–58
gastrointestinal infections *9*, 12,
    61–72, 149–50
Gram-negative 21, *25*
Gram-positive 21, *25*
growth 24–6
    in food 41–2, 43, 44, 45–58
    in the laboratory 29–35
heat resistance *44*
history of microbiology 6–8
internal contents 23
intoxications 10–11, 36, *83*,
    85–9, *109*
microaerophiles 26
parasitization by viruses *see*
    bacteriophages
reservoirs of infection 95, *109*,
    111
routes of infection 95–8
shapes 21, *23–4*
size 20, *21*
spoilage of food 41, 42, 43, 108
spores *see* spores, bacterial
surface structures 22
surveillance of food poisoning
    119
taxonomy 19
transmission cycles 162
see also specific bacteria
bacterial dysentery 69
bacterial viruses (phages) 20, 37
bacteriology, definition 8
bacteriophages 20, 37
bakeries 225–8, *251*
barbecues 184
beef patties *see* hamburgers
beetles *273*
beverages *see* drinks
bias, statistical association 123
biofilms 19, 181
biotyping 37
birds, control of 267, 269

blanching 43–4
boiling, water safety 341–2
boiling foods 183
bottle feeds *see* infant feeds
bottled water 156–7, 340
botulism 10–11, 85–6
　cooking 182
　food retail operations 222, 225
　food types and 107, *109*, 111,
　　112
　in history 6
　history of microbiology 7
　outbreak examples 136–7, 139
　specialist tests 383
bovine spongiform
　　encephalopathy (BSE) 13, 90,
　　91, 376
Bradford Hill Criteria 129–30
bratt pans 255
bread 43
broths, enrichment 29, *32*
Brucella spp. 12, *21*, 99, 107, 191
Budd, W 7
burden of disease 14, 114, 132
　developing countries 148–9,
　　327–8
　water and 148–9
bushcraft 343
bushmeat 333
butchers 135, 217–20
butter *50*, 105, 106–7

cake mixes 193
cakes 226–7, 228
Campden and Chorleywood Food
　　Research Association 322, 379
Campylobacter spp.
　burden of disease *14*, 132
　control measures 47, 49, *51*, 52,
　　66
　food contamination routes 12,
　　99, 162
　food handlers *176*
　food retail operations 217
　food types 101, *103*, 105, *109*,
　　110, *111*
　gastrointestinal infection 12, *62*,
　　65–6
　infection transmission through
　　water 150
　laboratory cultures *32*, *33*
　outbreak involvement 133, *134*
　reporting pyramid *60*
　reservoirs of infection 99, 100,
　　109
　routes of infection *96*
　shape *21*, 24

surveillance of food poisoning
　　119
　trends in laboratory reports *61*
　very large outbreaks of infection
　　15
　wilderness travel 337
canned foods 52, 102, 199, 236
carbon dioxide 54, 56
case-control studies 126, 127–8,
　　396
case definitions 118
case finding 125
catering education 314–16, *318*,
　　322
catering equipment 256–61
catering premises 246–55, 261,
　　267, *268*, 355
catering sector 351–3
catering waste 255–6
ceilings 249, 252
cells 17, 18, 19, 21–6
cereals 111
chaconine 9
challenge testing 203
Chartered Institute of
　　Environmental Health
　　(CIEH) 314–15, 366
cheese *50*, 105, 107–8, 135, 222,
　　223
chi-square test 123
children
　diarrhoeal disease 3, 327–9
　education 321
chilled foods 48, 108, 186–7, 194,
　　195–7
　commercial kitchens 259–60
　retail trade
　　delicatessen products 224
　　fish 220–1
　　home delivery 230
　　meat *218*, 219
　　plant-derived foods 215
　　transport 213
chlorine, water disinfection *338*,
　　342
chloroplasts 19
cholera 70–1
　food handlers *176*
　history of microbiology 7, 70
　outbreak example 142
　pandemics 148
　statutory notification 116
　street foods 329–30
　transmission through water
　　149–50
chopping boards 181, 236–7,
　　258–9

ciguatera poisoning 9, 10, 28, *82*,
　　84–5, 108, *109*, 176
Claviceps purpurea 6
cleaning 234, 236–43
　cooking equipment 257
　equipment for 260–1
　food retail operations 217–18,
　　221, 223–4, 229
　practice of 239–41
　purpose 233
climatic factors, food hygiene
　　326–7
clones *384*
Clostridium botulinum
　control measures 47, *49*, *51*, 52,
　　85–6, 236
　food handlers *176*
　food retail operations 216,
　　219–20, 222, 225, 227
　food storage 197, 198
　food types 85–6, 107, 110, 111,
　　112
　heat resistance (D value) *44*
　history of microbiology 7
　intoxications 10, *15*, *82*, 85–6,
　　107, 136–7, 139
　see also botulism
　shape *21*, 23
　special tests 383
Clostridium perfringens
　bakery products 227
　burden of disease *14*, 132
　control measures 26, 47, *49*, *51*,
　　52, 66, 67, 101
　cooking and 185, 188, 189–90
　detection 66–7
　food contamination routes 12,
　　13, *99*
　food handlers *176*
　food storage 197, 198
　food types 101, *103*, 105, *109*,
　　110, 111
　gastrointestinal infection 12, *62*,
　　66–7, 139–40
　history of microbiology 8
　laboratory cultures *33*
　outbreak involvement 133, *134*
　pH range *51*
　reservoirs of infection *96*, 98,
　　100, *109*
　shape *21*, 23
　spoilage of food 43
　statutory monitoring 98
　street foods 330
　typing 383
　water standards 156
Clostridium spores 26, *44*, 219–20

clothing 175, 261
cloths 238, 260
cockroaches 269–70
coconut 193–4
codes of practice 291–2, 294, 299,
    355, 391
Codex Alimentarius 201, 205,
    284, 302, 304, 330
cohort studies 125–7, 396
cold storage 196–7, 198–9,
    259–60
commercial laboratories 377–9
communicable disease legislation
    116, 297–9, 372
  see also infectious disease
    control
communicable disease surveillance
    386–8
Community Network for the
    Epidemiological Surveillance
    and Control of
    Communicable Diseases
    298
confidence interval (CI) 123
confounders 123
consultant medical microbiologists
    (CMMs) 372–3
Consultants in Communicable
    Disease Control (CCDC)
    115, 297, 369, 372, 373,
    394
consumers
  education 317, 319, 320–2
  food hygiene 204
contamination of food see food
    contamination
convection ovens 183–4
cook-chill systems 186, 187, 194,
    259, 352
cook-freeze systems 187–8, 259,
    352
cook-serve systems 352
cooking 180, 181–94
  food retail operations 211,
    218–19, 221, 228
cooking equipment 183–6, 257,
    258
cooking vessels 238, 257–8
cooling 42, 180, 194–6
  commercial kitchens 259–60
  food retail operations 211, 213,
    219
counter tops 217–18, 223–4, 238
counting methods, cultures 31,
    309
cream 105, 106, 191, 226–7, 286
crisis management 280–1

critical control points 14
  see also Hazard Analysis and
    Critical Control Points
Cryptosporidium 27, 28
  at risk foods 163
  detection 163
  food handlers 176
  food types 105
  gastrointestinal infection 12, 62,
    72–3, 136, 152, 162–4
  ozone treatment 55
  reservoirs of infection 96, 99,
    100
  seafood contamination 109
  surveillance of food poisoning
    119, 164
  treatment processes 163
  trends in laboratory reports 61
  very large outbreaks of infection
    15
  water standards 155, 156, 162
  wilderness travel 341, 342
culture media 29–31, 32–4
culturing bacteria 29–35, 309
culturing fungi 29, 30
curing of foods 42, 56, 101, 102
cuts, food handlers 170
cutting boards 181, 236–7, 258–9
cyanides 9
Cyclospora 27, 28
  food handlers 176
  gastrointestinal infection 62,
    72–3, 141
  water and 152
cysticercosis 331
  see also tapeworm

D values 44, 181
dairy products 105–8
  attribution of illness 131
  cooking 190–1
  food hygiene legislation 286
  food preservation strategies
    57–8
  gases in preservation of 54
  outbreak examples 107, 136–8
  water activity 50
  see also milk
deep-fat fryers 258, 262
deep freeze storage 197–9, 259,
    260
Defra 294, 296, 370
dehydrated foods 50–1
  milk 106, 137
  wilderness travel 344
delicatessen counters 222–5
deliveries, retail trade 229–30

deoxyribose nucleic acid (DNA)
    17, 20, 23, 35–6, 37
Department of Health 394
dermatitis 170
descriptive studies 115, 125, 395–6
detergents 239–40, 241, 242–3
developing countries 326–33
  bacterial gastrointestinal
    infections 69, 70, 71
  bush meat 333
  contamination of foods by water
    153–5
  enteric fever 79
  extra-gastrointestinal viral
    infections 80, 81
  food preparation 194
  infections transmitted through
    water 149–50, 151
  intoxications 89–90
  lactic acid fermentation 328–9
  mycotoxins 330–1
  parasites 331–2
  significance of disease 148–9,
    327–8
  street foods 329–30
  surveillance of food poisoning
    119
  water-related burden of disease
    148–9
  see also wilderness travel
diarrhoea
  developing countries 327–30
  food handlers 170, 171, 175,
    176, 223
  wilderness travel 336–7, 344
  see also gastrointestinal
    infections
diarrhoeal syndrome 83, 87–8,
    142
diarrhoetic shellfish poisoning
    (DSP) 9–10, 28, 81, 82, 84,
    108, 109, 110
  outbreak example 138
  toxin heat resistance 45
dieticians 317, 318
dinoflagellates 28, 84, 108, 153
  see also red tide associated algal
    toxins
Diphyllobothrium 108, 109
dishwashing 229, 234, 241, 242,
    254
disinfectants 234–6, 261
  for hands 171, 236
disinfection 233–6
  water in wilderness travel
    338–9, 341–3
  see also cleaning

display cases, heated 258
distribution systems 204, 210,
    213–14
domestic catering 353
domestic kitchens
    cold storage 198
    cooking 182, 183
    cooling 194–5, 196
    reservoirs of infection 97–8
doors 250, 271, *272*
drains 237, 254–5
dried foods *42*
    environmental monitoring 378
    gases in preservation of 55
    meats 102
    milk 106, 137, 190–1, 378
    outbreak examples 137, 142
    storage 199, 260
    water activity *50*
    wilderness travel 344
drinking utensils 238
drinking water *see* water, drinking
drinks
    gases in preservation of 54
    gastrointestinal parasites 73
    mycotoxins 90
    outbreak examples 142
    preservation strategies 57
    reservoirs of infection 112
due diligence 291, 313, 314
Durand, P 7
dustbins 256
dye tests 309

Early Warning and Response
    System (EWRS) 298
eating utensils 238
ECHO viruses 151
education and training 178,
    313–24
    children 321
    developing countries 330
    keeping up to date 322–3
    legislation on 366
    open access information 323
    postgraduate 31
    professional 314–16, *318*, *319*,
        322–3, 381
    of the public 317, *319*, 320–2
    public analysts 317
    reference laboratories 385
    retail trade *212*
    sources *318–19*
    university 316–17, *318*, *319*
eggs 103–5
    allergens 227
    attribution of illness 130, *131*

contamination routes *99*
cooking 193
food poisoning surveillance 121,
    126–7
gases in preservation of 54
outbreak examples 135–6, 193
pH of foods containing 52
salmonellosis 64–5
water activity *50*
electricity 252
electron microscopy 36
electrophoresis 37, *38*
ELISA 35, 36
emergencies 280, 290–1, 391–2
emetic syndrome *83*, 87, 88, 142,
    190, 194
end product testing 13–14
endospores *see* spores
energy requirements (cells) 18
energy sources (kitchens) 252
enrichment broths 29, *32*
Entamoeba
    food handlers *176*
    infection transmission through
        water 152
    pattern of infection 12
    routes of infection *96*
    wilderness travel 337
enteral feeds 192
enteric fever 78–9, 116, 150, *177*,
    297
Enterobacter sakazakii 106, 191–2,
    378
enumeration methods, cultures
    31, 309
environmental health practitioners
    (EHPs) 116, 364–6
    education 314, *318*, 322
environmental monitoring 378
environmental sampling 380–1
enzyme-linked immunosorbent
    assay (ELISA) 35, 36
enzymes 17–18, 35–6
epidemiology 114–43
    bacterial infections
        extra-gastrointestinal 77, 79
        gastrointestinal 64, 66, 67, 68,
            70, 71, 72, 103
    burden of disease 132
    definition 8, 114
    factors in food poisoning
        outbreaks 133
    intoxications 84, 85–6, 87, 88, 89
    measurements used in 122–3
    outbreak examples 126–7,
        133–42
    reference laboratories 384–5

surveillance and 112–24
    analytical studies 125–9, 396
    attribution of illness 129–31
    communication of findings
        128–9
    descriptive studies 125
    evaluation 131
    field investigations 124–5
    policy development 131–2
    terminology used in 121–2, *384*
    viral infections 80, 81
ergot poisoning 6
Escherichia coli 0157 68
    burden of disease *14*, *132*
    cooking 189
    food types *111*
    infection transmission through
        water 150–1
    laboratory cultures *32*, *33*
    outbreak examples 135, 138,
        142
    outbreak involvement 133, *134*
    pH range *51*
    trends in laboratory reports *61*
    very large outbreaks of infection
        15, 101, 135
    wilderness travel 337
Escherichia coli
    control measures 68
    culturing 30
    enteroaggregative (EAggEC) 69
    enteroinvasive (EIEC) 69
    enteropathogenic (EPEC) 69,
        96
    enterotoxigenic (ETEC) 69, *96*,
        99
    food contamination routes *99*,
        101
    food handlers *176*
    food types 101, 102, *103*, 105,
        106, 107, *111*
    heat resistance *44*
    infection transmission through
        water 150–1
    microbiological criteria 308
    reservoirs of infection 99
    routes of infection *96*
    shape *21*, *24*
    street foods 330
    verocytotoxin producing
        (VTEC) *62*, 67–8, 99
    cooking 184, 189
    food handlers *176*
    food types 101, 102, *103*,
        105, 106, 107, *111*
    veterinary public health 376
    see also Escherichia coli 0157

veterinary public health 376
water activity *49*
water standards 155, 156, 157
ethylene oxide 55
eukaryotic cells 19, *20*
  see also algae; fungi; parasites
European Centre for Disease
  Prevention and Control
  (ECDC) 298, 388
European Food Safety Authority
  (EFSA) 276, 279, 298, 388
European Union
  aircraft 356
  allergens 227
  communicable disease 298
  emergencies 391
  environmental monitoring 378
  fish 221, 222
  fitness to work 175
  food alert system 279–81, 391,
    397
  food hygiene *45*, 282–90, 292,
    295, 311, 313–14
  food poisoning surveillance
    119–20, 387–8, 389
  food premises 245–6, 264, 355
  food safety 210, 245, 276–82,
    356, 369
  home delivery 230
  imported food 369
  infestations 264
  kitchen equipment 256
  microbiological criteria 288,
    290, 301–2, 303–5, 308
  official food controls 283,
    286–7, 293–4, *295*
  ships 356
  transport of foods 213
  types of 275
  veterinary contribution 375–6
  water 155–6
expedition food 343–4
extraction systems 250–1

faeces
  food contamination routes 12,
    99, 100–1, 105, 110–11,
    162
  reservoirs of infection 95–6, 98
  routes of infection *96*, *97*
  stool testing 178
  waste management 161
  water contamination 149–50,
    151, 158, 160
  water standards 155
  wilderness travel 337, 344–5
  see also sewage

fan ovens 183–4
Fasciola hepatica 27, *99*, *109*,
  151–2
fermentation *42*, 51, 102, 328–9
field investigations *115*, 124–5
filtration, water *339*, 340–1, 342–3
fingerprinting *see* typing
  techniques
fire prevention 262
first aid 261–2
fish 108–10
  ciguatera poisoning 9, 10, 28,
    82, 84–5, 108, *109*, *176*
  food hygiene legislation 220,
    221, 222, 287
  outbreak examples 138–40
  preservation strategies *57*
  retail trade 220–2
  scombrotoxin poisoning *see*
    scombrotoxin poisoning
  see also shellfish
Fisher's exact test 123
fishmongers 220–2
flatworms *see* helminths
flies 100, 162, 216, 228, 270–1
floors 237, 248
food, legal definition 276–7
Food and Agriculture
  Organization (FAO) 201, 330
food alert systems 279–81, 391,
  396–7
food business operators, definition
  277
food businesses
  definition 245–6, 277
  registration 289–90
food contamination
  definition 41
  food hygiene legislation 290–1
  in-store restaurants 228–9
  retail trade 214, 215, *216*,
    217–18, 221, 223–4,
    226–7, 228–9
  routes 12–13, 94, *99*
  take-away food 228–9
food emergencies 280, 290–1,
  391–2
food examiners 292, 380–1
  education 317, *318*, 381
food handlers
  attribution of illness *131*
  fitness to work 175–8, 223, 297
  food contamination routes 12
  food storage 197
  outbreak example 134
  personal hygiene 169–79, 202
  retail trade *212*, *218*, 223, 226

routes of infection 95–6, 97,
  101
sanitary facilities 253–4
training 178, *212*, *318*
  see also education and
    training
washing facilities 253–4
water for hand washing 164
food hygiene
  cleaning 233, 234, 236–43
    retail operations 217–18, 221,
      223–4, 229
  Codex principles 201, 202
  cooking 180, 181–94, 218–19,
    228
  cooling 180, 194–6, 213, 219,
    259–60
  definition 5
  developing countries 326–33
  disinfection 233–6
  education 313–24
  food handlers 169–79
  in food manufacturing 201–7
  history 5–8
  infestation *see* pests
  legislation 275, 282–92, *295*,
    301–4, 311
  premises 202–3, 245–55, 264,
    315
  preparation 180–1
  retail trade 209–31, 352–3
  sterilization 233, 236
  storage 180, 196–9
  training 178
  in the wilderness 336–45
food inspectors *318*
food law *see* laws and regulations
Food Law Code of Practice 291–2
food manufacturing
  commercial laboratories 377–9
  critical control points 14
  food hygiene 201–7
  in-process control 14
  outbreak examples 134–5, 137
  traditional methods 15
food poisoning
  agents of 7–13, 59–91
    attribution of illness 129–31
    factors contributing to 133
    food types and 100–12
    outbreak examples 133–42
  burden of disease *14*, 132
  communicable disease
    legislation 297
  definition 5
  environmental health
    practitioners 366

food poisoning – *contd*
  epidemiological investigation
      114–43
  growth of micro organisms in
      food 41–2
  control of *see* food
      preservation
  history 6, 7–8
  mechanisms 8–13
      see also infections;
          intoxications; prion
          diseases
  outbreak conclusion 397
  outbreak control 396–7
  outbreak investigation 393–6
  outbreak management 396–7
  prevention *see* food hygiene;
      food preservation
  public sector laboratories 381
  recognition 393–4
  reference laboratories 384–5
  reservoirs of infection 95–100,
      109
  spoilage of food 41, 43
  surveillance systems 115–24
  survival of micro organisms in
      food 41–2
  very large outbreaks *15*, 101,
      108, 135
food premises
  definition 245, 355
  hygiene 202–3, 245–55, 264,
      315
  rodent access 251–2, 267,
      268
  see also aircraft; ships
food preparation 180–1
  hand washing during 164
  wilderness travel 344
food preservation 41, 42
  controlling microbial growth
      45–58
  definition 41
  developing countries 328–9
  heating 43–6
  history 6, 7
  meats 101, 102
food retail operations *see* retail
    trade
food safety
  aircraft 355–6, 357–9, 368
  education 313–24
  environmental health
      practitioners 364–6
  food service sector 351–3
  food trade associations 361–3
  imported foods 367, 369

legislation 210, 245, 262, 275,
    276–82, 290–1, 296–7,
    313–14, 369
  medical practitioners 371–3
  ships 355–7, 359, 368
  veterinarians' role 374–6
food safety criteria 303, 304, 305,
    308
food safety objectives (FSOs)
    309–11
food sampling
  commercial laboratories 378–9
  environmental health
      practitioners 365–6
  microbiological criteria 292,
      303, 304, 305, 306–8, 311
  public sector laboratories 380,
      381–2
food scientists *318*
food service sector 351–3
food spoilage 41, 42–3, 45, 50,
    108
  prevention *see* food preservation
Food Standards Agency (FSA)
    262, 281–2, 289, 296, 390–2
  aircraft 355
  communicable disease
      surveillance 387
  consumer education 320, 321
  emergency control orders 290–1
  environmental health
      practitioners 365
  food alerts 396–7
  food hygiene campaign 321
  Food Law Code of Practice
      291–2
  food trade associations 362
  guidance documents 288, 289
  imported foods 369
  microbiological food
      surveillance 388
  official food controls 294
  professional education 322
  role *394*
  ships 355, 357
  small retail businesses 352–3
food storage 180, 196–9
  commercial kitchens 256–7,
      259–60
  containers 238
  retail operations *211*, 213
  wilderness travel 344
food trade associations (FTAs)
    361–3
food types 100–12
forced air convection ovens 183–4
freeze dried foods 50

freezing
  cook-freeze systems 187
  food storage 197–8
  to control microbial growth *42*,
      48, *49*
frozen foods
  cooking 188
  cooling 195–6
  retail trade 213, 221, 230
  storage 197–8, 259, 260
fruits 110, 111
  attribution of illness *131*
  gases in preservation of 54
  mycotoxins 90, 111
  outbreak examples 140–1, 142
  preparation 194
  preservation strategies 57
  retail trade 214–17
  safe sludge matrix *158*
  storage 197
  washing 157, 216
  water activity *50*
frying 182, 262
frying equipment 258
fungi 26, 27, 28–9
  detection 29, *30*, *34*, 36
  food preservation 44, 46–7
  food storage 197, 198
  food types 89, 90, 107, 111
  growth 41
      controlling 44, 47, 48, 53
  intoxications 11, 27, *83*, 89–90,
      153, 330–1
  mycotoxin heat resistance *44*,
      182
  size 20, *21*
  spoilage of food 41
  water activity *49*

game *see* wild animals
gas, commercial kitchens 252
gases, preservative 54–5, 56
gastroenteritis
  infectious *see* gastrointestinal
      infections
  intoxication-related *see*
      intoxications
gastrointestinal infections 9, 11–12
  bacterial 9, 12, 61–72
  burden of disease *14*, 132
  food handlers 170, 171, 175,
      223
  parasitic 9, 12, 72–3
  very large outbreaks *15*, 101,
      135
  viral 9, 12, 62, 73–5
gelatine 193

general practitioners (GPs) 371–2
genetics 8, 17, 23
genotype 31, 37, *384*
genus 18–19
geographical data 122, 127–8
Giardia 27, *28*
    food handlers *176*
    gastrointestinal infection 12, *62*,
        72–3
    infection transmission through
        water 152, 153
    reservoirs of infection *96, 100*
    seafood contamination *109*
    wilderness travel 337
gloves 175, 239
gluten 227
good practice guides 292, 315
grains 89, 110, 111
    alimentary toxic aleukia 153
    pests *251*
    safe sludge matrix *158*
Gram-negative bacteria 21, *25*
    see also specific bacteria
Gram-positive bacteria 21, *25*
    see also specific bacteria
grease traps 254
grilling 182, 184
gullies 237, 255

H antigens 22
haemagglutinin 9, 186
haemolytic uraemic syndrome
    (HUS) 67, 68
hamburgers 101, 182, 184, 189
hands 169–70, 238–9
    disinfectants 171, 236
    drying 254
    food poisoning organisms on
        95–6, 97, 169, 171, 238–9
    gloves 175, 239
    washing 164, 166, 170, 171–3,
        174, 253–4, 345
Hazard Analysis and Critical
    Control Points (HACCP) 14,
    135, 201–2, 205–6, *207*
    contamination of food by water
        153–4
    drinking water safety plans 159
    education 315
    food hygiene legislation 282,
        283, 284, 314
    food preparation 180
    FSA's role 391
    microbiological criteria 301,
        302, 305
    street foods 330
hazards

categories *307*
degrees *307*
risk assessment 131–2
Health Protection Agency Centre
    for Infections (HPA CfI)
    386–7
Health Protection Agency (HPA)
    115, 116–17, *296*
    communicable disease
        legislation 297–8
    environmental health
        practitioners 366
    food handlers 175–8
    medical practitioners 373
    microbiological criteria 306
    microbiological food
        surveillance 388, 389
    outbreak surveillance
        questionnaires 124
    public sector laboratories 380
    role *394*
    update training 322, 323
health protection units (HPUs)
    373
heat resistance
    micro-organisms 44, 181
    toxins 44–5
heat treatments *42*, 43–6, 101–2,
    234
    see also cooking; pasteurization
heating, workrooms 251
helminths 26, 27, *28*, 99, *109*,
    151–2, 331–3
hepatitis viruses
    communicable disease
        legislation 297
    hepatitis A *20, 22, 76*, 80, *109*
        food handlers *176*, 226
        infection transmission
            through water 151
        outbreak example 140–1
        wilderness travel 341–2
    hepatitis E *76*, 80–1, *109*, 151
    infection caused by 12, *76*, 80–1
    routes of infection *96*
herbs 110
histamine 10, 88–9, 140, 220–1
histidine 10, 88
Home Authority (HA) principle
    355, 357–8, 359
home caterers 353
home delivery 229–30
honey *86*, 112
horizontal sectors 362
hoses 261
hospital clinicians 372
hospitals 351–2

enteral feeds 192
infant feeds 191
nasogastric feeds 192
outbreak control teams 373
outbreak example 137–8
hot cabinets 258
hotel bars 262
Houston, A 7
human reservoirs of infection 95–8
    see also food handlers
hurdle concept 203
hurdle technology 46
hydrostatic pressure *42*
hygiene *see* food hygiene
hygiene improvement notices 291
hygiene prohibition notices 291

ice-cream 107
IID study 371
immunoassays 35, 36
immunology, definition 8
imported food safety 367, 369
incidence rate 122
incident management 362
infant botulism 86, 112
infant feeds 191–2, 378
    see also infant formula milk
infant formula milk 106, 154,
    191–2
    environmental monitoring 378
    outbreak example 137
infants, breast-feeding 154, 328
infection control doctors 373
infections 8, 9, 11–13, 61–81
    annual numbers of 14
    bacterial extra-gastrointestinal
        9, 12, 75–9
    bacterial gastrointestinal 9, 12,
        61–72
    outbreak examples 134–6,
        137–8, 139–42, 193
    parasitic extra--gastrointestinal
        9, 12, 79
    parasitic gastrointestinal 9, 12,
        62, 72–3
    reporting pyramid *60*
    reservoirs of 60, 95–100, *109*,
        111
    role of GPs 371–2
    routes of 94, 95–8
    very large outbreaks *15*, 101,
        108, 135
    viral extra-gastrointestinal 9, 12,
        80–1
    viral gastrointestinal 9, 12, *62*,
        73–5
    water and 148–53

infectious disease control 368–9, 372
    see also communicable disease legislation; communicable disease surveillance
infestation see pests
infra-red cooking 182, 184
insects 269–73
    disease transmission 100, 162
    food retail operations 212, 213–14, 228
    insectocutors 250, 272
in-store restaurants 228–9
Institute of Food Science and Technology 323
insulated containers 196
International Health Regulations (IHR) 299, 368
international surveillance 119–20, 387–8, 389
international travel 367, 368–9
    see also wilderness travel
intoxications 8–11, 81–90
    outbreak examples 107, 136–7, 138, 139, 140, 141–2
    very large outbreaks 15
    water and 153
    see also toxins
iodine, water disinfection 338, 342
ionizing radiation 55
irradiation 42, 55
irrigation water 157–8

juices see drinks

K antigens 22
kitchen waste 255–6
kitchens 247–53, 254–5
    cleaning 236–8
    domestic 97–8, 182, 183, 194–5, 196, 198
    equipment 255–61
Koch, R 6, 70, 129
Koch's postulates 129
Kuru 13, 91

laboratories
    commercial 377–9
    official food control 293–4
    public sector 380–2
    reference 381, 383–5
    reports 116–17
lactic acid fermentation 42, 51, 328–9
latrines 344–5
laws and regulations 245, 275–99
    aircraft 355–6, 368

animal feedstuffs 98, 277–81, 293, 294
animals 282, 283, 285–7, 293, 294, 298–9
communicable disease 297–9, 372
    eggs 104
    emergencies 280, 290–1, 391–2
    environmental health practitioners 365
    environmental monitoring 378
    fire prevention 262
    first aid 261–2
    food handlers 173, 175, 297
    food hygiene 275, 282–92, 295, 301–4, 311
    food premises 245–6, 251, 254, 264, 355
    food retail operations
        allergens 227
        bakery products 227–8, 229
        fish 220, 221, 222
        home delivery 230
        meat 135, 217, 219
        transport of foods 213, 230
    food safety 210, 245, 262, 275, 276–82, 290–1, 296–7, 313–14, 356, 369
    Food Standards Agency's role 390
    historical 6, 364
    imported food safety 369
    infestations 264
    kitchen equipment 256
    kitchen layout 247
    lighting 249
    marine biotoxins 84, 138, 370
    meat 135, 217, 219, 286–7
    microbiological criteria 288, 290, 301–6, 308
    official food controls 283, 286–7, 293–7
    pest birds 269
    port health authorities 368, 370
    port health officers 355
    Salmonella 98, 136, 298
    sanitary facilities 253
    shellfish harvesting waters 75, 159, 370
    ships 355–6, 368
    surveillance of food poisoning 115–16, 117, 298
    training 366
    treatment of milk 45, 286, 289
    types of 275–6
    veterinary contribution 375–6
    water 155–60, 162

Leatherhead Food International 322–3, 379
Legionnaires' disease 252
legislation see laws and regulations
licensed trade 262
lighting
    kitchens 249–50
    toilet areas 253
Linnaeus 18
Lister, J 6
Listeria monocytogenes
    burden of disease 14, 132
    commercial kitchens 252
    consumer education 320
    control measures 47, 48, 49, 51, 77–8
    environmental monitoring 378
    extra-gastrointestinal infection 12, 75–8, 102, 106–8, 119, 134–5, 320
    food contamination routes 99
    food handlers 176
    food retail operations 216, 217, 219, 221, 222, 223–4, 225, 228
    food storage 197
    food types 77, 102, 105, 106–8, 109, 110, 111
    heat resistance 44
    laboratory cultures 30, 32, 33
    microbiological criteria 311
    outbreak examples 134–5
    routes of infection 96
    shape 21, 23
    surveillance of food poisoning 119
    taxonomy 19
listeriosis 75, 77–8, 102, 106–8, 119, 134–5
liver flukes 27, 99, 109, 151–2, 332–3
local authorities 294, 296, 297, 352, 369, 370, 372, 373
    food emergencies 391–2
    microbiological food surveillance 388
    public sector laboratories 380–1
    role 394
longitudinal integrated safety assurance schemes (LISAs) 375
luciferin-luciferase biochemicals 18

mad cow disease see bovine spongiform encephalopathy
mail-order foods 230

malnutrition infection cycle 328
marine algae *see* algae
Maritime and Coastguard Agency
    (MCA) 357, 368
mathematical models 131–2
meat 100–3
    attribution of illness 130, *131*
    contamination routes *99*, 100–1
    cooking 182, 184, 185, 186,
        188–90, 192, 218–19
    cooling 195, 219
    curing 56, 101, 102
    food hygiene legislation 286–7
    gases in preservation of 54
    HACCP implementation *207*
    hepatitis E infection 81
    infant feeds 192
    microbiological criteria 304
    outbreak examples 134–5
    packaging 56
    pH changes 52
    preparation 181
    preservation 56, *57*, 101, 102
    prion disease 90, 91
    reservoirs of infection 98
    retail trade 213, 214, 217–20,
        222, 223, 225
    storage 197, 198, 199
    street foods 330
    transport 213, 214
    veterinary public health 376
    water activity 50
meat hygiene inspectors 316, *318*,
    323
Meat Training Council (MTC) 316
medical microbiologists 372–3
medical practitioners *318*, 371–3
mice *see* rodents
microaerophiles 26, 52
microbial morphology 17
microbial physiology 17
microbiological criteria 288, 292,
    301–11
    application 304
    appropriate level of protection
        309, 310
    definition 301
    development 301–4
    food businesses' responsibility
        304–5
    food safety objectives 309–11
    limits 308
    microbiological methods 309
    role of authorities 305–6
    sampling plans 306–8, 311
microbiological food surveillance
    388–9

microbiological guideline 301
microbiological risk assessment
    (MRA) 131
microbiological specification 301
microbiological standard 301
microbiologists 372–3
microbiology 17–39
    agents of food poisoning 7–13,
        59–91
        attribution of illness 129–31
        factors contributing to 133
        food types and 100–12
        outbreak examples 133–42
    algae 26, 27–8
    commercial laboratories 377–9
    criteria *see* microbiological
        criteria
    definition 17
    detection of microbes 29–39,
        120–1
    divisions of 8, 18
    examination of foods 13–14,
        292
    food hygiene legislation 288,
        292, 301–6
    food surveillance 120–1,
        129–32, 386–9
    food types 100–12
    fungi 26, 27, 28–9
    history of 5–8
    identification of microbes
        29–39, 121
    in-process control 14
    infections *see* infections
    intoxications *see* intoxications
    micro-organism building blocks
        17–18
    micro-organism groupings 19,
        20
    micro-organism growth
        in food 41–2, 45–8
        in the laboratory 29–35
    micro-organism naming 18–19
    official food controls 293–4
    parasites 26–7
    predictive 203
    professional societies 323
    public sector laboratories
        380–2
    reference laboratories 381,
        383–5
    reservoirs of infection 60,
        95–100, *109*, 111
    size of micro-organisms 20, *21*
    spoilage of food 41, 42–3, 45
    viruses 20–1
    water 146–65

microscopy 6, 36
microwave cooking 182, 184–5
military ships and aircraft 359
milk 105–6
    attribution of illness *131*
    contamination routes *99*
    control of microbial growth
        57–8
        pasteurization 7, 43, *45*, 137,
            182–3, 190, 237
    cooking 190–1
    environmental monitoring 378
    food hygiene legislation *45*, 286,
        289
    outbreak examples 136, 137,
        138
    packaging 57, 58
    storage 197, 199
    tuberculosis transmission 12
    veterinary public health 376
Millbank filters 340, *341*
mincing machines 259
mineral waters 156–7
mites *251*
mitochondria 19, *20*
mixing machines 259
moisture content of food *see* water
    content of food
most probable number (MPN)
    counts 31, 309
moulds *see* fungi
Mycobacterium spp. 12, *21*
mycology, definition 8
    see also fungi
mycotoxins 11, 27, *83*, 89–90
    cheese 107
    developing countries 330–1
    plant-derived foods 111
    water activity *49*
    water and 153

nasal passages 97, 170, 239
nasogastric feeds 192
national control plans 293
national surveillance 116–17,
    119
nematodes 26, 27
    developing countries *332*
    food contamination routes *99*
    food preservation *49*
    infection transmission through
        water 151–2
    outbreak example 134
    routes of infection *96*
    seafood contamination 108,
        109
nested case-control studies 126

norovirus *20, 22,* 73–4
  burden of disease *14, 132*
  control measures 74–5
  food contamination routes 12
  food types *103, 110, 111*
  gastrointestinal infection 12, *62,*
      74
  infection transmission through
      water 151
  level of outbreak involvement
      133
  outbreak examples 134, 138
  outbreak involvement *134*
  reporting pyramid *60*
  routes of infection *96*
  surveillance of food poisoning
      119
  wilderness travel 337
nose 97, 170, 239
notifiable diseases 116, 297, 299,
      372
nuclease activity 35
nucleic acids 17, 20, 23, 35–6, 37
nutritionists 317, *318*
nuts 89, 110, 111
  allergens 227
  outbreak example 107, 136–7

O antigens 22
ochratoxins *83,* 90, 153
odds ratio (OR) 122
Official Food Control laboratories
      380, 381, 382
official food controls 283, 286–7,
      293–7
ohmic heating 185
oils
  flavoured 225
  frying 258
opisthorchiasis 332–3
organoleptic changes 42, 43
outbreak conclusion 397
outbreak control 396–7
outbreak control teams (OCTs)
      164, 373, 392, 393–5, 397
outbreak examples 126–7,
      133–42, 193
outbreak investigations 123–4,
      128–9, 393–6
  see also surveillance
outbreak management 396–7
outbreak surveillance 120
ovens 183–5, 186
oxygen
  microbial growth 26, 52–4
  redox potential 53, 309
ozone, water treatment 55

packaging of foods 42, 54, 56–7,
      58
paralytic shellfish poisoning (PSP)
      9–10, 28, 45, 81, *82,* 84, 108,
      109
parasites 26–7, *28*
  detection 36
  developing countries 331–2
  food preservation 44, *49*
  growth 41
  outbreak examples 134, 141
  reservoirs of infection *96, 99,*
      100, 108, 109
  seafood contamination *109*
  size 20, *21*
  see also parasitic infections;
      specific parasites
parasitic infections
  burden of disease *14*
  extra-gastrointestinal *9,* 12,
      79
  food contamination routes 13
  gastrointestinal *9,* 12, *62,* 72–3,
      136
  transmission through water
      151–3
  very large outbreaks *15,* 73
parasitology, definition 8, 18
paratyphoid fever 78, 116, 150,
      177, 297
pasta 142
Pasteur, L 6
pasteurization 234
  coconut 193–4
  eggs 104
  milk 7, 43, *45,* 105–6, 137,
      182–3, 190, 237
  outbreak example 137–8
pasties 102, 189, 229
pathogens
  definition 17
  requirements to be classed as
      11
patulin *83,* 90, 153
PCR (polymerase chain reaction)
      35–6
Penicillium spp. 90, 153
performance criteria (PCs) 309,
      310, 311
performance objectives (POs)
      309, 310
personal hygiene 169–79, 202
pests 100, 264–74
  food retail operations *212,*
      213–14, 216, 228
  insectocutors 250, *272*
  service ducts 251–2

pets 98, 99–100
pH of foods *42,* 51–2
  see also acidity of foods
phages 20, 37
Phaseolus vulgaris (red kidney
      beans) 9, 185–6
phenotype 31, 35, 37, *384*
phycology, definition 18
pickled cured meats 102
pies 102, 188, 193, *207,* 225,
      227–8, 229
plant-derived foods 110–11
  agricultural land for 157, 158
  attribution of illness *131*
  case-control study 128
  gases in preservation of 54
  infant feeds 192
  mycotoxins 89, 153, 330–1
  outbreak examples 136–7,
      140–2
  preparation 180–1, 194
  retail trade 214–17
  storage 197
  washing 157–8, 216
  water activity *50*
plate counts 31, 309
policy development *115,* 131–2
poliomyelitis virus 12, *20,* 81,
      341, *342*
polymerase chain reaction (PCR)
      35–6
port health authorities (PHAs)
      355, 367, 368–70
positive release systems 378
postgraduate training 316–17
potassium permanganate 342
potatoes 9, 111
poultry meat 100–3
  attribution of illness 130, *131*
  contamination routes *99*
  cooking 182, 184, 185, 188,
      189–90, 218–19
  cooling 195, 219
  gases in preservation of 54
  HACCP implementation *207*
  retail trade 217, 218
  water activity *50*
poultry meat inspectors 316, *318*
precautionary principle 277
predictive microbiology 203
premises
  food hygiene 202–3, 245–55,
      264, 315
  rodent access 251–2, 267, *268*
  see also aircraft; ships
preparation of food 164, 180–1,
      344

prerequisite programmes 201–5
preservation of food *see* food
    preservation
pressure cooking 182, 183, 189
prevalence, definition 122
prion diseases 13, 18, 90–1,
    376
process control 14, 204, 309
process hygiene criteria 303–4,
    305, 308
product design 203–4
product distribution 204
product information 204
product recalls 391
professional education 314–16,
    318, *319*, 322–3
prokaryotic cells 19, *20*
    see also bacteria
propylene oxide 55
protective clothing 175, 261
proteins
    denatured 240–1
    detection of micro-organisms
        35, 36
    prion disease 90–1
protozoan parasites 12, *15*, 26, 27,
    28
    detection, microscopy 36
    developing countries *332*
    extra-gastrointestinal infections
        9, 12, 79
    food preservation *49*
    gastrointestinal infections 9, 12,
        62, 72–3, 136, 141
    growth 41
    infection transmission through
        water 152–3
    ozone treatment 55
    reservoirs of infection *96*, 99,
        100, *109*
    seafood contamination *109*
    see also Cryptosporidium;
        Cyclospora; Giardia;
        Toxoplasma
public, the *see* consumers
public analysts 317
public health legislation 297–9,
    368, 370, 372
public houses 262
public sector catering 351–2
public sector laboratories 380–2
pulsed field gel electrophoresis
    (PFGE) 37, *38*
purifiers, water 342–3

quantitative microbiological risk
    assessment (QMRA) 131–2

quaternary-ammonium
    compounds (QACs) 235–6
questionnaires 124

Rapid Alert System for Food and
    Feed (RASFF) 279–81, 391,
    397
rapid methods, micro-organism
    detection 35
rats *see* rodents
raw materials, food hygiene 203
red kidney beans (*Phaseolus
    vulgaris*) 9, 185–6
red tide-associated algal toxins
    9–10, 28, 81, 84, 153
redox potential (Eh) 53, 309
reference laboratories 381, 383–5
refrigeration 46–8, 194–6, 197,
    198–9
    commercial kitchens 259–60
    fish counters 220, 221
    food transport 213, 230
refuse disposal 255–6
regulations *see* laws and
    regulations
relative risk (RR) 122, 123
reservoirs of infection 60, 95–100,
    109, 111
residential care homes 351–2
responsibility, food law 278,
    281–2, 304–5
restaurants, in-store 228–9
retail trade
    food hygiene 204, 209–31,
        352–3
    bakery 225–8
    delicatessen counters 222–5
    education 322
    fish 220–2
    home delivery 229–30
    in-store restaurants 228–9
    key hazards *211–12*
    meat 135, 213, 214, 217–20
    plant-derived foods 214–17
    take-away food 228–9
    transportation 210, 213–14,
        230
    ventilation guidelines *251*
ribose nucleic acid (RNA) 17, 20
rice 87, 88, 194
    attribution of illness *131*
    outbreak example 142
risk analysis 201–2
    food law 277
    veterinary role 376
risk assessment
    food hygiene legislation 284

international surveillance 387
    policy development 131–2
risk management 131, 201–2
risk ratio 122, 123
rodenticides 267
rodents 264–7
    food retail operations *212*,
        213–14, 228
    as reservoirs of infection 99, 100
    service ducts 251–2
rotavirus 20, 22, 75
    infection transmission through
        water 151
    pattern of gastrointestinal
        infection 12
    reporting pyramid *60*
    routes of infection *96*
    surveillance of food poisoning
        119
roundworms *see* nematodes
Royal Institute of Public Health
    (RIPH) 314, 315–16
Royal Society for the Promotion
    of Health (RSPH) 314, 316,
    317

Safer Food, Better Business
    (SFBB) 322, 352–3
salads 110, 111
    agricultural land for 157, *158*
    case-control study 128
    outbreak example 141
    preparation 180–1, 194
    retail trade 214–17
    washing *216*
Salmonella spp.
    bacteriophage typing 37
    burden of disease *14*, 132
    control measures 47, 48, *49*, *51*,
        52, 64–5, 79, 103–5
    cooking and 189–90, 191,
        193–4
    extra-gastrointestinal infection
        12, *76*, 78–9, 116, 150,
        177, 297
    food contamination routes 12,
        13, *99*
    food handlers *176*
    food retail operations 217, 221,
        226
    food storage 197, 198
    food types 101, 103–5, 106,
        107, *109*, *110*, *111*
    gastrointestinal infection 12,
        61–5, 108
    outbreak examples 135–6,
        137, 138–9, 141, 193

Salmonella spp. – *contd*
  heat resistance *44*
  history of microbiology 6, 7
  infection transmission through
    water 150
  laboratory cultures *30, 32, 33*
  legislation 98, 136, 298
  microbiological criteria 308
  outbreak involvement 133, *134*
  pulsed field gel electrophoresis
    38
  reporting pyramid *60*
  reservoirs of infection 95, 98,
    99, 100
  routes of infection *96*
  shape *21, 24*
  statutory monitoring 98
  street foods 330
  surveillance of food poisoning
    119, 121, 126–7, 128
  taxonomy 19
  trends in laboratory reports *61*
  very large outbreaks of infection
    15, 108
  wilderness travel 337
salmonellosis 63–5, 108, 135–6,
    141, 226
salting 56, 101, 102
sampling *see* food sampling
sandwiches 226, 228
sanitary conditions, history 6–7
sanitary facilities 253–4
sanitary and phytosanitary (SPS)
    agreement 309
sapovirus 151
Sarcocystis 152–3
sausages *50*, 101, 102
schools 351–2
scombrotoxin poisoning 10, *83*,
    88–9, 109, *110*
  food handlers *176*
  levels of outbreak involvement
    133
  outbreak examples 140
  outbreak involvement *134*
'Score on the Doors' scheme
    353
scrapie 13, 90
seafood 71, 74, 108–10
  animal waste and 161
  attribution of illness *131*
  ciguatera poisoning 9, 10, 28,
    82, 84–5, 108, *109*, *176*
  food hygiene legislation *75*, 84,
    138, 159, 220, 221, 222,
    287
  microbiological criteria 308

  outbreak examples 138–40
  port health authorities 370
  regulations 74, *75*, 159, 221,
    370
  retail trade 220–2
  scombrotoxin poisoning *see*
    scombrotoxin poisoning
  shellfish *see* shellfish
seaport health 367–70
seaweed, as food 110
serotypes 19, 37
Serratia marcescens 43
service ducts 251–2
sewage 160–2
  flies 100
  history of microbiology 7
  management 160, 161
  safe sludge matrix 157, *158*
  seafood 108–9
  see also faeces
shelf life
  food manufacture 378
  food retail operations *212*
    bakery products 227–8
    delicatessen products 224–5
    fish 221–2
    in-store restaurant foods
      229
    meat 219–20
    plant-derived foods 216–17
    stock control 214
    take-away food 229
    transport 213
shelf-stable foods 46
shellfish 74, 108–9
  animal waste and 161
  depuration 159
  microbiological criteria 308
  poisoning 9–10, 28, 81, *82*, 84,
    108, *109*, 110
    outbreak examples 138–9
    toxin heat resistance 45
  port health authorities 370
  regulations 74, *75*, 159, 221,
    370
  retail trade 220, 221, 222
Shigella spp. 69–70
  food handlers *177*
  infection transmission through
    water 150
  routes of infection *96*, 111
  shape *21*
  wilderness travel 337
ships 290, 355–7, 359, 368
signage 250
silver, water disinfection 342
sinks 254

skin
  damage to food handlers' 170,
    175
  food poisoning organisms on
    95–6, 97, 169–70, 238–9
slicing machines 259
slow cooking 185–6
slow viral diseases *see*
    transmissible spongiform
    encephalopathies (TSEs)
smoking of foods 56, 101
Snow, J 7
Society for Applied Microbiology
    (SfAM) 323
Society of Food Hygiene
    Technology (SOFHT) 317,
    323
Society for General Microbiology
    (SGM) 323
socio-economic factors, food
    hygiene 327
soil
  cleaning 239–42
  food poisoning agents in 111
  safe sludge matrix 157, *158*
solanine 9
sores, food handlers 170, 175
sous vide food processing 186–7
species 18, 19
spices 88, 110
spit-roasting 190
spoilage of food *see* food spoilage
spores 19
  bacterial 19, *25, 26*
    freezing *49*
    heat treatment 43, 44
    spoilage of food 43
staff rooms 261
Staphylococcus aureus
  control measures 47, *49, 51*, 87
  cooking 190
  detection 30, *34, 35*, 87
  food contamination routes *99*
  food handlers 169, 170, 171,
    177, 223, 239
  food storage 197, 198
  food types 86–7, 102, *103*, 105,
    106, 107, *109*
  heat resistance *44*, 182
  history of microbiology 8
  intoxication 11, *15*, 44–5, *83*,
    86–7, 141–2
  level of outbreak involvement
    133
  microbiological criteria 308
  routes of infection *96*, 97, *98*
  shape *21, 23*

street foods 330
statistical tests 123
statutory requirements *see* laws and regulations
steam cooking 182, 183
steam ovens 184
sterilization 43, *45*, 236
  cooking 182, 183, 191
  purpose 233
sterilized milk 190
stock control 214
stool testing 178
storage
  of equipment 256–7
  of food *see* food storage
street foods 329–30
streptococci 170
sulphur dioxide 54–5
sunlight 326–7
surrogate surveillance 117–18
surveillance 112–24
  analytical studies 125–9, 396
  attribution of illness 129–31
  communicable disease 386–8
  communication of findings 128–9, 389, 396–7
  descriptive studies 125, 395–6
  field investigations *115*, 124–5
  legislation 115–16, 117, 298
  microbiological food 388–9
  policy development 131–2
  reference laboratories 384–5
syndromic surveillance 117

Taenia see tapeworm
take-away food 228–9
tapeworm (*Taenia*) 27, *28*
  developing countries 331, *332*
  food contamination routes *99*
  food handlers *177*
  infection transmission through water 151–2
  life cycles 160
  routes of infection *96*
  size 20, *21*
Taq polymerase 36
taxonomy 17, 18–19
temperature control
  cook-chill systems 186
  food hygiene legislation 289
  food retail operations
    delicatessen products 224
    fish 220–1, 222
    in-store restaurants 228, 229
    meat 218–19

plant-derived foods 215
  take-away food 228
  transport 213, 230
  outbreak examples 138–40, 142
thread worm *177*
3-class attribute plans 306, 307, 308
throat organisms 170
tilting bratt pans 255
time, epidemiological analysis 121–2
time control, outbreak examples 138–40
toasting 182, 184
toilets 253, 254, 344–5
toxins 8
  algal 9–10, 26, 81, 84, 108, 153
  detection 36
  E. coli produced 67–8, 69
  heat resistance 44–5, 84
  microbiological 8, 9–11, 27–8, 81–90
  non-microbiological 8–9
  outbreak examples 107, 136–7, 138, 139, 140, 141–2
  spoilage of food 43
  very large outbreaks of intoxication *15*
Toxoplasma 12, *14*, 79
  infection transmission through water 152
  reservoirs of infection *96*, *99*, *100*, 101
toxoplasmosis 12, 79
traceability, food law 278–9, 285
Trading Standards Officers *318*
training *see* education and training
transmissible spongiform encephalopathies (TSEs) 13, 18, 90–1, 376
transparency, food law 277
transport of food 210, 213–14, 230
travel *see* international travel; wilderness travel
trematode infections 331–3
Trichinella britovi 134
Trichinella spiralis 12, 27, *96*, *99*, 101
tuberculosis 12, 105
2-class attribute plans 306, 308
typhoid fever 7, 78, 116, 150
  communicable disease legislation 297
  food handlers *177*, 223

typing techniques 37–8
  food poisoning surveillance 120–1
  public sector laboratories 381–2
  secondary tests 383
  terms *384*

ultra heat treated (UHT) milk 190
ultraviolet (UV) light
  food preservation 55
  insectocutors 250, *272*
umbrella organizations 362
university training 316–17
utensils, cleaning 217–18, 221, 223–4, 237–8, 254
utility tests 307

vacuum packaging *42*, 54
Van Leeuwenhoek, A 6
variant Creutzfeldt–Jacob disease (vCJD) 13, 90–1
vegetables 110, 111
  agricultural land for 157, *158*
  attribution of illness *131*
  gases in preservation of 54
  infant feeds 192
  in oil 225
  preparation 194
  retail trade 214–17
  washing 157, 216
  water activity *50*
ventilation systems 250–1, 253, 262
vermin *see* pests
verocytotoxin producing *E. coli* (VTEC) *see Escherichia coli*, verocytotoxin producing
vertical sectors 362
veterinarians 374–6
  education *318*
  food hygiene legislation 287
Vibrio cholerae 70–1
  control measures *72*
  food handlers *176*
  food types *109*
  outbreak example 142
  routes of infection *96*
  shape *21*, *24*
  transmission through water 149–50
Vibrio parahaemolyticus 71–2
  control measures *47*, *49*, *51*, 72
  food types 71, *109*
  laboratory cultures *34*
  routes of infection *96*
  shape *21*

viral infections
  burden of disease *14*, 132
  extra-gastrointestinal *9*, 12,
    80–1
  food contamination routes 12,
    13, 21
  food handlers 170, 171
  food types *103*, *110*
  gastrointestinal *9*, 12, *62*, 73–5
  level of outbreak involvement
    133
  outbreak examples 134, 138,
    140–1
  outbreak involvement *134*
  reporting pyramid *60*
  surveillance 119
  transmission through water 151
  utensil cleanliness 238
  see also viruses
virology, definition 8
virulence factors 11
viruses 20–1
  detection 35–6
  food preservation 44
  growth 41
  routes of infection *96*
  size 20, *21*
  taxonomy 19
  wilderness travel 337, 341–2
  see also viral infections
vomiting, food handlers 134, 170,
    171, 175, *223*
  see also gastrointestinal
    infections

walls 248–9, 252
washbasins 171, 173, 253, 254
washing facilities 253–4
wasps 272–3
waste disposal 255–6
waste management 160, 161

water 146–65
  animals and 149
  commercial kitchens 252–3
  contamination of foods by
    153–5, 160, 161
  disinfection by sunlight 326–7
  drinking
    burden of disease 148–9
    gastrointestinal parasites 73
    infection transmission 150–1,
      152, 153
    standards 155, 156, 159, 160,
      162
    wilderness travel 337–43
    see also Cryptosporidium
  flies and 100
  in food production 164
  in foods see water content of
    food
  hardness 240, 241
  history of microbiology 7
  household use 164
  infections related to *147*
  infections transmitted through
    149–53
  microbial toxins related to *147*
  ozone treatment 55
  private supplies 160
  retail use 164
  sampling 380–1
  sources of pollution *159*
  standards 155–60, 162
  waste management 161
water activity 49–50, 181
water content of food 49–51
Water Safety Plans (WSPs) 155,
    159
water systems 252
weevils *251*
wild animals
  bush meat 333

food contamination routes 110,
    162
food hygiene legislation 285–6
food safety education 316
management 160, 161
as reservoirs of infection 98, 99,
    100, 162
see also pests
wilderness travel 336–45
  see also international travel
windows 250, 271, *272*
work surfaces 256
  cleaning 217–18, 221, 223–4,
    238
World Health Organization
  (WHO) 155, 201, 299, 302,
    309
  developing countries 327, 328,
    330
  education 321–2, 323
  silver disinfection 342
wounds, skin 170, 175

yeasts 29
  control measures 44, 47, 48, *49*,
    54
  food storage 198
  heat resistance *44*
  laboratory cultures *34*
Yersinia enterocolitica 72
  control measures 47, *49*, *51*, 72
  food contamination routes *99*
  food storage 197
  laboratory cultures *34*
  routes of infection *96*
  shape *21*
yoghurt 51, 105, 107
  outbreak example 107, 136–7

zoonoses 12, 161, 162, 298–9,
    333, 367, 374